Breastfeeding Management
for the Clinician
USING THE EVIDENCE

Second Edition

Marsha Walker

Executive Director
National Alliance for Breastfeeding Advocacy Board of Directors

Massachusetts Breastfeeding Coalition
Weston, Massachusetts

JONES AND BARTLETT PUBLISHERS
Sudbury, Massachusetts
BOSTON   TORONTO   LONDON   SINGAPORE

World Headquarters

Jones and Bartlett Publishers
40 Tall Pine Drive
Sudbury, MA 01776
978-443-5000
info@jbpub.com
www.jbpub.com

Jones and Bartlett Publishers
Canada
6339 Ormindale Way
Mississauga, Ontario L5V 1J2
Canada

Jones and Bartlett Publishers
International
Barb House, Barb Mews
London W6 7PA
United Kingdom

Jones and Bartlett's books and products are available through most bookstores and online booksellers. To contact Jones and Bartlett Publishers directly, call 800-832-0034, fax 978-443-8000, or visit our website, www.jbpub.com.

Substantial discounts on bulk quantities of Jones and Bartlett's publications are available to corporations, professional associations, and other qualified organizations. For details and specific discount information, contact the special sales department at Jones and Bartlett via the above contact information or send an email to specialsales@jbpub.com.

The authors, editor, and publisher have made every effort to provide accurate information. However, they are not responsible for errors, omissions, or for any outcomes related to the use of the contents of this book and take no responsibility for the use of the products and procedures described. Treatments and side effects described in this book may not be applicable to all people; likewise, some people may require a dose or experience a side effect that is not described herein. Drugs and medical devices are discussed that may have limited availability controlled by the Food and Drug Administration (FDA) for use only in a research study or clinical trial. Research, clinical practice, and government regulations often change the accepted standard in this field. When consideration is being given to use of any drug in the clinical setting, the health care provider or reader is responsible for determining FDA status of the drug, reading the package insert, and reviewing prescribing information for the most up-to-date recommendations on dose, precautions, and contraindications, and determining the appropriate usage for the product. This is especially important in the case of drugs that are new or seldom used.

Production Credits

Publisher: Kevin Sullivan
Acquisitions Editor: Emily Ekle
Acquisitions Editor: Amy Sibley
Associate Editor: Patricia Donnelly
Editorial Assistant: Rachel Shuster
Production Editor: Amanda Clerkin
Marketing Manager: Rebecca Wasley

V.P., Manufacturing and Inventory Control: Therese Connell
Composition: Arlene Apone
Cover Design: Scott Moden
Cover Image Credit: © Anastasia Bobrova/ShutterStock, Inc.
Printing and Binding: Malloy, Inc.
Cover Printing: Malloy, Inc.

Library of Congress Cataloging-in-Publication Data
Walker, Marsha.
 Breastfeeding management for the clinician : using the evidence / Marsha Walker. — 2nd ed.
   p. ; cm.
 Includes bibliographical references and index.
 ISBN-13: 978-0-7637-6651-1 (alk. paper)
 ISBN-10: 0-7637-6651-8 (alk. paper)
 1. Breastfeeding. 2. Infants—Nutrition. 3. Evidence-based medicine. I. Title.
 [DNLM: 1. Breast Feeding. 2. Evidence-Based Medicine. 3. Lactation—physiology. WS 125 W182b 2011]
 RJ216.W346 2011
 649'.33—dc22
                        2009033393

6048

Printed in the United States of America
13 12 11 10 09   10 9 8 7 6 5 4 3 2 1

✍ *Dedication* ✍

As always, my work is dedicated to my growing family: Hap, my husband, for his unlimited patience and support (especially with IT); Shannon, my daughter, wife to Tom, and mother of breastfed Haley, Sophie, and Isabelle; Justin, my son, husband to Sarina and father of Ella. I can't ask for more than this.

✐ Contents ✑

✆ *Preface* ✇

It is the goal of *Breastfeeding Management for the Clinician* to provide current and relevant information on breastfeeding and lactation, blended with clinical suggestions for best outcomes in the mothers and infants entrusted to our care. Although lactation is a robust process, predating placental gestation, it has become fraught with barriers: Human lactation is only occasionally taught in nursing and medical schools, leaving a gap in healthcare providers' ability to provide appropriate lactation care and services.

With minimal staffing on maternity units, short hospital stays, delays in community follow-up, and the resulting time crunches, breastfeeding often falls through the cracks. Absent or inappropriate care results in reduced initiation, duration, and exclusivity of breastfeeding. This book is intended to provide busy clinicians with options for clinical interventions and the rationale behind them.

Designed as a practical reference rather than a thick textbook, it is hoped that this approach provides quick access to—and help with—the more common as well as some less frequently seen conditions that clinicians are called on to address. It is my sincere desire that the use of this book as a clinical tool results in the best outcomes for all breastfeeding mothers and infants the reader encounters.

The Context of Lactation and Breastfeeding

Influence of the Biospecificity of Human Milk

Introduction

Effective breastfeeding management requires a general understanding of the structure and function of human milk itself. Many of the recommendations for successful breastfeeding and optimal infant health outcomes are based on using what the clinician knows about the components of human milk, what they do, and how they work. This chapter and Appendix 1 provide an overview of the components of breastmilk and of breastfeeding management based on milk composition.

Human milk is a highly complex and unique fluid that is strikingly different from the milks of other species, including the cow. Aggressive marketing of infant formula has blurred the public's perception of the differences between human milk and infant formula. Data from the HealthStyles survey, an annual national mail survey to U.S. adults, were examined to understand changes in public attitudes toward breastfeeding. The 1999 and 2003 HealthStyles surveys (Li et al., 2007) included four breastfeeding items related to public attitudes toward breastfeeding in public and toward differences between infant formula and breastmilk. The percentage of respondents in agreement with the statement, "Infant formula is as good as breastmilk," increased significantly from 14.3% in 1999 to 25.7% in 2003 (Li et al., 2007). Hundreds of human milk components interact synergistically to fulfill the dual function of breastmilk, nourishing and protecting infants and young children who are breastfed or who receive human milk. The addition of ingredients into infant formula derived from nonhuman sources and pre- and probiotics cannot duplicate the health, cognitive, and developmental outcomes seen in infants fed human milk, no matter what formula advertising might claim.

Lactation is an ancient process that is thought to predate placental gestation. Milk composition and the length of lactation have been modified and adapted to meet the needs of each particular species. Generally, the protein content of milk varies with the rate of growth of the offspring. In many species, including humans, low-solute milk with relatively low concentrations of protein is related to a pattern of frequent feedings. Researchers often refer to species that manifest or practice this concept as a "continuous contact" species. Calorie-dense milk with a high fat concentration can be associated with both the size of the species and low environmental temperatures. For example, marine mammals have fat concentrations of 50% or more in their milk to enable their young to lay down a thick insulating layer of fat. Each species has features (e.g., an organ, a behavior, a body system) that serve as major focal points for determining the type, variety, and interactions of the milk components fed to the young. In humans, these focal points include the brain, the immune system, and the acquisition of affiliative behavior.

Human milk composition is not static or uniform like infant formula. Breastmilk is a living dynamic fluid that represents an elegant interplay between the needs and vulnerabilities of the infant and the rapid adaptability of the mother's body to provide milk components to meet those needs and support those vulnerabilities:

- Colostrum (1–5 days) evolves through transitional milk (6–13 days) to mature milk (14 days and beyond).
- During early lactation, a few hours can show a significant change in milk composition. Lactoferrin, for example, decreases significantly over the first 3 days of lactation.
- Milk composition changes during each feeding as the breast drains and the fat content rises.
- Milk composition changes during each day and over the course of the entire lactation.
- Milk of preterm mothers differs from that of mothers delivering at term.
- More than 200 components have been identified, with some having still unknown roles.

- Infant formula is an inert nutritional medium with no growth factors, hormones, or live cells like those found in breastmilk.
- Human milk is a biological mediator, carrying a rich variety of bioactive substances intended to grow a brain, construct an immune system, and facilitate affiliative behavior.

Colostrum

Colostrum, the first milk, is present in the breasts from about 12–16 weeks of pregnancy onward. This thick fluid's yellowish color comes from beta-carotene. It differs from mature milk both in the nature of its components and in their relative proportions. Colostrum has a mean energy value of 67 kcal/dL (18.76 kcal/oz) compared with mature milk's mean energy value of 75 kcal/dL (21 kcal/oz). The volume of colostrum per feeding during the first 3 days ranges from 2 to 20 mL. Colostrum is higher in protein, sodium, chloride, potassium, and fat-soluble vitamins such as vitamin A (three times higher on day 3 than in mature milk), vitamin E (three times higher than in mature milk), and carotenoids (10 times higher than in mature milk). It is lower in sugars, fat (2%), and lactose. Colostrum is rich in antioxidants, antibodies, and immunoglobulins, especially secretory immunoglobulin A (sIgA). Colostrum contains a high concentration of sIgA, approximately 10 g/L compared with approximately 1 g/L in mature milk. It contains interferon, which has strong antiviral activity, and fibronectin, which makes certain phagocytes more aggressive so that they ingest microbes even when not tagged by an antibody. Colostrum contains pancreatic secretory trypsin inhibitor (PSTI), a peptide found in the pancreas that protects it from damage by the digestive enzymes that it produces. PSTI is also found in mature breastmilk, but it is 7 times more concentrated in colostrum. Marchbank et al. (2009) found that PSTI stimulated cell migration and proliferation by threefold and reduced apoptosis (cell death) in damaged intestinal cells by 70–80%. PSTI both protects and repairs the delicate intestines of the newborn, readying the organ for processing future foods. Feeding infants colostrum establishes and maintains gut integrity, an important advantage over infant formula, because PSTI is not found in artificial milks. Not only is colostrum replete with anti-infective properties, but the colostrum of mothers delivering preterm is more highly enriched with potent disease protectors than the colostrum of mothers delivering at term.

Preterm infants consuming their own mother's colostrum can benefit from ingestion of up to twice as many macrophages, lymphocytes, and total cells compared with that which is present in term colostrum (Mathur et al., 1990). They also receive more IgA, lysozymes, lactoferrin, and neutrophils than seen in term colostrum. Infant formula contains none of these formidable fighters of infection, leaving infants who are not fed colostrum or human milk vulnerable to infections and diseases preventable or reduced by breastfeeding or the provision of expressed colostrum and milk. Colostrum contributes to the establishment of bifidus flora in the digestive tract. The composition and volume of colostrum are in keeping with the needs and stores of a newborn human baby. Its primary function is anti-infective, but its biochemical composition has a laxative effect on meconium. It also provides a concentrated dose of certain nutrients such as zinc.

Clinical Implications: Allergy and Disease

The gastrointestinal (GI) tract of a normal fetus is sterile. The neonatal GI tract undergoes rapid growth and maturational change after birth (Figure 1-1). It is important to note that the type of delivery has an effect on the development of the intestinal microbiota. Vaginally born infants are colonized with their mother's bacteria. In contrast, cesarean-born infants' initial exposure is more likely to be from environmental microbes in the air, other infants, and the nursing staff, all of which serve as vectors for transfer. The gut flora of infants born by cesarean delivery is characterized by the widespread presence of the pathogen *Clostridium difficile* (Penders et al., 2006) and a substantial absence of *Bifidobacterium* species as opposed to the large numbers of *Bifidobacterium* species seen in vaginally delivered infants (Biasucci et al., 2008). The composition of the first bacterial colonizers of the newborn gut could have long-lasting effects. Intestinal bacteria play an important role in the development of the infant's immune system. If intestinal flora develop on an alternate trajectory as caused by a cesarean delivery and/or feeding with infant formula, the development of the immune system might also be different, leaving it vulnerable to a number of diseases and conditions including autoimmune disorders. For example, atopic diseases appear more often in infants who have experienced a cesarean delivery compared with those delivered vaginally. One meta-analysis found a 20% increase in the subsequent risk of asthma in children who had been delivered by cesarean section (Thavagnanam et al., 2008). Cardwell et al. (2008) showed a 20% increase in the risk of childhood type 1 diabetes after cesarean delivery.

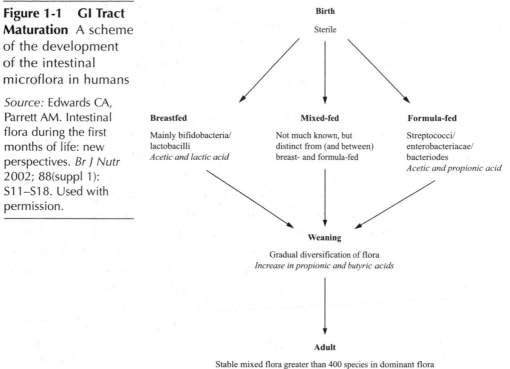

Figure 1-1 GI Tract Maturation A scheme of the development of the intestinal microflora in humans

Source: Edwards CA, Parrett AM. Intestinal flora during the first months of life: new perspectives. *Br J Nutr* 2002; 88(suppl 1): S11–S18. Used with permission.

Birth
Sterile

Breastfed
Mainly bifidobacteria/ lactobacilli
Acetic and lactic acid

Mixed-fed
Not much known, but distinct from (and between) breast- and formula-fed

Formula-fed
Streptococci/ enterobacteriacae/ bacteriodes
Acetic and propionic acid

Weaning
Gradual diversification of flora
Increase in propionic and butyric acids

Adult
Stable mixed flora greater than 400 species in dominant flora
Acetic/propionic/butyric acid

The primary gut flora in cesarean-born infants may be disturbed for as long as 6 months after birth (Gronlund et al., 1999). Coinciding with cesarean deliveries is the delayed onset of lactogenesis II (Dewey, 2003; Evans et al., 2003; Scott et al., 2007), leaving these infants without the early support of breastmilk for the colonization and physiological development of their intestinal flora. Infants at highest risk of colonization by undesirable microbes, or when transfer from maternal sources cannot occur, are cesarean-delivered babies, preterm infants, full-term infants requiring intensive care, or infants separated from their mothers. Infants requiring intensive care acquire intestinal organisms slowly and the establishment of bifidobacterial flora is retarded. Such a delayed bacterial colonization of the gut with a limited number of bacterial species tends to be virulent.

Control and manipulation of the neonatal gut with human milk can be used as a strategy to prevent and treat intestinal diseases (Dai & Walker, 1999). Major ecological disturbances are observed in newborn infants treated with antimicrobial agents. If several infants in a hospital nursery are treated with antibiotics, the intestinal colonization pattern of other infants in the same nursery may be disturbed, with the intestinal microflora returning to normal after several weeks (Tullus & Burman, 1989). One way of minimizing ecological disturbances in the neonatal intensive care unit (NICU) is to provide these infants with fresh breastmilk (Zetterstrom et al., 1994).

Breastfed and formula-fed infants have different gut flora (Mountzouris et al., 2002). Breastfed infants have a lower gut pH (acidic environment) of approximately 5.1–5.4 throughout the first 6 weeks, which is dominated by *Bifidobacterium* with reduced pathogenic (disease-causing) microbes such as *Escherichia coli*, bacteroides, clostridia, and streptococci. Flora with a diet-dependent pattern are present from the fourth day of life, with breastmilk-fed guts showing a 47% *Bifidobacterium* level and formula-fed guts showing a 15% level. In comparison, enterococci prevail in formula-fed infants (Rubaltelli et al., 1998). Infants fed formula have a high gut pH of approximately 5.9–7.3 characterized by a variety of putrefactive bacterial species. In infants fed breastmilk and formula supplements, the mean pH is approximately 5.7–6.0 during the first 4 weeks after birth, falling to 5.45 by the sixth week. When formula supplements are given to breastfed infants during the first 7 days of life, the production of a strongly acidic environment is delayed and its full potential may never be reached. Breastfed infants who receive supplements develop gut flora and behavior like those of formula-fed infants. Another bacterial group found in breastfed infants that is almost as widespread as bifidobacteria is the genus *Ruminococcus* (Morelli, 2008). *Ruminococcus* has a protective function because it produces ruminococcin, which inhibits the development of many of the pathologic species of *Clostridium* (Dabard et al., 2001). One notable difference between the microflora of breastfed and formula-fed infants is the low presence of clostridia in breastfed infants as compared with formula-fed infants. New molecular biology techniques have detected the presence of the genus *Desulfovibrio* mainly in formula-fed infants (Hopkins et al., 2005; Stewart et al., 2006). These organisms have been linked with the development of inflammatory bowel disease.

Differences in intestinal microbiota may precede the development of overweight and obesity, as data are accumulating that implicate systemic low-grade inflammation and local gut microbiota as contributing factors to overnutrition (Backhed et al., 2004; Fantuzzi, 2005). High levels of *Bacteroides* in the gut microbiota in animal models were shown to predispose toward increased energy storage and obesity (Backhed et al., 2004; Ley et al., 2005). Alteration of gut microbiota in infants during a critical developmental window has been linked to a number of inflammatory conditions (Kalliomaki et al., 2001), creating an environment ripe with the potential for the acquisition of health challenges with inflammatory origins. Kalliomaki and coworkers (2008) demonstrated that bifidobacterial numbers were higher in infancy and *Staphylococcus aureus* was lower in infancy for children remaining at normal weight at 7 years than in children developing overweight. This implies that high numbers of bifidobacteria and low numbers of *S. aureus* during infancy as seen in breastfed infants may confer a degree of protection against overweight and obesity. Because adiposity is characterized by low-grade inflammation, the provision of breastmilk with its control of inflammatory pathways contributes to the protection of infants from the development of overweight and obesity.

Food intolerances during infancy are common and thought to be related to the failure of adequately developed tolerance to antigens (Field, 2005). Tolerance contributes to reduced incidences of food-related allergies in breastfed infants (van Odijk et al., 2003) as a result of an active process whereby dietary antigens present in breastmilk coupled with immunosuppressive cytokines combine to induce tolerance to dietary and microflora antigens (Brandtzaeg, 2003). Specific deviations of the gut flora such as atypical composition and decreased numbers of bifidobacteria (Kalliomaki et al., 2001) can predispose infants to allergic disease (Salminen et al., 2005), inflammatory gut disease, and rotavirus diarrhea (Lee & Puong, 2002).

Infants have a functionally immature and immunonaive gut at birth. The tight junctions of the GI mucosa take many weeks to mature and close the gut to whole proteins and pathogens. Intestinal permeability decreases faster in breastfed infants than in formula-fed infants (Catassi et al., 1995), with human milk accelerating the maturation of the gut barrier function while formula does not (Newburg & Walker, 2007). Feeding of infant formula denies the newborn gut the trophic effects of human milk while imposing direct damage to the integrity of gut epithelium (Weaver et al., 1987). The open junctions and immaturity of the GI tract's mucosal barrier play a role in the acquisition of necrotizing enterocolitis (NEC), diarrheal disease, and allergy. Preterm infants experience a high risk for acquiring NEC due to their lower gastric acid production, reduced ability to break down toxins, and low levels of sIgA, which increases bacterial adherence to the intestinal mucosa. Preterm infants cannot fully digest carbohydrates and proteins. Undigested casein, the protein in infant formula, can function as a chemoattractant for neutrophils, exacerbating the inflammatory response and opening the tight junctions between intestinal epithelial cells, disrupting the integrity of the epithelium barrier, and allowing the delivery of whole bacteria, endotoxin, and viruses directly into the bloodstream (Claud & Walker, 2001). Feeding preterm infants with infant formula may produce colonization of the intestine with pathogenic bacteria, resulting in an exaggerated inflammatory response. The sIgA from colostrum, transitional milk, and mature milk coats the gut, passively providing immunity during a time of reduced neonatal gut immune function. Mothers' milk sIgA is antigen specific; that is, the antibodies are targeted against pathogens in the infant's immediate surroundings. The mother synthesizes antibodies when she ingests, inhales, or otherwise comes in contact with disease-causing microbes. When the mother is exposed to a pathogen, M cells of the Peyer's patch in her gut-associated lymphoid tissue or tracheobronchial tree mucosa acquire the pathogen after which the M cell presents its antigen to the B cell. The B cell migrates to the mammary epithelial cell, which secretes IgA with the antibody to the particular pathogen. The IgA enters the breastmilk and is consumed by the infant. The sIgA binds the pathogen in the infant's intestine, inhibiting its ability to infect the infant. These antibodies ignore useful bacteria normally found in the gut and ward off disease without causing inflammation.

It is important to keep the mother and her newborn baby together during their hospital stay. This practice allows the mother to enrich her milk with antibodies against bacteria and viruses to which both she and her baby are exposed. Separating mother and baby interferes with this disease defense mechanism. Feeding artificial baby milk to a newborn infant removes this protection.

The prudent clinician can avoid giving the baby infant formula in the hospital or before gut closure occurs. Once dietary supplementation begins, the bacterial profile of breastfed infants resembles that of formula-fed infants; namely, bifidobacteria are no longer dominant and obligate anaerobic bacterial populations develop (Mackie et al., 1999). Breastmilk ingestion creates and maintains a low intestinal pH and a microflora in which bifidobacteria are predominant and gram-negative enteric organisms are almost completely absent. Relatively small amounts of formula supplementation of breastfed infants (one supplement per 24 hours) result in shifts from a breastfed to a formula-fed gut flora pattern (Bullen et al., 1977). With the introduction of supplementary formula, the flora becomes almost indistinguishable from normal adult flora within 24 hours (Gerstley et al., 1932). If breastmilk were again given exclusively, it would take 2–4 weeks for the intestinal environment to return to a state favoring the gram-positive flora (Brown & Bosworth, 1922; Gerstley et al., 1932). Interestingly, optimal microflora in the infant might have long-term benefits if the flora of the adult is determined by events occurring in the critical period of gut colonization (Edwards & Parrett, 2002).

Other events and exposures that occur during the critical window of immune system development may combine to increase the risk and incidence of allergic disease later in life, such as cesarean delivery, prolonged labor, and infant multivitamin supplementation (Milner & Gergen, 2005). A higher incidence of atopy and allergic rhinitis was observed in adults who had received vitamin D supplementation during their first year of life (Hypponen et al., 2004). These data provide additional support for the importance of exclusive breastfeeding (Host & Halken, 2005) during the first half year of life and the avoidance of adding solid foods, infant formula, additives, supplements, or beverages to an infant's diet before maturation of the gut.

In susceptible families, breastfed infants can be sensitized to cow's milk protein by the giving of "just one bottle" (inadvertent supplementation, unnecessary supplementation, or planned supplementation) in the newborn nursery during the first 3 days of life (Cantani & Micera, 2005; Host 1991; Host et al., 1988). As early as 1935, Ratner recommended that isolated exposure to cow's milk be avoided in infants fed breastmilk (Ratner, 1935). Small doses of allergens can serve to sensitize an infant to subsequent challenges compared with large doses, which induce tolerance. Infants' risk of developing atopic disease has been calculated as 37% if one parent has atopic disease and as 62–85% if both parents are affected, dependent on whether the parents have similar or dissimilar clinical disease. Those infants showing elevated levels of IgE in cord blood irrespective of family history are also considered to be at high risk (Chandra, 2000). The incidence of cow's milk protein allergy is lower in exclusively breastfed infants compared with formula-fed or mixed-fed infants, with about 0.5% of exclusively breastfed infants showing reproducible clinical reactions to cow's milk protein (Vandenplas et al., 2007). In breastfed infants at risk, exclusive breastfeeding for at least 4 months or breastfeeding with hypoallergenic formulas if medically needed to supplement breastfeeding decreases the risk of atopic dermatitis (Greer et al., 2008).

If atopic disease associated with cow milk allergy occurs, partially hydrolyzed formula is not recommended because it contains potentially allergenic cow milk peptides. Different hydrolysates have differing effects on atopic disease. Extensively hydrolyzed casein-based formula may be more advantageous if needed as a supplement for infants at risk for allergy development (von Berg et al., 2003). Miniello et al. (2008) recommend that if supplemental feeding is needed, infants from atopic families should be supplemented with a hydrolyzed infant formula for the first 6 months of life. High-risk infants without a history of eczema in a primary relative may receive a protective effect from less expensive partially hydrolyzed formula. Those infants who have first-degree relatives with eczema should receive an extensively hydrolyzed formula. Soy formula is not recommended for the prevention of atopy in infants at high risk of developing allergy (Osborn & Sinn, 2006). Rozenfeld et al. (2002) demonstrated that a monoclonal antibody specific to casein (a bovine milk protein) displayed affinity to a component of glycinin, an ingredient in soy-based formulas.

Cross-sensitization between protein sources is well established. Among infants with cow's milk protein allergy, 13% to 20% have allergies to beef (Martelli et al., 2002). Solid foods should not be introduced until 6 months of age; the introduction of dairy products should be delayed until 1 year of age; and the mother should consider eliminating peanuts, tree nuts, cow's milk, eggs, and fish from her diet (American Academy of Pediatrics [AAP], 2000; Zeiger, 1999). A 7-day washout of milk proteins is required when instituting a restricted diet, delaying the expected clinical response by the infant (Brill, 2008). A maternal elimination diet may also need to include the elimination of beef and may need to be continued for at least 2 weeks, and up to 4 weeks in cases of atopic dermatitis or allergic colitis. If symptoms improve or disappear during the elimination diet, one food per week can be reintroduced to the mother's diet. If symptoms do not reappear upon reintroduction of a particular food, the mother should begin consuming it again. If symptoms reappear, it should continue to be eliminated from her diet during the course of breastfeeding.

In susceptible families, early exposure to cow's milk proteins or the absence of breastfeeding can increase the risk of the infant or child developing insulin-dependent diabetes mellitus (type 1 or IDDM) (Karjalainen et al., 1992; Mayer et al., 1988) and type 2 diabetes mellitus (Young et al., 2002). The human insulin content in breastmilk is significantly higher than the content of bovine insulin in cow's milk. Insulin content in infant formulas is extremely low to absent. Insulin supports gut maturation. In animal models, oral administration of human insulin stimulates the intestinal immune system, thereby generating active cellular mechanisms that suppress the development of autoimmune diabetes. The lack of human insulin in infant formulas may break the tolerance to insulin and lead to the development of type 1 diabetes (Vaarala et al., 1998). The avoidance of cow's milk protein during the first several months of life may reduce the later development of IDDM or delay its onset in susceptible individuals (AAP, 1994). Infants who are exclusively breastfed for at least 4 months have a lower risk of seroconversion leading to beta-cell autoimmunity. Short-term breastfeeding (less than 2–3 months) and the early introduction of cow's milk–based infant formula may predispose young children who are genetically susceptible to type 1 diabetes to progressive signs of beta-cell autoimmunity (Kimpimaki et al., 2001). Holmberg and coworkers (2007) concluded that positivity for beta-cell autoantibodies in children from the general population was associated with a short duration of both total and exclusive breastfeeding as well as an early introduction of formula. Sensitization and development of immune memory to cow's milk protein is the initial step in the etiology of IDDM (Kostraba et al., 1993). Sensitization can occur with very early exposure to cow's milk before gut cellular tight junction closure takes place. It can also occur with exposure to cow's milk during an infection-caused GI alteration when the mucosal barrier becomes compromised, allowing antigens to cross and initiate immune reactions. Sensitization can take place if the presence of cow's milk protein in the gut damages the mucosal barrier, inflames the gut, or destroys binding components of cellular junctions or if another early insult with cow's milk protein leads to sensitization (Savilahti et al., 1993). Of further importance is the fact that exposure to infant cereal during the first 3 months of life in genetically predisposed infants significantly increases the risk of developing diabetes (Norris et al., 2003; Ziegler et al., 2003).

In the hospital it is important to ensure 8–12 feedings each 24 hours. Avoid giving the infant extra formula, water, or sugar water in an attempt to influence bilirubin levels. Bilirubin levels correlate inversely with the number of feedings during the first 24 hours (Table 1-1) (Yamauchi & Yamanouchi, 1990). Bilirubin levels also correlate inversely with the number of feedings over the first 3 days of life (DeCarvalho et al., 1982), as in the following examples:

- If the average number of feedings per day is 6, third-day bilirubin levels would be at 11 mg/dL.
- If the average number of feedings per day is 6.8, third-day bilirubin levels would be at 9.3 ± 3.5 mg/dL.
- If the average number of feedings per day is 10.1, third-day bilirubin levels would be at 6.5 ± 4.0 mg/dL.
- If the average number of feedings per day is 11, third-day bilirubin levels would be at 5 mg/dL.

TABLE 1-1 Correlation of Number of Feedings in First 24 Hours and Bilirubin Levels

Number of Feedings	Bilirubin Levels at 6 Days of Age
4 times in first 24 h	26% with elevated bilirubin levels on day 6 (12–14 mg/dL)
7–8 times in first 24 h	12% with elevated bilirubin levels on day 6
>9 times in first 24 h	None with elevated bilirubin levels on day 6

Source: Yamauchi Y, & Yamanouchi H. Breastfeeding Frequency During the First 24 Hours After Birth in Full Term Neonates. *Pediatr.* 1990;86:171–175.

As well, bilirubin levels correlate inversely with the amount of water or glucose water given to breastfed newborns (Nicoll, Ginsburg, & Tripp, 1982). The more water or sugar water given to breastfed infants, the higher the bilirubin levels on day 3. Bilirubin functions as an antioxidant to protect cell membranes. Breastfed infants have higher levels of bilirubin than formula-fed infants because they are supposed to. Artificially lowering normally elevated bilirubin levels when feeding babies infant formula has not been shown to be beneficial.

Nutritional Components

Water

Water makes up the majority (87.5%) of human milk. All other components are dissolved, dispersed, or suspended in water. An infant receiving adequate amounts of breastmilk will automatically consume his or her entire water requirement. Even in hot arid or humid climates, human milk provides 100% of water needs (Ashraf et al., 1993).

Clinical Implications

Because human milk with its low solute load provides all the water an infant needs, breastfed infants do not require additional water. Consuming more water than needed can suppress the infant's appetite (especially if the water contains dextrose) and reduce the number of calories the infant receives, placing him or her at risk for hyperbilirubinemia and early weight loss. Sterile water has no calories; 5% dextrose water has 5 calories per ounce, whereas colostrum has 18 calories per ounce. An infant receiving an ounce of sugar water in place of an ounce of colostrum will experience a two-thirds deficit in calories.

Large amounts of low-solute water given to an infant over a short period of time can contribute to oral water intoxication, swelling of the brain, and seizures (Keating et al., 1991). Oral water intoxication is more commonly seen in formula-fed infants whose caregivers use water bottles to extend the time between feedings or dilute formula supplies to make them last longer. This condition, however, can also occur in breastfed infants. A combination of factors can place the infant at risk for water intoxication, such as administration of large amounts of hypotonic intravenous solutions to laboring mothers (Tarnow-Mordi et al., 1981), addition of intravenous oxytocin (Singhi et al., 1985), and a large oral intake of fluid during labor (Johansson et al., 2002). A fluid shift to the fetus plus the birth-related surge in circulating vasopressin (the antidiuretic hormone) in the infant (Leung et al., 1980) can contribute to a water-sparing reaction or water retention in the infant. Excessive water in the infant can artificially inflate the birth weight, causing undue concern about large weight losses as the infant experiences diuresis or eliminates this water.

The mistaken belief that breastfed infants need supplemental water to prevent dehydration, hyperbilirubinemia, hypoglycemia, and weight loss disrupts breast-feeding and is often offered simply for convenience (Williams, 2006). Glover and Sandilands (1990) reported that infants who received glucose water supplementation in the hospital lost more weight and stayed in hospital longer than infants who did not receive supplementation. Ruth-Sanchez and Greene (1997) described a 3-day-old breastfed infant who was given 675 mL (22.5 oz) of dextrose water by nurses and the mother in the 24 hours before NICU admission for resulting seizure activity. Breastfed infants do not require additional water, even in hot or arid climates (Almroth & Bidinger, 1990; Cohen et al., 2000; Sachdev et al., 1991).

Despite data to the contrary, the practice of giving water or sugar water to breastfed infants persists. In 2007, to characterize maternity practices related to breastfeeding, the Centers for Disease Control and Prevention (2008) conducted the first national Maternity Practices in Infant Nutrition and Care Survey. Survey responses were received from 2,687 hospitals and birthing facilities. When asked whether healthy, full-term, breastfed infants who receive supplements are given glucose water or water, 30% of facilities reported giving feedings of glucose water and 15% reported giving water, practices that are not supportive of breastfeeding. Data from the Infant Feeding Practices Study II (a survey of mother-reported infant feeding patterns) revealed that 13% of infants received sugar water while in the hospital and 10% of the infants were receiving plain water at the age of 1 month (Grummer-Strawn et al., 2008), even when findings show that infants who do not consume solid foods have no need of solute-free water (Centers for Disease Control and Prevention, 1994; Scariati et al., 1997b). Mothers with low confidence levels with regards to their ability to breastfeed are vulnerable to the plethora of advice that is offered to them, even if it is misguided or incorrect, such as suggestions to offer supplementary or complementary water feedings (Blyth et al., 2002). If they perceive this advice as an indication of insufficient milk, they are significantly more likely to wean.

Healthcare providers must clearly understand the danger of excessive water supplementation and adequately convey these concerns to parents. An approach to help eliminate water supplementation is as follows:

- Teach and assess proper positioning, latch, and milk transfer.
- Document swallowing and ensure that the mother knows when her baby is swallowing milk.
- Avoid using sterile water or dextrose water. If a breastfed infant requires supplementation, use expressed colostrum/milk.
- Educate the parents and extended family regarding the hazard of giving young breastfed babies bottles of water, even in hot weather.
- Avoid placing water bottles in the infant's bassinet in the hospital.
- Remind mothers that babies also nurse at the breast for thirst, frequently coming off the breast after only a few minutes of nursing.
- If a baby is latched but not swallowing adequately, have the mother use alternate massage (massage and compress the breast during pauses between sucking bursts) to sustain sucking and swallowing.
- Maternal consumption of water in excess of thirst does not increase milk production and can cause the mother to produce less milk (Dusdieker et al., 1985).

Lipids

Milk lipids (among other components) have generated intense interest from numerous studies showing that formula-fed infants and children demonstrate less advanced cognitive development and poorer psychomotor development compared with breastfed children (Table 1-2). A number of components found in human milk but absent in unsupplemented formulas are thought to contribute to these deficits, including particular long-chain polyunsaturated fatty acids (LCPUFAs).

TABLE 1-2 Artificially Fed Infants Demonstrate Different Neurodevelopment and Cognitive Outcomes

- A different brain composition than breastfed infants (Uauy, 1990)
- Reduced concentrations of brain sialic acid, leading to potential deficits in neuro-development and cognition (Wang et al., 2003)
- Poorer neurobehavioral organization at 1 week of age (Hart et al., 2003)
- Lower neurodevelopmental response at 4 months of age (Agostoni et al., 1995)
- Lower cognitive development observed from 6 months through 16 years (Anderson et al., 1999)
- Lower mental development and psychomotor development scores at 12 months (Agostoni et al., 2001)
- Less mature nervous systems at 1 year of age and attainment of near-adult values of central and peripheral conduction later than breastfed infants (Khedr et al., 2004)
- Lower mental development scores at 18 months (Florey et al., 1995)
- Poorer developmental outcome of very-low-birth-weight infants at 18 months of age (Vohr et al., 2006)
- Lower mental development scores at 2 years of age (Morrow-Tlucak et al., 1988)
- Lower cognitive development at 3 years of age (Bauer et al., 1991; Johnson & Swank, 1996)
- Lower cognitive function of very-low-birth-weight infants at 5 years of age (Tanaka et al., 2008)
- Lower IQ scores at 6.5 years (Kramer et al., 2008)
- Lower IQ scores at 7 years (Lucas et al., 1992)
- Twice the rate of minor neurological dysfunction at 9 years (Lanting et al., 1994)
- Lower IQ scores at 11–16 years (Greene et al., 1995)
- Lower IQ and lower attainment in school at 18 years (Horwood & Fergusson, 1998)
- Lower cognitive development when born small for gestational age (Rao et al., 2002; Slykerman et al., 2005)
- Increased risk for specific language impairment (Tomblin et al., 1997)
- Half the DHA as the brain of a breastfed infant (Cunnane et al., 2000)
- Significantly lower DHA in the gray and white matter of the cerebellum (coordinates movement and balance) (Jamieson et al., 1999)
- Slower brainstem maturation in preterm infants (Amin et al., 2000)
- Increased abnormalities in neurobehaviors of preterm infants (Brown et al., 2006)

(continues)

TABLE 1-2 Artificially Fed Infants Demonstrate Different Neurodevelopment and Cognitive Outcomes *(continued)*

- Poorer stereoacuity at 3.5 years and at 6 years of age (Singhal et al., 2007; Williams et al., 2001)
- Suboptimal quality of general movements that correlate with poorer neurobehavioral condition of children at school age (Bouwstra et al., 2003)
- Increased gross motor delay (Sacker et al., 2006)
- Poorer speech processing with the potential for less optimal linguistic and cognitive development (Ferguson & Molfese, 2007)
- Lower IQ scores in young adults (Mortensen et al., 2002)

Many classes of lipids and thousands of subclasses exist. The fat content of human milk ranges from 3.5% to 4.5% and is influenced by a number of factors (Table 1-3).

Lipids provide a well-tolerated energy source, contributing approximately 50% of the calories in milk. They provide essential fatty acids and cholesterol. Triacylglycerols account for more than 98% of the lipids in milk. The composition of triacylglycerols is usually shown in terms of the kinds and amounts of fatty acids. A shorthand notation is commonly used when discussing fatty acids that abbreviates the chemical formula by stating the number of carbons to the left of the colon and the number of double bonds to the right of the colon:

16:0 palmitic acid

18:2 linoleic acid

20:4 arachidonic acid (AA)

22:6 docosahexaenoic acid (DHA)

Unlike breastmilk, unsupplemented infant formula does not contain the LCPUFAs DHA and AA. These two fatty acids are found in abundance as structural lipids in the infant's brain, retina, and central nervous system. Because the animal butterfat of cow's milk formula is replaced with plant oils, human milk and formula have quite different fatty acid profiles. Infant formulas typically contain soy oil, corn oil, and tropical oils such as palm and coconut oils, which may be well absorbed but are not used by the brain in the same way LCPUFAs are from human milk.

TABLE 1-3 Factors Influencing Human Milk Fat Content and Composition

Factor	Influence
During a feeding	Rises over the course of a feeding. This was further explained when the fat content of the milk was measured before and after every feed for 24 hours. Rather than fat content being related to the presence of foremilk or hindmilk, the fat content was related to the degree of fullness of the breast. As the breast is progressively drained, the fat content in the milk increases (Daly et al., 1993).
Volume	Lower milk fat content with higher volumes of milk
Number of days postpartum	Phospholipid and cholesterol levels are highest in early lactation.
Diurnal rhythm	Varies
Length of gestation	LCPUFA secretion increases with shortening length of gestation.
Parity	Endogenous fatty acid synthesis decreases with increased parity.
Maternal diet	Can change the LCPUFA profile as well as medium-chain fatty acids (increases with a low-fat diet)
Length of time between feeds	The shorter the interval, the higher the fat concentration.
Maternal energy status	A high weight gain in pregnancy is associated with increased milk fat.
Smoking	Maternal smoking decreases the fat content.

Source: Picciano MF. Nutrient composition of human milk. *Pediatr Clin North Am.* 2001;48, 53–67.

LCPUFAs have been added to term and preterm formulas in an attempt to provide infants with an exogenous source of these fully formed fatty acids. Concentrations of DHA and AA in human milk are highly variable and depend on the amount of these preformed fatty acids in the mother's diet and their biosynthesis from precursors (Brenna et al., 2007). Higher DHA values have been identified in preterm mothers' milk compared with that found in term human milk, underscoring the importance of using the mother's own milk to feed her preterm infant (Bokor et al., 2007). Infant formulas are supplemented with differing amounts of DHA and AA that are typically based on the average amount found in term human milk. Because there appears to be a higher concentration of DHA in preterm milk, preterm infant formula supplemented with DHA may not contain high enough levels compared with preterm human milk.

The source of the DHA and AA varies. Infant formulas in the United States use DHA from fermented microalgae (*Crypthecodiunium cohnii*) and AA from soil fungus (*Mortierelle alpina*). These ingredients are new to the food chain and in animal studies showed side effects such as fat loss through stool, oily soft stools (steatorrhea) in acute toxicity tests, higher liver weights in male rats, and increased fetal and neonatal undeveloped renal papilla and dilated renal pelvicies (LSRO Report, 1998). Little evidence exists showing that supplementing formula with LCPUFAs confers any significant long-term benefit to term or preterm infants (Raiten et al., 1998; Simmer, 2002a, 2002b). The results of most of the well-conducted, randomized, controlled trials have not shown beneficial effects of LCPUFA supplementation of infant formula on the physical, visual, and neuro-developmental outcomes of term or preterm infants. Routine supplementation of infant formula with LCPUFA to improve the physical, neurodevelopmental, or visual outcomes of term or preterm infants cannot be recommended based on the current evidence (Simmer et al., 2008a, 2008b).

Because of concerns regarding the safety and effectiveness of the DHA/AA additive, the U.S. Food and Drug Administration and Health Canada commissioned the Institute of Medicine to evaluate the process used to determine the safety of new ingredients added to infant formulas. The Institute of Medicine's subsequent report noted a number of shortcomings, including the absence of a structured approach to monitoring side effects after the new formula was on the market (see Additional Readings for information on the full report).

The bioactive fatty acids DHA and AA, when consumed in human milk, are part of a complex matrix of other fatty acids. Important physiological considerations related to this matrix are not accounted for by the simple addition of LCPUFAs to infant formula. Many concerns have been raised about these additives (Heird, 1999):

- Supplementation with highly unsaturated oils increases the susceptibility of membranes to oxidant damage and disrupts the antioxidant system. Damage from oxygen radicals can provoke diseases thought to be related to oxidant damage, such as NEC, bronchopulmonary dysplasia, and retrolental fibroplasia (Song et al., 2000; Song & Miyazawa, 2001). LCPUFA administration has effects on retinol and alpha-tocopherol metabolism (Decsi & Koletzko, 1995).

- Higher levels of PUFAs in muscle cell membranes have been related to increased insulin sensitivity (Pan et al., 1994).

- There is a possible effect on gene transcription (Clarke & Jump, 1996).

- High-fat supplementation of formula and commercial jarred baby foods has raised the question that these additives may contribute to the obesity epidemic (Massiera et al., 2003).

- Increasing DHA fortification of commercial baby food adds to the concerns about excessive intake and/or imbalanced ratios of n-6 and n-3 fatty acids.

- Imbalanced ratios of fatty acids can result in altered growth patterns (Carlson et al., 1992, 1993).

- Many studies have insufficient sample sizes to determine any functional benefit or safety profile; comparison of research results is confounded by the use of different sources of DHA and AA, different amounts and ratios of these fatty acids, different compositions of the base formulas, and different lengths of time the study formulas were consumed (Koo, 2003).

- Most studies compare supplemented versus unsupplemented formulas to each other but lack a control group of exclusively breastfed infants; many have high attrition rates.

- The accuracy and reliability of the tests used to determine visual and cognitive effects of LCPUFAs during the first 2 years are controversial.

- Enrollment criteria for most studies typically excluded sick infants, twins and higher order multiples, and most infants with any type of problem. This population choice may leave doubts about the suitability of fatty acid supplemented formula for these infants, regardless of the source of the LCPUFAs.

- Meta-analysis of randomized trials suggests that any functional benefit in visual or neurodevelopment from LCPUFA supplementation of infant formula is likely to be of minor clinical significance, at least for the term infant (Koo, 2003).

- Little evidence indicates that LCPUFA-containing infant formula provides clinically significant improvements in vision and intelligence in healthy term infants. The 25% higher cost can place a significant burden on a family's budget and on public nutrition programs.

- Human milk contains LCPUFAs other than DHA and AA that can be converted to DHA and AA and affects the conversion of alpha-linolenic and linoleic acid to DHA and AA. Their presence may partially explain the apparent need for greater amounts of DHA and AA in formula to achieve the same plasma lipid content of these fatty acids observed in human milk-fed infants (Clandinin et al., 1997).

- Breastmilk contains lipases that enhance fat digestion in breastfed infants; it is a complex matrix, containing numerous bioactive components, hormones, and live cells not found in infant formula. Important physiological considerations relative to the matrix are not accounted for by the simple addition of LCPUFAs to infant formula (Office of Food Additive Safety, 2001).

Clinical Implications

The provision of breastmilk during the period of brain development is important for several reasons:

- IQ studies are remarkably consistent in their demonstration of higher IQ scores that are dose dependent relative to the number of months a child has been breastfed.

- The brain composition of formula-fed infants is measurably and chemically different; namely, DHA levels remain static in formula-fed infants but rise in breastfed infants (Farquharson et al., 1992).

- Unsupplemented formula contains no DHA or AA, just their precursors, linolenic and linoleic acid. Infants must rely on an immature liver to synthesize enough of these LCPUFAs to meet the needs of the developing brain.

- Supplemented formulas have unknown side effects:
  1. Fermented microalgae and soil fungus could contain contaminants from the fermentation and oil extraction process, such as hexane residue.
  2. Positional distributions of plant-based LCPUFAs on triacylglycerols are different from those of human milk triglycerides. Triacylglycerols or triglycerides are the form in which the body stores fat. They consist of a glycerol spine with three attached fatty acids. The location of the fatty acid

on the glycerol spine is identified by stereospecific numbering (sn). Certain fatty acids have preferences for binding at certain positions.

a. Infant formula strives to match the overall fatty acid composition of human milk, but it cannot duplicate the triacylglycerol structure that alters lipid metabolism in infants not fed human milk (Nelson & Innis, 1999). Even though the formula is supplemented with DHA and AA, the shape of the molecule is different from that of the DHA and AA found in human milk.

b. AA and DHA in human milk are present in the sn-1 or sn-2 positions but can be present in all three positions in the single cell oils (Myher et al., 1996). In human milk 55% of DHA is found in the sn-2 position.

c. Human milk triglycerides usually contain no more than one molecule of DHA or AA, whereas some single-cell triglycerides contain two or even three such molecules. Most of the LCPUFAs in formula are located in the outer positions of the triacylglycerol molecule, placing them at potential risk for slow and low absorption (Straarup et al., 2006).

d. DHA and AA added to infant formula can act differently in the body from human DHA and AA, depending on where and in what proportion they are found on the triglyceride molecule. It is unknown how these differences in molecular shape and triglyceride positioning could affect their metabolism and functioning.

- Fungal sources of AA pose a risk of introducing mycotoxins that could act as opportunistic pathogens in an immunocompromised host.

- Fungal and microalgal oil supplements have been shown to cause a dose-dependent increase in excess gas and belching in adults (Innis & Hansen, 1996).

- The National Alliance for Breastfeeding Advocacy has received numerous complaints of infants experiencing watery explosive diarrhea, diaper rash, excessive foul-smelling gas, and abdominal cramping from ingesting infant formula with the highest levels of LCPUFA supplementation. Also reported was obesity in 6-month-old infants who initially breastfed but had DHA/AA-supplemented formula added to their diet as a supplement, followed by infant cereal at 4 months of age.

- The U.S. Food and Drug Administration has received approximately 100 reports from healthcare providers and parents describing adverse reactions to DHA/AA-supplemented formulas. Reports state that numerous side effects such as vomiting and diarrhea disappeared as soon as the infant was switched to a formula without these additives (Vallaeys, 2008). Some infants may have more difficulty digesting triglycerides with multiple DHA molecules occupying two or three places on the glycerol spine. Also, a possible contributor to variations in how infants handle these oils is the fact that they contain 40–50% DHA and AA, with the remaining components being high-oleic sunflower oil, diglycerides, and nonsaponifiable materials.

- Studies on LCPUFA-supplemented formula have shown no consistent beneficial outcomes (Follett et al., 2003).

- Neural maturation of formula-fed preterm infants shows a deficit compared with those fed human milk.

- Delayed maturation in visual acuity can occur in both term and preterm formula-fed infants. This delay may affect other mental and physical functions linked to vision in later development (Birch et al., 1993).

The sterol content of human milk ranges from 10 to 20 mg/dL, rising over the course of the lactation, with cholesterol as the major component. Cholesterol is an essential part of all membranes and is required for normal growth and functioning. Breastfed infants' serum cholesterol levels are higher than those of formula-fed infants. This difference may have a long-term effect on the ability of the adult to metabolize cholesterol. Cholesterol is part of and necessary for the laying down of the myelin sheath that is involved in nerve conduction in the brain. Formula contains little to no cholesterol. Information for parents pertinent to the fat component of human milk includes the following:

- Inform parents of the developmental and cognitive differences between infants fed formula or breastmilk. The average eight-point IQ score elevation in breastfed infants can be the difference between optimal and suboptimal functioning, especially in disadvantaged environments. Eight points is one-half of a standard deviation and is thought to provide a buffer to the neonatal brain from such detrimental factors as maternal smoking, maternal polychlorinated biphenol (PCB) ingestion, and lead ingestion in infancy. One IQ point has been estimated to be worth

$14,500.00 in economic benefits from improved worker productivity (Grosse et al., 2002).

- The fatty acid composition of breastmilk can be altered by the maternal diet. Lowering the amounts of trans-fatty acids from hydrogenated fats and increasing the amounts of omega-3 fatty acids from eggs and fish are both beneficial.

- Teach mothers to allow the baby to finish the first side before switching to the second breast. This allows the baby to self-regulate his or her intake, receive the maximum amount of calories (from fat levels that rise at the end of a feeding), and avoid low-calorie, high-lactose feedings that result from placing time limits on the first breast "so the baby will take the second side."

- For infants experiencing slow weight gain, mothers can be guided to finish the first side by using alternate massage before offering the second side and to shorten the intervals between daytime feeds to increase the fat content of the milk.

- When breastmilk is stored in the refrigerator or freezer, the fat rises to the top of the container. This can be skimmed off and given to a slow-gaining or preterm infant for extra calories. This milk can be quite calorie dense at 26–28 calories per ounce.

- Smoking decreases the fat content of breastmilk. Vio and colleagues (1991) described milk volume, fat content, and infants' average weight gain over a 14-day study of maternal smokers and nonsmokers. Mean milk volume of nonsmokers was 961 ± 120 g/day, whereas the mean volume of maternal smokers was 693 ± 110 g/day. Fat concentrations of nonsmokers were 4.05%, whereas that for smokers was 3.25%. Infants' average weight increase over the 14-day study period was 550 ± 130 g (19.6 oz) for children of nonsmokers and 340 ± 170 g (12.1 oz) for children of smokers. Infants whose mothers smoke need careful follow-up and frequent weight checks.

Protein

Human milk proteins, like so many other milk components, exert multiple physiological activities that include enhancement of the immune system; defensive duties against pathogenic bacteria, viruses, and yeast; and the development of the gut. The protein concentration of human milk is high during the colostrum period, leveling off to about 0.8–1.0% in mature milk. It is also higher in preterm milk initially than in term milk. Milk proteins have classically been divided into casein and whey proteins. A third group of proteins, called mucins, surrounds the lipid globules in milk and contributes only a small percentage of the total protein content.

Caseins of human milk constitute 10–50% of the total protein, with this percentage rising over the course of the lactation. Colostrum and preterm milk either do not contain or are very low in casein. Casein gives milk its characteristic white appearance. This easily digested protein provides amino acids and aids in calcium and phosphorus absorption in the newborn. Bovine casein is less easily digested in human infants and may not exert the same effect that human milk casein does. The casein protein that predominates in cow's milk forms a tough rubbery curd in the stomach of an infant and requires a longer time to break down and digest. The whey-to-casein ratio in human milk changes over the course of lactation from 90:10 in the early milk, to 60:40 in mature milk, and to 50:50 in late lactation, and as a consequence of the continually changing ratio there is really no fixed ratio of casein to whey in human milk (Lonnerdal, 2003). By comparison, these ratios do not change in infant formula and can, in fact, be directly opposite that of human milk.

Maternal dietary intake of protein can influence differing protein fractions in human milk (Lopez Alvarez, 2007). In a well-nourished population of mothers with widely varying differences in protein and energy intake, the nitrogen component as well as the protein fraction in their breastmilk remained unaffected (Boniglia et al., 2003). However, in a malnourished sample of Colombian mothers, those who did not receive sufficient protein intake experienced a two-thirds reduction in protein content of early milk and diminished C4 complement, IgA, and IgG (Picciano, 1998). In a study that sought to improve the quality of breastmilk through protein supplementation, Chao et al. (2004) supplemented mothers with a protein-rich chicken extract from the 37th week of gestation until 3 days postpartum. Total protein in colostrum did not significantly change; however, dietary supplementation resulted in up to a 35% increase in breastmilk lactoferrin, a 62% increase in epidermal growth factor, and a 196% increase in transforming growth factor-beta 2.

Whey proteins are very diverse. Alpha-lactalbumin and lactoferrin are the chief fractions. Human alpha-lactalbumin has a high nutritional value and has been shown to have antitumor activity (Hakansson et al., 1995). Alpha-lactalbumin can appear as a large complex in human milk and is modified in the infant's stomach into a molecular complex called HAMLET (human alpha-lactalbumin made lethal to tumor cells) and in this form has been shown to kill transformed cells (Gustafsson et al., 2005; Newburg, 2005) as well as 40 different carcinoma and lymphoma cell lines (Svensson et al., 2000). HAMLET has been suggested as a possible reason why breastfeeding results in lower rates of childhood leukemia and a reduced incidence of breast cancer (Hanson, 2004). Lactoferrin is an iron-binding protein. Colostrum contains 5–7 g/L of lactoferrin, which gradually decreases over time. A 1-month-old infant consumes about 260 mg/kg/day of lactoferrin and at 4 months about 125 mg/kg/day (Butte et al., 1984). Lactoferrin promotes the growth of intestinal epithelium and has been thought to exert its bacteriocidal effect through withholding iron from iron-requiring pathogens. This type of inhibition can be reversed by the addition of iron in excess of the binding capacity of lactoferrin. It may, however, have a more important effect, which is to alter the properties of the bacterial cell membrane, making it more vulnerable to the killing effects of lysozyme. Immunoglobulins are part of the whey protein fraction, as are enzymes.

Immunoglobulins are members of the defense agent team in breastmilk. The predominant immunoglobulin in human milk is immunoglobulin A (IgA). Concentrations of IgA are highest in colostrum and gradually decline to a plateau of about 1 mg/mL for the duration of lactation. The infant's approximate mean intake of IgA is 125 mg/kg/day at 1 month and 75 mg/kg/day by 4 months (Butte et al., 1984). Breastfeeding actively stimulates and directs the immune response of the breastfed infant. Vaccine responses to oral polio virus vaccine and parenteral tetanus and diphtheria toxoid vaccines are enhanced by breastfeeding, with formula-fed infants sometimes showing lower antibody levels to their immunizations (Hahn-Zoric et al., 1990; Pickering et al., 1998).

Human milk also contains numerous enzymes. Some function in the mammary gland, some act in the infant, and some have unknown functions. Many are involved in the digestive process, whereas others function in defense against disease. For example, lysozyme is active against the human immunodeficiency virus and plays a role in the antibacterial activity of human milk, showing the most effect against gram-positive bacteria. High concentrations are present throughout lactation, whereas concentrations are several orders of magnitude lower in bovine milk. Whereas secretory IgA and lactoferrin levels decrease after the early period of lactation, lysozyme levels remain higher during the 6-month to 2-year period of lactation than they were during the first month of breastfeeding.

Platelet-activating factor acetylhydrolase (PAF-AH) plays an important role in the prevention of NEC, an often fatal bowel disease in preterm infants. PAF is a potent ulcerative agent in the GI tract. NEC can be induced within hours after administration of PAF in experimental animals. PAF-AH hydrolyzes PAF to produce an inactive form, thereby helping to prevent the development of NEC in infants receiving breastmilk (Furukawa et al., 1993). It is interesting to note that among the species studied, the only one devoid of milk PAF-AH was bovine milk; thus, cow's milk cannot substitute for human milk (Park et al., 1983).

The nonprotein nitrogen fraction of human milk accounts for 20–25% of the total nitrogen found in human milk. It is made up of peptides, urea, uric acid, ammonia, free amino acids, creatine, creatinine, nucleic acids, nucleotides, polyamines, carnitine, choline, amino alcohols of phospholipids, amino sugars, peptide hormones, and growth factors. Nucleotides have received increased attention because some infant formulas have been supplemented with them. Human milk has a specific content of free nucleotides that differs from the mix found in cow's milk. Nucleotides are involved in the modulation of the immune system, the intestinal microenvironment, and the absorption and metabolism of nutrients. The total nucleotide content of human milk, if nucleic acid content is included, greatly exceeds the levels found in formula supplemented with nucleotides. Although nucleotide-supplemented formula is marketed as "being closer to breastmilk," it remains unproven whether this contributes to decreased morbidity or increased revenues.

Clinical Implications

Cow's milk serves as the base of most infant formulas. The prevalence of cow's milk allergy has been placed at between 2% and 5% of infants (Host et al., 1995). Risk factors include a family history of atopy and early dietary exposure to cow's milk. The age at onset is directly correlated with the time of introduction of infant formula (Oski et al., 1994). Even exclusively breastfed infants can develop symptoms of cow's milk protein intolerance that may respond to elimination of the offending agent from the mother's diet.

Because of the high cross-reactivity to soy protein, the potential for soy allergy is 10–14% and is not used for infants with documented cow's milk allergy. Soy formula neither reduces allergic symptoms nor delays allergies (Chandra & Hamed, 1991). Soy formula has no advantage as a supplement to breastmilk, has no proven value in the prevention or management of infant colic or fussiness, and is only indicated for infants with galactosemia, hereditary lactase deficiency (extremely rare), or when the family prefers a vegetarian diet (Bhatia & Greer, 2008). Although cow's milk protein–based lactose-free formulas are available, they have not been shown to have any clinical impact on colic, growth, or development, and they are not recommended for infants with diarrhea (Heyman, 2006). Breastfed infants should be continued on human milk during episodes of diarrhea. Human milk proteins play a critical role in directing the construction of the immune system. Infants fed soy formula have the lowest antibody titers to their vaccines, whereas those fed cow milk–based formula are still below breastfed infants both in antibody titers and incidence of illness (Zoppi et al., 1983). Some soy formula–fed infants have had to be reimmunized after soy formula feeding. It is recommended that the clinician take the following steps:

- Prenatally, help parents understand the importance of exclusive breast-feeding for about 6 months, especially those with a family history of allergies and diabetes.

- Avoid giving bottles of formula (cow milk based or soy based) in the hospital. Even one bottle can sensitize a susceptible infant and provoke an allergy later when challenged again.

- Encourage frequent breastfeeding, 8–12 times every 24 hours right from the start. Colostrum contains large amounts of protein, especially the sIgA that helps protect the infant against disease. These protein levels in colostrum also serve to prevent hypoglycemia.

Carbohydrates

The principal carbohydrate in human milk is lactose (galactose + glucose), with other carbohydrates occurring in smaller amounts, such as oligosaccharides, monosaccharides, and peptide-bound and protein-bound carbohydrates. Lactose is thought to have several functions:

- Lactose favors the colonization of the infant's intestine with microflora that competes with and excludes pathogens.

- Infants undergo rapid brain development during the nursing period. Myelination requires large amounts of galactosylceramide (galacto-cerebrosides) and other galactolipids that are major components of this growth. The infant liver may be unable to synthesize all the galactolipids needed at this time. Milk galactose is most likely present to ensure an adequate supply of galactocerebrosides for optimal brain development. Brain growth and development during this time is known to be vulnerable to many types of nutrient deficiencies. This vulnerability has important ramifications for infants on artificial diets, especially when lactose is removed from their sole source of nutrition, as with soy formula or cow milk–based formula that has had the lactose removed.

- Lactose enhances calcium absorption. Infants fed cow milk–based formula with the lactose removed show reduced calcium absorption (Abrams et al., 2002). Lactose levels are quite stable, showing little or no change in response to a wide variety of environmental or dietary challenges. Infants are well suited to use lactose because lactase, a brush border intestinal enzyme that digests lactose, is present by 24 weeks of fetal life. Lactase levels increase throughout the last trimester of fetal life, reaching concentrations at term that are two to four times the levels seen at 2–11 months of age. One hypothesis suggests that a relationship exists between the relative size of the brain and the level of lactose in a species' milk. Humans with their large brains have very high lactose levels in their milk compared with other species.

Oligosaccharides are biologically active carbohydrates. More than 200 neutral and acidic oligosaccharides have been identified to date at levels of approximately 12–14 g/L (1.2–1.4 g/dL), making them collectively the third largest solid component of human milk. An individual mother's milk can contain anywhere from a few dozen to more than a hundred different oligosaccharides. The concentration of oligosaccharides in cow's milk is about 20-fold lower than that found in human milk (Veh et al., 1981). Oligosaccharides have water-soluble cell surface analogs that can inhibit enteropathogen binding to host cell receptors. Oligosaccharides can inhibit the binding to their receptors of such bacteria as *Streptococcus pneumoniae*, *Haemophilus influenzae*, *E. coli*, and *Campylobacter jejuni*. Milk oligosaccharides also contain human blood group antigens, with women from different blood group types exhibiting distinct patterns.

Lactating mothers may differ genetically in their ability to produce protective oligosaccharides and thus may influence their breastfed infant's susceptibility to enteric disease (Morrow et al., 2004; Uauy & Araya, 2004). Infant formulas have an oligosaccharide-bound sialic acid content that is 10–27 times lower than that of human milk because the manufacturing process for infant formulas has virtually eliminated this component from the finished product (Martin-Sosa et al., 2003). Formula-fed infants have a reduced intake of and fewer oligosaccharides than human milk–fed infants in their stool and urine, which also differ in composition from those of breastfed infants (Hanson, 2004). Many infant formulas have been supplemented with plant-based oligosaccharides in an effort to mimic their function and outcome as seen in breastfed infants, such as inducing softer stools and creating gut flora patterns similar to breastfed infants. One potential side effect of this type of supplementation is the possibility of bacterial translocation. The term "bacterial translocation" is used to describe the passage of viable resident bacteria from the GI tract to normally sterile tissues such as the mesenteric lymph nodes and other internal organs. Barrat et al. (2008) reported that in a study of rats fed a formula with added oligosaccharides and inulin, an increase in bacterial translocation occurred in the immature gut. This side effect may pose a potential infectious risk and requires further study.

Human milk oligosaccharides are an important source of sialic acid for the infant. Sialic acid is an integral part of the plasma membranes of nerve cells concentrated in the region of nerve endings and dendrites in the brain. The brains of breastfed infants have higher amounts of sialic acid than formula-fed infants (Wang et al., 2003). Formula-fed infants derive less than 25% of the amount of sialic acid that is supplied to breastfed infants through mature human milk. Formula-fed infants have a lower dietary source of sialic acid and are unable to synthesize the difference (McVeagh & Miller, 1997). Soy formulas have almost undetectable amounts of sialic acid (Wang et al., 2001). In animal models, an exogenous source of sialic acid increased learning performance as well as the concentration of sialic acid in the frontal cortex of the brain (Wang et al., 2007). Large amounts of sialylated oligosaccharides may be one mechanism by which breastfeeding promotes higher cognitive performance in children.

Clinical Implications

Human milk provides several tiers of protection from pathogens, and those tiers have the potential to work synergistically. The processing of infant formulas based on cow's milk utilizes procedures that exclude from the final product colostrum, milk-fat globule membranes, and fractions that contain DNA. Milk oligosaccharides from other species confer protection to the young of that species. Random additions of a few oligosaccharides to infant formula would not be expected to generate a tier of disease protection because those oligosaccharides in breastmilk are unique to human milk and have not be replicated synthetically. Reassure parents that it is uncommon for infant fussiness to be related to lactose intolerance. Primary lactose intolerance (lactase deficiency) is extremely rare. Weaning a breastfed infant to a lactose-free formula removes all layers of disease protection and changes the nature of the nutrient supply to the brain. There is a 10-fold difference in sialic concentrations among different types of formulas, with none containing more than 25% of the brain builders found in human milk.

Vitamins

The water-soluble vitamins in human milk are ascorbic acid (vitamin C), thiamin (vitamin B1), riboflavin (vitamin B2), niacin, pyridoxine (vitamin B6), folate, pantothenate, biotin, and vitamin B12. The concentration of water-soluble vitamins in human milk shows variations reflecting the stage of lactation, maternal intake, and delivery before term. The breast cannot synthesize water-soluble vitamins, so their origins lie in the maternal plasma, derived from the maternal diet. Concentrations are generally lower in the early days of breastfeeding compared with those found in mature milk. In mothers who are adequately nourished, maternal supplementation in higher than physiological doses either has no effect or is transient. Maternal vitamin supplementation generally shows benefits only when the mother herself is malnourished. Storage and handling of expressed human milk can alter some of the vitamin components in it. Total ascorbic acid (vitamin C) levels decreased on average by one-third after 24 hours of storage at 4°C, with wide variations between individual mothers (Buss et al., 2001). Francis and coworkers (2008) found that various bottle systems showed measurable decreases in the mean concentration of ascorbic acid over a 20-minute sampling period (the approximate time of a feeding). Those bottles with the largest milk-to-air interface had the greatest decreases in mean concentration of ascorbic acid over time. The air moving through the milk and the formation of bubbles on the surface of the milk could be factors in the observed decreases of ascorbic acid concentration. Ascorbic acid is also degraded by exposure to light, suggesting that tinted bottles for expressing, storing, and feeding human milk might be appropriate. Those infants who are solely dependent on bottle feeds for their total ascorbic acid intake by formula or breastmilk, especially high-risk or preterm infants, may need their ascorbic acid status evaluated. Caregivers (parents and health professionals) should avoid shaking the bottle, may wish to use bottle systems with lower milk-to-air surface interfaces, and may wish to consider using tinted bottles for expressing, storing, and feeding purposes.

Vitamin B12 is needed by the infant's developing nervous system. This vitamin occurs exclusively in animal tissue, is bound to protein, and is minimal to absent in vegetable protein. A mother consuming a vegan diet, without meat or dairy products, may have milk deficient in vitamin B12.

The fat-soluble vitamins are A, D, E, and K. Vitamin A and its precursors, known as carotenoids (beta-carotene), occur at twice the levels in colostrum as in mature human milk. The level of vitamin A in the milk of well-nourished mothers delivering prematurely is even higher. This vitamin is important in infant growth and development. An inverse relationship exists between the risk of morbidity and mortality and vitamin A status. Even after breastfeeding is discontinued, it appears to confer a protective effect due to some of the vitamin A provided by breastmilk being stored in the child's liver.

Vitamin D comprises a group of related fat-soluble compounds with antirachitic (rickets) activity. Vitamin D is not actually a vitamin or a nutrient but a precursor of a steroid hormone formed when the skin is directly exposed to ultraviolet B radiation in sunlight. It is essential for the normal absorption of calcium from the gut. There are two forms of vitamin D, D2 (ergocalciferol that is synthesized by plants) and D3 (cholecalciferol) synthesized by mammals. The main source of vitamin D for humans is through its synthesis in the skin when exposed to ultraviolet B radiation in the range of 290–315 nm, with less than 10% derived from dietary sources. The most common food source of vitamin D is the plant steroid ergosterol, the liver and oils of some fatty fish, and foods fortified with vitamin D such as milk, orange juice, margarine, and cereals. Although vitamin D is synthesized in the skin upon exposure to sunlight, many people derive much of their vitamin D from foods that are supplemented or enriched with it. Levels of this vitamin vary in breastmilk and are often reported as being inadequate (Box 1-1).

Human milk is actually not deficient in vitamin D. Infants suffering from vitamin D deficiency and rickets do so from a deficit of exposure of the skin to sunlight or may be born deficient if their mother was also deficient during the pregnancy. Attaining sufficient and safe sunlight exposure for infants has been complicated by the recommendation from the AAP to keep infants less than 6 months of age out of direct sunlight and to use sunscreen on older infants and children (AAP, 1999). Rickets and poor bone mineralization are rare in breastfed infants but do occur. Incidents of vitamin D insufficiency and its extreme form, rickets, are still reported. Rickets is primarily associated with dark-skinned children on vegetarian diets, dark-skinned infants exclusively breastfed beyond 3 to 6 months of age, premature infants, and infants born to mothers who are vitamin-D deficient themselves (Misra et al., 2008). Greer and associates (1982) randomized infants into a group receiving a placebo and a group receiving a supplement of 10 μg of vitamin D daily. The bone-mineral content of the placebo group was

BOX 1-1 Details on Vitamin D

- Breastmilk contains an average vitamin D content of 26 IU/L (range, 5–136 IU) in a vitamin D–sufficient mother.[1]
- Infant formula contains 400 IU (10 μg) per liter.[2]
- If an infant consumes an average of 750 mL/day of breastmilk, exclusive breastfeeding without sun exposure would provide a range of 11–38 IU/day of vitamin D, which is below the recommended minimum intake of 400 IU/day.[3]
- An adequate intake level of vitamin D for infants with some sunlight exposure has not been established, but breastfed infants with limited sunlight exposure have not been shown to develop rickets.
- The cost of averting a single case of rickets by universally dosing infants with vitamin D could be between $252,614 and $958,293 per case.[4]
- The cost to breastfeeding initiation and duration rates has not been accounted for, nor has the concern that formula manufacturers will promote their products in such a way as to imply that breastmilk is inadequate and that their products should be used to prevent a condition caused by the use of "deficient" breastmilk.[5]

1. Institute of Medicine, Food and Nutrition Board, Standing Committee on the Evaluation of Dietary Reference Intakes. (1997). Vitamin D. In: Dietary Reference Intakes for Calcium, Phosphorous, Magnesium, Vitamin D and Fluoride. Washington, DC: National Academy Press; pp. 250–287.
2. Life Sciences Research Office Report. (1998). Assessment of nutrition requirements for infant formulas. *J Nutr.* 128:2059S–2293S.
3. Wagner, C.L., Greer, F.R., and the Section on Breastfeeding and Committee on Nutrition. (2008). Prevention of rickets and vitamin D deficiency in infants, children, and adolescents. *Pediatrics.* 122:1142–1152.
4. Vitamin D Expert Panel, Centers for Disease Control and Prevention. Final report. Retrieved June 15, 2005, from www.cdc.gov/nccdphp/dnpa/nutrition/pdf/Vitamin_D_Expert_Panel_Meeting.pdf
5. Heinig, M.J. (2003). Vitamin D and the breastfed infant: controversies and concerns. *J Hum Lact.* 19:247–249.

significantly lower in the first few months after birth but at the end of the first year was actually higher than that in the supplemented group.

Exclusive breastfeeding results in normal infant bone-mineral content when maternal vitamin D status is adequate (Greer & Marshall, 1989), when neonatal stores are normal, and when the infant is regularly exposed to sunlight. Specker et al. (1985) reported that 30 minutes of sun exposure per week for infants wearing only a diaper and 2 hours of sun exposure per week for fully clothed infants without a hat maintained vitamin D levels of greater than 27.5 nmol/L. However, the duration of sun exposure that is necessary for infants to maintain vitamin D levels at greater than 50 nmol/L, the currently accepted level for vitamin D sufficiency in children, is undetermined. Darkly pigmented infants require a greater exposure to sunshine to initiate the synthesis of vitamin D in the skin (Clemens et al., 1982). It has been shown that 400 IU/day of vitamin D maintains serum concentrations at greater than 50 nmol/L in exclusively breastfed infants (Wagner et al., 2006). Reports in the literature of confirmed rickets in breastfed infants (Kreiter et al., 2000; Shah et al., 2000) have led to a recommendation by the AAP that all breastfed infants be supplemented with 400 IU of vitamin D per day beginning in the first few days of life (Wagner et al., 2008). Controversy has been generated by this recommendation and the concomitant urging by the AAP that people limit their exposure to sunlight to reduce the incidence of skin cancer. Vitamin D status in infants also depends on numerous factors:

- Is the infant being exclusively breastfed? Is he or she being given medications, other foods, or drinks that could interfere with nutrient absorption such as calcium? Chronic calcium deficiency increases vitamin D metabolism with secondary vitamin D deficiency (Clements et al., 1987).

- What was the vitamin D status of the mother during her pregnancy? Maternal vitamin D concentrations largely determine the vitamin D status of the fetus and newborn infant. A mother deficient in vitamin D during her pregnancy will give birth to a vitamin D–deficient infant or an infant who will reach vitamin D deficiency more quickly than an infant born to a vitamin D–sufficient mother. Was the infant preterm? Preterm infants lack the necessary time to accumulate vitamin D stores. What is the mother's current vitamin D intake and exposure to sunlight?

- Is the infant's skin deeply pigmented? Approximately 90% of all reported cases of nutritional rickets have occurred in African-American children, identifying a population of infants at higher risk for rickets and for whom maternal supplementation or direct supplementation of vitamin D may be more important (Hirsch, 2007). Is he or she from a poor socioeconomic background? Is he or she malnourished or does the infant have fat malabsorption? How old is the infant? Overt rickets is more common in children older than 6 months of age (Pugliese et al., 1998; Sills et al., 1994).

A number of environmental, genetic, hormonal, nutritional, and cultural factors interact and/or overlap, putting some susceptible children at risk for rickets (Mojab, 2002):

- Maternal deficiency (prenatal and postpartum)
- Daylight hours spent indoors
- Living conditions such as residence in high latitudes and urban areas with buildings or pollution that block sunlight
- Dark skin pigmentation
- Use of sunscreen
- Covering the body when outside (cold climate, fear of skin cancer, cultural dress customs)

The antirachitic activity in human milk varies by season, maternal vitamin D intake, sun exposure, and race. Various levels of maternal vitamin D supplementation have been studied in an attempt to delineate how much is necessary to increase an infant's vitamin D levels to a mid-range of normal through the consumption of breastmilk. Researchers have supplemented lactating mothers with 2,000–4,000 IU vitamin D/day for 3 months, causing a significant rise in maternal vitamin D levels as well as improving vitamin D levels in breastmilk and in the recipient infants (Basile et al., 2006; Hollis & Wagner, 2004). Such a dose is much higher than the current Dietary Reference Intake for lactating mothers (400 IU/day). Concern has been raised regarding the safety of this practice; however, Vieth et al. (2001) and Heaney et al. (2003) show that vitamin D intakes of 10,000 IU/day (250 mg) or more are safe for periods up to 5 months. Further research is necessary to determine optimal vitamin D intakes for pregnant and lactating women from both sunlight and supplements.

Delineating high-risk groups of infants suitable for supplementation such as dark-skinned, exclusively breastfed infants who spend much time indoors has been suggested as a means of providing supplemental vitamin D appropriately, while avoiding the implication that breastmilk is deficient in this substance (Weisberg et al., 2004). High-dose vitamin D supplementation in nursing mothers may be a workable strategy for improving the vitamin D status of both the mothers and their exclusively breastfeeding infants. Welch et al. (2000) recommend viewing vitamin D supplementation as a mechanism to ensure an adequate substrate for a hormone whose normal production has been adversely affected by the realities of modern living conditions—not as a treatment for nutritional inadequacy of human milk.

Vitamin E (alpha-tocopherol) functions as an antioxidant. It protects cell membranes and is required for muscle integrity. This vitamin's concentration in colostrum is higher than in mature milk because vitamin E levels are low in the newborn and absorption is inefficient. Human milk supplies more than adequate amounts of vitamin E to the infant.

Vitamin K is essential for the formation of several proteins required for blood clotting. It is produced by the intestinal flora but takes several days in the previously sterile neonatal gut to be effective. Vitamin K stores at birth are very low, so newborns are immediately dependent on an external source for the vitamin. A deficiency of vitamin K increases the risk of a syndrome called hemorrhagic disease of the newborn. The early onset form occurs at 2–10 days of age in 1 of every 200 to 400 newborns who do not receive additional vitamin K. The late onset form occurs around 1 month of age in 1 of every 1,000 to 2,000 unsupplemented newborns. The most dependable method of preventing hemorrhagic disease of the newborn is an injected or oral dose of vitamin K at birth (Kleinman, 2004). Vitamin K levels in human milk respond to maternal supplements, but this response is variable and has not been well studied. Vitamin K is localized in the milk-fat globule, with hindmilk containing twofold higher vitamin K concentrations than milk collected from a full breast pumping.

Minerals and Trace Elements

The most prevalent monovalent ions in human milk are sodium, potassium, and chloride; the most prevalent divalent ions are calcium, magnesium, citrate, phosphate, and sulfate. Numerous factors affect the levels of these minerals in human milk. During pregnancy, involution, and mastitis, the junctions between the alveolar cells remain open, allowing sodium and chloride to enter the milk space, drawing water along with them. Lactose and potassium are also thought to move from the milk space to the blood. The net result is that under these conditions, milk has greatly increased concentrations of sodium and chloride and decreased concentrations of lactose and potassium. The presence of high sodium concentrations in human milk is diagnostic of either mastitis or low milk-volume secretion. Colostrum has much higher concentrations of sodium and chloride than does mature milk because the gland is undergoing the transition between pregnancy, when the junctions are open, and full lactation, when they are closed. Preterm milk shows lower concentrations of sodium and chloride that rise to normal levels approximately 30 days postpartum.

The concentrations in milk of the major divalent ions are species specific. The calcium level increases markedly during the first few days postpartum but then decreases gradually over the course of the lactation. Citrate and phosphate concentrations rise in parallel with the sharp increase in milk volume between 2 to 4 days postpartum. The calcium-to-phosphorus ratio is lower in cow's milk (1:4) than in human milk (2:2). Lactation also affects the mother's calcium movement. Calcium uptake in the maternal duodenum is enhanced during lactation. After weaning, women who have lactated show significantly more bone in the lumbar spine than women who have not lactated (Kalkwarf et al., 1996).

Microminerals

Microminerals (trace minerals or trace elements) can be classified into four categories:

1. Essential: required in the diet, such as iron, zinc, copper, manganese, molybdenum, cobalt, selenium, iodine, and fluorine

2. Possibly essential: chromium, nickel, silicon, tin, and vanadium

3. Toxic in excess: aluminum, arsenic, cadmium, lead, and mercury

4. All other elements

Because infants typically receive their entire nutrition from a single type of food, it is important that the proper trace elements are present and occur in the appropriate concentrations.

The iron concentration in human milk is highest during the first few days after birth and diminishes with the progression of lactation. Compared with the calculated requirements for the growing infant (8–10 mg/day), human milk appears as if it is relatively low in iron at a concentration of 0.2–0.8 mg/L. In reality, the full-term infant is born with large physiological stores in the liver and hemoglobin, which, along with the iron in breastmilk, are sufficient to meet requirements for about 6 months if infants are exclusively breastfed. Approximately 50% of the iron from human milk is absorbed by the infant compared with 2–19% from iron-fortified formula and 4% from fortified infant cereals. Iron concentrations increase during the weaning period and when women produce less than 300 mL/day after 7 months (Dewey et al., 1984). The iron concentration in milk is not influenced by the maternal iron status.

The infant who is exclusively breastfed for the first 6 months of life is not at risk for iron-deficiency anemia (Duncan et al., 1985). Caution has been advised with supraphysiological iron supplementation, however, because it can cause as much as a 40-fold increase in iron retention (Schulz-Lell et al., 1987). Lactose, which promotes iron absorption, is present in higher concentrations in breast-milk, especially compared with commercial formulas, some of which contain no lactose at all. Breastfed infants do not suffer microhemorrhages of the bowel as some formula-fed infants do, so they will not have iron depletion through blood loss. Pisacane and coworkers (1995) studied the iron status of infants breastfed for 1 year who were never given cow's milk, supplemental iron, or iron-enriched formula. None who were exclusively breastfed for 7 months was anemic. Those breastfed exclusively for 6½ months versus 5½ months were less likely to be anemic. Iron supplementation of normal, healthy, full-term infants in the first 6 months therefore appears unnecessary and, in fact, increases the risk of disease by saturating lactoferrin. Supplementary foods reduce the intake of human milk and may impair iron absorption.

Zinc is an essential component of more than 200 enzymes that have both catalytic and structural roles. This nutrient appears to play a critical role in gene expression. Many DNA-binding proteins are zinc complexes. Zinc concentration in colostrum ranges from 8 to 12 µg/mL and in mature milk from 1 to 3 µg/mL. The zinc in human milk is more efficiently utilized by infants than the zinc in cow's milk or formulas. Zinc bioavailability from soy formulas is considerably lower than that from milk-based formulas due to the phytate content of soy protein isolates. The full-term breastfed infant is at little risk for zinc deficiency. Only in rare cases have breastfed infants experienced such a deficiency, usually because of defective zinc uptake by the mammary gland. Human milk has therapeutic value in treating infants suffering from a hereditary zinc deficiency disease called acrodermatitis enteropathica, whereas cow's milk and formulas do not. In general, symptoms of the disease arise when the affected infant is weaned from human milk to bovine milk. The molecular localization of zinc differs between the two milks, affecting the degree to which this micromineral is absorbed.

Copper, selenium, chromium, iodide, manganese, nickel, fluorine, molybdenum, and cobalt all appear in adequate amounts in human milk. Healthy, full-term, breastfed infants require no supplementation of any of these minerals, including fluoride. However, the iodine content of the breastmilk of mothers who smoke cigarettes is lower than that of nonsmokers. Mothers who smoke have been reported to have higher levels of thiocyanate, which may reduce iodide transport into breastmilk. Infants of mothers who smoke may need to have their iodine levels monitored and to be given iodine supplements if appropriate (Laurberg et al., 2004).

Clinical Implications

Continued research has revealed the highly complex nature of human milk. Many of the ingredients in breastmilk participate in multiple functions (Table 1-4). The interrelationships among the various components may be more significant than the amounts present or their levels of uptake. The ability of human milk and the act of breastfeeding to promote affiliative behavior, protect infant health, and support normal growth and development is unmatched by any other feeding system. Normal, healthy, full-term infants who are exclusively breastfed do not

TABLE 1-4   Multiple Functions of the Major Nutrients of Human Milk in the Infant

Nutrients	Amount	Function
Protein		
sIgA	50–100 mg/dL	Immune protection
IgM	2 mg/dL	Immune protection
IgG	1 mg/dL	Immune protection
Lactoferrin	100–300 mg/dL	Anti-infective, iron carrier
Lysozyme	5–25 mg/dL	Anti-infective
Alpha-lactalbumin	200–300 mg/dL	Ion carrier (Ca^{2+}), part of lactose synthase
Casein	200–300 mg/dL	Ion carrier, inhibits microbial adhesion to mucosal membranes
Carbohydrate		
Lactose	6.5–7.3 g/L	Energy source
Oligosaccharides	1.0–1.5 g/L	Microbial ligands
Glycoconjugates	—	Microbial and viral ligands
Fat		
Triglyceride	3.0–4.5 g/L	Energy source
LCPUFA	—	Essential for brain and retinal development and for infant growth
FFA	—	Anti-infective

FFA, free fatty acids, produced from triglycerides during fat digestion in the stomach and intestine.

Source: Reprinted from Hamosh M. Bioactive factors in human milk. *Pediatric Clinics of North America.* Volume 48 (1): © 2001; 69–86. With permission from Elsevier, Inc.

need vitamin or mineral supplements with the exception of some who may need additional vitamin D.

Lactating mothers rarely need supplemental vitamins and minerals because most supplements do not appreciably affect milk nutrient concentrations. However, vegetarian mothers may need either a vitamin B12 supplement or consultation regarding acceptable food sources of this vitamin in their diet. Mothers who have undergone gastric bypass surgery will also need a source for vitamin B12 supplementation.

Although diet can affect the composition of fatty acids in the mother's milk, no definitive data support the practice of supplementing the mother with additional DHA to raise DHA levels in her milk or indicate that doing so results in any long-term benefits to her infant (Follett et al., 2003). The association between maternal supplementation with DHA and infant status is a saturable curve (Gibson et al., 1997). As Follett et al. (2003) state, "Increasing supplementation of mothers is not associated with increased infant erythrocyte DHA if a level of 0.8% has been reached. Therefore, higher levels of DHA do not result in higher stores or improved function in the infant." Mitoulas (2000) advises that maternal supplementation of particular medium- or long-chain fatty acids may adversely affect other fatty acids such that the proportions of various fatty acids may become unbalanced, decreasing the proportion of some when others are increased. It is unknown what effect altered fatty acid profiles have on other human milk components or the recipient infant.

Fluoride supplementation is no longer recommended for infants younger than 6 months of age and only thereafter for infants living in communities with suboptimally fluoridated water supplies. Adding solid foods or infant formula before about 6 months of age may interfere with iron uptake in the breastfed infant and saturate the iron-binding capacity of lactoferrin, increasing the infant's risk of GI disease. Some commercially available bottled baby water contains added fluoride. Parents should be advised that breastfed infants do not require additional water or fluoride and told to check with their primary healthcare provider about the safety of such products advertised for young infants.

Defense Agents

The immune system of human milk is a complex interplay between milk factors, the matrix of human milk, synergistic activities of defense components, differences in resident gut microflora of the infant, and individual differences in mothers and infants. Defensive characteristics of human milk are potent inhibitors of numerous diseases. As little as 2 weeks of exclusive breastfeeding reduces enterovirus infections in infants for up to 1 year (Sadeharju et al., 2007). Although breastmilk is often referred to as the infant's first immunization, it has been shown that breastfed infants also show a better developed response to a number of vaccines such as *H. influenzae* and pneumococcal (Silfverdal et al., 2007). Human milk provides the recipient infant with several tiers of protection against pathogens, resulting in the reduced incidence of a number of acute and chronic diseases and conditions long after breastfeeding has ceased (Hanson et al., 2002). These include the following:

- Nutrients that facilitate optimal development of the infant, including the immune system and intestinal mucosa (Table 1-5)
- Antibodies in the milk to specific environmental pathogens
- Broad-spectrum protective agents such as lactoferrin and fatty acids that provide a third layer of defense (see Table 1-4)
- Glycoconjugates and oligosaccharides
- Live cells
- Anti-inflammatory agents (Table 1-6)
- Immunostimulating agents

Jensen (1995) described common features of the biochemically diverse defense agents in human milk:

- An inverse relationship often exists between the production of these factors in the breast and their production by the infant over time.
- As lactation progresses, the concentrations of many of these factors in human milk decline. At the same time, the production at the mucosal sites of those very factors increases in the developing infant.
- Most components of the immunological system in human milk are produced throughout lactation and during gradual weaning.
- The factors are usually common to other mucosal sites.
- They are adapted to resist digestion in the GI tract of the recipient infant.
- They offer protection via noninflammatory mechanisms.
- The agents act synergistically with one another or with defense agents produced by the body.

TABLE 1-5   Protective Components in Human Milk

Immune Protection	Function
sIgA, G, M, D, E	Specific antigen-targeted anti-infective activity
Nonspecific protection	Antibacterial, antiviral, and antimicrobial-toxin, enhancing newborn's immune system maturation
Major nutrients	See Table 1-4
Minor nutrients	
Nucleotides	Enhance T-cell maturation, natural killer cell activity, antibody response to certain vaccines, intestinal maturation, and repair after diarrhea
Vitamins	
A (beta-carotene)	Anti-inflammatory (scavenging of oxygen radicals)
C (ascorbic acid)	Anti-inflammatory (scavenging of oxygen radicals)
E (alpha-tocopherol)	Anti-inflammatory (scavenging of oxygen radicals)
Enzymes	
Bile salt–dependent lipase	Production of FFA with antiprotozoan and anti-bacterial activity
Catalase	Anti-inflammatory (degrades H_2O_2)
Glutathione peroxidase	Anti-inflammatory (prevents lipid peroxidation)
PAF acetylhydrolase	Protects against NEC (hydrolysis of PAF)
Hormones	
Prolactin	Enhances the development of B and T lymphocytes, affects differentiation of intestinal lymphoid tissue
Cortisol, thyroxine, insulin, and growth factors	Promote maturation of the newborn's intestine and development of intestinal host-defense mechanism
Cells	
Macrophages, PMNs, and cytokines	Microbial phagocytosis, production of lymphokines and lymphocytes, interaction with and enhancement of other protective agents
Cytokines	Modulate functions and maturation of the immune system

PAF, platelet-activating factor; PMN, polymorphonuclear.

Source: Reprinted from Hamosh M. Bioactive factors in human milk. *Pediatric Clinics of North America.* Volume 48 (1). 2001: 69–86. With permission from Elsevier, Inc.

TABLE 1-6   Anti-Inflammatory Components of Human Milk

Component	Function
Vitamins	
A	Scavenges oxygen radicals
C	Scavenges oxygen radicals
E	Scavenges oxygen radicals
Enzymes	
Catalase	Degrades H_2O_2
Glutathione peroxidase	Prevents lipid peroxidation
PAF-acetylhydrolase	Degrades PAF, a potent ulcerogen
Antienzymes	
Alpha$_1$-antitrypsin	Inhibits inflammatory proteases
Alpha$_1$-antichymotrypsin	Inhibits inflammatory proteases
Prostaglandins	
PGE$_1$	Cytoprotective
PGE$_2$	Cytoprotective
Growth factors	
EGF	Promotes gut growth and functional maturation
TGF-alpha	Promotes epithelial cell growth
TGF-beta	Suppresses lymphocyte function
Cytokines	
IL-10	Suppresses function of macrophages and natural killer and T cells
Cytokine receptors	
TGF-alpha; RI, RII	Bind to and inhibit TGF-alpha

EGF, epidermal growth factor; IL, interleukin; PAF, platelet-activating factor; PGE, prostaglandin E; TGF, transforming growth factor.

Source: Reprinted from Hamosh M. Bioactive factors in human milk. *Pediatric Clinics of North America.* Volume 48 (1). 2001: 69–86. With permission from Elsevier, Inc.

Types of Defense Agents

Human milk contains a potent mixture of agents that work synergistically to form an innate immune system that allows the nursing mother to protect her infant from a host of diseases.

Direct-Acting Antimicrobial Agents

- Oligosaccharides and glycoconjugates: These agents inhibit toxin binding from *Vibrio cholerae* and *E. coli* and interfere with the attachment of *H. influenzae*, *S. pneumoniae*, and *C. jejuni*.

- Proteins: Many of the whey proteins have direct antimicrobial actions. Lactoferrin competes with bacteria for ferric iron and disrupts their proliferation. A concentration of approximately 5–6 mg/mL is found in colostrum, with the concentration decreasing to 2 mg/mL at 4 weeks and to 1 mg/mL in milk thereafter. Lysozyme lyses susceptible bacteria. The approximate mean intake of milk lysozyme per day in healthy full-term infants is about 3–4 mg/kg/day at 1 month and 6 mg/kg/day at 4 months. Fibronectin facilitates the actions of mononuclear phagocytic cells. Complement components are present as well. Immunoglobulins represent important defensive agents. The predominant immunoglobulin in human milk is sIgA. IgE, the principal type of antibody responsible for immediate hypersensitivity reactions, is absent from human milk. Mucins defend against *E. coli* and rotavirus. Nucleotides are thought to enhance the growth of beneficial bacteria in the gut.

- Bifidus growth promoter.

- Defense agents: These are created from partially digested substrates from human milk. Fatty acids and monoglycerides are able to disrupt enveloped viruses (Isaacs, 2005) with lipid-induced active antiviral activity apparent in the infant's stomach within 1 hour of feeding (Isaacs et al., 1990).

- Leukocytes: These are living white cells present in human milk in highest concentrations during the first 2–4 days of lactation. The leukocyte component of human milk is made up of lymphocytes, macrophages, and polymorphonuclear leukocytes (neutrophils and eosinophils). Neutrophils and macrophages are the most abundant in human milk. Lymphocytes are found in human milk, with 80% of them appearing as T cells. They synthesize IgA antibody. Milk lymphocytes manufacture several chemicals, including gamma-interferon, migration inhibition factor, and monocyte chemotactic factor, all of which augment the body's own immune response.

- Anti-inflammatory agents:
  1. Factors that promote the growth of epithelium
     a. Cortisol
     b. Epithelial growth factor
     c. Polyamines
     d. Lactoferrin
  2. Antioxidants
     a. Ascorbate-like compound
     b. Uric acid
     c. Beta-carotene
  3. Prostaglandins
  4. PAF-AH
  5. Immunomodulators
     a. Alpha-tocopherol.
     b. Cytokines regulate many epithelial cell functions and are at their highest in human milk when they are at their lowest in the recipient infant. Most of the cytokines that are known to be deficient in the neonate are found in significant amounts in breastmilk. Cytokines have been shown to be higher in milk samples from Asian mothers compared with African mothers and may vary according to race (Chirico et al., 2008). Some of these are interleukin-1B, IL-6, IL-8, and IL-10.
     c. Granulocyte-colony stimulating factor.
     d. Macrophage-colony stimulating factor.
     e. Tumor necrosis factor-alpha, interferon, epithelial growth factor, transforming growth factor-alpha, and transforming growth factor-beta 2.

Human Milk Fortification

Whereas the immunological factors in breastmilk are important for all infants, they are essential to preterm or ill infants whose immune systems may be immature or challenged by other health conditions. Nutrient fortification of preterm mother's milk is seen in NICUs when an infant's needs exceed the capacity of breastmilk to provide selected nutrients in amounts that support a particular growth velocity. Most NICUs do not use single-nutrient fortification but rely on multinutrient commercial fortifiers of differing composition. Preterm mothers' milk inhibits the growth of many bacteria, including *E. coli, Staphylococcus, Enterobacter sakazakii,* and group B *Streptococcus;* however, the addition of a cow's milk protein–based powdered human milk fortifier high in iron can neutralize the ability of human milk to kill these bacterial species (Chan, 2003). The addition to human milk of an older formulation of the same product decreased the IgA levels to *E. coli* and resulted in a 19% decrease in lysozymal activity in human milk, a measure of bacterial lysis (Jocson et al., 1997). The addition of a relatively large amount of iron directly into human milk may interfere with the ability of lactoferrin to bind iron and lyse bacterial cell walls. Quan et al. (1994) reported significant decreases in lysozyme content and IgA specific for *E. coli* when commercial fortifiers were added to fresh frozen milk. Chan and coworkers (2007) compared the antibacterial activity of preterm milk that had a commercial cow's milk–based high iron fortifier added to it or a human milk–based fortifier that was lower in iron. The commercial fortifier sample was shown to almost completely eliminate the bacterial inhibitory actions of the milk compared with the human milk fortifier sample that retained its bacteriocidal activity. Fortifiers can be added to expressed hindmilk when the rate of weight gain is low. Some fortifiers can increase the osmolality of the milk, increasing the risk for GI irritation and intolerance (Fenton & Belik, 2002; Srinivasan et al., 2004). They may also contain cow's milk protein and soy, which presents allergy as a potential side effect. The addition of human milk fortifier may temporarily delay gastric emptying and cause a short-term increase in gastric residuals and emesis.

Lessaris et al. (2000) showed that human milk fortifier differentially altered the biochemical profile of human milk with regard to transforming growth factor-alpha (a gut peptide that exerts a maturational effect on the neonatal gut) concentration and molecular mass profile. What effect this alteration in human milk biochemistry has on neonatal gut function remains unknown. The addition of iron and vitamin C to preterm human milk was shown to increase oxidative stress and reduce the content of mono- and polyunsaturated fatty acids (Friel et al., 2007).

Powdered infant formula is not sterile, including powdered human milk fortifiers. Powdered infant formula has been found to harbor *E. sakazakii* (Baker, 2002). Caution should be exercised when adding a preparation to human milk, such as a fortifier, that neutralizes the milk's ability to destroy harmful bacteria, especially if the potential for bacterial contamination is contained in the fortifier itself. Fortified human milk can be stored in a refrigerator at 35–40°F (2–4°C) for no longer than 24 hours. Once fortified human milk is prepared, it can remain at room temperature for 4 hours (Telang et al., 2005). The American Dietetic Association recommends a hang time for fortified breastmilk of no longer than 4 hours at room temperature (25°C/77°F) (Robbins & Becker, 2004). Fortified human milk should not be used if it is unrefrigerated for more than a total of 2 hours. After a bottle feeding begins, it must be used within 1 hour or discarded.

Milk Treatment and Storage

The antioxidant activity of human milk is diminished by both refrigeration and freezing and over the course of time; however, it remains significantly higher than infant formula in antioxidant capacity despite how it is stored or when it is collected or ingested by the infant (Ezaki et al., 2008; Hanna et al., 2004). This is extremely important to preterm infants who are born before their antioxidant defense system is fully developed and functional (Baydas et al., 2002; Georgeson et al., 2002).

Preterm infants can experience oxidative stress from conditions such as infection and chronic lung disease and from interventions such as mechanical ventilation, oxygen therapy, intravenous nutrition, and blood transfusions. Some of the conditions and diseases common to preterm infants, such as NEC and retinopathy of prematurity, are often attributed to a profusion of oxidative stress and a deficiency in the oxidative defense system. Ingesting human milk rapidly increases antioxidant concentrations (Ostrea et al., 1986; Sommerburg et al., 2000; Zoeren-Grobben et al., 1993), partially explaining the reduced incidence of NEC and retinopathy of prematurity in infants protected by the consumption of human milk (Hylander et al., 2001). Preterm infants below 1,000-g birthweight and a gestational age below 30 weeks may be at high risk of acquiring a symptomatic cytomegalovirus (CMV) infection through their mother's milk if she is CMV positive. Refrigeration and freezing of milk from preterm mothers may reduce the risk of transferring CMV to the infant but does not eliminate it (Hamprecht et al., 2008). Inactivation of CMV can be accomplished by Holder pasteurization (heating to 62.5°C/144.5°F for 30 minutes) but can decrease the immunological components in breastmilk. Rapid high-temperature treatment of human milk (72°C/161.6°F for 5 or 15 seconds) has been shown to eliminate CMV infectivity without destroying many of the anti-infective capabilities of the milk (Lawrence, 2006).

The goal of milk treatment and storage is to preserve the nutrient and protective properties of the milk. Heat treatment includes the following processes:

- Microwaving. Refrigerated or frozen breastmilk is often microwaved by parents to quickly thaw or heat it, but microwaving for 50 seconds destroys 30.5% of the milk's IgA. Quan and coworkers (1992) found that microwaving breastmilk at 72–98°C (162–208°F) decreases the activity of lysozyme by 96% and that of total IgA by 98%. Treatment at low temperatures, 20–53°C (68–127°F), did not affect total IgA but decreased lysozyme by 19%. Subsequent *E. coli* growth 3.5 hours after treatment was 5.2 times greater than in the control at low microwave temperatures and 18 times greater at the high temperatures, showing dramatic loss of anti-infective factors. Microwaving bottles of expressed breastmilk also poses a risk of injury to the infant from hot spots in the milk, which could burn the tongue, mouth, and throat as well as cause scalding and full thickness burn injuries to the body from exploding bottles and nipples. Advise parents to place the bottle of expressed breastmilk under warm running water or in a bowl of warm water. Human milk is delivered to the baby at body temperature leaving little reason to heat milk beyond 36.9°C (98.6°F).

- Pasteurization. Human milk is most often pasteurized by milk banks for use as donor milk for preterm or ill infants, in special situations where the unique defense properties in human milk would be therapeutic, when infants cannot tolerate artificial baby milks, and so forth. Banked donor human milk can be obtained by prescription from any of the human milk banks listed in Appendix 1-2. Heat treatment can reduce the effectiveness of some of the defense factors in milk such as the B- and T-cell components of milk, lactoferrin, and IgA. The Human Milk Banking Association of North America (2008) requires the use of Holder pasteurization (62.5°C for 30 minutes) to eliminate viral contaminants such as human immunodeficiency virus, human T-cell lymphotropic virus-1, and CMV as well as common bacterial contaminants. High-temperature, short-time processing can also be done with human milk at 70° or 75°C for 15 seconds. Silvestre et al. (2008b) noted that the temperature applied is more important than the duration of application for preserving the bactericidal capacity of pasteurized human milk. They found that when comparing untreated milk, milk pasteurized at 63°C for

30 minutes, and milk pasteurized at 75°C for 15 seconds, a reduction in the growth of *E. coli* of 70.10%, 52.27%, and 36.9%, respectively, occurred. The lower milk processing temperature was preferable for preserving more bactericidal capacity. Refrigeration of this pasteurized milk did not further reduce its antibacterial properties. Holder pasteurization also preserves the effects of human milk oligosaccharides (Bertino et al., 2008). Pasteurization can reduce the antioxidant capacity of expressed breastmilk (Silvestre et al., 2008a). A newer high-temperature, short-time form of pasteurization has been developed that better maintains the immunological quality of the milk (Chen & Allen, 2001).

- Evaporation. In an effort to engineer human milk as an appropriate fortifier for preterm milk, Braga and Palhares (2007) evaporated pasteurized human milk samples by removing 30% of the water. The pasteurized evaporated human milk met the recommended requirements of sodium, potassium, magnesium, protein, fat, and lactose but not calcium and phosphorus requirements. Further studies are needed to see if this type of human milk manipulation is appropriate for preterm infants, especially if calcium and phosphorus were added.

- Refrigeration and freezing. Human milk can be safely stored under appropriate conditions to ensure infants receive their mother's or banked milk under a variety of conditions (Lawrence, 1999; Ogundele, 2000). Recommendations for storage times and temperatures vary. Storage of milk overnight results in formation of a cream layer on top containing about 20% fat and a skim layer below it containing about 1% fat. These layers are generally mixed before being fed to the infant. However, in special situations, such as a slow-gaining or preterm infant, the top high-fat layer can be skimmed off and given to infants as physiological high-calorie supplements. Few data are available on storage times and conditions for fortified preterm human milk. Refrigerated fortified human milk should generally be used within 24 hours of when it was prepared (Jocson et al., 1997). Martínez-Costa et al. (2007) showed that refrigeration for 48 hours did not cause significant modifications in antibacterial properties of human milk, but storage beyond 72 hours significantly lowered the degree of bacteriolysis versus fresh milk. Ogundele (2002) reported that although the bactericidal activities of refrigerated samples diminished rapidly, up to two-thirds of the original activity level was maintained by freezing for up to 3 months. The ability of milk fat globule membrane to adhere to suspended bacteria was gradually lost in frozen milk samples, whereas it was greatly enhanced during the first few days in refrigerated samples, before declining sharply. This study shows that loss of bactericidal activity in refrigerated milk is well compensated for by enhanced bacteria sequestration activity.

Human milk also contains bacteria that represent an important factor in the initiation and development of the normal and proper neonatal gut microbiota (Collado et al., 2009). While concern about the growth of pathological bacteria in stored human milk is valid, consideration needs to be given to whether cold storage effects the natural bacterial composition of human milk. Marin et al. (2009) found that cold storage of human milk at –20°C (–4°F) for 6 weeks did not significantly affect either the quantitative or qualitative natural bacterial composition of the milk. However, it was interesting that bacterial counts in milk expressed with a mechanical breast pump were higher than in samples obtained by manual expression.

Human milk contains two lipases (enzymes that digest fat) that do not change the lipid structure during refrigeration. However, when milk is frozen, lipolysis can occur. As this process continues, soaps form that can change the taste and smell of the milk. It is speculated that some mothers have more lipase activity than others, which can lead to a more rancid milk that some infants reject. If this occurs, these mothers can be advised to heat their milk to a scald (not boiling) after expressing it, then immediately cool and freeze it to stop the fat from being broken down (Jones & Tully, 2005). Hamosh and colleagues (1996) studied the stability of protein and lipids as well as bacterial growth in expressed milk of employed mothers and generated the recommendations for short-term milk storage included in Table 1-7.

Breastmilk can be stored in a number of ways (Table 1-8) (Arnold, 1995; Arnold & Tully, 1992; Manohar et al., 1997; Tully, 2000; Williamson & Murti, 1996). Because human milk is a live fluid, capable of engaging in biological processes, it is important to understand that it remains active during storage. The defense agents in human milk allow it to be stored under a number of conditions and in a variety of containers. When discussing storage conditions and containers, it is also important to differentiate between the needs and tolerances of a healthy full-term infant and those of a sick or preterm infant (Jones & Tully, 2005). Parents may wish to use glass or polypropylene bottles for feeding and storage of breastmilk (Environmental Working Group, 2007). Polycarbonate bottles have been shown to contain bisphenol A (BPA), a plasticizer that mimics estrogen. BPA

TABLE 1-7   Storage of Breastmilk for Healthy Infants

38°C (100°F) room air—safe storage for less than 4 hours

25°C (77°F) room air—safe storage for as long as 4 hours

15°C (59°F)—safe storage for 24 hours (equivalent to a Styrofoam box with blue ice)

4°C (39°F)—in a refrigerator 72 hours and probably longer

   Previously thawed milk in a refrigerator—24 hours

   Freezer inside refrigerator compartment—2 weeks

–20°C (–4°F) freezer separate from refrigerator—3 to 6 months, or up to 12 months (milk should not be stored in shelves on the door but in the back of the freezer. Storage containers should be placed on a rack above the floor of the freezer to avoid warming during the automatic defrost cycle in freezers above the refrigerator compartment.)

–70°C deep freezer—longer than 12 months

Sources: Hamosh, Ellis, Pollock, et al., Breastfeeding and the working mother. *Pediatr* 1996; Williams-Arnold LD. Human Milk Storage for Health Infants and Children. *Health Education Associates*, 2000.

has been shown to be a developmental, neural, and reproductive toxicant that can interfere with healthy growth and body function (Gibson, 2007). The amount of BPA that leaches from heated baby bottles is within the range shown to cause harm in animal studies (Workgroup for Safe Markets, 2008). Infant formula itself can be contaminated with BPA. Liquid formula packaged in metal cans often contains BPA from the BPA-based epoxy resin coating that lines the formula cans (Cao et al., 2008).

Clinical Implications

Raw cow's milk contains numerous antimicrobial agents, primarily in colostrum, that are beneficial to the calf. These, however, are of little significance to the human infant consumer of a cow's milk product. Bovine colostrum is not used in the milk supply, and the effectiveness of any defense agent is neutralized by the removal of all cells, pasteurization, and homogenization. Bovine milk is intended to be consumed unaltered by the calf and conveys no disease defense to the human infant. In contrast, the immunological composition of human milk has evolved and adapted to offset the postnatal delays in the development of the human immune system. The thymus is the central organ of the immune system in an infant. Within this organ, T lymphocytes mature and multiply, including

TABLE 1-8 Selected Characteristics of Various Breastmilk Storage Containers

Container Type	Description	Advantages	Disadvantages	Effect on Milk	Healthy Full Term	Child in Day Care	Preterm, Ill, Hospitalized
Polyethylene bags	thin bottle liner, freezer bags, bags for storage, doubled bags	inexpensive, do not require washing	fragile, compromised by expansion of milk during freezing, easily punctured, leak, hard to pour, need support, volume marks inaccurate	fat loss, easily contaminated, photodegradation of nutrients, loss of sIgA	OK	No	No
Hard plastic (bottles, urine specimen cups, graduated feeders, centrifuge tubes)	polypropylene (cloudy, semi-flexible)	good for short-term storage of colostrum in a refrigerator (retains good cell count and viability)	can become scratched if frequently reused, increasing chance of bacterial buildup in scratches in stored milk	small loss of cellular components	OK	OK	OK with tight-fitting lids, short storage times
	polycarbonate (clear, hard plastic)	more durable, less prone to scratching					
Glass	bottles, canning jars, sterile water bottles	best for preserving immune components of milk	can break or chip	possible photodegradation, cellular components adhere to walls of container but drop back into the milk sooner than with plastic	OK	OK	OK with tight-fitting lids, better for longer storage, less loss of immune components
Stainless steel	not typically used in the United States			No data	OK		
Other containers	ice cube trays, popsicle molds	handy items found around the house			OK	No	No

Table data compiled from the following sources: Arnold LDW. Storage containers for human milk: An issue revisited. *J Hum Lact.* 1995;11:325–328; 2006 Human Milk Banking Association of North America. Best Practice for Expressing, Storing and Handling of Mother's Own Milk in Hospital and at Home. Raleigh, NC: 2006; Manohar AA, Williamson M, Koppikar GV. Effect of storage of colostrum in various containers. *Indian Pediatr.* 1997;34:293–295; Tully MR. Recommendations for handling of mother's own milk. *J Hum Lact.* 2000;16:151–159; Williamson MT, Murti PK. Effects of storage, time, temperature, and composition of containers on biologic components of human milk. *J Hum Lact.* 1996;12:31–35.

killer cells that are important for defense and regulatory T cells that are important for the prevention of autoimmune diseases (Wing et al., 2002). The thymus of a fully breastfed infant is twice the size of a formula-fed infant's thymus (Ngom et al., 2004). The thymic index has been correlated to the percentage of CD8+ cells, with a higher CD8 percentage seen in breastfed compared with formula-fed infants at 8 months of age (Jeppesen et al., 2004). The infant is exposed to micro-bial immunogens while receiving protective agents in human milk. This process creates an attenuated immunization, in that the pathogenicity of the microbial agent is reduced by the accompanying immune factors. Human milk also prepares the recipient infant to resist certain immune-mediated diseases and a host of other acute and chronic diseases and conditions.

Because formula-fed infants have higher rates of illness, artificial feeding results in higher costs to the healthcare system. Ball and Wright (1999) calculated the costs to the healthcare system associated with three common childhood dis-eases: otitis media, lower respiratory tract illness (bronchiolitis, croup, bron-chitis, pneumonia), and GI illness. The excess total direct medical costs incurred by never-breastfed infants during the first year of life for these three illnesses alone ranged between $331 and $475 per infant, more than the costs incurred by breastfed infants. The authors reported 2,033 excess office visits, 212 excess days of hospitalization, and 609 excess prescriptions for these illnesses per 1,000 never-breastfed infants compared with 1,000 infants exclusively breastfed for at least 3 months. The family of a formula-fed infant incurs direct costs for care if uninsured or for copayments if insured, as well as nonmedical costs such as family care and transportation to and from the physician's office and/or hospital. Missed days of work are costly to both employee and employer. If a parent misses 2 hours of work for the excess illnesses attributable to formula feeding, then more than 2,000 hours, the equivalent of 1 year of employment, are lost per 1,000 never-breastfed infants.

It is recommended that clinicians take the following steps to educate mothers:

1. Ensure that infants receive colostrum and human milk as the preferred food and first immunization.

2. Avoid actions that dilute the anti-infective properties of human milk such as maternal smoking, mixing human milk with formula in the same container, and microwaving expressed milk.

3. Become familiar with data on the effects of heat treatment, refrigeration, freezing, and storage container on the defense agents in human milk (Table 1-9).

TABLE 1-9   Results of Various Treatments on Human Milk

Treatment	Results
Refrigerated storage	
4°C (39°F), 72 hours	Creaming, decrease in bacterial growth, possible lipolysis
–20°C (–4°F), 12 months	Lipolysis, possible demulsification and protein denaturation when thawed
–70°C (–94°F), indefinite	Possible demulsification and protein denaturation when thawed
Pasteurization	
56°C (132.8°F), 30 min	Inactivation of enzymes and antimicrobial proteins, partial loss of some vitamins, destruction of microorganisms
62.5°C (149.36°F), 30 min	Inactivation of enzymes and antimicrobial proteins, partial loss of some vitamins, destruction of microorganisms
70°C (158°F), 15 seconds	Inactivation of enzymes and antimicrobial proteins, partial loss of some vitamins, destruction of microorganisms
Microwave treatment	Decrease in IgA and lysozyme, substantial increase in coliforms
Sonication	Homogenization of milk-fat globules
Selection	Selection of high-protein milks, use of high-fat hindmilk
Supplementation	Addition of nutrients for preterm infants
Processing	Treatment of milk to isolate fats, proteins, and other components; fractions then added to milk
Manipulation of mother's diet	Change the fatty acid profile

Source: Jensen RG, Jensen GL. Specialty lipids for infant nutrition. I. Milks and formulas. *J Pediatr Gastroenterol Nutr*. 1992;15:232–245.

Summary: The Design in Nature

Lactation is an ancient physiological process, dating back almost 200 million years. Human lactation and human milk have evolved to meet the needs and address the vulnerabilities of the human young. Milk intended for a four-legged, cud-chewing, nonverbal species may cause human infants to grow, but their growth and development will take a different trajectory than that of their breastfed counterparts. Infant formula and human milk components are not interchangeable. Artificial diets are not the same as human milk. The immuno-nutrition provided by human milk has no equal.

References

Abrams, S. A., Griffin, I. J., Davila, P. M. (2002). Calcium and zinc absorption from lactose-containing and lactose-free infant formulas. *Am J Clin Nutr*. 76, 442–446.

Agostoni, C., Marangoni, F., Giovannini, M., et al. (2001). Prolonged breastfeeding (six months or more) and milk fat content at six months are associated with higher developmental scores at one year of age within a breastfed population. *Adv Exp Med Biol*. 501, 137–141.

Agostoni, C., Trojan, S., Bellu, R., et al. (1995). Neurodevelopmental quotient of healthy term infants at 4 months and feeding practice: the role of long-chain polyunsaturated fatty acids. *Pediatr Res*. 38, 262–265.

Almroth S, Bidinger PD. (1990). No need for water supplementation for exclusively breast-fed infants under hot and arid conditions. *Trans R Soc Trop Med Hyg*. 84, 602–604.

American Academy of Pediatrics [AAP], Committee on Environmental Health. (1999). Ultraviolet light: a hazard to children. *Pediatrics*. 104, 328–333.

American Academy of Pediatrics [AAP], Committee on Nutrition. (2000). Hypoallergenic formulas. *Pediatrics*. 106, 346–349.

American Academy of Pediatrics [AAP], Work Group on Cow's Milk Protein and Diabetes Mellitus. (1994). Infant feeding practices and their possible relationship to the etiology of diabetes mellitus. *Pediatrics*. 94, 752–754.

Amin, S. B., Merle, K. S., Orlando, M. S., et al. (2000). Brainstem maturation in premature infants as a function of enteral feeding type. *Pediatrics*. 106, 318–322.

Anderson, J. W., Johnstone, B. M., Remley, D. T. (1999). Breastfeeding and cognitive development: A meta-analysis. *Am J Clin Nutr*. 70, 525–535.

Arnold, L. D. W. (1995). Storage containers for human milk: An issue revisited. *J Hum Lact*. 11:325–328.

Ashraf, R. N., Jalil, F., Aperia, A., et al. (1993). Additional water is not needed for healthy breastfed babies in a hot climate. *Acta Paediatr Scand*. 82, 1007–1011.

Backhed, F., Ding, H., Wang, T., et al. (2004). The gut microbiota as an environmental factor that regulates fat storage. *Proc Natl Acad Sci USA*. 101, 15718–15723.

Baker, R. D. (2002). Infant formula safety. Pediatrics. 110:833–835.

Ball, T. M., Wright, A. L. (1999). Health care costs of formula-feeding in the first year of life. *Pediatrics*. 103, 870–876.

Barrat, E., Michel, C., Poupeau, G., David-Sochard, A., Rival, M., Pagniez, A., Champ, M., Darmaun, D. (2008). Supplementation with galactooligosaccharides and inulin increases bacterial translocation in artificially reared newborn rats. *Pediatr Res*. 64, 34–39.

Basile, L. A., Taylor, S. N., Wagner, C. L., Horst, R. L., Hollis, B. W. (2006). The effect of high-dose vitamin D supplementation on serum vitamin D levels and milk calcium concentration in lactating women and their infants. *Breastfeeding Med*. 1, 27–35.

Bauer, G., Ewald, S., Hoffman, J., Dubanoski, R. (1991). Breastfeeding and cognitive development of three-year-old children. *Psych Reports*. 68, 1218.

Baydas, G., Karatas, F., Gursu, M. F., et al. (2002). Antioxidant vitamin levels in term and preterm infants and their relation to maternal vitamin status. *Arch Med Res* 33, 276–280.

Bertino E, Coppa GV, Giuliani F, et al. (2008). Effects of Holder pasteurization on human milk oligosaccharides. *Int J Immunopathol Pharmacol.* 21, 381–385.

Bhatia, J., Greer, F. (2008). Committee on Nutrition. Use of soy protein-based formulas in infant feeding. *Pediatrics.* 212, 1062–1068.

Biasucci, G., Benenati, B., Morelli, L., Bessi, E., Boehm, G. (2008). Cesarean delivery may affect the early biodiversity of intestinal bacteria. *J Nutr.* 138, 1796S–1800S.

Birch, E. E., Birch, D. G., Hoffman, D. R., et al. (1993). Breastfeeding and optimal visual development. *J Pediatr Ophthal Strabismus.* 30, 33–38.

Blyth, R., Creedy, D. K., Dennis, C. L., Moyle, W., Pratt, J., DeVries, S. (2002). Effect of maternal confidence on breastfeeding duration: An application of breastfeeding self-efficacy theory. *Birth.* 29, 278–284.

Bokor, S., Koletzko, B., Decsi, T. (2007). Systematic review of fatty acid composition of human milk from mothers of preterm compared to full-term infants. *Ann Nutr Metab.* 51, 550–556.

Boniglia, C., Carratu, B., Chiarotti, F., Giammarioli, S., Manzini, E. (2003). Influence of maternal protein intake on nitrogen fractions of human milk. *Int J Vitam Nutr Res.* 73, 447–452.

Bouwstra, H., Boersma, E. R., Boehm, G., et al. (2003). Exclusive breastfeeding of healthy term infants for at least 6 weeks improves neurological condition. *J Nutr.* 133, 4243–4245.

Braga, L. P. M., Palhares, D. B. (2007). Effect of evaporation and pasteurization in the biochemical and immunological composition of human milk. *J Pediatr (Rio J).* 83, 59–63.

Brandtzaeg, P. (2003). Mucosal immunity: integration between mother and the breastfed infant. *Vaccine.* 21, 3382–3388.

Brenna, J. T., Varamini, B., Jensen, R. G., Diersen-Schade, D. A., Boettcher, J. A., Arterburn, L. M. (2007). Docosahexaenoic and arachidonic acid concentrations in human breast milk worldwide. *Am J Clin Nutr.* 85, 1457-1464.

Brill H. (2008). Approach to milk protein allergy in infants. *Can Fam Physician.* 54, 1258–1264.

Brown, E. W., Bosworth, A.W. (1922). Studies of infant feeding SVI. A bacteriological study of the feces and the food of normal babies receiving breastmilk. *Am J Dis Child.* 23, 243.

Brown, N. C., Doyle, L. W., Bear, M. J., Inder, T. E. (2006).Alterations in neurobehavior at term reflect differing exposures in very preterm infants. *Pediatrics.* 118, 2461–2471.

Bullen, C. L., Tearle, P. V., Stewart, M. G. (1977). The effect of humanized milks and supplemented breast feeding on the faecal flora of infants. *J Med Microbiol.* 10, 403–413.

Buss, I. H., McGill, F., Darlow, B. A., Winterbourn, C. C. (2001).Vitamin C is reduced in human milk after storage. *Acta Paediatr.* 90, 813–815.

Butte, N. F., Goldblum, R. M., Fehl, L. M., et al. (1984). Daily ingestion of immunologic components in human milk during the first four months of life. *Acta Paediatr Scand.* 73, 296–301.

Cantani, A., Micera, M. (2005). Neonatal cow milk sensitization in 143 case-reports: role of early exposure to cow's milk formula. *Eur Rev Med Pharmacol Sci.* 9, 227–230.

Cao, X. L., Dufresne, G., Belisle, S., Clement, G., Falicki, M., Beraldin, F., Rulibikiye, A. (2008). Levels of bisphenol A in canned liquid infant formula products in Canada and dietary intake estimates. *J Agric Food Chem.* 56, 7919–7924.

Cardwell CR, Stene LC, Joner G, et al. (2008). Caesarean section is associated with an increased risk of childhood-onset type 1 diabetes mellitus: a meta-analysis of observational studies. *Diabetologia.* 51, 726–735.

Carlson, S. E., Cooke, R. J., Werkman, S. H., et al. (1992). First year growth of preterm infants fed standard compared to marine oil n-3 supplemented formula. *Lipids.* 27, 901–907.

Carlson, S. E., Werkman, S. H., Peeples, J. M., et al. (1993). Arachidonic acid status correlates with first year growth in preterm infants. *Proc Natl Acad Sci USA.* 90, 1073–1077.

Catassi, C., et al. (1995). Intestinal permeability changes during the first month: effect of natural versus artificial feeding. *J Pediatr Gastroenterol Nutr.* 21, 383–386.

Centers for Disease Control and Prevention. (2007). Breastfeeding-Related Maternity Practices at Hospitals and Birth Centers—United States, 2007. *MMWR. 57*(23), 621–625.

Centers for Disease Control and Prevention.(1993). Hyponatremic seizures among infants fed with commercial bottled drinking water: Wisconsin, 1993. *MMWR.* 43:641–643.

Chan, G. (2003). Effects of powdered human milk fortifiers on the antimicrobial actions of human milk. *J Perinatol.* 23, 620–623.

Chan, G.M., Lee, M. L., Rechtman, D. J. (2007). Effects of a human milk-derived human milk fortifier on the antibacterial actions of human milk. *Breastfeeding Med.*2, 205–208.

Chandra, R. K. (2000). Food allergy and nutrition in early life: implications for later health. *Proc Nutr Soc.* 59, 273–277.

Chandra, R. K., Hamed, A. (1991). Cumulative incidence of atopic disorders in high risk infants fed whey hydrolysate, soy, and conventional cow milk formulas. *Ann Allerg.* 67, 129–132.

Chen, H.-Y., Allen, J. C. (2001). Human milk antibacterial factors: the effect of temperature on defense systems. *Adv Exp Med Biol.* 501, 341–348.

Chirico, G., Marzollo, R., Cortinovis, S., Fonte, C., Gasparoni, A. (2008). Antiinfective properties of human milk. *J Nutr.* 138, 1801S–1806S.

Clandinin, M. T., van Aerde, J. E., Parrot, A., et al. (1997). Assessment of the efficacious dose of arachidonic and docosahexaenoic acids in preterm infant formulas: fatty acid composition of erythrocyte membrane lipids. *Pediatr Res.* 42, 819–825.

Chao, J. C. J. Tseng, H. P., Chang, C. W., Chien, Y. Y., Au, H. K., Chen, J. R., Chen, C. F. (2004). Chicken extract affects colostrum protein composition in lactating women. *J Nutr Biol.* 15, 37–44.

Clarke, S. D., Jump, D. B. (1996). Polyunsaturated fatty acid regulation of hepatic gene transcription. *J Nutr.* 126(Suppl), 1105–1109.

Claud, E. C., Walker, W. A. (2001). Hypothesis: inappropriate colonization of the premature intestine can cause neonatal necrotizing enterocolitis. *FASEB J.* 15, 1398–1403.

Clemens, T. L., Adams, J. S., Henderson, S. L., Holick, M. F. (1982). Increased skin pigment reduces capacity of skin to synthesize vitamin D3. *Lancet.* 1, 74–76.

Clements, M. R., et al. (1987). A new mechanism for induced vitamin D deficiency in calcium deprivation. *Nature.* 325, 62–65.

Cohen, R. J., Brown, K. H., Rivera, L. L., Dewey, K. G. (2000). Exclusively breastfed, low birthweight infants do not need supplemental water. *Acta Paediatr.* 89, 550–552.

Collado, M. C., Delgado, S., Maldonado, A., Rodriguez, J. M. (2009). Assessment of the bacterial diversity of breast milk of healthy women by quantitative real-time PCR. *Lett Appl Microbiol.* 48, 523-528.

Cunnane, S. C., Francescutti, V., Brenna, J. T., et al. (2000). Breastfed infants achieve a higher rate of brain and whole body docosahexaenoate accumulation than formula-fed infants not consuming dietary docosahexaenoate. *Lipids.* 35, 105–111.

Dabard, J., Bridonneau, C., Phillipe, C., et al. (2001). A new lantibiotic produced by a *Ruminococcus gnavus* strain isolated from human feces. *Appl Environ Microbiol.* 67, 4111–4118.

Dai, D., Walker, W. A.(1999). Protective nutrients and bacterial colonization in the immature human gut. *Adv Pediatr.* 46, 353–382.

Daly, S. E. J., Di Rosso, A., Owens, R. A., Hartmann, P. E. (1993). Degree of breast emptying explains changes in the fat content, but not fatty acid composition, of human milk. *Exp Phys.* 78, 741–755.

DeCarvalho, M., Klaus, M. H., Merkatz, R. B. (1982). Frequency of breastfeeding and serum bilirubin concentration. *Am J Dis Child.* 136, 737–738.

Decsi, T., Koletzko, B. (1995). Growth, fatty acid composition of plasma lipid classes, and plasma retinol and alpha-tocopherol concentrations in full-term infants fed formula enriched with n-6 and n-3 long-chain polyunsaturated fatty acids. *Acta Paediatr Scand.* 84, 725–732.

Dewey, K. (2003). Is breastfeeding protective against childhood obesity? *J Hum Lact.* 19:9–18.

Dewey, K. G., Finley, D. A., Lonnerdal, B. (1984). Breastmilk volume and composition during late lactation (7–20 months). *J Pediatr Gastroenterol Nutr.* 3, 713–720.

Duncan, B., Schifman, R. B., Corrigan, J. J., et al. (1985). Iron and the exclusively breastfed infant from birth to six months. *J Pediatr Gastroenterol Nutr.* 4:421.

Dusdieker, L. B., Booth, B. M., Stumbo, P. J., et al. (1985). Effect of supplemental fluids on human milk production. *J Pediatr.* 106, 207.

Edwards, C. A., Parrett, A. M. (2002). Intestinal flora during the first months of life: new perspectives. *Br J Nutr.* 88(Suppl 1), S11–S18.

Environmental Working Group. EWG's Guide to Infant Formula and Baby Bottles. Retrieved October 30, 2008 from http://www.ewg.org/book/export/html/25570

Evans, K. C., Evans, R. G., Royal, R., Esterman, A. J., James, S. L. (2003). Effect of cesarean section on breastmilk transfer to the normal term newborn over the first week of life. *Arch Dis Child Fetal Neonat Ed.* 88, F380–F382.

Ezaki, S., Ito, T., Suzuki, K., Tamura, M. (2008). Association between total antioxidant capacity in breastmilk and postnatal age in days in premature infants. *J Clin Biochem Nutr.* 42, 133–137.

Fantuzzi, G. (2005). Adipose tissue, adipokines, and inflammation. *J Allerg Clin Immunol.* 115:91, –919.

Farquharson, J., Cockburn, F., Patrick, W. A., et al. (1992). Infant cerebral cortex phospholipid fatty-acid composition and diet. *Lancet.* 340, 810.

Fenton, T. R., Belik, J. (2002). Routine handling of milk fed to preterm infants can significantly increase osmolality. *J Pediatr Gastroenterol Nutr.* 35:298–302.

Ferguson, M., Molfese, P. J. (2007). Breastfed infants process speech differently from bottle-fed infants: evidence from neuroelectrophysiology. *Dev Neuropsychol.* 31, 337–347.

Field, C. J. (2005). The immunological components of human milk and their effect on immune development in infants. *J Nutr.* 135, 1–4.

Florey, C., du,V., Leech, A. M., Blackhall, A. (1995). Infant feeding and mental and motor development at 18 months of age in first born singletons. *Intl J Epidemiol.* 24(Suppl 1), S21–S26.

Follett, J., Ishii, K. D., Heinig, M. J.(2003). The Role of Long-Chain Fatty Acids in Infant Health: Helping Families Make Informed Decisions About DHA. Independent Study Workbook 50301. Davis, CA: UC Davis Human Lactation Center. Retrieved June 12, 2005 from http://lactation.ucdavis.edu

Francis, J., Rogers, K., Brewer, P., Dickton, D., Pardini, R. (2008). Comparative analysis of ascorbic acid in human milk and infant formula using varied milk delivery systems. *Int Breastfeeding J.* 3, 19. Retrieved October 30, 2008 from http://www.internationalbreastfeedingjournal.com/content/3/1/19

Friel, J. K., Diehl-Jones, W. L., Suh, M., Tsopmo, A., Shirwadkar, V. P. (2007). Impact of iron and vitamin C-containing supplements on preterm human milk: in vitro. *Free Radic Biol Med.* 42, 1591–1598.

Furukawa, M., Lee, E. L., Johnston, J. M. (1993). Platelet-activating factor-induced ischemic bowel necrosis: the effect of platelet-activating factor acetylhydrolase. Pediatr Res. 34, 237–241.

Georgeson, G. D., Szony, B. J., Streitman, K., et al. (2002). Antioxidant enzyme activities are decreased in preterm infants and in neonates born via cesarean section. *Eur J Obstet Gynaecol Reprod Biol.* 103, 136–139.

Gerstley, J. R., Howell, K. M., Nagel, B. R. (1932). Some factors influencing the fecal flora of infants. *Am J Dis Child.* 43:555.

Gibson, L. (2007). Toxic baby bottles. Environment California Research & Policy Center. Retrieved October 30, 2008 from http://www.environmentcalifornia.org/reports/environmental-health/environmental-health-reports/toxic-baby-bottles

Gibson, R. A., Neumann, M. A., Makrides, M. (1997). Effect of increasing breastmilk docosahexaenoic acid on plasma and erythrocyte phospholipid fatty acids and neural indices of exclusively breastfed infants. *Eur J Clin Nutr.* 51, 578–584.

Glover J, Sandilands M. (1990). Supplementation of breastfeeding infants and weight loss in hospital. *J Hum Lact.* 6, 163–166.

Greene, L. C., Lucas, A., Barbara, M., et al. (1995). Relationship between early diet and subsequent cognitive performance during adolescence. *Biochem Soc Trans.* 23, 376S.

Greer, F. R., Marshall, S. (1989). Bone mineral content, serum vitamin D metabolite concentrations and ultraviolet B light exposure in infants fed human milk with and without vitamin D2 supplements. *J Pediatr.* 114, 204–212.

Greer, F. R., Searcy, J. E., Levin, R. S., et al. (1982). Bone mineral content and serum 25-hydroxyvitamin D concentrations in breastfed infants with and without supplemental vitamin D: one year follow-up. *J Pediatr.* 100:919–922.

Greer, F. R., Sicherer, S. H., Burks, A.W. (2008).Committee on Nutrition and Section on Allergy and Immunology. Effects of early nutritional interventions on the development of atopic disease in infants and children: the role of maternal dietary restriction, breastfeeding, timing of introduction of complementary foods, and hydrolyzed formulas. *Pediatrics.* 121:183–191.

Gronlund, M. M., et al. (1999). Fecal microflora in healthy infants born by different methods of delivery: permanent changes in intestinal flora after cesarean delivery. *J Pediatr Gastroenterol Nutr.* 28, 19–25.

Grosse, S. D., Matte, T. D., Schwartz, J., Jackson, R. J. (2002). Economic gains resulting from the reduction in children's exposure to lead in the United States. *Environ Health Perspect.* 110:563–569.

Grummer-Strawn, L. M., Scanlon, K. S., Fein, S. B. (2008). Infant feeding and feeding transitions during the first year of life. *Pediatrics.* 122, S36-S42.

Gustafsson, L., Hallgren, O., Mossberg, A.-K., et al. (2005). HAMLET kills tumor cells by apoptosis: structure, cellular mechanisms, and therapy. *J Nutr.* 135, 1299–1303.

Hahn-Zoric, M., Fulconis, F., Minoli, I., et al. (1990). Antibody responses to parenteral and oral vaccines are impaired by conventional and low protein formulas as compared to breastfeeding. *Acta Paediatr Scand.* 79, 1137–1142.

Hakansson, A., Zhivotovsky, B., Orrenius, S., et al. (1995). Apoptosis induced by a human milk protein. *Proc Natl Acad Sci USA.* 92, 8064–8068.

Hamosh, M., Ellis, L. A., Pollock, D. R., et al. (1996). Breastfeeding and the working mother: effect of time and temperature of short-term storage on proteolysis, lipolysis, and bacterial growth in milk. *Pediatrics.* 97, 492–498.

Hamprecht K, Maschmann J, Jahn G, Poets CF, Goelz R. (2008). Cytomegalovirus transmission to preterm infants during lactation. *J Clin Virol.* 41,198–205.

Hanna, N., Ahmed, K., Anwar, M., et al. (2004). Effect of storage on breastmilk antioxidant activity. *Arch Dis Child Fetal Neonatal Ed.* 89,F518–F520.

Hanson, L. A. (2004). Immunobiology of Human Milk: How Breastfeeding Protects Babies. Amarillo, TX: Pharmasoft Publishing.

Hanson, L. A., Korotkova, M., Haversen, L., et al. (2002). Breastfeeding, a complex support system for the offspring. *Pediatr Int.* 44, 347–352.

Hardell, L., Dreifaldt, A. C. (2001). Breastfeeding duration and the risk of malignant diseases in childhood in Sweden. *Eur J Clin Nutr.* 55, 179–185.

Hart, S., Boylan, L. M., Carroll, S., et al. (2003). Brief report: breast-fed one-week-olds demonstrate superior neurobehavioral organization. *J Pediatr Psychol.* 28,529–534.

Heaney, R. P., Davies, K. M., Chen, T. C., et al. (2003). Human serum 25-hydroxycholecalciferol response to extended oral dosing with cholecalciferol. *Am J Clin Nutr.* 77, 204–210.

Heird, W. C. (1999). Biological effects and safety issues related to long-chain polyunsaturated fatty acids in infants. *Lipids.* 34,103–224.

Heyman, M.B. (2006). Lactose intolerance in infants, children, and adolescents. Pediatrics. 118,1279–1286.

Hirsch, D.S. (2007). Vitamin D and the breastfed infant. In: Hale TW, Hartmann PE. Textbook of Human Lactation. Amarillo, TX: Hale Publishing, pp. 425–461.

Hollis, B.W., Wagner, C.L. (2004). Assessment of dietary vitamin D requirements during pregnancy and lactation. *Am J Clin Nutr.* 79,717–726.

Holmberg H, Wahlberg J, Vaarala O, Ludvigsson J, ABIS Study Group. (2007). Short duration of breast-feeding as a risk-factor for beta-cell autoantibodies in 5-year-old children from the general population. *Br J Nutr.* 97,111–116.

Hopkins, M. J., Macfarlane, G. T., Furrie, E., Fite, A., Macfarlane, S. (2005). Characterisation of intestinal bacteria in infant stools using real-time PCR and northern hybridization analyses. *FEMS Microbiol Ecol.* 54,77–85.

Horwood, L. J., Fergusson, D. M. (1998). Breastfeeding and later cognitive and academic outcomes. *Pediatrics.* 101(1),e9. Retrieved August 16, 2005 from www.pediatrics.org/cgi/content/full/101/1/e9

Host, A. (1991). Importance of the first meal on the development of cow's milk allergy and intolerance. *Allerg Proc.* 10, 227–232.

Host, A., Halken, S. (2005). Primary prevention of food allergy in infants who are at risk. *Curr Opin Allerg Immunol.* 5,255–259.

Host, A., Husby, S., Osterballe, O. (1988). A prospective study of cow's milk allergy in exclusively breastfed infants. *Acta Paediatr Scand.* 77,663–670.

Host, A., Jacobsen, H. P., Halken, S., Holmenlund, D. (1995). The natural history of cow's milk protein allergy/intolerance. *Eur J Clin Nutr.* 49(Suppl 1),S13-S18.

Human Milk Banking Association of North America. (2008). In: Tully MR, ed. Guidelines for the Establishment and Operation of a Donor Human Milk Bank. Raleigh, NC: Human Milk Banking Association of North America.

Hylander, M. A., Strobino, D. M., Pezzullo, J. C., et al. (2001). Association of human milk feedings with a reduction in retinopathy of prematurity among very low birthweight infants. *J Perinatol.* 21,356–362.

Hypponen, E., Sovio, U., Wjst, M., et al. (2004). Infant vitamin D supplementation and allergic conditions in adulthood: northern Finland birth cohort 1966. *Ann N Y Acad Sci.* 1037:84–95.

Innis, S. M., Hansen, J. W. (1996). Plasma fatty acid responses, metabolic effects, and safety of microalgal and fungal oils rich in arachidonic and docosahexaenoic acids in healthy adults. *Am J Clin Nutr.* 64,159–167.

Isaacs, C. E.. (2005).Human milk inactivates pathogens individually, additively and synergistically. *J Nutr.* 135,1286–1288.

Isaacs, C. E., Kashyap, S., Heird, W. C., Thormar, H. (1990). Antiviral and antibacterial lipids in human milk and infant formula feeds. *Arch Dis Child.* 65,861–864.

Jamieson, E. C., Farquharson, J., Logan, R. W., et al. (1999). Infant cerebellar gray and white matter fatty acids in relation to age and diet. *Lipids.* 34,1065–1071.

Jensen, R. G., ed. (1995). Handbook of Milk Composition. San Diego, CA: Academic Press, Inc.

Jeppesen, D. L., Hasselbalch, H., Lisse, I. M., Ersboll, A. K., Engelmann, M. D. (2004). T-lymphocyte subsets, thymic size and breastfeeding in infancy. *Pediatr Allergy Immunol.* 15,127–132.

Jocson, M. A. L., Mason, E. O., Schanler, R. J. (1997). The effects of nutrient fortification and varying storage conditions on host defense properties of human milk. *Pediatrics.* 100,240–243.

Johansson, S., Lindow, S., Kapadia, H., Norman, M. (2002). Perinatal water intoxication due to excessive oral intake during labour. *Acta Paediatr.* 91,811–814.

Johnson, D. L., Swank, P. R. (1996). Breastfeeding and children's intelligence. *Psych Rep.* 79,1179–1185.

Jones, F., Tully, M. R.. (2005). Best Practice for Expressing, Storing and Handling Human Milk in Hospitals, Homes and Child Care Settings. Raleigh, NC: Human Milk Banking Association of North America.

Kalkwarf, H. J., Specker, B. L., Heubi, J. E., et al. (1996). Intestinal calcium absorption of women during lactation and after weaning. *Am J Clin Nutr.* 63,526.

Kalliomaki, M., Collado, M. C., Salminen, S., Isolauri, E. (2008). Early differences in fecal microbiota composition in children may predict overweight. *Am J Clin Nutr.* 87,534–538.

Kalliomaki, M., Kirjavainen, P., Eerola, E., Kero, P., Salminen, S., Isolauri, E. (2001). Distinct patterns of neonatal gut microflora in infants developing or not developing atopy. *J Allergy Clin Immunol.* 107,129–134.

Karjalainen, J., Martin, J. M., Knip, M., et al. (1992). A bovine albumin peptide as a possible trigger of insulin-dependent diabetes mellitus. *N Engl J Med.* 327,302–307.

Keating, J. P., Shears, G. J., Dodge, P. R. (1991). Oral water intoxication in infants, an American epidemic. *Am J Dis Child.* 145,985–990.

Khedr, E. M.H., Farghaly. W. M. A., El-Din Amry, S., Osman, A. A. A . (2004). Neural maturation of breastfed and formula-fed infants. *Acta Paediatr.* 93,734–738.

Kimpimaki, T., et al. (2001). Short-term exclusive breastfeeding predisposes young children with increased genetic risk of type 1 diabetes to progressive beta-cell autoimmunity. *Diabetologia.* 44,63–69.

Kleinman, R. E., ed. (2004). Pediatric Nutrition Handbook. 5th ed. Elk Grove Village, IL: American Academy of Pediatrics.

Koo, W. W. K. (2003). Efficacy and safety of docosahexaenoic acid and arachidonic acid addition to infant formulas: can one buy better vision and intelligence? *J Am Coll Nutr.* 22,101–107.

Kostraba, J. N., Cruickshanks, K. J., Lawler-Heavner, J., et al. (1993). Early exposure to cow's milk and solid foods in infancy, genetic predisposition, and risk of IDDM. *Diabetes.* 42,288–295.

Kramer, M. S., Aboud, F., Mironova, E., et al. (2008). Breastfeeding and child cognitive development: new evidence from a large randomized trial. *Arch Gen Psychiatry.* 65,578–584.

Kreiter, S. R., Schwartz, R. P., Kirkman, H. N. Jr, et al. (2000). Nutritional rickets in African American breast-fed infants. *J Pediatr.* 137,153–157.

Lanting, C. I., Fidler, V., Huisman, M., et al. (1994). Neurological differences between 9 year old children fed breastmilk or formula milk as babies. *Lancet.* 344,1319–1322.

Laurberg, P., Nohr, S. B., Pedersen, K. M., Fuglsang, E.(2004). Iodine nutrition in breast-fed infants is impaired by maternal smoking. *J Clin Endocrinol Metab.* 89,181–187.

Lawrence, R. A. (1999). Storage of human milk and the influence of procedures on immunological components of human milk. *Acta Paediatr* 88(Suppl.),14–18.

Lawrence, R. M. (2006). Cytomegalovirus in human breastmilk: Risk to the premature infant. *Breastfeeding Med.* 1,99–107.

Lee, Y. K., Puong, K. Y. (2002). Competition for adhesion between probiotics and human gastrointestinal pathogens in the presence of carbohydrate. *Br J Nutr.* 88(Suppl 1),S101–S108.

Lessaris, K. J., Forsythe, D. W., Wagner, C. L. (2000). Effect of human milk fortifier on the immunodetection and molecular mass profile of transforming growth factor-alpha. *Biol Neonate.* 77,156–161.

Leung, A. K., McArthur, R. G., McMillan, D. D., et al. (1980). Circulating antidiuretic hormone during labour and in the newborn. *Acta Paediatr Scand.* 69,505–510.

Ley, R., Backhed, F., Turnbaugh, P., Lozupone, C., Knight, R., Gordon, J. (2005). Obesity alters gut microbial ecology. *Proc Natl Acad Sci USA.* 102,11070–11075.

Li R, Rock VJ, Grummer-Strawn L. (2007). Changes in public attitudes toward breastfeeding in the United States, 1999–2003. *J Am Diet Assoc.* 107,122–127.

Lonnerdal, B. (2003). Nutritional and physiologic significance of human milk proteins. *Am J Clin Nutr.* 77,1537S–1543S.

Lopez Alvarez, M. J. (2007). Proteins in human milk. Breastfeeding Rev. 15,5–16.

LSRO (Life Sciences Research Office) (1998). Report: assessment of nutrient requirements for infant formulas. *J Nutr.*128,2059S–2293S.

Lucas, A., Morley, R., Cole, T. J., et al. (1992). Breastmilk and subsequent intelligence quotient in children born preterm. *Lancet.* 339,261–264.

Mackie, R. I., Sghir, A., Gaskins, H. R. (1999). Developmental microbial ecology of the neonatal gastrointestinal tract. *Am J Clin Nutr.* 69(Suppl),1035S–1045S.

Manohar, A. A., Williamson, M., Koppikar, G. V. (1997). Effect of storage of colostrum in various containers. *Ind Pediatr.* 34,293–295.

Marchbank, T., Weaver, G., Nilsen-Hamilton, M., Playford, R. J. (2009). Pancreatic secretory trypsin inhibitor is a major motogenic and protective factor in human breast milk. *Am J Physiol Gastrointest Liver Physiol.* 296,G697-G703.

Marin, M. L., Arroyo, R., Jimenez, E., Gomez, A., Fernandez, L., Rodriguez, J. M. (2009). Cold storage of human milk: effect on its bacterial composition. *J Pediatr Gastroenterol Nutr.* May 25. [Epub ahead of print]

Martelli, A., De Chiara, A., Corvo, M., Restani, P., Fiocchi, A. (2002). Beef allergy in children with cow's milk allergy: cow's milk allergy in children with beef allergy. *Ann Allerg Asthma Immunol.* 89(6 Suppl 1):38–43.

Martínez-Costa C, Silvestre MD, López MC, Plaza A, Miranda M, Guijarro R. (2007). Effects of refrigeration on the bactericidal activity of human milk: a preliminary study. *J Pediatr Gastroenterol Nutr.* 45,275–277.

Martin-Sosa, S., Martin, M. J., Garcia-Pardo, L. A., Hueso, P. (2003). Sialyloligosaccharides in human milk and in infant formulas: variations with the progression of lactation. *J Dairy Sci.* 86,52–59.

Massiera, F., et al. (2003). Arachidonic acid and prostacyclin signaling promote adipose tissue development: a human health concern? *J Lipid Res.* 44,271–279.

Mathur NB, Dwarkadas AM, Sharma VK, Saha K, Jain N. (1990). Anti-infective factors in preterm human colostrum. *Acta Paediatr Scand.* 79,1039–1044.

Mayer, E. J., Hamman, R. F., Gay, E. C., et al. (1988). Reduced risk of IDDM among breastfed children. *The Colorado IDDM Registry. Diabetes.* 37,1625–1632.

McKinney, P. A., Parslow, R., Gurney, K. A., et al. (1999). Perinatal and neonatal determinants of childhood type I diabetes. A case-control study in Yorkshire, UK. *Diabetes Care.* 22,928–932.

McVeagh, P., Miller, J. B. (1997). Human milk oligosaccharides: only the breast. *J Paediatr Child Health.* 33,281–286.

Milner, J. D., Gergen, P. J. (2005). Transient environmental exposures on the developing immune system: implications for allergy and asthma. *Curr Opin Allerg Clin Immunol.* 5,235–240.

Miniello VL, Francavilla R, Brunetti L, et al. (2008). Primary allergy prevention: partially or extensively hydrolyzed infant formulas? *Minerva Pediatr.* 60,1437–1443.

Misra, M., Pacaud, D., Petryk, A., Collett-Solberg, P. F., Kappy, M. (2008). Vitamin D deficiency in children and its management: review of current knowledge and recommendations. *Pediatrics.* 122,398–417.

Mitoulas, L. R. (2000). Short- and long-term variation in the production and content and composition of human milk fat. Unpublished PhD dissertation. Perth: University of Western Australia.

Mojab, C. G. (2002). Sunlight deficiency and breastfeeding. *Breastfeeding Abstr.* 22,3–4.

Morelli, L. (2008). Postnatal development of intestinal microflora as influenced by infant nutrition. *J Nutr.* 138:1791S–1795S.

Morrow, A. L., Ruiz-Palacios, G. M., Altaye, M., et al. (2004). Human milk oligosaccharides are associated with protection against diarrhea in breastfed infants. *J Pediatr.* 145:297–303.

Morrow-Tlucak, M., Haude, R. H., Ernhart, C. B. (1988). Breastfeeding and cognitive development in the first 2 years of life. *Soc Sci Med.* 26,635–639.

Mortensen, E. L., Michaelsen, K. F., Sanders, S. A., et al.(2002). The association between duration of breastfeeding and adult intelligence. *JAMA.* 287,2365–2371.

Mountzouris, K. C., McCartney, A. L., Gibson, G. R. (2002). Intestinal microflora of human infants and current trends for its nutritional modulation. *Br J Nutr.*87,405–420.

Myher, J. J., Kuksis, A., Geher, K., et al. (1996). Stereospecific analysis of triacylglycerols rich in long-chain polyunsaturated fatty acids. *Lipids.* 31,207–215.

Nelson, C. M., Innis, S. M. (1999). Plasma lipoprotein fatty acids are altered by the positional distribution of fatty acids in infant formula triacylglycerols and human milk. *Am J Clin Nutr.* 70:62–69.

Newburg, D. S. (2005). Innate immunity and human milk. *J Nutr.* 135,1308–1312.

Newburg, D. S., Walker, W. A. (2007). Protection of the neonate by the innate immune system of developing gut and of human milk. *Pediatr Res.* 61,2–8.

Ngom, P. T., Collinson, A. C., Pido-Lopez, J., Henson, S. M., Prentice, A. M., Aspinall, R. (2004). Improved thymic function in exclusively breastfed infants is associated with higher interleukin 7 concentrations in their mothers' breastmilk. *Am J Clin Nutr.* 80,722–728.

Nicoll, A., Ginsburg, R., Tripp, J. H. (1982). Supplementary feeding and jaundice in newborns. *Acta Paediatr Scand.* 71,759–761.

Norris, J., Barriga, K., Klingensmith, G., et al. (2003). Timing of initial cereal exposure in infancy and risk of islet autoimmunity. *JAMA.* 290,1713–1720.

Office of Food Additive Safety. (2001).GRAS Notice No. GRN 000041. Washington, DC: US Food and Drug Administration, May 17, 2001.

Ogundele MO. (2000). Techniques for the storage of human breastmilk: implications for anti-microbial functions and safety of stored milk. *Eur J Pediatr.* 159,793–797.

Ogundele MO.(2002). Effects of storage on the physicochemical and antibacterial properties of human milk. *Br J Biomed Sci.* 59,205–211.

Osborn, D. A., Sinn, J. (2006). Soy formula for the prevention of allergy and food intolerance in infants. *Cochrane Database Syst Rev.* Oct 18;(4),CD003741.

Oski, F. A., DeAngeles, C. D., Feigin, R. D., McMillan,J. A. (1994). Principles and Practice of Pediatrics. Philadelphia, PA: Lippincott.

Ostrea, E. M. Jr, Balun, J. E., Winkler, R., et al. (1986). Influence of breastfeeding on the restoration of the low serum concentration of vitamin E and beta-carotene in the newborn infant. *Am J Obstet Gynecol.* 154,1014–1017.

Pan, D.A., Hylbert, A. J., Storlien, L. H. (1994). Dietary fats, membrane phospholipids and obesity. *J Nutr.* 124,1555–1565.

Park, D. A., Bulkley, G. B., Granger, D. N. (1983). Role of oxygen-derived free radicals in digestive tract disease. Surgery.94,415–422.

Penders, J., Thijs, C., Vink, C., et al. (2006). Factors influencing the composition of the intestinal microbiota in early infancy. *Pediatrics.*118,511–521.

Picciano, M. F. (1998). Human milk: nutritional aspects of a dynamic food. *Biol Neonate.* 74,84–93.

Pickering, L. K., Granoff, D. M., Erickson, J. R., et al. (1998). Modulation of the immune system by human milk and infant formula containing nucleotides. *Pediatrics.* 101,242–249.

Pisacane, A., DeVizia, B., Valiante, A., et al. (1995). Iron status in breastfed infants. *J Pediatr.* 127,429.

Pugliese, M.F., Blumberg, D. L., Hludzinski, J., Kay, S. (1998). Nutritional rickets in suburbia. *J Am Coll Nutr.* 17,637–641.

Quan, R., Yang, C., Rubinstein, S., et al. (1992). Effects of microwave radiation on anti-infective factors in human milk. *Pediatrics.* 89,667.

Quan R, Yang C, Rubinstein S, Lewiston NJ, Stevenson DK, Kerner JA Jr. (1994). The effect of nutritional additives on anti-infective factors in human milk. *Clin Pediatr (Phila).* 33,325–328.

Raiten, D. J., Talbot, J. M., Waters, J. H., eds. (1998). Assessment of nutrient requirements for infant formulas. *J Nutr.* 128(Suppl 11S),2059S–2293S.

Rao, M. R., Hediger, M. L., Levine, R. J., et al. (2002). Effect of breastfeeding on cognitive development of infants born small for gestational age. *Acta Paediatr.* 91,267–274.

Ratner, B. (1935). The treatment of milk allergy and its basic principles. *JAMA.* 105,934–939.

Robbins, S. T., Beker, L. T., eds. (2004). Infant Feedings: Guidelines for Preparation of Formula and Breastmilk in Healthcare Facilities. Chicago: American Dietetic Association.

Rozenfeld, P., Docena, G. H., Añón, M. C., Fossati, C. A. (2002). Detection and identification of a soy protein component that cross-reacts with caseins from cow's milk. *Clin Exp Immunol*. 130,49–58.

Rubaltelli, F. F., et al. (1998). Intestinal flora in breast and bottle-fed infants. *J Perinatol Med*. 26,186–191.

Ruth-Sanchez, V., Greene, C. V. (1997). Water intoxication in a three day old: a case presentation. *Mother Baby J*. 2,5–11.

Sachdev, H. P. S., Krishna, J., Puri, R. K., Satyanarayana, L., Kumar, S. (1991). Water supplementation in exclusively breastfed infants during summer in the tropics. *Lancet*. 337,929–933.

Sacker, A., Quigley, M. A., Kelly, Y. J. (2006). Breastfeeding and developmental delay: findings from the Millennium Cohort study. *Pediatrics*. 118,e682-e689.

Sadeharju, K., Knip, M., Virtanen, S. M., et al. (2007), Maternal antibodies in breastmilk protect the child from enterovirus infections. *Pediatrics*. 119,941–946.

Salminen, S. J., Gueimonde, J., Isolauri, E. (2005). Probiotics that modify disease risk. *J Nutr*. 135,1294–1298.

Savilahti, E., Tuomilehto, J., Saukkonen, T. T., et al. (1993). Increased levels of cow's milk and b-lactoglobulin antibodies in young children with newly diagnosed IDDM. *Diabetes Care*. 16,984–989.

Scariati, P. D., Grummer-Strawn, L. M., Fein, S. (1997b).Water supplementation of infants in the first month of life. *Arch Pediatr Adolesc Med*. 151,830–832.

Schulz-Lell, G., Buss, R., Oldigs, H. D., et al. (1987). Iron balances in infant nutrition. *Acta Paediatr Scand*. 76,585.

Scott JA, Binns CW, Oddy WH. (2007). Predictors of delayed onset of lactation. *Matern Child Nutr*. 3,186–93.

Shah, M., Salhab, N., Patterson, D., Seikaly, M. G. (2000)Nutritional rickets still afflict children in North Texas. *Texas Med*. 96,64–68.

Silfverdal SA, Ekholm L, Bodin L. (2007). Breastfeeding enhances the antibody response to Hib and pneumococcal serotype 6B and 14 after vaccination with conjugate vaccines. *Vaccine*. 25,1497–1502.

Sills, I. N., Skuza, K. A., Horlick, M. N., et al. (1994). Vitamin D deficiency rickets. Reports of its demise are exaggerated. *Clin Pediatr (Phila)*. 33,491–493.

Silvestre D, Miranda M, Muriach M, Almansa I, Jareño E, Romero FJ. (2008a). Antioxidant capacity of human milk: effect of thermal conditions for the pasteurization. *Acta Paediatr*. 97,1070–1074.

Silvestre, D., Ruiz, P., Martinez-Costa, C., Plaza, A., Lopez, M. C. (2008b). Effect of pasteurization on the bactericidal capacity of human milk. *J Hum Lact*. 24,371–376.

Simmer, K. (2002a).Longchain polyunsaturated fatty acid supplementation in infants born at term (Cochrane Review). In: The Cochrane Library, 1. Oxford: Update Software.

Simmer K. (2002b).Longchain polyunsaturated fatty acid supplementation in preterm infants (Cochrane Review). In: The Cochrane Library, 1. Oxford: Update Software.

Simmer K, Patole SK, Rao SC. (2008a). Longchain polyunsaturated fatty acid supplementation in infants born at term. *Cochrane Database Syst Rev*. Jan 23;(1),CD000376.

Simmer K, Schulzke SM, Patole S. (2008b). Longchain polyunsaturated fatty acid supplementation in preterm infants. *Cochrane Database Syst Rev*. Jan 23;(1),CD000375.

Singhal, A., Morley, R., Cole.T.J., et al. (2007). Infant nutrition and stereoacuity at age 4–6 y. *Am J Clin Nutr*. 85,152–159.

Singhi, S., Chookang, E., Hall, J. S., Kalghangi, S. (1985). Iatrogenic neonatal and maternal hyponatremia following oxytocin and aqueous glucose infusion during labour. *Br J Obstet Gynaecol*. 92,356–363.

Slykerman, R. F., Thompson, J. M. D., Becroft, D. M. D., et al. (2005). Breastfeeding and intelligence of preschool children. *Acta Paediatr*. 94,832–837.

Sommerburg, O., Meissner, K., Nelle, M., et al. (2000). Carotenoid supply in breastfed and formula-fed neonates. *Eur J Paediatr*. 159,86–90.

Song, J. H., Miyazawa, T. (2001). Enhanced level of n-3 fatty acid in membrane phospholipids induces lipid peroxidation in rats fed dietary docosahexaenoic acid oil. *Atherosclerosis*. 155,9–18.

Song, J. H., et al. (2000). Polyunsaturated (n-3) fatty acids susceptible to peroxidation are increased in plasma and tissue lipids of rats fed docosahexaenoic acid-containing oils. *J Nutr.* 130,3028–3033.

Specker, B. L., Valanis, B., Hertzberg, V., et al. (1985). Sunshine exposure and serum 25-hydroxyvitamin D concentrations in exclusively breastfed infants. *J Pediatr.* 107,372–376.

Srinivasan, L., Bokiniec, R., King, C., Weaver, G., Edwards, A. D. (2004). Increased osmolality of breast-milk with therapeutic additives. *Arch Dis Child Fetal Neonatal Ed.* 89,F514–F517.

Stewart, J. A., Chadwick, V. S., Murray, A. (2006). Carriage, quantification, and predominance of methanogens and sulfate-reducing bacteria in fecal samples. *Lett Appl Microbiol.* 43,58–63.

Straarup, E. M., Lauritzen, L., Faerk, J., et al. (2006). The stereospecific triacylglycerol structures and fatty acid profiles of human milk and infant formulas. *J Pediatr Gastroenterol Nutr.* 42,293–299.

Svensson, M., Hakansson, A., Mossberg, A. K., et al. (2000). Conversion of alpha-lactalbumin to a protein inducing apoptosis. *Proc Natl Acad Sci USA.* 97,4221–4226.

Tanaka K, Kon N, Ohkawa N, Yoshikawa N, Shimizu T. (2009). Does breastfeeding in the neonatal period influence the cognitive function of very-low-birth-weight infants at 5 years of age? *Brain Dev.* 31,288-293.

Tarnow-Mordi, W. O., Shaw, J. C., Liu, D., et al. (1981). Iatrogenic hyponatremia of the newborn due to maternal fluid overload: a prospective study. *Br Med J Clin Res Ed.* 283,639–642.

Telang, S., Berseth, C. L., Ferguson, P. W., et al. (2005). Fortifying fresh human milk with commercial powdered human milk fortifiers does not affect bacterial growth during 6 hours at room temperature. *J Am Diet Assoc.* 105,1567–1572.

Thavagnanam S, Fleming J, Bromley A, Shields MD, Cardwell CR. (2008). A meta-analysis of the association between caesarean section and childhood asthma. *Clin Exp Allerg.* 38,629–633.

Tomblin, J. B., Smith, E., Zhang, X. (1997). Epidemiology of specific language impairment: prenatal and perinatal risk factors. *J Commun Disord.* 30,325–344.

Toschke, A. M., Vignerova, J., Lhotska, L., et al. (2002). Overweight and obesity in 6- to 14-year-old Czech children in 1991: protective effect of breast-feeding. *J Pediatr.* 141,764–769.

Tullus, K., Burman, L. G. (1989). Ecological impact of ampicillin and cefuroxime in neonatal units. *Lancet.*1,1405–1407.

Tully, M. R. (2000). Recommendations for handling of mother's own milk. *J Hum Lact.* 16,149–151.

Uauy, R. (1990). Are omega-3 fatty acids required for normal eye and brain development in the human? *J Pediatr Gastroenterol Nutr.* 11,296–302.

Uauy, R., Araya, M. (2004). Novel oligosaccharides in human milk: understanding mechanisms may lead to better prevention of enteric and other infections. *J Pediatr.* 145,283–285.

Vaarala, O., et al. (1998). Cow milk feeding induces antibodies to insulin in children—a link between cow milk and insulin-dependent mellitus? *Scand J Immunol.* 47,131–135.

Vallaeys, C. (2008). Replacing mother-imitating human breastmilk in the laboratory. Novel oils in infant formula and organic foods: safe and valuable functional food or risky marketing gimmick? Cornucopia, WI: Cornucopia Institute. Retrieved October 26, 2008 from http://www.cornucopia.org/2008/01/replacing-mother-infant-formula-report/

Vandenplas, Y., Brueton, M., Dupont, C., et al. (2007). Guidelines for the diagnosis and management of cow's milk protein allergy in infants. *Arch Dis Child.* 92,902–908.

van Odijk, J., Kull, I., Borres, M. P., et al. (2003). Breastfeeding and allergic disease: a multidisciplinary review of the literature (1996–2001) on the mode of early feeding in infancy and its impact on later atopic manifestations. *Allergy.* 58,833–843.

Veh, R. W., Michalski, J. C., Corfiend, A. P., et al. (1981). New chromatographic system for the rapid analysis and preparation of colostrum sialyl oligosaccharides. *J Chromatogr.* 212,313–322.

Vieth, R., Chan, P. C. R., MacFarlane, G. D. (2001). Efficiency and safety of vitamin D3 intake exceeding the lowest observed adverse effect level (LOAEL). *Am J Clin Nutr*. 73,288–294.

Vio, F., Salazar, G., Infante, C. (1991). Smoking during pregnancy and lactation and its effects on breast-milk volume. *Am J Clin Nut*. 54,1011–1016.

Vohr, B. R., Poindexter, B. B., Dusick, A. M., McKinley, L. T., Wright, L. L., Langer, J. C., Poole, W. K. (2006).NICHD Neonatal Research Network. Beneficial effects of breastmilk in the neonatal intensive care unit on the developmental outcome of extremely low birth weight infants at 18 months of age. *Pediatrics*. 118,e115–e123.

Von Berg, A., Koletzko, S., Grubl, A., et al. (2003). The effect of hydrolyzed cow's milk formula for allergy prevention in the first year of life: the German Infant Nutritional Intervention Study, a randomized double-blind trial. *J Allergy Clin Immunol*. 111,533–540.

Wagner CL, Greer FR; American Academy of Pediatrics Section on Breastfeeding; American Academy of Pediatrics Committee on Nutrition. (2008). Prevention of rickets and vitamin D deficiency in infants, children, and adolescents. *Pediatrics*. 122,1142-1152.

Wagner, C. L., Hulsey, T. C., Fanning, D., Ebeling, M., Hollis, B. W. (2006). High dose vitamin D3 supplementation in a cohort of breastfeeding mothers and their infants: a six-month follow-up pilot study. *Breastfeeding Med*. 1,59–70.

Wang, B., Brand-Miller, J., McVeagh, Petocz, P. (2001). Concentration and distribution of sialic acid in human milk and infant formulas. *Am J Clin Nutr*. 74,510–515.

Wang, B., McVeagh, P., Petocz, P., Brand-Miller, J. (2003). Brain ganglioside and glycoprotein sialic acid in breastfed compared with formula-fed infants. *Am J Clin Nutr*. 78,1024–1029.

Wang, B., Yu, B., Karim, M., et al. (2007).Dietary sialic acid supplementation improves learning and memory in piglets. *Am J Clin Nutr*. 85,561–569.

Weaver, L. T., Laker, M. F., Nelson, R., Lucas, A. (1987). Milk feeding and changes in intestinal permeability and morphology in the newborn. *J Pediatr Gastrointest Nutr*. 6,351-358.

Weisberg, P., Scanlon, K. S., Li, R., Cogswell, M. E. (2004). Nutritional rickets among children in the United States: review of cases reported between 1986 and 2003. *Am J Clin Nutr*. 80(Suppl),1697S–1705S.

Welch, T. R., Bergstrom, W. H., Tsang, R. C. (2000). Vitamin D-deficient rickets: the reemergence of a once-conquered disease. *J Pediatr*. 137,143–145.

Williams, C., Birch, E. E., Emmett, P. M., et al. (2001). Stereoacuity at age 3.5 years in children born full-term is associated with prenatal and postnatal dietary factors: a report from a population-based cohort study. *Am J Clin Nutr*. 73:316–322.

Williams, H. G. (2006). "And not a drop to drink"—why water is harmful for newborns. *Breastfeeding Rev*. 14,5–9.

Williams-Arnold, L. D. (2000). Human Milk Storage for Healthy Infants and Children. Sandwich, MA: Health Education Associates.

Williamson, M. T., Murti, P. K. (1996). Effects of storage, time, temperature, and composition of containers on biologic components of human milk. *J Hum Lact*. 12,31–35.

Wing, K., Ekmark, A., Karlsson, H., et al. (2002). Characterization of human CD25+ CD4+ T cells in thymus, cord and adult blood. *Immunology*. 106,190–199.

Workgroup for Safe Markets. Baby's toxic bottle: bisphenol A leaching from popular baby bottle. Retrieved October 30, 2008 from http://www.chej.org/BPA_Website.htm

Yamauchi, Y., Yamanouchi, H. (1990). Breastfeeding frequency during the first 24 hours after birth in full term neonates. *Pediatrics*. 86,171–175.

Young, T. K., Martens, P. J., Taback, S. P., et al. (2002). Type 2 diabetes mellitus in children. *Arch Pediatr Adolesc Med*. 156,651–655.

Zeiger, R. (1999). Prevention of food allergy in infants and children. *Immunol Allerg Clin North Am.* 19, 619–646.

Zetterstrom, R., et al. (1994). Early infant feeding and micro-ecology of the gut. *Acta Paediatr Jpn.* 36, 562–571.

Ziegler, A., Schmid, S., Huber, D., et al. (2003).Early infant feeding and risk of developing type I diabetes-associated antibodies. *JAMA.* 290,1721–1728.

Zoeren-Grobben, D., Moison, R. M., Ester, W. M., et al. (1993). Lipid peroxidation in human milk and infant formula: effect of storage, tube feeding and exposure to phototherapy. *Acta Paediatr.* 82,645–649.

Zoppi, G., Gasparini, R., Mantovanelli, F., et al. (1983). Diet and antibody response to vaccinations in healthy infants. *Lancet.* 2,11–14.

Additional Reading

Institute of Medicine. Evaluation of the Safety of New Ingredients in Infant Formula. Available at http://books.nap.edu/catalog/10935.html or www.nap.edu

Summary Interventions Based on the Biospecificity of Breastmilk

1. Promote breastfeeding as the normal and best way to feed an infant.
   - Educate parents regarding
     a. The components of breastmilk and formula, reminding them that the two are not the same and that health and developmental outcomes can be different
     b. Defense factors in breastmilk protect the infant from acute and chronic diseases, resulting in fewer days of missed work; formula cannot duplicate the health protective factors in human milk and increases the risk of acute and chronic disease, autoimmune disease, and conditions such as overweight, obesity, asthma, and diabetes
   - Inform parents of the developmental and cognitive differences when infants are fed formula, such as lower IQs and poorer school performance.
   - Assist parents to critically evaluate infant formula marketing by helping them understand that formula is not equivalent to human milk.

2. Keep mother and baby together during their hospital stay.
   - If separated, have the mother spend time in the baby's environment (nursery, special care).

3. Avoid giving the baby infant formula in the hospital or before gut closure occurs.
   - In breastfed infants at risk, hypoallergenic formulas can be used to supplement breastfeeding if medically necessary.

4. Ensure 8–12 feedings each 24 hours starting in the hospital.

5. Teach and assess proper positioning, latch, and milk transfer.

   • Document swallowing and ensure that the mother knows when her baby is swallowing milk.

   • If a baby is latched but not swallowing adequately, have the mother use alternate massage (massage and compress the breast during pauses between sucking bursts) to sustain sucking and swallowing.

6. Avoid using sterile water or dextrose water. If used, chart the amount and reason for use.

   • Educate the parents and extended family regarding the hazard of giving young breastfed infants bottles of water, even in hot weather.

   • Avoid placing water bottles in the infant's bassinet in the hospital.

   • Remind mothers that babies also nurse at the breast for thirst, frequently coming off the breast after only a few minutes of nursing.

7. Mothers simply need to drink to quench thirst.

   • Maternal consumption of water in excess of thirst does not increase milk supply and can decrease milk production.

8. Teach mothers to allow the baby to finish the first side before switching to the second breast.

   • For infants experiencing slow weight gain, mothers can be guided to finish the first side using alternate massage before offering the second side and to shorten the intervals between daytime feeds to increase the fat content of the milk.

   • When breastmilk is stored in the refrigerator or freezer, the fat rises to the top of the container; it can be skimmed off and given to slow gaining or preterm infants for extra calories.

   • Avoid vigorously shaking stored breastmilk to redistribute the fat layer. This can damage some of the cellular components and inject air into the milk.

   • Infants whose mothers smoke need to be carefully monitored and to have frequent weight checks.

9. Prenatally, help parents understand the importance of exclusive breastfeeding for about 6 months, especially those with a family history of allergies and diabetes.

10. Reassure parents that it is uncommon for infant fussiness to be related to lactose intolerance. Primary lactose intolerance (lactase deficiency) is extremely rare.

11. Lactating mothers rarely need supplemental vitamins and minerals.

    • Fluoride supplementation is no longer recommended for infants younger than 6 months of age and only thereafter for infants living in communities with suboptimally fluoridated water supplies.

    • Mothers can maintain good vitamin D status by consuming vitamin D–fortified food and through exposure to sunlight.

    • Child care providers should be instructed to take infants outside for short periods each day.

        a. Breastfed infants require 30 minutes of exposure to sunlight each week if wearing only a diaper or 2 hours per week if fully clothed without a hat to maintain normal vitamin D levels. Darkly pigmented infants require a greater exposure to sunshine to initiate the synthesis of vitamin D in the skin. Some infants may require additional vitamin D supplements, especially if they are dark skinned, experience reduced sunlight exposure, or demonstrate signs of suboptimal vitamin D intake.

    • Vegetarian mothers may either need a vitamin B12 supplement or consultation regarding acceptable food sources of this vitamin in their diet.

12. Adding solid foods or infant formula before about 6 months of age may interfere with iron uptake in the breastfed infant and saturate the iron-binding capacity of lactoferrin, increasing the risk of gastrointestinal disease.

13. Some commercially available bottled baby water contains added fluoride. Parents should be advised that breastfed infants do not require additional water or fluoride and to check with their primary healthcare provider about the safety of products advertised for young infants.

14. Microwaving bottles of expressed breastmilk can interfere with the disease-protective factors in breastmilk and poses an injury hazard to the infant. Advise parents to place the bottle of expressed breastmilk under warm running water or in a bowl of warm water.

15. Human milk can be safely stored under appropriate conditions.

Human Milk Banks in North America

California

Mothers' Milk Bank
751 South Bascom Ave.
San Jose, CA 95128
Phone (408) 998-4550
FAX (408) 297-9208
mothersmilkbank@hhs.co.santa-clara.ca.us
www.milkbanksj.org

Indiana

Indiana Mothers' Milk Bank, Inc.
Methodist Medical Plaza II
6820 Parkdale Place, Suite 109
Indianapolis, IN 46254
Phone (317) 329-7146
FAX (317) 329-7151
inmothersmilkbank@clarian.org
www.immilkbank.org

Iowa

Mother's Milk Bank of Iowa
Department of Food and Nutrition Services
University of Iowa Hospitals and Clinics, Room C330 GH
200 Hawkins Drive
Iowa City, IA 52242
Phone (319) 356-2652
FAX (319) 356-8674
jean-drulis@uiowa.edu
www.uihealthcare.com/milkbank/

Michigan

Bronson Mothers' Milk Bank
601 John Street
Suite N1300
Kalamazoo, MI 49007
Phone (269) 341-8849
FAX (269) 341-8918
Duffc@bronsonhg.org

New England

Mothers' Milk Bank of New England
PO Box 600091
Newtonville, MA 02460
info@milkbankne.org
www.milkbankne.org

North Carolina

WakeMed Mothers' Milk Bank and Lactation Center
3000 New Bern Ave.
Raleigh, NC 27610
Phone (919) 350-8599
FAX (919) 350-8923
BMoore@wakemed.org
Suevans@wakemed.org
MBradshaw@wakemed.org
www.wakemed.com/body.cfm?id=135

Ohio

Mothers' Milk Bank of Ohio
Grant Medical Center @
Victorian Village Health Center
1087 Dennison Avenue
Columbus, OH 43201
Phone (614) 544-0810
FAX (614) 544-0812
gmorrow@ohiohealth.com

Oregon

Northwest Mothers Milk Bank (developing)
3439 NE Sandy Blvd #130
Portland, OR 97232
info@nwmmb.org
www.nwmmb.org

Texas

Mothers' Milk Bank at Austin
900 E. 30th St., Suite 214
Austin, TX 78705
Phone (512) 494-0800
Toll-free 1 (877) 813-MILK (6455)
FAX (512) 494-0880
info@mmbaustin.org
www.mmbaustin.org

Mothers' Milk Bank of North Texas
1300 W. Lancaster Suite 108
Ft. Worth, TX 76102
Phone (817) 810-0071
Toll-free 1 (866) 810-0071
FAX (817) 810-0087
mmbnt@hotmail.com
www.mmbnt.org

CANADA

British Columbia

BC Women's Milk Bank
C & W Lactation Services
4500 Oak Street, IU 30
Vancouver, BC V6H 3N1
Phone (604) 875-2282
FAX (604) 875-2871
fjones@cw.bc.ca

Influence of the Maternal Anatomy and Physiology on Lactation

Introduction

The mammary gland, or breast, and its ability to produce milk for the young of a species are the common links between all mammals. The breast grows and develops over time, as it is not a fully functional organ at birth. It reaches its full functional capacity during pregnancy and childbirth. The breast performs through an elegant interplay occurring among all of the body's systems. There is a typical progression of growth and development, sometimes with deviations that may affect either the breast's ability to synthesize milk or the infant's ability to remove it. Breast development first occurs in several stages during the embryonic and fetal periods. Prenatal breast developmental stages can be described using gestational week or the 10 stages relative to embryonic and fetal length (Table 2-1).

Small amounts of milk secretion (colostrum) are present in the breasts of the newborn under the influence of circulating maternal hormones. This secretion, which is referred to as "witch's milk," ceases once the maternal hormones have cleared the infant's system, usually within 3–4 weeks. The lactiferous ducts communicate with a small depression known as the mammary pit that later elevates, forming the nipple and areola. A true inverted nipple occurs because of the failure of the pit to elevate.

Usually, one pair of glands develops along each milk line; when fully developed they lie between the second to sixth rib arches. However, accessory or supernumerary nipples and breast tissue can develop anywhere along the milk lines (Figure 2-1). The prevalence of accessory nipples is approximately 2–10%, with white Europeans and black Americans having frequencies of 0.2% and 1.6%, respectively, and Jewish women, 2.5% (Mathes et al., 2006). Approximately 20% of ectopic breast tissue occurs in the axillae (Surajit et al., 2007) and results when the mammary ridge fails to resolve during embryonic development. These extra nipples and breast tissue occasionally swell and secrete milk during lactogenesis II. Although the enlargement and activity of accessory breast tissue and nipples have no physiological significance, they do have the potential to significantly

TABLE 2-1   Stages of Fetal Breast Development

Stage by Fetal Length	Stage by Gestational Age
1: Ridge stage— embryo less than 5 mm	5–6 wk; milk line appears (ectodermal ridge)
2: Milk hill stage– embryo more than 5.5 mm	7–8 wk; mammary disc appears; primitive blood vessels form
3: Mammary disc stage— embryo 10–11 mm	10–12 wk; epithelial buds form
4: Lobule type stage— embryo 11.0–25.0 mm	12–16 wk; smooth musculature of areola and nipple are formed
	16 wk; vascular system completely formed
5: Cone stage— embryo 25–30 mm	13–20 wk; parenchymal branching
6: Budding stage— embryo 30–68 mm	20 wk; 15–20 ductal structures formed
7: Indentation stage— embryo 68 mm to 10 cm	32 wk; canalization forms primary milk ducts
8: Branching stage— fetus 10 cm	32 wk to term; lobulo-alveolar development; increased periductal stroma; lobules show single layer of epithelium
9: Canalization stage— 20–32 wk gestation	
10: End-vesicle stage with vesicles composed of a single layer of epithelium and containing colostrum	

Sources: Russo J, Russo IH. Development of the human breast. *Maturitas.* 2004;49:2–15; Geddes DT. Gross anatomy of the lactating breast. In: Hale TW, Hartmann PE. *Textbook of human lactation.* Amarillo, TX: Hale Publishing, 2007 Ch.2, pp 19–34.

grow during pregnancy and lactation and become painful or make breastfeeding awkward. No special management is necessary, but if axillary tissue becomes significantly enlarged and painful, warm compresses may provide symptomatic relief. Some ectopic tissue may be differentiated enough to actually secrete milk. Faridi and Dewan (2008) reported a mother who chose to express milk from ectopic tissue in the axilla, but most mothers simply allow the tissue to involute and do not remove milk. Breast development during childhood is a quiescent period of time with mammary growth simply reflecting general body growth.

Puberty

Hormones such as estrogen and growth hormone stimulate the growth of mammary ducts, whereas progesterone secreted by the ovary results in modest lobular-alveolar development. About 11 alveolar buds form in clusters around each terminal duct to create a lobule. The areola enlarges and darkens, and the breasts increase to the adult size, mostly through the deposition of adipose tissue. Each ovulatory or menstrual cycle facilitates a little more mammary development that continues until about age 35.

Figure 2-1 Areas for Possible Accessory Breast/Nipple Tissue Growth

Source: Reprinted with permission from Cadwell, et al., *Maternal and Infant Assessment for Breastfeeding and Human Lactation: A Guide for the Practitioner.* Sudbury, MA: Jones and Bartlett Publishers; 2002.

Pregnancy

The breast completes the majority of its growth and maturation during pregnancy under the influence of a number of hormones such as progesterone, prolactin, human placental lactogen, growth hormone, and insulin-like growth factor. By 16–20 weeks of gestation, the breast is capable of secreting its first milk: colostrum. Lactose appears in the blood and urine, heralding the stage called lactogenesis I. Preterm delivery (<28 weeks gestation) interrupts the development of the breast but does not preclude breastfeeding. Mothers delivering very preterm infants may see a delay in lactogenesis II, the onset of copious milk production, and experience diminished amounts of milk in the early week or two postpartum. Note that breast growth and accompanying change in the size of the breasts varies greatly from woman to woman. The greatest rate of breast growth usually occurs during the first 5 months of pregnancy, but such growth can also occur gradually throughout the entire pregnancy. The increase in breast volume can range from 12 to 227 mL. Some women, however, experience minimal breast enlargement during pregnancy, defined by Neifert et al. (1990) as an increase of less than one cup size.

No relationship has been found between breast growth in pregnancy and milk production at 1 month in mothers breastfeeding as frequently as desired or needed (Cox et al., 1999). Indeed, the human mammary glands may have the ability to increase secretory tissue during lactation in response to increased demand for milk. Hytten (1954) reported that the breast volume of one mother who reported no breast growth during pregnancy rose 160% by the seventh day postpartum. Irrespective of the size of their breasts before pregnancy, an increase in size of up to 200 mL or one bra cup size either during pregnancy or the first month postpartum usually indicates sufficient secretory tissue proliferation for ample milk production (Czank et al., 2007). Russo and Russo (2004) discussed the effects that breast changes during pregnancy have on increasing the protectiveness against breast cancer. They postulate that the mammary gland's differentiation activates specific genes that imprint the breast epithelia to subsequent hormonal milieu, providing protection against neoplastic changes.

It is not unusual for a woman to have breasts that are slightly different in size and shape from each other. About one in five women have breasts that differ in volume by more than 25% (Loughry et al., 1989). Breast size is generally not related to overall milk-making capacity. Nevertheless, breasts that are significantly asymmetrical, tubular, or cone shaped may be at a higher risk for producing insufficient milk. Breast abnormalities that could be predictive of insufficient milk-making capacity include those in the hypoplastic (underdevelopment) categories described by Heimburg et al. (1996) and adapted by Huggins and coworkers (2000) into four breast types of concern (Figure 2-2):

- Type 1: round breasts, no hypoplasia in the lower medial or lateral quadrants
- Type 2: hypoplasia of the lower medial quadrant
- Type 3: hypoplasia of both the lower medial and lateral quadrants
- Type 4: severe constriction with a minimal breast base

Other aspects of concern include breasts with exceptionally large areolas relative to the size of the breast, herniation of breast tissue into the nipple/areolar complex, marked asymmetry of the breast, hypoplastic breasts that point down and sideways, and an intramammary distance of more than 1.5 inches (indicating medial breast hypoplasia). In a study of 34 women with varying types of hypoplastic breasts, most women produced less than 50% of the milk necessary for their infants during the first week postpartum. Many reported little to no growth during pregnancy, with a finding that the more severe the hypoplasia, the poorer the milk production in the first week postpartum (Huggins et al., 2000).

Figure 2-2 Breast Classifications

Source: Reprinted with permission from Walker, *Core Curriculum for Lactation Consultant Practice.* Sudbury, MA: Jones and Bartlett Publishers; 2002.

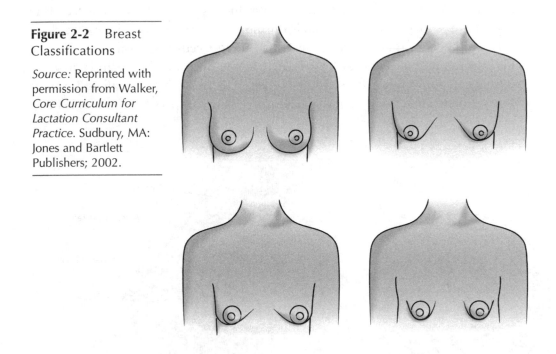

Functional Anatomy of the Breast

Breast imaging modalities have improved over recent years and are providing new insights and data on the inner workings of the mammary glands (Geddes, 2009). The breast is composed of glandular tissue, embedded in fatty tissue (the fatty patterns in the breast vary from woman to woman), and supported by fibrous connective tissue and suspensory ligaments (Cooper's ligaments) (Figure 2-3). Some mammary glandular tissue projects into the axilla (tail of Spence) and is connected to the normal duct system. Some 5–10 or so main ducts branch and extend from the nipple in a complex and intertwined pattern. Lobules extend from these ducts; they are composed of branching ductules that terminate in alveolar clusters. The alveolus, the milk-secreting unit, is lined with alveolar milk-secreting epithelial cells surrounded by supporting structures, a rich vascular supply, and myoepithelial cells. Although the size and number of alveolar units increase during pregnancy, the high circulating levels of estrogen and progesterone during pregnancy suppress most alveolar function until delivery of the placenta. Relatively large gaps exist between the milk-secreting cells during the first 4 days postpartum, enhancing the passage into milk of components such as immunoglobulins, cells such as lymphocytes and macrophages, and most drugs (Figure 2-4). After this time, the alveolar cells swell under the influence of prolactin, which closes these gaps. As a consequence, drug entry into milk may occur more readily during the early days until these gaps close.

Myoepithelial cells are smooth muscle contractile cells responsible for ejecting milk into the ductules under the influence of the hormone oxytocin (known as the milk ejection reflex or the letdown reflex). Ducts can be as small as 2 mm or less in diameter, tend to be superficial, and are easily compressed (Geddes 2007b).

Figure 2-3   Side View of Lactating Breast

- Fatty tissue
- Alveolar cluster
- Lactiferous duct
- Nipple
- Areola
- Ductule

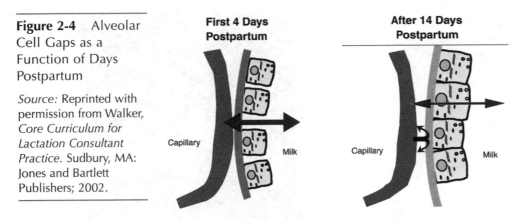

Figure 2-4   Alveolar Cell Gaps as a Function of Days Postpartum

Source: Reprinted with permission from Walker, *Core Curriculum for Lactation Consultant Practice.* Sudbury, MA: Jones and Bartlett Publishers; 2002.

Under ultrasound, an average 79% increase in duct diameter can be shown when milk ejection occurs, usually within 54 seconds after the infant goes to breast (Hartmann, 2000).

The nipple sits in the center of the areola and contains many nerve fiber endings, 5–10 main milk ducts and 10–15 other pores, smooth muscle fibers, and a rich blood supply. Most investigations have shown between 17 and 27 ducts within the nipple and five to nine orifices or actual openings at the tip (Going & Moffat, 2004; Taneri et al., 2006). Although older textbooks describe 15–25 ductal openings on the nipple, direct observation, three-dimensional modeling, ultrasound, ductography, and actual dissections of the nipple have helped clarify its internal structure (Geddes, 2007a). Five to 10 true mammary or lactiferous ducts transport milk from the lobules they drain (Going & Moffat, 2004; Love & Barsky, 2004; Ramsay et al., 2005) to the nipple tip, even though there are many more ducts within the nipple. This is in agreement with the classic work on breast anatomy conducted by Sir Ashley Cooper in 1840 (Cooper, 1840) showing 7–12 patent nipple ducts in cadaver dissections (Figure 2-5). Rusby et al. (2007) found a mean of 24 ducts within sectioned nipples with a range of 5–50 ducts. Although Ramsey et al. (2005) found approximately nine ducts in the nipple, it must be remembered that ultrasound cannot identify ducts of less than 0.5 mm.

Several ducts can arise from the same cleft in the nipple tip, accounting for the discrepancy between the number of ducts in the nipple and the number of openings that can be counted externally. The shared opening of multiple ducts on the surface of the nipple tip can be seen in Figure 2-6. There is usually a group of central orifices with peripheral ductal openings surrounding the central openings in a somewhat concentric pattern. Rusby et al. (2007) described the spatial arrangement of ducts within the nipple. Most ducts are arranged in a central bundle that narrows to a "waist" approximately 2 mm beneath the skin (Figure 2-7). This

Figure 2-5   Wax-Injected Ductal System in Cadaver Dissection

Source: Cooper AP. *Anatomy of the breast.* London: Longman, Orme, Green, Browne and Longmans,1840.

E. Ducts with common orifice

D. Narrow ducts at tip

C. Ducts arising from the areola

B. Waist

A. Duct bundle

Figure 2-6   Three dimensional reconstruction of a nipple from sectioned nipple specimens
A, B: Two sections of the nipple tip. Many small ducts in upper left quadrant of section A arise from a cleft in section B, 100 micrometers nearer the tip.
C, D: three dimensional reconstruction of a nipple tip.

Source: Rusby et al. Breast duct anatomy in the human nipple: three-dimensial patterns and clinical implications. *Breast Cancer Res Treat.* 2007;106:171–179.

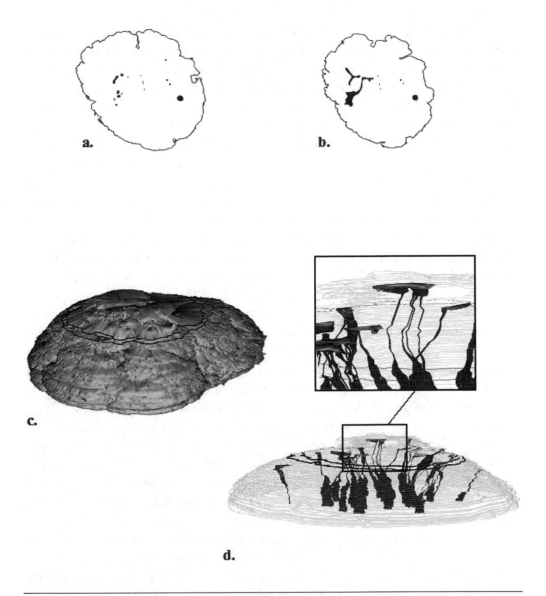

Figure 2-7   Pattern of ducts within the nipple. The ducts are arranged in a central bundle. The bundle narrows to a waist just beneath the skin. Some ducts originate on the areola or part way up the nipple. Most ducts narrow as they approach the tip of the nipple. Many of the ducts originate from a few clefts.

Source: Rusby et al. Breast duct anatomy in the human nipple: three-dimensial patterns and clinical implications. *Breast Cancer Res Treat.* 2007;106:171–179.

central bundle occupies 21–67% of the cross-sectional area of the nipple. Multiple ducts may branch and end within the nipple, whereas others end as lobular tissue or as a blind-ending sinus. Other ducts originate at the base of the nipple and on the areola and are morphologically different from the ducts within the central bundle. At 1 and 1.5 mm beneath the tip of the nipple, the average duct diameter was 0.06 mm. However, this increased more than 10-fold to 0.7 mm at a 3-mm depth. There was no relationship between the size of the duct and whether it ended within the nipple or passed deeper into the breast. The other types often disappear into a skin appendage and are most likely tubercles, tubes, sebaceous (oil-secreting) gland orifices, and sweat gland openings that lie superficial to the areola but do not communicate with the milk-secreting and transporting apparatus. Duct diameters greater than 2–3 mm are considered enlarged and may indicate ductal ectasia or mastalgia, but ductal diameters can range from 0.6 to 4.4 mm with no evidence of pathology (Ballesio et al., 2007; Peters et al., 2003; Tedeschi et al., 1963).

Under ultrasound examination Ramsey et al. (2005) was unable to visualize the commonly describe lactiferous sinus or dilated sac under the areola. Because the internal workings of the breast are dynamic, the frequently drawn "lactiferous sinus" could possibly be attributed to graphic renderings of a dilated duct immediately below the areola after a milk ejection or the convergence and branching of two ducts. Separate ductal systems of varying extent and differing lobe sizes may be present in the same breast quadrant with or without being connected. Ohtake et al. (2001) showed that different lobular systems could be connected to each other (anastomoses between ducts of different lobes) and demonstrated connections within the same lobular system. Going and Moffat (2004) described an autopsied breast through the use of 2-mm sections that showed one main collecting duct and its branches drained up to 23% of the total breast volume; the largest three systems drained 50%, and the largest six systems drained 75% of the breast. They liken the human breast to not one gland but many, with the lobes or ductal systems as separate domains. Some preliminary data indicate that hormone levels differ in different ductal systems, possibly representing diverse microenvironments among various lobes in the same breast (Elia et al., 2002). Murase et al. (2009) showed that milk synthesis differs in each mammary lobe, even within the same breast. The degree of fullness in each mammary lobe seems to play the most important role in the fat content. The protein content in the milk from each mammary lobe is also different and presumably determined by the feedback inhibitor of lactation, accumulated in the corresponding mammary lobe.

The areola is a circular pigmented area that frequently enlarges and darkens during pregnancy. There is a wide variation in the size of the nipple–areola complex among mothers. The mean diameter of the areola is 4 cm (range, 2.0–7.0 cm) (Mathes et al., 2006). Its skin does not contain fat but does contain smooth muscle and elastic tissues in radial and circular arrangements. Between 1 and 15 Montgomery's tubercles or glands become prominent during pregnancy and can secrete substances, including a small amount of milk. These glands may be functional during lactation, serving as a communication conduit with the infant through odor. Doucet et al. (2007) showed that infants behaved differently when faced with a breast covered in a plastic film versus a breast with either the nipple, areola, or whole breast revealed. When exposed to volatile compounds originating in areolar secretions or milk itself, infants demonstrated a delayed onset of crying, stimulation of eye opening, and mouthing behaviors. Infants exposed to the breast covered in a plastic film cried earlier and longer and opened their eyes less.

Increased numbers of Montgomery glands have been associated with increased infant weight gain during the first 3 days, improved latching and sucking activity, and a quicker onset of lactation in primiparous women (Schaal et al., 2005). When the nipple is stimulated, the muscular fibroelastic system in the nipple and areola contracts, decreasing the surface area of the areola and producing nipple erection. This results in the nipple becoming smaller, firmer, and more prominent. Nipples vary in size and shape, with some variations carrying the potential for a difficult latch such as those that are flat, inverted, dimpled, bulbous, bifurcated, exceptionally large, or double (Figure 2-8). In a study of 300 Japanese women (600 breasts), Sanuki and colleagues (2008) classified nipples as type I when the nipple height was greater than the diameter, type II when the nipple height was shorter than the diameter, type III when the nipple was inverted, and type IV when the nipple was of other shapes such as multiple or divided. They also subclassified types I and II according to the location of strictures (Figure 2-9). The mean diameter of the nipple was 1.3 cm (range, 0.6–2.3 cm) and the mean height of the nipple was 0.9 cm (range, 0–2.0 cm). Type II without constriction was the most common type of nipple (60.2%) followed by type II with constriction (25.3%). Inverted nipples were found in 3.5% of the breasts.

The breast is highly vascular, with 60% of the blood supply carried by the internal mammary artery and about 30% supplied by the lateral thoracic artery. During pregnancy, mammary blood flow increases to double the prepregnancy levels by 24 weeks and remains constant thereafter (Thoresen & Wesche, 1988; Vorherr, 1974). The 24-hour mammary blood flow necessary to produce 1 L of milk is about 500:1. Mammary blood flow, however, is markedly reduced in a breast that is synthesizing relatively small amounts of milk compared with one producing a normal volume. Blood flow to the breast decreases by 40–50% just before milk ejection, increasing in the next 1–2 minutes (Janbu et al., 1985). The

Figure 2-8   The Five Basic Types of Nipples

Type of Nipple	Before Stimulation	After Stimulation
The majority of mothers have what is referred to as a **common nipple**. It protrudes slightly when at rest and becomes erect and more graspable when stimulated. A baby has no trouble finding and grasping this nipple to pull in a large amount of breast tissue and stretch it to the roof of his or her mouth.		
The **flat nipple** has a very short shank that makes it less easy for the baby to find and grasp. In response to stimulation, slight movement inward or outward may be present, but not enough to aid the baby in finding and initially grasping the breast on center.		
An **inverted-appearing nipple** may appear inverted but becomes erect and easily graspable after stimulation.		
The **retracted nipple** is the most common type of inverted nipple. On stimulation it retracts, making attachment difficult.		
The truly **inverted nipple** is retracted both at rest and when stimulated. Such a nipple is very uncommon and more difficult for the baby to grasp.		

Source: Reprinted with permission from Lauwers & Shinskie, *Counseling the Nursing Mother: A Lactation Consultant's Guide, Third Edition.* Sudbury, MA: Jones and Bartlett Publishers; 2000.

Figure 2-9 Nipple Classification System by Type

Source: Sanuki et al. Morphologic study of nipple-areola complex in 600 breasts. *Aesth Plast Surg.* 2008. DOI 10.1007/s00266-008-9194-y.

diameter of nipple (d)

height of nipple (h)

diameter of areola

			600 breasts (%)
I s	d$\leq$h		39 (6.5%)
I sp	d$\leq$h constriction+		25 (4.2%)
II s	d>h		361 (60.2%)
II sp	d>h constriction+		152 (25.3%)
III	inverted nipple		21 (3.5%)
IV	unclassified		2 (0.3%)

lymphatic system of the breast is quite extensive—collecting excess fluid, bacteria, and cast-off cell parts—with the main drainage channeled to the axillary nodes. The breast is innervated mainly from branches of the fourth, fifth, and sixth intercostal nerves. The fourth intercostal nerve becomes more superficial as it approaches the areola, where it divides into five branches. The lowermost branch penetrates the areola at the 5 o'clock position on the left breast and the 7 o'clock position on the right breast. If this lowermost branch experiences trauma or is severed (during surgery), loss of sensation to the nipple and areola could result.

Clinical Implications

Lactation can be sustained within wide variations of breast size, shape, and appearance because the basic anatomical structure and physiological functioning are remarkably adept at performing under diverse conditions. A number of breast changes are commonly experienced during pregnancy, including breast enlargement, increased tenderness, darkening and/or enlargement of the areola, small amounts of colostrum leakage, increased visibility of veining on the chest, prominence of the glands of Montgomery, protrusion of the nipple, and appearance of stretch marks on the breasts. Absence of such changes may cause concern in both mothers and healthcare providers and may signal a need for closer follow-up after birth. Even so, mothers should still be encouraged to breastfeed.

Nipple Preparation

Nipple preparation techniques such as wearing breast shells or pulling on or manipulating the nipple have not been shown to improve nipple protractility and are no longer recommended (Alexander et al., 1992; MAIN Trial Collaborative Group, 1994). The nipple (including its attachment to the areola) is an elastic structure, capable of stretching two to three times its resting length (Smith et al., 1988). Infant suckling and/or mechanical pumping after birth usually cause a protrusive response in flat nipples. Accessory nipples may secrete milk, generally do not interfere with breastfeeding, and may be associated with urinary tract anomalies. Some mothers are not aware that what looks like a mole to them is actually a nipple and may be surprised if it secretes drops of milk. Because there is usually little underlying ductal or glandular tissue, these nipples tend to cease secreting milk soon after lactogenesis II. However, some mothers report continuous milk secretion from accessory nipples that are much more developed.

Hypoplastic breasts require close follow-up and monitoring of infant weight postpartum. Every effort should be made to help such breasts maximize their milk production within the early days and weeks of lactation. Insufficient glandular tissue may present as a flaccid breast with only patchy areas of glandular tissue evident upon palpation. Subsequent transillumination of the breast or ultrasound imaging may confirm the reduced amount of functional tissue (Neifert et al., 1985). Endocrine pathologies such as polycystic ovary syndrome may also contribute to insufficient mammary tissue, increasing the risk of delayed or failed lactogenesis II, reduced weight gain in infants, and the need for intense lactation support (Marasco et al., 2000).

Breast Augmentation

Surgical procedures to the breasts such as augmentation mammaplasty or reduction mammaplasty have the potential to affect lactation and milk production. Augmentation is accomplished with the insertion of saline-filled or silicone implants either under the chest muscle (submuscular) or on top of the muscle and under the glandular tissue (subglandular) (Figure 2-10). The implants may be inserted through either an axillary incision (under the arm), inframammary incision (under the breast), or periareolar incision (along the edge of the areola) (Figure 2-11). Some mothers may have silicone implants that were placed before they were withdrawn from the market in 1992. However, on November 17, 2006, the U.S. Food and Drug Administration (FDA) approved the use of silicone gel–filled implants, stating that there was no association between silicone implants and connective tissue disease. A number of complications can occur from breast augmentation and potentially impact the normal functioning of the breasts (FDA, 2000):

- Capsular contracture occurs when the scar tissue or capsule that normally forms around the implant tightens and squeezes the implant. With greater degrees of contracture, the breast may present as hard and painful and appear visibly distorted. Surgery is usually required to remedy this problem. Engorged breasts are also hard, painful, and swollen and may exacerbate the capsular contracture.

- Deflation or rupture of the implant may occur due to capsular contracture, mammography, physical manipulation, trauma, or normal aging of the implant. Affected women may notice decreased breast size, pain, tingling, swelling, numbness, burning, or changes in sensation. With silicone implants, silicone gel may migrate away from the implant, causing hard knots in the breast and lumps (granulomas) in the chest wall, armpit, arm, or abdomen. In such cases the implant needs to be surgically removed.

Figure 2-10
Location of
Breast Implants
(a) Implant *between*
breast and muscle.
(b) Implant *under*
muscle

Source: Reprinted with permission from Riordan, *Breastfeeding and Human Lactation, Third Edition*. Sudbury, MA: Jones and Bartlett Publishers; 2005.

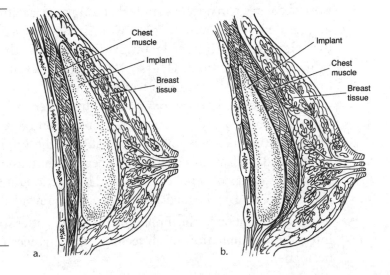

Figure 2-11 Breast Augmentation Incisions: through the armpit, under the areola, under the breast

Source: Reprinted with permission from Riordan, *Breastfeeding and Human Lactation, Third Edition.* Sudbury, MA: Jones and Bartlett Publishers; 2005.

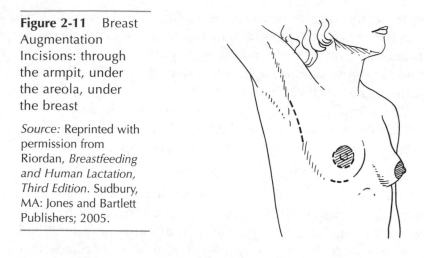

- Pain may occur at any time with implants.

- Breast infections may occur at any time and are more difficult to treat because the bacteria may not respond to common antibiotics.

- Necrosis (formation of dead tissue around the implant) may occur and require surgical correction or removal.

- Tissue atrophy occurs when pressure from the implant causes the breast tissue to thin and shrink. It has also been speculated that pressure from the implant on milk-secreting cells may diminish milk secretion (Hurst, 1996).

- The periareolar incision site is associated with the highest risk of inability to breastfeed. In a retrospective study that compared lactation outcomes between augmented and nonaugmented women, 64% of 42 augmented women experienced insufficient lactation compared with less than 7% of 42 nonaugmented women (Hurst, 1996). Strom et al. (1997) reported on breastfeeding outcomes of 28 women from a study on 292 cosmetic saline implant patients, 46 of whom had children after the procedure. Of the 28 women who breastfed, 11 reported problems and 8 reported breastfeeding problems they perceived as being related to the implants. Seven of the 8 women had implants placed through a periareolar incision. Nerves innervating the nipple and areola are best protected if resections at the base of the breast and skin incisions at the medial areolar border are avoided (Schlenz et al., 2000).

- Ranges of sensation in the nipple and breast vary after surgery from increased intensity to elimination of all feeling. Such changes can be temporary or permanent.

- Concern has been expressed over the possibility of silicone leaking into tissues and milk from ruptured silicone implants. No data exist that contraindicate breastfeeding with silicone implants, nor do mothers need to have these devices removed before lactating or have milk levels checked during lactation (FDA, 2000). When silicon was used as a proxy measure for silicone, Semple et al. (1998) found that silicon levels were significantly higher in infant formula than in either the blood or breastmilk of mothers with implants.

- Breast implants are not lifetime devices and will not last forever. Revisions are done frequently due to breast ptosis (drooping), desired size change, saline implants that deflate, to repair capsular contraction, and for scar revision. The average time from initial implant to the need for a revision is 7 years (Spear et al., 2003). If implants are removed and not replaced, the breasts may become excessively droopy and have a dimpled and/or puckered appearance. Revisions to the initial breast augmentation procedure, especially for capsular contracture, can further damage nerves and functional breast tissue, increasing the risk of insufficient milk production (Michalopoulos, 2007).

- Mothers may not be informed that their breasts could actually be hypoplastic, with only small amounts of functional tissue or that augmentation mammaplasty has the potential to reduce lactation ability.

Breast implants are regulated by the FDA as medical devices. Brown et al. (2006) accessed 339 adverse event reports on breast implants between 1968 and 2002 from the FDA database on adverse event reports of medical devices. Almost half (46%) mentioned problems with breastfeeding, such as inadequate milk supply, pain from the implant, rupture or contracture of the implant, silicone measured or seen in the mother's milk, and unspecified breastfeeding problems. Most reports also mentioned anxiety regarding the health of the infant and the safety of breastfeeding with silicone implants. Anxiety on the part of the mother regarding the integrity of the implant, whether breastfeeding will ruin the implant, and safety issues of breastfeeding with implants need to be discussed with mothers to prevent the avoidance of breastfeeding.

Breast Reduction

Indications for breast reduction surgery include musculoskeletal stress from large, heavy breasts, pain, poor body image, and restrictions on physical activities. Older surgical techniques that involved the "free nipple graft" technique or the complete removal of the nipple–areolar complex and reattachment often resulted in impaired or impossible lactation. Nipple sensation is usually greatly diminished in these women but not necessarily absent (Ahmed & Kolhe, 2000). A number of newer surgical techniques are able to preserve the attachment of the nipple–areola to underlying tissue as well as improve the vascular supply to the nipple with less disruption of sensory nerves (Gonzalez et al., 1993; Hallock, 1992; Nahabedian & Mofid, 2002). Certain types of reduction mammaplasty may result in much less of a compromise to lactation (Mottura, 2002; Ramirez, 2002), making it important to inform women before reduction surgery about the procedure's potential effect on lactation. Because of the intermixing of adipose tissue and glandular tissue, breast reduction surgery cannot be accomplished by a simple removal of "fat deposits" (Nickell & Skelton, 2005). Preserving the glandular tissue within the first 30 mm of the nipple and using a surgical technique that keeps the pedicle supporting the nipple–areolar complex as thick as possible may maximize the potential for optimal milk production (Nickell & Skelton, 2005; Ramsay et al., 2005). If a woman has only five or six main milk ducts, removal or destruction of just a few of those central ducts could permanently impair the milk production potential of that breast (Ramsay et al., 2005).

Mothers who have had reduction surgery should be encouraged to breastfeed with proper infant follow-up. The breastfeeding practices of a series of postpartum women who had undergone prior reduction mammaplasty by means of an inferior pedicle approach were reported in a retrospective study by Brzozowski et al. (2000), who also examined the factors that influenced the decision to breastfeed postoperatively. Successful breastfeeding was defined as the ability to feed for a duration equal to or greater than 2 weeks. Seventy-eight patients had children after their breast reduction surgery. Fifteen of the 78 patients (19.2%) breastfed exclusively, 8 (10.3%) breastfed with formula supplementation, 14 (17.9%) had an unsuccessful breastfeeding attempt, and 41 (52.6%) did not attempt breastfeeding. Of the 41 patients not attempting to breastfeed, 9 patients did so as a direct consequence of discouragement by a healthcare professional. Of the 78 women who had children postoperatively, a total of 27 were discouraged from breastfeeding by medical professionals, with only 8 of the 27 (29.6%) subsequently attempting to do so despite this recommendation. In comparison, 26 patients were encouraged to breastfeed; 19 (73.1%) of them did subsequently attempt breastfeeding. Postpartum breast engorgement and lactation was experienced by 31 of the 41 patients not attempting to breastfeed. Of these 31 patients, 19 believed they would have been able to breastfeed due to the extent of breast engorgement and lactation experienced. Studies examining successful lactation outcomes after breast reduction surgery show varying results, with approximately 50% reported as successfully breastfeeding depending on the type of surgery performed. The studies typically define successful breastfeeding as breastfeeding (with or without supplementation) for 2–3 weeks (Table 2-2). Mothers and infants require close follow-up in the early weeks with frequent infant weight checks.

Some mothers who have undergone surgical procedures on their breasts may complain of breast pain during lactation. This may be due to the formation of scar tissue. Clinicians will need to rule out other causes of breast pain, such as infection or improper latch. West and Hirsch (2008) noted that postsurgical mothers often experience nipple blanching or vasospasm of the nipple. Blanching may be due to a blood supply interruption or nerve trauma to the nipple–areola during the surgery, although the true cause is unknown. Mothers may find some relief from this painful condition by compressing the areola and mechanically squeezing blood back into the nipple (West & Hirsch, 2008). Clinicians can refer mothers to the additional readings and resources at the end of this chapter.

Other types of surgery, such as placement of chest drains during infancy, can also affect the development and functioning of the breasts. Skin incisions for chest drains can be misplaced, resulting in breast deformity from dermal adhesions and

TABLE 2-2 Successful Breastfeeding After Breast Reduction Mammaplasty

Study	Comments
Hefter et al. (2003)	Showed a 54% rate of successful breastfeeding (without supplementation)
Cruz-Korchin & Korchin (2004)	Reported a 60% successful breastfeeding rate where a medial pedicle reduction was performed
Cherchel et al. (2007)	Found a 44% successful breastfeeding rate (2 weeks with or without supplementation) with a superior pedicle reduction mammaplasty
Chiummariello et al. (2008)	Examined multiple techniques finding successful lactation rates of 60% after superior pedicle, 55.1% after lateral pedicle, 48% after medial pedicle, and 43.5% after inferior pedicle as defined by breastfeeding for 3 weeks without supplementation
Cruz & Korchin (2007)	Compared successful lactation outcomes of superior, inferior, and medial pedicle reduction with each other and with matched control subjects. A 60% success rate was found in each group, which was defined as breastfeeding for 2 weeks with or without supplementation

underdevelopment of the breast. This situation should be corrected when breast development begins at adolescence to allow unrestricted growth of the entire breast. Severe, uncorrected cases may result in the inability to breastfeed (Rainer et al., 2003). A number of aspects of the breast and nipple anatomy of lactating mothers may need closer observation and follow-up when present or absent.

Breast Anomalies

Visually assess the conformation of both breasts, checking for size, symmetry, distortions, scars, accessory breast tissue in the axilla, edema, and erythema (redness). Ask whether the breasts underwent changes during pregnancy. Check the origin of all scars.

- Mothers with breasts that are significantly hypoplastic, that have a wide intramammary space, or that have been augmented or reduced need intense lactation support. Infants should be breastfed 8–12 times each 24 hours, or pumping should be commenced in the absence of a vigorously suckling infant. Infant weights should be closely monitored (as frequently as every 2–3 days in the beginning) to ensure adequate intake. Mothers who have undergone a significant breast reduction may need to be advised that supplementation could be necessary if the breasts are unable to increase their production to meet the growing needs of the infant. Some mothers produce adequate amounts of colostrum in the hospital and early days but do not report lactogenesis II. Skin incisions on the medial borders of the areola or under the breast may result in diminished sensation to the nipple–areolar complex, with mothers being unable to feel whether the infant is latched correctly. This factor increases the risk for not only insufficient milk production but also nipple and areolar damage.

- Mothers who have had breast augmentation should be asked whether the intent was to cosmetically enhance the breasts or to compensate for a lack of development of normal breast tissues during adolescence. Augmentation will obviously not improve milk production if insufficient glandular tissue was present initially. Breast augmentation, as well as the underlying reason for the procedure, has the potential to alter breastfeeding outcomes through a number of factors: use of a periareolar incision, severing of milk ducts, altered nipple sensation, lack of functional breast tissue, little or no breast changes during pregnancy, and minimal postpartum engorgement (Hill et al., 2004). Mothers should be asked whether they experienced any previous hormonal aberrations that would have affected normal breast development.

- Medications to enhance milk production are usually ineffective if breast tissue is absent or significantly underdeveloped.

- Some mothers may not self-report augmentation or reduction mammaplasty. This information should be ascertained during telephone contacts if mothers call for help with insufficient milk or slow infant weight gain or weight loss.

- Mothers with anatomical breast problems can be offered the option of using a tube-feeding device at the breast to optimize breastmilk production, deliver a supplement if necessary, and enjoy the close contact and pleasure of feeding at the breast.

- Breasts that are edematous may be engorged—a normal event, but one that is managed by frequent breastfeeding (or pumping/hand expression if necessary) to prevent overfullness, reduced milk production, nipple trauma, and insufficient milk later on. Accessory breast tissue in the tail of Spence can swell and become engorged during lactogenesis II. Cold compresses may help reduce the edema. Care should be taken that a tight brassiere or underwires do not curtail drainage from this area.

- Red patches on the breast usually indicate areas of inflammation where milk is not draining adequately. Proper positioning, latch, suck, and swallow need to be ensured, with alternate massage being added to help the affected areas drain more efficiently. Alternate massage involves massaging and compressing the breast during the pause between the infant's sucking bursts to encourage the infant to sustain sucking and manually increase the internal pressure in the breast to improve milk transfer (Bowles et al., 1987; Stutte et al., 1988). Some mothers also benefit from taking anti-inflammatory medication.

Nipple Anomalies

Accessory breast tissue or extra nipples may look like moles or may be more developed with the appearance of small nipples and/or areolae. Occasionally, a mother may have an ectopic duct that drains milk to the skin surface but is located on the areola or even farther back on the breast tissue. Some nipples are not symmetrical and may have the appearance of a raspberry or even look like two nipples are present on the areola. Extra nipples and ectopic ducts may leak milk upon letdown but usually cause no problems during breastfeeding.

Flat, retracted, or "inverted" nipples are not unusual. A true inverted nipple—that is, one that fails to elevate from the mammary pit—may be visibly assessed. In contrast, flat or retracted nipples are typically discovered either when the infant has difficulty latching on or prenatally if the mother or healthcare provider compresses the tissue behind the nipple to see whether it protrudes (somewhat comparable with the infant latching on). The nipple should protrude, not retract, when this manipulation is performed. In older texts this is referred to as the "pinch test." To successfully transfer milk, the infant must be able to grasp the nipple and one-half inch or so of the areola and pull it back almost to the junction of the hard and soft palates. The nipple–areola complex stretches to two or three times its resting length during this maneuver. A nipple that pulls back from the infant when he or she grasps the breast may make latch-on more difficult for some infants and damage the nipple. Engorgement may cause the areola and nipple to flatten out and lose their elasticity. If the infant cannot latch in this situation, a mother can apply a cold compress and hand express or pump some milk to soften the areola.

Some mothers given large amounts of intravenous fluids during labor and/or whose labors have been induced or augmented with Pitocin have been anecdotally reported to experience edematous areolae that envelop the nipple, causing latch problems and pain. These nipples are not flat, just difficult to access. Cold compresses, cabbage leaves, and foods with a diuretic effect (watermelon) have all been anecdotally recommended to help decrease the swelling. Placing a breast pump and applying vacuum to an edematous areola may exacerbate the problem because nipples typically swell after pumping (Wilson-Clay & Hoover, 2005). Areolar compression that shifts excess fluid away from the areola should be considered before placing a pump on an areola already distended with fluid (Miller & Riordan, 2004). A technique called "reverse pressure softening" mechanically displaces areolar interstitial fluid inward, temporarily increasing elasticity and permitting an easier latch (Cotterman, 2004).

Hormones of Lactation

A remarkable procession of hormones, summarized in Table 2-3, is involved in facilitating the process of lactation.

TABLE 2-3 Hormonal Regulation of Breast Development and Function

Phase/Stage	Hormones	Function	Local Control
Pregnancy	Progesterone	Lobular formation	
	Prolactin	Completes lobular/alveolar development; stimulates glandular production of colostrum	
	Placental lactogen	Increases prolactin	
	Estrogen	Ductular sprouting	
Birth	Removal of progesterone	Allows prolactin to exert its effect	
Lactogenesis II	Prolactin	Lactogenic trigger	
	Removal of progesterone	Supportive and/or permissive	
	Glucocorticoids	Assists in milk production	
	Insulin	Supports milk production	
	Cortisol		
Maintenance of lactation (lactogenesis III)	Prolactin	Along with cortisol and insulin, acts to stimulate transcription of genes that encode milk proteins	Feedback inhibitor of lactation ([FIL] a whey protein) Stretch Back pressure Degree of drainage Frequency of feeds Infant appetite Milk storage capacity of breasts
	Oxytocin	Facilitates milk transfer	
	Thyroid hormone	↑ responsiveness of mammary cells to prolactin	
	Parathyroid hormone		
	Growth hormone		
Suckling	Prolactin	Stimulates milk synthesis	
	Oxytocin	Responsible for milk ejection and mothering behavior	
	Prolactin-inhibiting factor	Depressed by suckling; controls release of prolactin from the hypothalamus	

Prolactin

Prolactin is a single-chain protein hormone secreted in the anterior pituitary and several other sites. This multifunctional hormone has more than 300 separate biological activities. Its receptors are found not just in the breast but also at many other sites throughout the body, including the ovaries, central nervous system, immune system, and a wide range of peripheral organs. Prolactin's effects have been linked to maternal behavior (Grattan et al., 2001), and the hormone even plays a role in the immune response. Most notable is the role that prolactin plays in the regulation of the humoral and cellular immune responses in normal physiological states as well as pathological conditions such as autoimmune diseases (Neidhart, 1998). Prolactin facilitates lobuloalveolar growth during pregnancy and promotes lactogenesis by acting together with cortisol and insulin to stimulate the transcription of the genes that encode for milk proteins.

The hypothalamus is the regulator of prolactin secretion, acting as a limiting agent on its expression until the restraint is removed. Dopamine is a major prolactin-inhibiting factor (i.e., brake on prolactin secretion). Agents, stimuli, or drugs that interfere with dopamine secretion or receptor binding lead to enhanced secretion of prolactin. Drugs can also inhibit release of prolactin from the pituitary, such as ergot alkaloids. Prolactin is positively regulated by a number of other hormones, including thyroid-releasing hormone, gonadotropin-releasing hormone, and vasoactive intestinal polypeptide. Prolactin is released when the nipple is stimulated during nursing due to a spinal reflex arc that causes release of prolactin-stimulating hormones from the hypothalamus (Figure 2-12).

Prolactin levels rise during pregnancy from about 10 ng/mL in the nonpregnant state to approximately 200 ng/mL at term. Baseline levels do not drop back to normal in a lactating woman but average about 100 ng/mL at 3 months and 50 ng/mL at 6 months. Prolactin levels can double with the stimulus of suckling. After about 6 months of breastfeeding, the prolactin rise with suckling amounts to only 5–10 ng/mL. This diminished level reflects the increased prolactin-binding capacity or sensitivity of the mammary tissue, which allows full lactation in the face of falling prolactin levels over time. The high levels of prolactin seen during pregnancy and early lactation may also serve to increase the number of prolactin receptors and depends on tactile input for stimulation and release. Despite its importance to lactation itself, prolactin does not directly regulate the short-term or long-term rate of milk synthesis (Cox et al., 1996). Once lactation is well established, prolactin is still required for milk synthesis to occur, but its role is permissive rather than regulatory (Cregan et al., 2000).

Figure 2-12
Hormone Pathways
During Suckling

Source: Reprinted with
permission from
Lauwers and Shinskie,
*Counseling the Nursing
Mother: A Lactation
Consultant's Guide,
Third Edition.* Sudbury,
MA: Jones and Bartlett
Publishers; 2000.

Prolactin concentration in the plasma is highest during sleep and lowest during the waking hours; it operates as a true circadian rhythm (Stern & Reichlin, 1990). The prolactin response is superimposed on the circadian rhythm of prolactin secretion, meaning that the same intensity of suckling stimulus can elevate prolactin levels more effectively at certain times of the day when the circadian input enhances the effect of the suckling stimulus (Freeman et al., 2000).

Prolactin is seen in the maternal cerebrospinal fluid from which it diffuses into various regions of the brain, with the hypothalamus itself showing increases in prolactin receptors. Prolactin influences numerous brain functions, including maternal behavior, feeding and appetite, and oxytocin secretion. Given the high circulating levels of prolactin during pregnancy and lactation and the increased expression of prolactin receptors in the hypothalamus, prolactin stands as a key player in the coordination of neuroendocrine and behavioral adaptations in the maternal brain (Grattan, 2001).

Prolactin secretion is affected by stress as well as a number of hormones, including oxytocin and vasopressin (the antidiuretic hormone). The most common disease related to vasopressin is diabetes insipidus, a condition that results from a deficiency in secretion of vasopressin from the posterior pituitary or the inability of the kidney to respond to the hormone. Although the major sign of diabetes insipidus is excessive urine output, this magnitude of disturbance in water and electrolyte regulation can impede suckling-induced prolactin release.

Oxytocin

Oxytocin is a nine-amino-acid peptide that is synthesized in the hypothalamus and then transported to the posterior pituitary, from which it is released into the blood. It is simultaneously released through a closed system into the brain. Oxytocin differs from vasopressin by just two of the nine amino acids from which it is composed. Actions of oxytocin cause contraction of the smooth muscle myoepithelial cells surrounding the mammary alveoli, moving milk into the collecting ducts, which dilates these ducts and propels milk toward the nipple. The resulting increase in intraductal pressure and duct dilatation increases the milk flow rate. Multiple milk ejections typically occur during both breastfeeding and milk expression (Mitoulas et al., 2002), with many mothers able to feel the first milk ejection but not subsequent ones. The amount of milk ingested by the infant is related to the number of milk ejections per feeding and is independent of the amount of time spent at the breast (Ramsay et al., 2004). Successful lactation depends on the milk ejection reflex as only small volumes of milk (1–10 mL) can be either expressed (Kent et al., 2003) or removed by the breastfeeding infant (Ramsay et al., 2004) before milk ejection.

Oxytocin also exerts effects on neuroendocrine reflexes, produces analgesic effects, reduces the stress and anxiety response, causes contractions of the uterus, and contributes to the establishment of social and bonding behaviors related to caring for offspring (Gimpl & Fahrenholz, 2001). Breastfeeding within an hour of birth, when oxytocin levels are very high, supports a close maternal–infant bond. Upon nipple stimulation, oxytocin is released in a pulsatile nature consisting of brief 3- to 4-second bursts of oxytocin into the bloodstream every 5–15 minutes. Oxytocin cells fire in bursts so that oxytocin is secreted in pulses. The breast responds to oxytocin only at relatively high concentrations, and it rapidly desensitizes in response to continued exposure, so pulsatile delivery of oxytocin is essential for efficient milk ejection. This pulse shortens and widens the lactiferous ducts, increasing the pressure inside the breast, and is essential for maximum removal of milk from the breast (Neville, 2001). Mothers who deliver by cesarean section may lack a significant rise in prolactin levels 20–30 minutes after the onset of breastfeeding and experience fewer oxytocin pulses than mothers who have a vaginal delivery.

Administration of oxytocin to women who labor with epidural analgesia may interfere with the release of endogenous oxytocin (Wiklund et al., 2009). Plasma levels of oxytocin are reduced in mothers who receive epidural analgesia (Rahm et al., 2002) and may play a role in the delayed onset of breastfeeding in the post-partum period. Correlations between oxytocin pulsatility on day 2 and the duration of exclusive breastfeeding suggest that the development of an early pulsatile oxytocin pattern is of importance for sustained exclusive breastfeeding (Nissen et al., 1996). Oxytocin can also be released before the infant is placed at breast and is not solely dependent on tactile stimulation for release.

Both drugs and a mother's emotional state can affect oxytocin secretion. Morphine administration to breastfeeding women can lower the oxytocin response to sucking (Lindow et al., 1999). Wright (1985) showed experimentally that the administration of morphine into the lumbar subarachnoid space inhibited the milk ejection reflex. In addition, ethyl alcohol is an inhibitor of oxytocin release that can act in a dose-dependent manner (Cobo, 1973). Pain and psychological stress can inhibit the milk ejection reflex by reducing the number of oxytocin pulses during suckling episodes (Ueda et al., 1994). Opiate and beta-endorphin release during stress can block stimulus-related oxytocin secretion (Lawrence & Lawrence, 2005).

Significant elevations of oxytocin occur 15, 30, and 45 minutes after delivery and are thought to enhance mother and child interactions by shaping maternal behavior (Nissen et al., 1995). Not only does a systemic release of oxytocin into the bloodstream occur with infant suckling, but a closed system exists within the brain whereby oxytocin is also secreted into areas of the brain responsible for affiliative behavior. This secretion may be functionally related to the initiation of maternal behavior after birth (Nelson & Panksepp, 1998). Lactation, through its oxytocin mediation within the maternal brain, reduces responses to stressful situations, may protect some women from mental disorders (Cowley & Roy-Byrne, 1989; Klein et al., 1995), and aids in the mother's ability to deal with the demands of child rearing. The effects of oxytocin and vasopressin indicate that lactation is associated with a reduction in anxiety, obsessiveness, and stress reactivity that may create an adaptive state that favors the interests of the infant over those of the mother (Carter et al., 2001). Bottle-feeding mothers experience a greater cardiovascular response to psychological stressors, have higher incidences of psychiatric and cardiovascular disorders (Mezzacappa et al., 1999), and have higher blood pressure (Light et al., 2000) than do breastfeeding mothers. Oxytocin release during stress is higher in lactating mothers, leading to suppressed stress responsivity in these women (Uvnas-Moberg & Eriksson, 1996). Research suggests that the hormonal milieu of lactation may diminish the physiological stress response as well as the psychological perceptions of stress (Groer & Davis, 2002). Some data suggest reason for concern regarding the effects of epidural analgesia on the blocking of oxytocin release at delivery (Goodfellow et al., 1983).

The hormonal environment of lactation can be disrupted by the ingestion of alcohol. Some mothers are still advised by their healthcare providers or cultural surroundings that alcohol will serve as a lactation aid or help calm a fussy baby. Consuming alcohol at a level of 0.4 g/kg resulted in a rise in prolactin and a depressed oxytocin release such that there was a delay in milk ejection and lower milk yields when pumping (Mennella et al., 2005). Prolactin and oxytocin normally behave in tandem, but consumption of alcoholic beverages disrupts this synchrony. Prolactin levels have been shown to increase when pumping immediately after alcohol consumption but decrease as blood alcohol levels fall over time. If women pumped within the hour of consuming alcohol, the prolactin response during the next pumping session, 1.5 hours later, was delayed by several minutes and milk yield was significantly lower (Mennella & Pepino, 2008). Infants have been shown to consume 20% less milk after their mothers' consumption of alcohol (Mennella & Beauchamp, 1991). Chien et al. (2008) studied Chinese lactating mothers who were given a traditional soup that contained rice wine. Milk ejection was delayed in these mothers, milk composition was altered, prolactin levels were raised, and milk yields were reduced. Although an occasional alcoholic beverage may have little effect on the overall lactation process, regular alcohol consumption may be problematic in terms of milk composition and infant weight gain.

Effects of Other Hormones Influenced by Suckling

Not only are prolactin and oxytocin released during infant suckling, but a simultaneous activation of 19 different maternal and infant gastrointestinal hormones also enhances the mother's and baby's digestive capacity as a mechanism against energy loss and as a way to ensure adequate energy supply for milk production and infant growth (Uvnas-Moberg et al., 1987) (Table 2-4). Bone mineral density is enhanced after weaning in lactating women (Polatti et al., 1999).

Clinical Implications
Alterations in prolactin secretion can affect lactogenesis II and III.

- Retained placental fragments can inhibit the withdrawal of progesterone and the subsequent prolactin release (Neifert et al., 1981). Other more uncommon conditions of the placenta that prolong the elevation of

TABLE 2-4 Selected GI Hormones Associated With Suckling

Hormone	Action	Effect From Suckling
Gastrin: released in response to protein intake	Stimulates acid secretion in the stomach and growth of gastric mucosa; trophic; promotes glucose-induced insulin release	Rise in maternal levels within 30 seconds of onset of breastfeeding
Cholecystokinin: released in response to fat intake	Stimulates contraction and growth of the gall bladder; promotes glucose-induced insulin release; induces satiety and postprandial sedation and sleep	Released in response to suckling in both mother and baby
Somatostatin: 90% released from stomach	Inhibits GI secretions, motility, blood flow, most GI hormones; released during stress; higher in sick infants	Decreases 1 hour after the onset of breastfeeding
Insulin	Metabolic regulator	Rises in response to suckling in both mother and baby; stabilizes blood sugar levels; promotes storage of ingested nutrients in infants

GI, gastrointestinal.

pregnancy hormones, such as placenta increta (invasion of the myometrium by the chorionic villi), may also interfere with lactogenesis II (Anderson, 2001).

- Sheehan syndrome is caused by such a severe postpartum hemorrhage that it leads to pituitary infarction, hypoperfusion, or other vascular injury to the pituitary. The pituitary gland is very vascular and becomes more sensitive to a decreased blood flow at the end of a pregnancy.

- Other conditions that affect prolactin secretion, such as hypothyroidism, diabetes insipidus, and polycystic ovary syndrome, may become evident during early lactation.

- Surgical interruption of sensory nerves to the nipple–areola may remove the tactile stimulation, leading to altered prolactin secretion.

- Pituitary surgery has the potential for diminishing total prolactin secretion as well as the normal prolactin surge during suckling. However, evidence has also shown that with early frequent suckling, adequate breast drainage, and close follow-up, lactation can successfully take place (DeCoopman, 1993).

- Certain medications may suppress prolactin secretion, usually dopamine agonists such as ergot alkaloids (cabergoline, ergotamine) and early use of oral contraceptives containing estrogens (Hale & Ilett, 2002).

Because prolactin concentrations are highest during sleep, recommendations to breastfeed at night become important in the early days and weeks when lactation is becoming established. Separating mother and baby in the hospital should be avoided, as should recommendations to stretch out feedings at night or have the father give a bottle at night so the mother can sleep.

Oxytocin is important to both mothering behavior and the delivery of milk to the infant. It also functions to contract the uterus so as to minimize bleeding from the placental attachment site. Mothers, especially multiparous mothers, feel this as uterine cramping (afterpains) during the milk ejection reflex. Oxytocin has a calming effect, lowers maternal blood pressure, and decreases anxiety. Women receiving magnesium sulfate and/or who are placed on seizure precautions due to pregnancy-induced hypertension may find that breastfeeding is therapeutic. Some mothers also report feeling a tingling or heavy sensation in the breasts upon letdown (albeit infrequently in the early days after birth), feeling thirsty, experiencing a warm or flushed feeling, sensing increased heat from the breasts, feeling sleepy (Mulford, 1990), or encountering headaches or nausea when the milk lets down. Many of these seemingly random feelings are generated in response to the complex interplay of oxytocin and a variety of metabolic hormones that are simultaneously released each time the infant goes to the breast. Mothers who experience nausea when breastfeeding often find that eating a cracker before nursing lessens this problem. Other mothers have found relief by wearing "sea bands," cuffs worn around the wrists that either place pressure on the nausea acupressure points or deliver small electrical charges to these areas.

Synthetic oxytocin has historically been recommended for mothers who experience difficulty with their letdown reflex. Use of oxytocin nasal spray to enhance letdown has been reported (Newton & Egli, 1958), as well as easier establishment of breastfeeding and improved milk output in puerperal women (Huntingford, 1961). When oxytocin nasal spray was used by a group of infrequently pumping preterm mothers, a 3.5 times increase in volume of milk pumped by those using oxytocin nasal spray before each pumping session was observed (Ruis et al.,

1981). A review in the Cochrane Database (Renfrew et al., 2000) reported that sublingual or buccal preparations of oxytocin were also associated with increased milk production, although most of these early studies suffer from methodology problems and samples of mothers with very restricted breastfeeding "schedules." Fewtrell et al. (2006) did not find significant differences in milk output of preterm pumping mothers when using oxytocin nasal spray. Because oxytocin nasal spray is not generally used to increase milk production but to aid in the milk ejection, this is not surprising. However, it was noted that many mothers in this study complained that their milk production decreased after they ceased using the spray. Using the spray may be beneficial in helping mothers through the early difficult days of breastfeeding or pumping milk for a preterm infant because milk output was increased during the first couple of days in the group using the spray. This may be enough of an encouraging sign for some mothers to continue pumping. Use of oxytocin nasal spray may give mothers a boost of confidence as they see milk issuing from their breasts. Since the commercial preparation of intranasal oxytocin was removed from the market, its use has diminished. However, the preparation can be created by a compounding pharmacy, and some mothers may benefit from its judicious use.

The hormonal milieu of lactation is usually taken for granted until a problem arises. In general, breastfeeding management guidelines should reflect the nature of and work with the process of lactation. The optimal functioning of the hormones involved in lactation starts with the earliest contact between mother and infant after birth.

- Newborn infants placed in uninterrupted skin-to-skin contact on their mother's chest immediately after birth engage in a prefeeding sequence of behaviors designed to locate and latch to the nipple. This process takes about an hour in infants from unmedicated labors (Widstrom et al., 1987). One behavior demonstrated by newborns is the stimulation and massage of the mother's breast before latch on. Oxytocin levels rise in response to this massage, causing nipple erection and stimulating the milk ejection reflex before it has become conditioned to the sucking stimulus (Matthiesen et al., 2001). These high levels of oxytocin persist when the infant suckles and flood the mothering center in the maternal brain, thereby enhancing maternal behavior (Widstrom et al., 1990). Early and extended contact has long been known to result in prolonged breastfeeding (Salariya et al., 1978). Newborns should be placed and left on the mother's chest to engage in this behavior immediately after birth.

- Mothers should be encouraged to breastfeed frequently according to infant behavioral feeding cues, helping to increase the number and sensitivity of prolactin receptors.

- Mothers should be encouraged to breastfeed at night when prolactin levels are highest and when suckling enhances prolactin's effects.

- Any medical history or observation of elements known to affect lactation should be charted and the mother encouraged to breastfeed. Close follow-up is needed in special situations.

Lactogenesis II

Lactogenesis II is described as the onset of copious milk production occurring between 32 and 96 hours postpartum. The timing of this event varies among mothers. Some women experience delayed lactogenesis II. Delayed lactogenesis II has been defined as milk transfer less than 9.2 g per feeding at 60 hours after birth and maternal perception of the lack of breast fullness, edema, and leaking at 72 or more hours postpartum (Chapman & Perez-Escamilla, 2000a). The rapid drop in maternal progesterone levels after expulsion of the placenta, in combination with the secretion of prolactin and other permissive hormones such as cortisol and insulin, triggers lactogenesis II. Milk synthesis occurs during the first 3 days postpartum even in the absence of infant suckling or milk expression. The composition of colostrum has been shown to be similar between breastfeeding and nonbreastfeeding women during the first 3 days after birth. Beginning on day 4, however, nonbreastfeeding women's milk reverts to the composition of colostrum, whereas the chemical composition of breastfeeding women's milk changes to that of more mature milk. This change illustrates that efficient milk removal is essential for continued lactation (Kulski & Hartmann, 1981).

Biochemical markers that are associated with lactogenesis II include an increase in concentration of breastmilk lactose, glucose, and citrate, with parallel decreases occurring in levels of protein, nitrogen, sodium, chloride, and magnesium that are mostly complete by 72 hours postpartum (Neville et al., 1991). These changes result from the closure of the gaps between the milk-secreting cells and generally precede the onset of the large increase in milk volume by about 24 hours (Neville et al., 2001).

Maternal perception of lactogenesis II follows the biochemical changes and varies widely, with mothers reporting breast fullness, heaviness, hardness, swelling, and leaking from 1 to 148 hours after birth (Chapman & Perez-Escamilla, 1999). No single indicator for lactogenesis II exists. Misunderstanding of this process can lead mothers and healthcare providers to unnecessarily use supplements and further compromise the process (Chapman & Perez-Escamilla, 2000b).

Within the first 24 hours after birth, 100 mL or less of colostrum is available to the infant. This amount increases approximately 36 hours after birth and reaches an average of 500 mL at 4 days (Neville et al., 1991). The large increase in volume between 36 and 96 hours postpartum is usually perceived by the mother as the milk coming in and is a reliable indicator for this event (Perez-Escamilla & Chapman, 2001). Women with delayed onset of lactogenesis II tend toward a lower level of milk output and their infants lose more weight during the early postpartum period. Edema further increases the feeling of fullness and swelling.

Factors Related to Delayed Lactogenesis II

Whereas delayed lactogenesis II refers to a longer than usual time to the onset of copious milk production, failed lactogenesis II describes either a primary inability to produce adequate milk volumes or secondary conditions that impede full milk production (Hurst, 2007). A variety of factors has been identified that can affect or delay lactogenesis II (Neville & Morton, 2001):

- Preglandular: hormonal causes such as
  - Retained placenta, that is, the failure of progesterone withdrawal or reduced prolactin release or other placental abnormalities such as placenta increta (Anderson, 2001; Betzold et al., 2004; Neifert et al., 1981)
  - Gestational ovarian theca lutein cysts that elevate testosterone levels, thereby suppressing milk production (Hoover et al., 2002)
- Glandular (Neifert et al., 1985): surgical procedures, insufficient mammary tissue
- Postglandular: ineffective or infrequent milk removal, cesarean delivery, primiparity (Scott et al., 2007), peripartum complications, and formula supplementation (Sievers et al., 2003)

Other factors that can influence lactogenesis II include preterm delivery, insulin-dependent diabetes mellitus (IDDM), obesity, and stress. Not all mechanisms involved are well understood. The breast is unique in that it is probably the only organ in the body that does not have a specific diagnostic test to measure its adequacy (Hartmann & Cregan, 2001). Because there is no test to determine whether or not the breast will lactate adequately, the clinician must use indirect or secondary measures to determine lactation sufficiency (Hurst, 2007).

Prematurity

Lactogenesis II and subsequent milk volumes can be compromised in mothers delivering prematurely (Cregan & Hartmann, 1999) for any number of reasons, including delayed initiation of pumping (Hopkinson et al., 1988) and ineffectiveness of pumps in removing milk (Hartmann et al., 2000). Chemical markers of lactogenesis II in milk samples of preterm mothers show delayed changes in concentrations relative to milk samples of full-term mothers, resulting in lower milk production (Cregan et al., 2000). Preterm mothers with chemical markers outside the range of markers observed in full-term mothers produced significantly lower amounts of milk than did preterm mothers with markers within the range for full-term women. Some speculation has been put forward that antenatal corticosteroid therapy given in high-risk pregnancies could unintentionally stimulate the breast, causing lactogenesis II to occur before delivery (Hartmann & Cregan, 2001). Henderson et al. (2008) showed that delivery at gestational ages less than 28 weeks caused a significant delay in the onset of lactogenesis II. The volume of milk was even more suppressed when antenatal corticosteroids were administered between 28 and 34 weeks of gestation and delivery occurred 3–9 days later. Mothers of premature infants who pumped less than six times a day also experienced a delay in lactogenesis II.

Insulin-Dependent Diabetes Mellitus

Lactogenesis II can be delayed in both mothers with IDDM and mothers with gestational diabetes. When milk levels of lactose and citrate were used as markers of lactogenesis II, Arthur and coworkers (1989) found a 15- to 28-hour delay in mothers with IDDM as well as a decrease in milk volume in the first 3 days postpartum. When the milk markers of lactose and total nitrogen were used, a delay of approximately 24 hours was confirmed (Neubauer et al., 1993). During the first postpartum week, serum prolactin levels were lower in mothers with IDDM and were related to elevated serum glucose concentrations (Ostrom & Ferris, 1993). Mothers with poor glycemic control should be encouraged to breastfeed very frequently during the early days of lactation. The breast contains insulin-sensitive tissue and requires insulin to initiate milk production. This delay in lactogenesis II may illustrate how the mother's body competes with the breasts for the available insulin. Less-optimal breastfeeding management may also contribute to the physiological delay in lactogenesis II in diabetic women. Mothers with IDDM have been observed to start breastfeeding an average of 24 hours later than non-diabetic women (Ferris et al., 1988). An increased number of breastfeeding episodes within the first 12 hours postpartum have been shown to be critical in stimulating lactogenesis II in mothers with IDDM (Ferris et al., 1993).

Obesity

Overweight (body mass index [BMI] of 26–29 kg/m^2) and obesity (BMI greater than 29 kg/m^2) have been shown to be risk factors for both delayed onset of lactation and shorter duration of breastfeeding. Mothers with a heavy or obese build have been identified as experiencing delayed onset of lactogenesis and demonstrating reduced milk transfer at 60 hours postpartum (Chapman & Perez-Escamilla, 1999, 2000b). Women who are overweight or obese are also less likely to be breastfeeding at hospital discharge (Hilson et al., 1997). Mothers with delayed lactogenesis (72 hours or later postpartum) were significantly more likely to have a higher prepregnant BMI than those mothers with earlier onset of lactogenesis II (Hilson, 2000; Rasmussen et al., 2001). Obese mothers demonstrate a lower prolactin response to suckling, especially during the early days of lactation when this response is more important than in later lactation (Rasmussen & Kjolhede, 2004).

A relationship between postpartum BMI and duration of breastfeeding has been established as well. When comparing BMI and breastfeeding duration, an inverse relationship is seen whereby breastfeeding duration decreases as BMI increases (Donath & Amir, 2000). In this dose-response pattern, overweight women have an increased risk of unsuccessful initiation and continuation of breastfeeding compared with normal weight mothers. Obese mothers have a further elevated risk. Rutishauser and Carlin (1992) reported that 18% of women with a BMI between 26 and 30 discontinued breastfeeding between 14 and 60 days postpartum, whereas 37% of women with a BMI greater than 30 ceased breastfeeding during this period. Forty-one percent of the failure in breastfeeding initiation in this study population was attributable to prepregnant overweight and obesity.

Data from a study involving 151 women showed that a 1-unit (1 kg/m^2) increase in prepregnant BMI was associated with a 0.5-hour delay in lactogenesis II (Hilson et al., 2004). The clinical implications of this calculation become apparent when comparing the difference in the onset of lactation between a mother with a BMI of 40 kg/m^2 and a mother with a BMI of 20 kg/m^2. A 10-hour delay in lactogenesis II for an obese mother can contribute to supplementation of the infant because the concerned mother becomes anxious about the delayed milk arrival (Hilson et al., 2004). Dewey et al. (2003) found that women with a BMI greater than 27 kg/m² were 2.5 times more likely to experience a delayed onset of lactation and their infants were 3 times more likely to demonstrate suboptimal breastfeeding on day 7. With as many as 34% of white American women being overweight (National Center for Health Statistics, 1997) and given the increasing obesity trend among young women in general (Flegel et al., 2002), higher BMIs may present continuing and increasing challenges to both the initiation and the duration of breastfeeding in this population.

A number of other mitigating factors might further contribute to the adverse breastfeeding outcomes seen in overweight and obese mothers:

- Obese women have a higher risk of cesarean delivery and of bearing a large infant:
    - This may result in a delay of the infant going to breast as well as discomfort or illness in the mother.
    - The infant may suffer birth trauma and/or unstable blood glucose values, resulting in formula supplementation and possible delay in early and frequent suckling.
- Gestational diabetes mellitus is more prevalent in obese women than in overweight women and may delay lactogenesis II.
- Mechanical difficulties may exist in positioning and latching an infant onto a large breast.
- Maternal obesity may be associated with metabolic or steroidal hormonal alterations that affect the breasts' ability to initiate and produce sufficient quantities of milk or particular nutrients. Rasmussen and Kjolhede (2004) demonstrated that obese women had a lower prolactin response to suckling. A blunted prolactin response to suckling in the early days when lactation is becoming established may not only delay lactogenesis II but may also establish low levels of milk production, leading to early supplementation and premature weaning.

Stress

A relationship between stress experienced during labor and delivery and delayed lactogenesis II has been observed in mothers experiencing long stage II durations and urgent cesarean sections. Chen et al. (1998) demonstrated that a number of markers of maternal and fetal distress during labor and delivery were associated with delayed breast fullness, smaller milk volume on day 5, and/or delayed casein appearance. Chapman and Perez-Escamilla (1999) reported that, among other risk factors, unscheduled cesarean section and prolonged stage II of labor were associated with delayed onset of breast fullness (more than 72 hours postpartum). Dewey et al. (2002) described delayed lactogenesis II as being more common if there was a long duration of labor (more than 14 hours), the mother had an urgent cesarean section, and the infant had a low sucking score on day 3. All these conditions are strongly related to the amount of stress experienced by both the mother and the infant during labor and delivery, can have a marked impact on lactogenesis II, and may be partially predictive of the magnitude of infant weight loss by day 3.

Complex interrelationships exist among the various factors that may affect lactogenesis, making it difficult to separate the effects of stress from those of other variables. When lactogenesis II is impaired, leading to delayed onset of milk production, insufficient milk volume, and/or infant weight loss, this problem can also be due to the combined result of stress with one or more maternal, infant, or environmental factors (Dewey, 2001). Chatterton et al. (2000) found a relationship between salivary amylase (a measure of stress) and decreased prolactin levels at 6 weeks postpartum in preterm mothers who were pumping their milk. This degree of suppression of prolactin levels could represent a declining responsiveness that results in inadequate milk production in mothers of some preterm infants.

Suckling and Suckling Frequency

The function of infant suckling (or mechanical milk removal) varies between lactogenesis II, the onset of copious milk production, and lactogenesis III, the maintenance of abundant milk production. Lactogenesis II occurs in the absence of milk removal over the first 3 days postpartum, but changes in milk composition and volume will not proceed along the continuum to maximum milk production and mature milk composition in the absence of frequent milk removal after that time. Although suckling (or mechanical milk removal) may not be a prerequisite for lactogenesis II, it is critical for lactogenesis III. Delayed suckling by the infant, whether due to premature delivery (Cregan et al., 2000), cesarean delivery (Sozmen, 1992), or other factors that necessitate mechanical milk removal, may affect the timing or delay the onset of lactogenesis II. Additional breast pumping after a couple of breastfeeds before the onset of lactogenesis II has not been shown to hasten the event or result in increased milk transfer to the baby at 72 hours

(Chapman et al., 2001). However, direct suckling at the breast during the first 24 hours postpartum interacts with maternal obesity status to determine milk transfer at 60 hours postpartum. Mothers who exclusively formula feed their infants perceive the onset of lactation as being significantly later than those who breastfeed (Chapman & Perez-Escamilla, 1999). Direct, early, and frequent suckling at the breast during the early days of lactation has the following effects:

- It prevents a delayed onset of lactogenesis II or conversely facilitates the normal timing for the onset of lactogenesis II.
- It properly hydrates the infant.
- It provides sufficient calories for infant growth.
- It prevents excessive infant weight loss.
- It stabilizes infant blood glucose levels.
- It moderates infant bilirubin levels.
- It may prime the breasts by increasing the number and sensitivity of prolactin receptors in milk-secreting cells, setting the stage for abundant milk synthesis following lactogenesis II.

Clinical Implications

Woolridge (1995) provided a practical identification of six separate stages in the lactation process:

1. Priming (changes of pregnancy).
2. Initiation (birth and the management of early breastfeeding).
3. Calibration (the concept that milk production gets under way without the breasts actually "knowing" how much milk to make in the beginning). Over the first 3 to 5 weeks after birth, milk output is progressively calibrated to the infant's needs, usually building up (up-regulation) but occasionally down-regulating to meet the infant's needs.
4. Maintenance (the period of exclusive breastfeeding).
5. Decline (the period after complementary foods or supplements are added).
6. Involution (weaning).

The second, third, and fourth time periods are crucial to ensuring abundant milk production and optimal weight gain in the infant. Dewey et al. (2003) identified a number of factors that can negatively affect lactogenesis II, infant breastfeeding behaviors, and excessive weight loss: primiparity, urgent cesarean section, long/stressful labor, labor pain medications, high maternal BMI, flat or inverted nipples, nonbreastmilk fluid supplementation in the first 48 hours, and pacifier use. Close attention must be given to any of the previously mentioned alterations that could affect the breasts' ability to calibrate their milk output to the needs of the infant.

Medications

Medications for lactation have mostly centered around preparations that are used to increase faltering milk volumes. Because prolactin is necessary for the initiation of lactation, a new treatment using recombinant human prolactin may be helpful in those mothers with prolactin deficiency or blunted prolactin responses (Page-Wilson et al., 2007). Future studies with recombinant human prolactin are looking at its use in mothers with Sheehan syndrome, adoptive mothers, and as an aid to induce lactation. Thyroid hormones are important for milk production and in animals are necessary for the mammary glands to be responsive to prolactin during lactation (Hapon et al., 2003). Insufficient lactation in women has been treated with nasal administration of thyrotrophin-releasing hormone, which has been shown to increase prolactin levels and daily milk volume (Peters et al., 1991).

Lactogenesis III

The maintenance of milk production is influenced by three levels of controls: endocrine, autocrine (local), and metabolic. The endocrine system is thought to set each individual woman's maximum potential to produce milk, but it is the local control mechanisms acting in concert that actually regulate the short-term synthesis of milk (Hartmann et al., 1998).

Autocrine or Local Control of Milk Synthesis

Local control of milk synthesis is governed by a number of factors:

1. Degree of breast fullness
   - Computerized breast measurements (Daly et al., 1992) have shown that the degree of fullness of the breast and the short-term rate of milk synthesis (between feeds) are inversely related; that is, the emptier the breast, the higher the rate of milk synthesis.

- There is a wide variability in the rate of milk synthesis, ranging from 11 to 58 mL/h; however, the infant does not drain the breasts to the same degree at consecutive feedings. The amount of milk available in the breasts does not necessarily determine the amount of milk the infant removes at each feeding.
- On average over a 24-hour period, infants remove approximately 76% of the available milk at a feeding (Daly et al., 1996). The breast can rapidly change the rate of milk synthesis from one feeding interval to the next.
- There is an inverse relationship between the breast volume and fat content of the milk. At the maximum breast volume when the breast is full of milk, minimum fat content is seen in the milk. When the breast is well drained and at minimum volume, the milk is seen with maximum fat content (Kent et al., 2006).
- As milk accumulates in the breast, the binding of prolactin to its membrane receptors is reduced, an event that occurs independently within each breast, facilitating an inhibitory effect on milk secretion rates (Cox et al., 1996). Prolactin uptake from the blood by the lactocytes (milk-secreting cells) depends on the fullness of the breast, such that prolactin uptake may be inhibited in full alveoli (Cregan et al., 2002).
- Each breast can control the rate of milk synthesis independently of the other, even though both are exposed to the same hormonal stimuli. Thus one breast may produce more milk than the other (Daly et al., 1993). In 7 of 10 mothers the right breast is more productive with no association between handedness or preferential offering to the infant (Kent et al., 2006). The differences between milk output appear early in the postpartum period and remain relatively constant throughout the day and over many weeks of lactation (Engstrom et al., 2007). Although the difference in output between breasts is normal, it is still important to recognize when reduced output in a breast signals a problem (blocked milk duct, mastitis, tight breast pump flange, or, more rarely, neoplastic changes). This is especially true if the onset of reduced production is sudden or appears as a significant discrepancy from previous milk production. Although the reason for milk output differences are unknown, it has been speculated that the right breast receives more blood flow

than the left breast, giving it an advantage in the mechanics of milk production (Aljazaf, 2004).

2. Infant appetite
   - Maternal milk supply is balanced to the infant's demand for or intake of milk because the average mother's potential for milk production exceeds the average infant's appetite (Daly & Hartmann, 1995a).
   - Approximately 29% of infants whose mothers have a high milk storage capacity choose to take smaller feeds even though more milk is available, whereas 40% of infants whose mothers have a low milk storage capacity choose to take larger feeds and drain the breast more thoroughly at each feeding (Kent, 2007).
   - If an infant's demand or need for milk increases, the infant may choose to feed at the same frequency but increase the amount of milk ingested at the feed. Thus the degree to which the breast is emptied may be the factor driving overall milk synthesis.
   - Frequency of breastfeeding may be critical in some mothers, especially those expressing milk in the absence of an infant at breast.

3. Storage capacity of the breasts
   - The size of the breast typically has no relationship to the overall amount of milk it is capable of synthesizing. However, larger breasts (that may contain more glandular tissue) may be able to store more milk between feedings, partially determining how the infant's demand for milk is met by the mother. Mothers with smaller storage capacities make similar amounts of milk over 24-hour periods but may need to feed their infant more frequently than mothers with larger breastmilk storage capacity (Daly & Hartmann, 1995b).

4. Feedback inhibitor of lactation
   - Feedback inhibitor of lactation is an active whey protein that inhibits milk secretion as alveoli become distended and milk is not removed (Prentice et al., 1989). Its concentration increases with longer periods of milk accumulation, down-regulating milk production in a chemical feedback loop.
   - The inhibition of milk secretion is reversible and depends on concentration; it does not affect the composition of the milk because it affects the secretion of all milk components simultaneously.

Volume of Milk Production Over Time

Milk production varies widely among breastfeeding mothers, and a number of factors may influence a woman's lactation capacity. The range of milk volumes varies among mothers from 500 mL/day to 1,200 mL/day, with calculations of breastmilk transfer to the infant gradually increasing from approximately 650 mL/day at 1 month, to 770 mL/day at 3 months, to 800 mL/day at 6 months, when it seems to level off (Neville et al., 1988). As solid foods are introduced around 6 months, milk production decreases to between 95 and 315 mL/day at 15 to 30 months (Hennart et al., 1981; Kent et al., 1999; Neville et al., 1991). The milk composition changes with decreases in the concentration of glucose, citrate, phosphate, and calcium and increases in the concentrations of fat, protein, lactose, and sodium. The amount of breast tissues remains constant between 1 and 6 months of lactation and decreases significantly between 6 and 9 months with only a small drop in milk production. The breasts return to their preconception size by 15 months of lactation (Kent et al., 1999). Mothers may become concerned during this time that their milk production is insufficient because of the change in breast size. Clinicians can assure mothers that this is part of the normal process of breast involution. Involution of the breast occurs in two stages. First the lactocytes (milk-producing cells) are removed by apoptosis (programmed cell death), and then the surrounding stroma (supporting tissue) is remodeled (Watson, 2006).

The Newborn Stomach

During the first few days after birth, the breasts secrete colostrum in amounts that seem small compared with what a formula-fed infant can be compelled to consume. The amounts and composition of colostrum and milk are synchronized to the newborn infant's anatomy, physiology, needs, and stores (Table 2-5). Misunderstanding of this unique matchup can lead to unnecessary supplementation.

The volume of a feeding in the early hours and days after birth is quite small. A number of factors contribute to this normal state (Table 2-6).

Clinical Implications

A newborn infant may show a delayed interest in feeding if the mother has been heavily medicated during labor and/or has received large quantities of fluid during labor, adding to the excess extracellular fluid burden that accompanies the transition to postnatal life. The newborn stomach is rather noncompliant and does not easily relax to accommodate a feeding during the early hours after birth. Over the

TABLE 2-5 Volume of Milk Production and Intake

Time Postpartum	Volume/ Day Average (range)	Volume/ Feed Average	Notes	References
Day 1 (0–24 h)	37 mL (7–123 mL) 6 mL/kg (vaginal) 4 mL/kg (cesarean)	7 mL	Matches the physiologic capacity of the newborn stomach	Casey et al., 1986; Evans et al., 2003; Houston, Howie, & McNeilly, 1983; Roderuck, Williams, & Macy, 1946; Saint, Smith, & Hartmann, 1984
Day 2 (24–48 h)	84 mL (44–335 mL) 25 mL/kg (vaginal) 13 mL/kg (c-sec)	14 mL		Evans et al., 2003; Houston, Howie, & McNeilly, 1983
24 hours 30 hours 36 hours 48 hours 60 hours 72 hours		4.2 mL ± 10.6 3.1 mL ± 6.6 3.1 mL ± 4.9 6.4 mL ± 6.8 14.0 mL ± 13.5 26.1 mL ± 26.6	Nonpumping cesarean mothers; multiparous mothers had ↑ milk volumes	Chapman et al., 2001
24–144 h	24 h milk intake increased from 82 mL to 556 mL between 24–144 hours postpartum			Arthur, Smith, & Hartmann, 1989
Day 3 (48–72 h)	408 mL (98–775) 66 mL/kg (vaginal) 44 mL/kg (c-sec)	38 mL	Lactogenesis II occurs in this time period	Casey et al., 1986; Evans et al., 2003; Houston, Howie, & McNeilly, 1983; Neville et al., 1988; Saint, Smith, & Hartmann, 1984
Day 4 (72–96 h)	625 mL (378–876) 106 mL/kg (vag) 82 mL/kg (c-sec)	58 mL	Delayed lactogenesis II results in ↓ milk volumes	Houston, Howie, & McNeilly, 1983; Saint, Smith, & Hartmann, 1984; Evans et al., 2003

(continues)

TABLE 2-5   Volume of Milk Production and Intake *(continued)*

Time Postpartum	Volume/ Day Average (range)	Volume/ Feed Average	Notes	References
Day 5	200–900 g 123 mL/kg (vag) 111 mL/kg (c-sec)		Milk output is calibrated to meet infant needs over 3–5 weeks	Woolridge, 1995; Evans et al., 2003
Day 6	138 mL/kg (vag) 129 mL/kg (c-sec)			Evans et al., 2003
Day 7	576 mL (mean) (200–1013)	65 mL	Multiparous women produced an average of 142 mL more milk each 24 hours	Ingram et al., 1999
4 weeks	750 mL (mean) (328–1127) 675 mL (600–950)	94 mL		Ingram et al., 1999
2–6 months 2.5 months	1680–3000 mL 3080 mL		Milk yields in mothers of twins; mothers of triplets	Saint, Maggiore, & Hartmann, 1986
3 months	750 mL (609–837) 720 mL (550–880)			Butte et al., 1984
5 months	770 mL (630–950)			
6 months	800 mL			Neville et al., 1988
1–6 months	750 mL ± 200 mL	71.8 mL ± 26.3mL	All infants were fully breastfed on demand; includes both multiparous and primiparous mothers	Mitoulas et al., 2002
9 months 12 months 18 months 24 months	740 mL 520 mL 218 mL 114 mL			Kent et al., 1999

Source: Adapted from Royal College of Midwives. *Successful Breastfeeding.* 3rd ed. London: Churchill Livingstone; 2002; p. 26.

TABLE 2-6   Factors Related to Feed Size/Frequency in the Early Hours and Days After Birth

Factor	Comment
Physiological diuresis of excess fluid	Lack of hunger or thirst (CNS depression, changing hormonal concentrations)
Immaturity of gastric function	Noncompliant, nonrelaxing stomach
Stomach capacity	Size related to birth weight
Physiological vs. anatomical capacity	The volume that fits comfortably as a feed vs. the amount that can be held to the point of discomfort and pain
Gastric emptying time	Generally delayed in the first 12 h of life; faster for breastmilk than for formula
Increasing age and number of feedings	Encourages the stomach to relax and stretch to better accommodate increasing volumes of milk

next 3 days of life, a reduction in the gastric tone and an increase in compliance allow the stomach to accept increasing volumes of milk per feeding (Zangen et al., 2001). Clinically, this change is seen as infants ingesting very small volumes of milk (5 mL = 1 teaspoon) and regurgitating milk or formula if they are persuaded to accept in excess of what their stomachs can physiologically accommodate.

There is a difference between the physiological and anatomical capacity of the newborn stomach (Tables 2-7 and 2-8). The physiological capacity is what an infant can comfortably ingest at a feeding (feeding volume as determined by pre- and post-feed weights), whereas the anatomical capacity is what the stomach will hold at its maximum fullness (as determined on autopsy). Physiological capacity (Scammon & Doyle, 1920) is considerably less than anatomical capacity during the early days. Physiological and anatomical stomach capacities begin to approximate each other around 4 days of age. The actual size of the newborn stomach has received little attention, especially in regards to the volume of what a "normal" feeding should be. Widstrom et al. (1988) studied gastric aspirates in newborns immediately after birth showing gastric contents of 0–11 mL. They suggested that the fetus typically drinks about 10-mL portions of amniotic fluid, which are gradually emptied from the stomach.

Using real-time ultrasound imaging, Nagata et al. (1994) calculated fetal stomach volume at 38 weeks to be approximately 9.9 mL, whereas Sase et al. (2005) using ultrasound calculated newborn stomach volumes at approximately

TABLE 2-7 Average Physiological Capacity of the Stomach in the First 10 Days of Life

Physiological stomach capacity birth weights 2.0–4.0+ kg (4.4–8.8 lbs) 14,571 feeding records of 323 breastfed newborns

Day of Life	mL	mL/kg
1	7	2
2	13	4
3	27	8
4	46	14
5	57	17
6	64	19
7	68	21
8	71	22
9	76	23
10	81	24

Source: Scammon RE, Doyle LO. Observations on the capacity of the stomach in the first ten days of postnatal life. *Am J Dis Child.* 1920;20:516–538.

TABLE 2-8 Average Anatomical Capacity of the Stomach in Newborns

Age/Weight	Average Capacity (mL)
Newborn 1.5–2.0 kg	22
Newborn 2.0–2.5 kg	30
Newborn 2.5–3.0 kg	30
Newborn 3.0–3.5 kg	35
Newborn 3.5–4.0 kg	35
Newborn 4.0+ kg	38
1 week, all weights	45
2 weeks, all weights	75

Source: Scammon RE, Doyle LO. Observations on the capacity of the stomach in the first ten days of postnatal life. *Am J Dis Child.* 1920;20:516–538.

10 mL. Naveed et al. (1992) calculated the anatomical stomach capacity at autopsy of 100 perinatal stillbirths and 37 deaths occurring in the first week. They found the larger the infant, the greater the anatomical capacity of the stomach. An infant over 5.5 lb (2,500 g) was shown to have an anatomical capacity of 18–21 mL.

Communicating the concept of the small stomach size and the need for small feedings and avoidance of large formula supplements during the early days led to the concept of a visual aid to illustrate the small size of the newborn stomach (Spangler et al., 2008). Objects such as marbles, ping pong balls, and eggs serve to illustrate the approximate breastmilk intake of infants at various ages and help parents and clinicians understand that encouraging infants to take volumes beyond their physiological capacity may be detrimental. The anatomical and physiological capacities of the newborn stomach vary widely and depend on gestational age and feeding history. There is really no single visual aid such as a walnut that accurately reflects the exact volume a specific infant can safely consume. Many clinicians use a teaspoon to represent an average feeding volume on day 1 because 5 mL is within the range of intakes of normal term breastfed infants.

Human milk is easily and rapidly digested. The mean gastric half-emptying time for formula is 65 minutes (range, 27–98 minutes), whereas the mean gastric half-emptying time for breastmilk is 47 minutes (range, 16–86 minutes) (Lambrecht et al., 1988; Van den Driessche et al., 1999). Thus breastfed infants can be hungry sooner than 2 or 3 hours after a feeding. Routine or capricious supplementation of a breastfed infant with water or formula after nursing is not supported by the data.

Summary: The Design in Nature

Lactation is a robust process that is organized to meet the nutritional, emotional, developmental, and health needs of the infant and young child. Breastfeeding is a dynamic coordination between the changing needs, stores, and capacities of a child and the delivery of appropriate nutrients, immune factors, and physical contact necessary to support the normal growth and development of a new person. Breastfeeding and lactation can occur within a wide range of anatomical and physiological parameters in both the infant and the mother. It is the clinician's responsibility to ensure that both happen (Appendix 2-1).

References

Ahmed, O. A., Kolhe, P. S. (2000). Comparison of nipple and areolar sensation after breast reduction by free nipple graft and inferior pedicle techniques. *Br J Plast Surg.* 53,126–129.

Alexander, J., Grant, A., Campbell, M. J. (1992). Randomized controlled trial of breast shells and Hoffman's exercises for inverted and non-protractile nipples. *Br Med J.* 304,1030–1032.

Aljazaf, KMNH. (2004). Ultrasound imaging in the analysis of the blood supply and blood flow in the human lactating breast. Dissertation. Medical Imaging Science, Curtin University of Technology, Perth, Australia.

Anderson, A. M. (2001). Disruption of lactogenesis by retained placental fragments. *J Hum Lact.* 17,142–144.

Arthur, P. G., Smith, M., Hartmann, P. E. (1989). Milk lactose, citrate, and glucose as markers of lactogenesis in normal and diabetic women. *J Pediatr Gastroenterol Nutr.* 9,488–496.

Ballesio, L., Maggi, C., Savelli, S., et al. (2007). Adjunctive diagnostic value of ultrasonography evaluation in patients with suspected ductal breast disease. *Radiol Med.* 112,354–365.

Betzold CM, Hoover KL, Snyder CL. (2004). Delayed lactogenesis II: a comparison of four cases. *J Midwif Womens Health.* 49,132–137.

Bowles, B. C., Stutte, P. C., Hensley, J. H. (1987). New benefits from an old technique: alternate massage in breastfeeding. *Genesis.* 9,5–9, 17.

Brown, S. L., Todd, J. F., Cope, J. U., Sachs, H. C. (2006). Breast implant surveillance reports to the US Food and Drug Administration: Maternal-child health problems. *J Long-Term Effects Med Implants.* 16,281–290.

Brzozowski, D., Niessen, M., Evans, H. B., Hurst, L. N. (2000). Breastfeeding after inferior pedicle reduction mammaplasty. *Plast Reconstr Surg.* 105,530–534.

Butte, N., Garza, C., O'Brien Smith, E., Nichols, B. L. (1984). Human milk intake and growth in exclusively breastfed infants. *J Pediatr.* 104:187–195.

Carter, C. S., Altemus, M., Chrousos, G. P (2001). Neuroendocrine and emotional changes in the postpartum period. *Prog Brain Res.* 133,241–249.

Casey, C., Neifert, M., Seacat, J., Neville, M. (1986).Nutrient intake by breastfed infants during the first five days after birth. *Am J Dis Child.* 140,933–936.

Chapman, D., Perez-Escamilla, R. (1999). Identification of risk factors for delayed onset of lactation. *J Am Diet Assoc.* 99,450–454.

Chapman, D. J., Perez-Escamilla, R. (2000a). Lactogenesis stage II: hormonal regulation, determinants, and public health consequences. *Recent Res Dev Nutr.* 3,43–63.

Chapman, D. J., Perez-Escamilla, R. (2000b). Maternal perception of the onset of lactation is a valid, public health indicator of lactogenesis state II. *J Nutr.*130,2972–2980.

Chapman, D. J., Young, S., Ferris, A. M., Perez-Escamilla, R. (2001). Impact of breast pumping on lactogenesis stage II after cesarean delivery: a randomized clinical trial. *Pediatrics.* 107(6). Retrieved May 8, 2005 from www.pediatrics.org/cgi/content/full/107/6/e94

Chatterton, R. T., Hill, P. D., Aldag, J. C., et al. (2000). Relation of plasma oxytocin and prolactin concentrations to milk production in mothers of preterm infants: influence of stress. *J Clin Endocrinol Metab.* 85,3661–3668.

Chen, D., Nommsen-Rivers, L., Dewey, K.G., Lonnerdal, B. (1998). Stress during labor and delivery and early lactation performance. *Am J Clin Nutr.* 68,335–344.

Cherchel A, Azzam C, De Mey A. (2007). Breastfeeding after vertical reduction mammaplasty using a superior pedicle. *J Plast Reconstr Aesthet Surg.* 60,465–70.

Chien, Y. C., Huang, Y. J., Hsu, C. S., Chao, J. C., Liu, J. F. (2008). Maternal lactation characteristics after consumption of an alcoholic soup during the postpartum "doing the month" ritual. *Public Health Nutr.* 22,1–7.

Chiummariello S, Cigna E, Buccheri EM, Dessy LA, Alfano C, Scuderi N. (2008). Breastfeeding after reduction mammaplasty using different techniques. *Aesthetic Plast Surg.* 32,294–297.

Cobo, E. (1973). Effect of different doses of ethanol on the milk-ejecting reflex in lactating women. *Am J Obstet Gynecol.*115,817–821.

Cooper, A. P. (1840). Anatomy of the Breast. London: Longman, Orme, Green, Browne and Longmans.

Cotterman, K. J. (2004). Reverse pressure softening: a simple tool to prepare areola for easier latching during engorgement. *J Hum Lact.* 20,227–237.

Cowley, D. S., Roy-Byrne, P. P. (1989). Panic disorder during pregnancy. *J Psychosom Obstet Gynaecol.* 10, 193–210.

Cox, D. B., Kent, J. C., Casey, T. M., et al. (1999). Breast growth and the urinary excretion of lactose during human pregnancy and early lactation: endocrine relationships. *Exp Physiol.* 84,421–434.

Cox, D. B., Owens, R. A., Hartmann, P. E. (1996). Blood and milk prolactin and the rate of milk synthesis in women. *Exp Physiol.* 81,1007–1020.

Cregan, M. D., De Mello, T. R., Hartmann, P. E. (2000). Pre-term delivery and breast expression: consequences for initiating lactation. *Adv Exp Med Biol.* 478,427–428.

Cregan,M. D., Hartmann, P. E. (1999). Computerized breast measurement from conception to weaning: clinical implications. *J Hum Lact.* 15,89–96.

Cregan, M. D., Mitoulas, L. R., Hartmann, P. E. (2002). Milk prolactin, feed volume and duration between feeds of women breastfeeding their full-term infants over a 24 h period. *Exp Physiol.* 87,207–214.

Cruz, N. I., Korchin, L. (2007). Lactational performance after breast reduction with different pedicles. *Plast Reconstr Surg.* 120,35–40.

Cruz-Korchin, N., Korchin, L. (2004). Breast-feeding after vertical mammaplasty with medial pedicle. *Plast Reconstr Surg.* 114,890–894.

Czank, C., Henderson, J. J., Kent, J. C., Lai, C. T., Hartmann, P. E. (2007). Hormonal control of the lactation cycle. In: Hale TW, Hartmann PE, eds. Textbook of Human Lactation. Amarillo, TX: Hale Publishing.

Daly, S. E. J., Hartmann, P. E. (1995a). Infant demand and milk supply. Part 1: Infant demand and milk production in lactating women. *J Hum Lact.* 1,:21–26.

Daly, S. E. J., Hartmann, P. E. (1995b). Infant demand and milk supply. Part 2: The short-term control of milk synthesis in lactating women. *J Hum Lact.* 11,27–37.

Daly, S. E. J., Kent, J.C., Huynh, D.Q., et al. (1992). The determination of short-term breast volume changes and the rate of synthesis of human milk using computerized breast measurement. *Exp Physiol.* 77,79–87.

Daly, S. E. J., Kent, J.C., Owens, R. A., Hartmann, P. E. (1996). Frequency and degree of milk removal and the short-term control of human milk synthesis. *Exp Physiol.* 81,861–875.

Daly, S. E. J., Owens, R. A., Hartmann, P. E. (1993). The short-term synthesis and infant-regulated removal of milk in lactating women. *Exp Physiol.* 78,209–220.

DeCoopman, J. (1993). Breastfeeding after pituitary resection: support for a theory of autocrine control of milk supply? *J Hum Lact.* 9,35–40.

Dewey, K. G. (2001). Maternal and fetal stress are associated with impaired lactogenesis in humans. *J Nutr.* 131,3012S–3015S.

Dewey, K. G., Nommsen-Rivers, L., Heinig, M. J., Cohen, R. J. (2002). Lactogenesis and infant weight change in the first weeks of life. *Adv Exp Med Biol.* 503,159–166.

Dewey, K. G., Nommsen-Rivers, L., Heinig, M. J., Cohen, R. J. (2003). Risk factors for suboptimal infant breastfeeding behavior, delayed onset of lactation, and excess neonatal weight loss. *Pediatrics.* 112,607–619.

Donath, S. M., Amir, L. H. (2000). Does maternal obesity adversely affect breastfeeding initiation and duration? *J Paediatr Child Health.* 36,482–486.

Doucet, S., Soussignan, R., Sagot, P., Schaal, B. (2007). The "smellscape" of mother's breast: effects of odor masking and selective unmasking on neonatal arousal, oral, and visual responses. *Dev Psychobiol.*49,129–138.

Elia, M., Handpour, S., Terranova, P., et al. (2002). Marked variation in nipple aspirate fluid (NAF), estrogen concentration and NAF/serum ratios between ducts in high risk women [abstract]. Presented at the 93rd annual meeting of the American Association for Cancer Research, San Francisco, Calif., April 6–10.

Engstrom, J. L., Meier, P. P., Jegier, B., Motykowski, J. E., Zuleger, J. L. (2007). Comparison of milk output from the right and left breasts during simultaneous pumping in mothers of very low birthweight infants. *Breastfeeding Med.* 2,83–91.

Evans, K. C., Evans, R. G., Royal, R., et al. (2003). Effect of caesarean section on breastmilk transfer to the normal term newborn over the first week of life. *Arch Dis Child Fetal Neonatal Ed.* 88,F380–F382.

Faridi, M. M. A., Dewan, P. (2008). Successful breastfeeding with breast malformations. *J Hum Lact.* 24, 446–450.

Ferris, A. M., Dalidowitz, C. K., Ingardia, C. M., et al. (1988). Lactation outcome in insulin-dependent diabetic women. *J Am Diet Assoc.* 88,317–322.

Ferris, A. M., Neubauer, S. H., Bendel, R. R., et al. (1993). Perinatal lactation protocol and outcome in mothers with and without insulin-dependent diabetes mellitus. *Am J Clin Nutr.* 58:43–48.

Fewtrell, M. S., Loh, K. L., Blake, A, Ridout, D. A., Hawdon, J. (2006). Ramdomised, double blind trial of oxytocin nasal spray in mothers expressing breast milk for preterm infants. *Arch Dis Child Fetal Neonatal Ed.* 91,F169–F174.

Flegel, K. M., Carroll, M. D., Ogden, C. L., Johnson, C. L. (2002). Prevalence and trends in obesity among U.S. adults, 1999–2000. JAMA. 288,1723–1727.

Freeman, M. E., Kanyicska, B., Lerant, A., Nagy, G. (2000). Prolactin: structure, function, and regulation of secretion. *Physiol Rev.* 80,1523–1631.

Geddes, D. T. (2007a). Gross anatomy of the lactating breast. In: Hale TW, Hartmann PE, eds. Textbook of Human Lactation. Amarillo, TX: Hale Publishing.

Geddes, D. T. (2007b). Inside the lactating breast: The latest anatomy research. *J Midwif Womens Health.* 52,556–563.

Geddes, D. T. (2009). Ultrasound imaging of the lactating breast: methodology and application. *Int Breastfeed J.* 4:4. Retrieved August 13, 2009 from http://www.internationalbreastfeedingjournal.com/content/pdf/1746–4358–4–4.pdf

Gimp, G., Fahrenholz, F. (2001). The oxytocin receptor system: structure, function, and regulation. *Physiol Rev.* 81,629–683.

Going, J. J., Moffat, D. F. (2004). Escaping from flatland: clinical and biological aspects of human mammary duct anatomy in three dimensions. *J Pathol.* 203,538–544.

Gonzalez, F., Brown, F. E., Gold, M. E., et al. (1993). Preoperative and postoperative nipple-areola sensibility in patients undergoing reduction mammaplasty. *Plast Reconstr Surg.* 92,809–814.

Goodfellow, C. F., Hull, M. G. R., Swaab, D. F., et al. (1983). Oxytocin deficiency at delivery with epidural analgesia. *Br J Obstet Gynaecol.* 90,214–219.

Grattan, D. R. (2001). The actions of prolactin in the brain during pregnancy and lactation. *Prog Brain Res.* 133,153–171.

Grattan, D. R., Pi, X. J., Andrews, Z. B., et al. (2001). Prolactin receptors in the brain during pregnancy and lactation: implications for behavior. *Horm Behav.* 40,115–124.

Groer, M. W., Davis, M. W. (2002). Postpartum stress: current concepts and the possible protective role of breastfeeding. *JOGNN.* 31,411–417.

Hale, T. W., Ilett, K. F. (2002). Drug Therapy and Breastfeeding: From Theory to Clinical Practice. New York: Parthenon.

Hallock, G. G. (1992). Prediction of nipple viability following reduction mammoplasty using laser Doppler flowmetry. *Ann Plast Surg.* 29,457–460.

Hapon, M. B., Simoncini, M., Via, G., Jahn, G. A. (2003). Effect of hypothyroidism on hormone profiles in virgin, pregnant and lactating rats, and on lactation. *Reproduction.* 126,371–382.

Hartmann, P. (2000). Human lactation: current research and clinical implications. Presented at ALCA 2000: 5th biennial conference of the Australian Lactation Consultants' Association, Melbourne, Australia.

Hartmann, P., Cregan, M. (2001). Lactogenesis and the effects of insulin-dependent diabetes mellitus and prematurity. *J Nutr.* 131,3016S–3020S.

Hartmann, P. E., Mitoulas, L. R,, Gurrin, L. C. (2000). Physiology of breast milk expression using an electric breast pump. Proceedings of the 10th International Conference of the Research on Human Milk and Lactation (ISRHML), Tucson, Arizona.

Hartmann, P. E., Sherriff, J. L., Mitoulas, L. R. (1998). Homeostatic mechanisms that regulate lactation during energetic stress. *J Nutr.* 128,394S–399S.

Hefter W, Lindholm P, Elvenes OP. (2003). Lactation and breast-feeding ability following lateral pedicle mammaplasty. *Br J Plast Surg.* 56,746–51.

Heimburg, D., Exner, K., Kruft, S., Lemperle, G. (1996). The tuberous breast deformity: classification and treatment. *Br J Plast Surg.* 49,339–345.

Henderson, J. J., Hartmann, P. E., Newnham, J. P., Simmer, K. (2008). Effect of preterm birth and antenatal corticosteroid treatment on lactogenesis II in women. *Pediatr.* 121,e92–e100.

Hennart, P., Delogne-Desnoeck, J., Vis, H., Robyn, C. (1981). Serum levels of prolactin and milk production in women during a lactation period of thirty months. *Clin Endocrinol.* 14,349–353.

Hill, P. D., Wilhelm, P. A., Aldag, J. C., Chatterton, R. T. (2004). Breast augmentation and lactation outcome: a case report. *MCN.* 29,238–242.

Hilson, J. A. (2000). Maternal obesity and breastfeeding success. PhD thesis, Cornell University, Ithaca, NY.

Hilson, J. A., Rasmussen, K. M., Kjolhede, C. L. (2004). High prepregnant body mass index is associated with poor lactation outcomes among white, rural women independent of psychosocial and demographic correlates. *J Hum Lact.* 20,18–29.

Hilson, J. A., Rasmussen, K. M., Kjolhede, C. L. (1997). Maternal obesity and breastfeeding success in a rural population of white women. *Am J Clin Nutr.* 66,1371–1378.

Hoover, K. L., Barbalinardo, L. H., Platia, M. P. (2002). Delayed lactogenesis II secondary to gestational ovarian theca lutein cysts in two normal singleton pregnancies. *J Hum Lact.* 18,264–268.

Hopkinson, J. M., Schanler, R. J., Garza, C. (1988). Milk production by mothers of premature infants. *Pediatrics.* 81,815–820.

Houston, M. J., Howie, P., McNeilly, A. S. (1983). Factors affecting the duration of breastfeeding: 1. Measurement of breastmilk intake in the first week of life. *Early Hum Dev.* 8,49–54.

Huggins, K. E., Petok, E. S., Mireles, O. (2000). Markers of lactation insufficiency: a study of 34 mothers. Current Issues in Clinical Lactation. Sudbury, MA: Jones and Bartlett, pp. 25–35.

Huntingford, P. J. H. (1961). Intranasal use of synthetic oxytocin in management of breast-feeding. *Br Med J.* 243,709–711.

Hurst, N. M. (1996). Lactation after augmentation mammoplasty. *Obstet Gynecol.* 87,30–34.

Hurst, N. M. (2007). Recognizing and treating delayed or failed lactogenesis II. *J Midwif Women's Health.* 52,588–594.

Hytten, F. E. (1954). Clinical and chemical studies in human lactation: VI The functional capacity of the breast. *Br Med J.* 1(4867),912–915.

Ingram, J. C., Woolridge, M. W., Greenwood, R. J., McGrath, L. (1999). Maternal predictors of early breast milk output. *Acta Paediatr.* 88,493–499.

Janbu, T., Koss, K. S., Thoresen, M., Wesche, J. (1985). Blood velocities t the female breast during lactation and following oxytocin injections. *J Dev Physiol.* 7,373–380.

Kent, J. C. (2007). How breastfeeding works. *J Midwif Womens Health.* 52,564–570.

Kent, J. C., Mitoulas, L. R., Cox, D. B., Owens, R. A., Hartmann, P. E. (1999). Breast volume and milk production during extended lactation in women. *Exp Physiol.* 84,435–447.

Kent, J. C., Mitoulas, L. R., Cregan, M. D., Ramsay, D. T., Doherty, D. A., Hartmann, P. E. (2006). Volume and frequency of breastfeeds and fat content of breast milk throughout the day. *Pediatrics.* 117,e387–e395.

Kent, J. C., Ramsay, D. T., Doherty, D., Larsson, M., Hartmann, P. E. (2003). Response of breasts to different stimulation patterns of an electric breast pump. *J Hum Lact.* 19,179–187.

Klein, D. F., Skrobala, A. M., Garfinkel, R. S. (1995). Preliminary look at the effects of pregnancy on the course of panic disorder. *Anxiety.* 1,227–232.

Kulski, J., Hartmann, P. (1981). Changes in human milk composition during initiation of lactation. *Aust J Exp Biol Med Sci.* 59,101–114.

Lambrecht, L., Robberecht, E., Deschynkel, K., Afschrift, M. (1988). Ultrasonic evaluation of gastric clearing in young infants. *Pediatr Radiol.* 18,314–318.

Lawrence, R. A., Lawrence, R. M. (2005). Breastfeeding: A Guide for the Medical Profession. Philadelphia: Elsevier Mosby.

Light, K., Smith, T., Johns, J., et al. (2000). Oxytocin responsivity in mothers of infants: a preliminary study of relationships with blood pressure during laboratory stress and normal ambulatory activity. *Health Psychol.* 19,560–567.

Lindow, S. W., Hendricks, M. S., Nugent, F. A., et al. (1999). Morphine suppresses the oxytocin response in breastfeeding women. *Gynecol Obstet Invest.* 48:33–37.

Loughry, C. W., Sheffer, D. B., Price, T. E., et al. (1989). Breast volume measurement of 598 women using biostereometric analysis. *Am Plast Surg.* 22,380–385.

Love, S. M., Barsky, S. H. (2004). Anatomy of the nipple and breast ducts revisited. *Cancer.* 101,1947–1957.

MAIN Trial Collaborative Group. (1994). Preparing for breastfeeding: treatment of inverted and non-protractile nipples in pregnancy. *Midwifery.* 10:200–214.

Marasco, L., Marmet, C., Shell, E. (2000). Polycystic ovary syndrome: a connection to insufficient milk supply? *J Hum Lact.* 16:143–148.

Murase, M., Mizuno, K., Nishida, Y., et al. (2009). Comparison of creamatocrit and protein concentration in each mammary lobe of the same breast: does the milk composition of each mammary lobe differ in the same breast? Breastfeed Med. doi:10.1089/bfm.2008.0124. Online Ahead of Print: April 15, 2009

Mathes, S. J., Seyfer, A. E., Miranda, E. P. (2006). Congenital anomalies of the chest wall. In: Mathes SJ, Hentz VR, eds. Plastic Surgery VI. Philadelphia: Elsevier, pp. 457–537.

Matthiesen, A.-S., Ransjo-Arvidson, A.-B., Nissen, E., Uvnas-Moberg, K. (2001). Postpartum maternal oxytocin release by newborns: effects of infant hand massage and sucking. *Birth.* 28:13–19.

Mennella, J. A., Beauchamp, G. K. (1991). The transfer of alcohol to human milk: effects on flavor and the infant's behavior. *N Engl J Med.* 325:981–985.

Mennella, J. A., Pepino, M. Y. (2008). Biphasic effects of moderate drinking on prolactin during lactation. *Alcohol Clin Exp Res.* 32:1899–1908.

Mennella, J. A., Pepino, M. Y., Teff, K. L. (2005). Acute alcohol consumption disrupts hormonal milieu of lactating women. *J Clin Endocrinol Metab.* 90:1979–1985.

Mezzacappa, E., Kelsey, R., Katlin, E. (1999). A preliminary study of maternal cardiovascular function and breastfeeding in the first year. Poster session at annual meeting, American Psychosomatic Society, Vancouver, BC, Canada.

Michalopoulos K. (2007). The effects of breast augmentation surgery on future ability to lactate. *Breast J.* 13:62–67.

Miller, V., Riordan, J. (2004). Treating postpartum breast edema with areolar compression. *J Hum Lact.* 20:223–226.

Mitoulas, L. R., Lai, C. T., Gurrin, L. C., et al. (2002). Efficacy of breast milk expression using an electric breast pump. *J Hum Lact.* 18:344–352.

Mottura, A. A. (2002). Circumvertical reduction mammaplasty. *Clin Plast Surg.* 29:393–399.

Mulford ,C. (1990). Subtle signs and symptoms of the milk ejection reflex. *J Hum Lact.* 6:177–178.

Nagata, S., Koyanagi, T., Fukushima, S., Akazawa, K., Nakano, H. (1994). Change in the three-dimensional shape of the stomach in the developing human fetus. *Early Hum Dev.* 37:27–38.

Nahabedian, M. Y., Mofid, M. M. (2002). Viability and sensation of the nipple-areolar complex after reduction mammaplasty. *Ann Plast Surg.* 49:24–31.

National Center for Health Statistics.(1997). Update: Prevalence of overweight among children, adolescents, and adults—United States, 1988–1994. *MMWR.* 46:199–202.

Naveed, M., Manjunath, C., Sreenivas, V. (1992). An autopsy study of relationship between perinatal stomach capacity and birth weight. *Indian J Gastroenterol.* 11:156–158.

Neidhart, M. (1998). Prolactin in autoimmune disease. *Proc Soc Exp Biol Med.* 217:408–419.

Neifert, M., DeMarzo, S., Seacat, J., et al. (1990). The influence of breast surgery, breast appearance, and pregnancy-induced breast changes on lactation sufficiency as measured by infant weight gain. *Birth.* 17,31–38.

Neifert, M. R., McDonough, S. L., Neville, M. C. (1981). Failure of lactogenesis associated with placental retention. *Am J Obstet Gynecol.* 140,477–478.

Neifert, M. R., Seacat, J. M., Jobe, W. E. (1985). Lactation failure due to insufficient glandular development of the breast. *Pediatrics.* 76,823–828.

Nelson, E. E., Panksepp, J. (1998). Brain substrates of infant-mother attachment: contributions of opioids, oxytocin, and norepinephrine. *Neurosci Biobehav Rev.* 22,437–452.

Neubauer, S. H., Ferris, A. M., Chase, C. G., et al. (1993). Delayed lactogenesis in women with insulin-dependent diabetes mellitus. *Am J Clin Nutr.* 58,54–60.

Neville, M. C. (2001). Anatomy and physiology of lactation. *Pediatr Clin North Am.* 48,13–34.

Neville, M. C., Allen, J. C., Archer, P., et al. (1991). Studies in human lactation: milk volume and nutrient composition during weaning and lactogenesis. *Am J Clin Nutr.* 54,81–93.

Neville, M., Keller, R., Seacat, J., et al. (1988). Studies in human lactation: milk volumes in lactating women during the onset of lactation and full lactation. *Am J Clin Nutr.*48,1375–1386.

Neville, M. C., Morton, J. (2001). Physiology and endocrine changes underlying human lactogenesis II. *J Nutr.* 131,3005S–3008S.

Neville, M. C., Morton, J. A., Umemora, S. (2001). Lactogenesis: the transition between pregnancy and lactation. *Pediatr Clin North Am.* 48:35–52.

Newton, M., Egli, G. E. (1958). The effect of intranasal administration of oxytocin on the let-down of milk in lactating women. *Am J Obstet Gynecol.* 76,103-107.

Nickell, W. B., Skelton, J. (2005). Breast fat and fallacies: more than 100 years of anatomical fantasy. *J Hum Lact.* 21,126–130.

Nissen, E., Lilja, G., Widstrom, A.-M., Uvnas-Moberg, K. (1995). Elevation of oxytocin levels early post partum in women. *Acta Obstet Gynaecol Scand.* 74:530–533.

Nissen, E., Uvnas-Moberg, K., Svensson, K., et al. (1996). Different patterns of oxytocin, prolactin but not cortisol release during breastfeeding in women delivered by cesarean section or by the vaginal route. *Early Hum Dev.* 45,103–118.

Ohtake, T., Kimijima, I., Fukushima, T., et al. (2001). Computer-assisted complete three-dimensional reconstruction of the mammary ductal/lobular systems. *Cancer.* 91,2263–2272.

Ostrom, K. M., Ferris, A. M. (1993). Prolactin concentrations in serum and milk of mothers with and without insulin dependent diabetes mellitus. *Am J Clin Nutr.* 58:49–53.

Page-Wilson, G., Smith, P. C., Welt, C. K. (2007). Short-term prolactin administration causes expressible galactorrhea but does not affect bone turnover: pilot data for a new lactation agent. *Int Breastfeed J.* 2,10.

Pérez-Escamilla, R., Chapman, D. J. (2001). Validity and public health implications of maternal perception of the onset of lactation: an international analytical overview. *J Nutr.* 131,3021S-3024S.

Peters, F., Diemer, P., Mecks, O., Behnken, L. J. (2003). Severity of mastalgia in relation to milk duct dilatation. *Obstet Gynecol*. 101,54–60.

Peters, F., Schulze-Tollert, J., Schuth, W. (1991). Thyrotrophin-releasing hormone—a lactation-promoting agent? *Br J Obstet Gynaecol*. 98,880–885.

Polatti, F., Capuzzo, E., Viazzo, F., Colleoni, R., Klersy, C. (1999). Bone mineral changes during and after lactation. *Obstet Gynecol*. 94,52–56.

Prentice, A., Addey, C. V. P., Wilde, C. J. (1989). Evidence for local feedback control of human milk secretion. *Biochem Soc Trans*. 17,122.

Rahm, V. A., Hallgren, A., Hogberg, H., et al. (2002). Plasma oxytocin levels in women during labor with or without epidural analgesia: a prospective study. *Acta Obstet Gyncaecol Scand*. 81,1033–1039.

Rainer, C., Gardetto, A., Fruhwirth, M., et al. (2003). Breast deformity in adolescence as a result of pneumothorax drainage during neonatal intensive care. *Pediatrics*. 111,80–86.

Ramirez, O. M. (2002). Reduction mammaplasty with the "owl" incision and no undermining. *Plast Reconstr Surg*. 109,512–522.

Ramsay, D. T., Kent, J. C., Hartmann, R. A., Hartmann, P. E. (2005). Anatomy of the lactating breast redefined with ultrasound imaging. *J Anat*. 206,525–534.

Ramsay, D. T., Kent, J. C., Owens, R. A., Hartmann, P. E. (2004). Ultrasound imaging of milk ejection in the breast of lactating women. *Pediatrics*. 113,361–367.

Rasmussen, K. M., Hilson, J. A., Kjolhede, C. L. (2001). Obesity may impair lactogenesis II. *J Nutr*. 131, 3009S–3011S.

Rasmussen, K. M., Kjolhede, C. L. (2004). Prepregnant overweight and obesity diminish the prolactin response to suckling in the first week postpartum. *Pediatrics*.113,e465–e471.

Renfrew, M. J., Lang, S., Woolridge, M. (2000). Oxytocin for promoting successful lactation (Cochrane Review). In: The Cochrane Library, Issue 3. Oxford, UK: Update Software.

Roderuck, C., Williams, H. H., Macy, I. G. (1946). Metabolism of women during the reproductive years. *J Nutr*. 32,267–283.

Ruis, H., Rolland, R., Doesburg, W., et al. (1981). Oxytocin enhances onset of lactation among mothers delivering prematurely. *Br Med J (Clin Res Ed)*. 283,340–342.

Rusby, J. E., Brachtel, E. F., Michaelson, J. S., Koerner, F. C., Smith, B. L. (2007). Breast duct anatomy in the human nipple: three-dimensional patterns and clinical applications. *Breast Cancer Res Treat*. 106,171–179.

Russo, J., Russo, I. H. (2004). Development of the human breast. *Maruritas*. 49,2–15.

Rutishauser, I. H. E., Carlin. J. B. (1992). Body mass index and duration of breastfeeding: a survival analysis during the first six months of life. *J Epidemiol Commun Health*. 46,559–565.

Saint, L., Maggiore, P., Hartmann, P. E. (1986). Yield and nutrient content of milk in eight women breastfeeding twins and one woman breastfeeding triplets. *Br J Nutr*. 56,49–58.

Saint, L., Smith, M., Hartmann, P. (1984). The yield and nutrient content of colostrum and milk from giving birth to one month postpartum. *Br J Nutr*. 52,87–95.

Salariya, E. M., Easton, P. M., Cater, J. I. (1978). Infant feeding: duration of breast-feeding after early initiation and frequent feeding. *Lancet*. 2,1141–1143.

Sanuki, J., Fukama, E., Uchida, Y. (2008). Morphologic study of nipple-areola complex in 600 breasts. *Aesth Plast Surg*. 33,295–297.

Sase, M., Miwa, I., Sumie, M., et al. (2005). Gastric emptying cycles in the human fetus. *Am J Obstet Gynecol* 193,1000–1004

Scammon, R. E., Doyle, L. O. (1920). Observations on the capacity of the stomach in the first ten days of postnatal life. *Am J Dis Child*. ;20,516–538.

Schaal, B., Doucet, S., Sagot, P., Hertling, E., Soussignan, R. (2005). Human breast areolae as scent organs: morphological data and possible involvement in maternal-neonatal adaptation. *Dev Psychobiol*. 48,100–110.

Schlenz, I., Kuzbari, R., Gruber, H., Holle, J. (2000). The sensitivity of the nipple-areola complex: an anatomic study. *Plast Reconstr Surg.* 105,905–909.

Scott, J. A., Binns, C. W., Oddy, W. H. (2007). Predictors of delayed onset of lactation. *Matern Child Nutr.* 3,186–193.

Semple, J. L., Lugowski, S. J., Baines, C. J., et al. (1998). Breast milk contamination and silicone implant: preliminary results using silicon as a proxy measurement for silicone. *Plast Reconstr Surg.* 102,528–533.

Sievers, E., Haase, S., Oldigs, H. D., Schaub, J. (2003). The impact of peripartum factors on the onset and duration of lactation. *Biol Neonate.* 83:246–252.

Smith, W., Erenberg, A., Nowak, A. (1988). Imaging evaluation of the human nipple during breast-feeding. *Am J Dis Child.* 142,76–78.

Sozmen, M. (1992). Effects of early suckling of cesarean-born babies on lactation. *Biol Neonate.* 62,67–68.

Spangler, A. K., Randenberg, A. L., Brenner, M. G., Howett, M. (2008). Belly models as teaching tools: what is their utility? *J Hum Lact.* 24,199–205.

Spear, S. L., Low, M., Ducic, I. (2003). Revision augmentation mastopexy: indications, operations, and outcomes. *Ann Plast Surg.* 51,540–546.

Stern, J. M., Reichlin, S. (1990). Prolactin circadian rhythm persists throughout lactation in women. *Neuroendocrinology* 51,31–37.

Strom, S. S., Baldwin, B. J., Sigurdson, A. J., Schusterman, M. A. (1997). Cosmetic saline breast implants: a survey of satisfaction, breastfeeding experience, cancer screening, and health. *Plastic Reconstruct Surg.* 100,1553–1557.

Stutte, P. C., Bowles, B. C., Morman, G. Y. (1988). The effects of breast massage on volume and fat content of human milk. *Genesis.* 10,22–25.

Surajit, N., Basanti, A., Basanti, D. (2007). Polymastia of the axillae. *Ind J Dermatol.* 52,118–120.

Taneri, F., Kurukahvecioglu, O., Akyurek, N., et al. (2006). Microanatomy of milk ducts in the nipple. *Eur Surg Res.* 38,545–549.

Tedeschi, L., Ahari, S., Byrne, J. (1963). Involutional mammary duct ectasia and periductal mastitis. *Am J Surg.* 106,517–521.

Thoresen, M., Wesche, J. (1988). Doppler measurements of changes in human mammary and uterine blood flow during pregnancy and lactation. *Acta Obstet Gynaecol Scand.* 67,741–745.

Ueda, T., Yokoyama, Y., Irahara, M., et al. (1994). Influence of psychological stress on suckling-induced pulsatile oxytocin release. *Obstet Gynecol.* 84,259–262.

U.S. Food and Drug Administration [FDA]. (2000). Breast implants: an information update—2000. Retrieved April 6, 2005 from www.fda.gov/cdrh/breastimplants/

Uvnas-Moberg, K., Eriksson, M.(1996). Breastfeeding: physiological, endocrine and behavioral adaptations caused by oxytocin and local neurogenic activity in the nipple and mammary gland. *Acta Paediatr.* 85,525–530.

Uvnas-Moberg, K., Widstrom, A. M., Marchini, G., Winberg, J. (1987). Release of GI hormones in mother and infant by sensory stimulation. *Acta Paediatr Scand.* 76,851–860.

Van den Driessche, M., Peeters, K., Marien, P., et al. (1999). Gastric emptying in formula-fed and breastfed infants measured with the 13C-octanoic acid breath test. *J Pediatr Gastroenterol Nutr.* 29,46–51.

Vorherr, H. (1974). The Breast: Morphology, Physiology and Lactation. London: Academic Press.

Watson, C. J. (2006). Involution: apoptosis and tissue remodeling that convert the mammary gland from milk factory to a quiescent organ. *Breast Cancer Res.* 8,203

West, D., Hirsch, E. M.. (2008). Breastfeeding After Breast and Nipple Procedures: A Guide for Healthcare Professionals. Amarillo, TX: Hale Publishing.

Widstrom, A. M., Christensson, K., Ransjo-Arvidson, A. B., Matthiesen, A. S., Winberg, J., Uvnas-Moberg, K. (1988). Gastric aspirates of newborn infants: pH, volume and levels of gastrin- and somatostatin-like immunoreactivity. *Acta Paediatr Scand.* 77,502–508.

Widstrom, A.-M., Ransjo-Arvidson, A.-B., Christensson, K., et al. (1987). Gastric suction in healthy new-born infants: effects on circulation and developing feeding behavior. *Acta Paediatr.* 76,566–572.

Widstrom, A.-M., Wahlberg, V., Matthiesen, A.S., et al. (1990). Short term effects of early suckling and touch of the nipple on maternal behavior. *Early Hum Dev.* 21,153–163.

Wiklund, I., Norman, M., Uvnas-Moberg, K., Ransjo-Arvidson, A.-B,.Andolf, E. (2009). Epidural analgesia: breastfeeding success and related factors. *Midwifery.* 25,e31–e38. .

Wilson-Clay, B., Hoover, K. (2005). The Breastfeeding Atlas. 3rd ed. Austin, TX: LactNews Press.

Woolridge, M. W. (1995). Breastfeeding: physiology into practice. In: Davies DP, ed. Nutrition in Child Health. Proceedings of conference jointly organized by the Royal College of Physicians of London and the British Paediatric Association. UK: RCPL Press; pp. 13–31.

Wright, D. M. (1985). Evidence for a spinal site at which opioids may act to inhibit the milk ejection reflex. *J Endocrinol.* 106,401–407.

Zangen, S., Di Lorenzo, C., Zangen, T., et al. (2001). Rapid maturation of gastric relaxation in newborn infants. *Pediatr Res.* 50,629–632.

Additional Reading and Resources

Breastfeeding After Breast Reduction website
    www.bfar.org
Low Milk Supply website
    www.lowmilksupply.org
Mothers Overcoming Breastfeeding Issues website
    www.mobimotherhood.org
West D. *Defining Your Own Success: Breastfeeding After Breast Reduction Surgery.* Schaumburg, IL: La Leche League International; 2001.
West D, Marasco L. *The Breastfeeding Mother's Guide to Making More Milk.* New York: McGraw-Hill; 2008.

Summary Interventions Based on the Maternal Anatomy and Physiology of Lactation

Recommendation

1. Breastfeeding can and should be recommended, even when alterations in breast appearance and function may be present. Precise management instructions are needed plus very close follow-up of infant weight gain.
   - Early, frequent feeds plus pumping after feedings during the early days to maximize output from whatever secretory tissue is present.
   - Infant weight checks approximately every 3 days after discharge until weight gain stabilizes.
   - Pumped breastmilk can be given as a supplement through a tube-feeding device at breast. If maximal milk production has been reached and is still insufficient for normal infant growth, supplemental infant formula can be provided through a tube-feeding device at breast.
   - Alternate breast massage can be performed by the mother on each breast at each feeding to maximize breast drainage and promote as much milk synthesis as possible (Bowles et al., 1987; Stutte et al., 1988).
   - Endocrine pathologies that result in marginal breast growth or milk output should be followed up by the primary healthcare provider and/or specialist.

2. Mothers with breast augmentation/reduction should be encouraged to breastfeed. Ascertain the location of the incisions. Ask the mother whether her breasts before augmentation were hypoplastic, had a wide intramammary gap, were asymmetrical, or herniated into the areola. These types of breasts may be at risk for insufficient milk production. Lack of sensation in the

areola and nipple also puts mothers at a significant risk for damage to the nipple because they may be unable to feel incorrect latch or sucking.

- Precise position, latch, suck, and swallow observations are necessary as well as frequent infant weight checks. Mothers should be able to state when the baby is swallowing milk and should be instructed to always check that the baby's mouth is wide open and properly latched to the breast.
- Breastmilk or formula supplements can be delivered to the baby at the breast through a tube-feeding device.

3. Assist mothers with achieving an optimal latch. Assess whether nipples are anomalous, flat, inverted, enveloped by an edematous areola, or supernumerary. Select an appropriate intervention if necessary.
- Ensure that the infant has a wide gape with at least a 150-degree angle of opening at the corner of his or her mouth, especially if the nipple is bulbous or unusually shaped.
- Flat nipples can be gently pulled out and rolled before latch-on to help them become erect. Mothers can use a modified syringe to evert flat or inverted nipples. Reverse pressure softening can be applied for an edematous areola.

4. Risk factors for delayed lactogenesis II should be identified as early as possible (Dewey et al., 2003).
- Mothers with IDDM should be encouraged to breastfeed their infant as many times as possible as soon after delivery as possible, especially during the first 12–24 hours.
- Obese mothers may need extra help in positioning their infant at breast and require close follow-up regarding milk production and infant weight gain. A rolled up towel or receiving blanket can be placed under the breast to support it and avoid the baby pulling down on the nipple or a heavy breast resting on the baby's chest if in a clutch or football hold.
- Mothers with long stage II labors or urgent cesarean sections should be encouraged to breastfeed frequently in the hospital and called or seen on day 3 or 4 to ensure adequate infant weight gain.
- Infants who fail to suck correctly or frequently enough will need a referral immediately upon discharge from the hospital with frequent weight checks.

5. Infants should be breastfed 8–12 times each 24 hours during the early weeks of breastmilk calibration.
- Avoid supplementing the breastfed infant unless medically indicated.

Chapter 3

Influence of the Infant's Anatomy and Physiology

Introduction

The newborn infant brings a unique set of anatomical structures, physiological activities, reflexive behaviors, and nutritional needs and stores to the breast-feeding relationship. The mechanical acts of latching, suckling, swallowing, and breathing must all occur in a synchronized interplay among anatomical structures, physiological parameters, and the infant's immediate environment. After birth, the fetus must transition to extrauterine life and undergo extraordinary changes in an amazingly short period of time. Some of these changes affect and are affected by breastfeeding. This chapter views breastfeeding from the perspective of the infant and the structures and functions that he or she brings to the breastfeeding process.

Functional Infant Anatomy and Physiology Associated With Breastfeeding

To breastfeed effectively, an infant must engage in and coordinate the three basic processes of suck, swallow, and breathe. Anatomical structures contributing to these processes are usually in close proximity to one another and may overlap in function (Figure 3-1). This topic is covered in depth by Wolf and Glass (1992) and Morris and Klein (2000). Knowledge of these structures, their functions, and their interrelatedness allows the clinician to assess the feeding process and to recognize anatomical or physiological deviations and how they affect the ability to breastfeed effectively (Box 3-1).

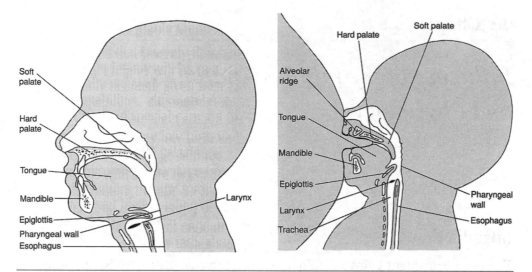

Figure 3-1   Swallowing Anatomy Midsagittal sections of the cranial and oral anatomy of an adult and an infant swallowing.

Source: Reprinted with permission from Riordan, *Breastfeeding and Human Lactation,* 3rd ed. Sudbury, MA: Jones and Bartlett; 2005.

BOX 3-1   Evaluation of Oral Structures

Tongue

Key Functions

  Assists in sealing oral cavity anteriorly and posteriorly
  Changes configuration to provide compression to nipple to increase volume of oral cavity for suction
  Bolus formation

Normal Position and Movement

  Position: Soft, with well-defined shape that is thin and flat with a rounded tip. Rests in the bottom of the mouth, and not seen when the lips are closed.
  Movement: Actively cups around the finger, forming a central groove. Movements should be rhythmic, wavelike, and in small excursions. Compression and suction should be present.

Abnormalities of Position and Movement

  Position: Protruding out of the mouth, retracting into the mouth, or humped/bunched with a thick feeling. Tip should not be elevated against the palate.
  Movement: Protrusion or thrusting during sucking, lack of central grooving, arrhythmic movements.

BOX 3-1   Evaluation of Oral Structures (continued)

Jaw

Key Functions

Provides a stable base for movements of the tongue

Helps create negative pressure by slight downward movement

Normal Position and Movement

Position: Upper and lower alveolar ridges are aligned, with loose opposition

Movement: Smooth, rhythmic movement in small excursions

Abnormalities of Position and Movement

Position: Hanging open, clenched tightly, or lower jaw retracted (micrognathia)

Movement: Wide or excessive jaw excursion, clenching or biting during sucking

Lips

Key Functions

Assist in forming anterior seal

Assist in stabilizing nipple position

Normal Position and Movement

Lips are soft, shape to the nipple, and provide slight pressure at corners.

Abnormal Position and Movement

Loose and floppy with poor seal around nipple, or tight and pursed

Cheeks

Key Functions

Provide stability to oral cavity

Aid in bolus formation

Normal Position and Movement

Fat pads visible, soft profile, with little movement during sucking

Abnormalities of Position and Movement

Floppy or stiff, pulling in during sucking

Palate

Key Functions

Hard palate: Helps compress nipple, maintains nipple position

Soft palate: Assists in creating posterior seal, elevates during swallow

Normal Position and Movement

Hard and soft palates should be intact with smooth contours.

Abnormalities of Position and Movement

Clefts of any portion of the palate, high arched hard palate, bifid uvula, decreased movement of soft palate

Oral Cavity

The oral cavity or the mouth consists of the lips, upper jaw (maxilla), lower jaw (mandible), cheeks, tongue, floor of the mouth, gum ridges, hard and soft palates, and uvula.

Lips and Cheeks

- The lips help locate the nipple and bring it into the mouth (not necessary with bottle-feeding).
- The lips stabilize the position of the nipple–areolar complex within the mouth.
- The lips help form the anterior seal around the nipple–areolar complex.
- The cheeks provide stability and maintain the shape of the mouth.
- In young infants the fat pads passively provide the majority of positional stability.
- As the infant grows the fat pads diminish and the cheek muscles provide active stability.
- The cheeks provide lateral boundaries for food on the tongue and help in bolus formation.
- The fat pads are visible through 6–8 months of age.
- Fat pads are considerably diminished in preterm infants.

The labial frenum (the terms "frenum" and "frenulum" are used interchangeably) attaches the upper lip to the upper gum. A tight labial frenum may create difficulty flanging the upper lip and maintaining a seal (Wiessinger & Miller, 1995), possibly resulting in sore nipples, decreased milk intake, and engorgement, and later creating a gap between the child's front teeth.

Mandible (Lower Jaw)

- The jaw is innervated by cranial nerve V, the trigeminal (motor).
- It provides a base for movements of the tongue, lips, and cheeks.
- Downward movement during sucking expands the size of the sealed oral cavity to create suction.
- A receding jaw positions the tongue posteriorly, where it can lead to obstruction of the airway.

- A receding jaw can contribute to sore nipples unless the chin is brought closer to the breast.
- Breastfeeding creates beneficial forces on the development of the jaws during a period of very rapid growth. The forward forces of suckling (as in breastfeeding) oppose the backward forces of sucking (as in bottle-feeding) (Page, 2001).

Tongue

- The tongue is innervated by
  - Cranial nerve VII, facial (sensory)
  - Cranial nerve IX, glossopharyngeal (taste)
  - Cranial nerve XII, hypoglossal (motor muscles of the tongue)
- During breastfeeding the tongue actively brings the nipple into the mouth, shapes the nipple and areola into a teat, and stabilizes the teat's position.
- During bottle-feeding the tongue is not needed to draw the artificial nipple into the mouth, but the tongue still helps stabilize the position of the nipple.
- The tongue helps seal the oral cavity (the anterior portion along with the lower lip seal against the nipple–areolar complex, while the posterior portion seals against the soft palate until the soft palate lifts for swallowing).
- By changing configuration the tongue is the primary means of increasing the volume of the oral cavity to create negative pressure/suction.
- The tongue provides compression against the nipple–areolar complex or teat (Bosma et al., 1990).
- The tongue forms a central groove to channel liquid toward the pharynx, whereas the lateral portions of the tongue elevate and curl to provide the framework or a cylindrical pathway for the movement of milk (Tamura et al., 1996).
- The neonatal tongue differs morphologically from the adult tongue in that it is specialized for suckling, especially in the adaptation that allows the curling of the lateral edges of the tongue (Iskander & Sanders, 2003).
- The tongue helps form a bolus and holds it in the oral cavity until swallowing is triggered.

- The lingual frenulum is a fold of mucous membrane that extends from the floor of the mouth to the midline of the undersurface of the tongue, anchoring the tongue to the base of the mouth. Tongue functioning can be impaired if the frenulum is tight or short.

Hard Palate

Wolf and Glass (1992) describe the hard palate's functions as assisting with the positioning and stability of the nipple when drawn into the mouth and working in conjunction with the tongue in the compression of the nipple–areolar complex. The contour of the palate is shaped in utero and after birth by the continuous pressure of the tongue against the palate when the mouth is closed. A palate with a high arch or one that is very narrow may be an indication of an abnormality or a restriction of tongue movement.

In the early stages of oral cavity development, Palmer (1998) described the palate as being almost as malleable as softened wax. The soft human breast in the infant's mouth contributes to a rounded U-shaped palatal configuration, because the flexible and supple breast flattens and broadens in response to the infant's tongue action. An appropriately shaped palate aligns the teeth properly and does not infringe upward, thus avoiding a contributing factor to reducing the size of the nasal cavity.

Snyder (1995) describes size parameters of the reference palate as being 0.75 inch (2 cm) in width (as measured from the lateral aspects of the alveolar ridges midway to the junction of the hard and soft palates) and approximately 1 inch from the anterior superior alveolar ridge to the hard and soft palates' junction. Wilson-Clay and Hoover (2002) measured the palates of 98 infants ranging in age from 35 weeks of gestation to age 3 months by inserting a gloved finger to a depth that triggered sucking. The length from lip closure to the hard and soft palates' juncture ranged from 0.75 to 1.26 inches (1.9–3.2 cm). Palatal variations have been described as narrow, grooved or channeled, high, flat, V-shaped, short, long, and bubble.

Soft Palate (Velum)

The soft palate is continuous and extends directly posterior to the hard palate. It does not have a bony core but rather a layer of fibrous tissue called the palatine aponeurosis to which all soft palate musculature is attached. The soft palate makes up the posterior third of the palate, is fleshy and moveable, and raises during swallowing so that food passes into the esophagus and not up into the nasal cavity. The boundary between the hard and soft palates has traditionally indicated how far back into the mouth the nipple should extend at maximum suction. However, Jacobs et al. (2007) demonstrated under ultrasound that only about 25% of infants in their study positioned the nipple at exactly the junction of the hard and soft palates. The mean distance from the tip of the nipple to the junction of the hard and soft palates was 5 mm in breastfeeding couples with no nipple pain or milk transfer issues, which illustrated that most infants did not draw the nipple–areola as far into the mouth as once thought. The nipple was not stationary during feedings with a 4.0 ± 1.3 mm movement. Hanging from the posterior edge of the soft palate is the uvula that contains some muscle fibers.

Nasal Cavity

Inspired air passes through the nasal cavity, where the palatine bone or hard palate separates the oral cavity from the nasal cavity. The opening to the eustachian tube is present in this area (nasopharynx). The nasal cavity is sealed off from the oropharynx and oral cavity when the soft palate is fully elevated.

Pharynx

The pharynx, a soft tube involved in swallowing, is divided into three regions: the nasopharynx; the oropharynx, which is the space between the elevated soft palate and the epiglottis; and the hypopharynx or laryngeal pharynx, which is the area and the structures between the epiglottis and the sphincter at the top of the esophagus. Changes in head position (flexion, extension, sideways movement) influence the diameter of the pharynx, which is thought to be related to protection of the airway.

Larynx

The larynx is composed primarily of cartilage and contains structures necessary for producing sounds and protecting the airway during swallowing. The epiglottis is a structure that rests at the base of the tongue and folds down during swallowing to close and seal off the inlet to the larynx and trachea, thereby preventing liquid and food from entering the airway. At rest, it is elevated and allows air to flow freely through the larynx into the trachea.

Trachea

The trachea is a semirigid tube composed of semicircular rings of cartilage connected to each other and to the larynx. As it descends, it branches into the two primary bronchi that go to each lung.

Hyoid Bone

The hyoid is a small, free-floating bone that is the nexus of connections between the structures involved in the anatomy and physiology of sucking, swallowing, and breathing as well as in head and neck control. The hyoid is held in position by seven connections: to the scapula, sternum, cervical vertebrae, laryngeal cartilage, tongue, mandible, and temporal bone. When the hyoid moves up and forward during swallowing, the appropriate connections help open the entry to the esophagus. The muscles attached to the hyoid are involved in the bulk of mechanical breastfeeding behaviors, and their ability to function optimally depends on the position of the head and neck.

Esophagus

The esophagus is the tube through which food passes on its way to the stomach, propelled by smooth and striated muscles that create peristalsis. It terminates at the stomach at the lower esophageal sphincter, which relaxes during peristalsis to allow food or fluid to enter the stomach. The lower esophageal sphincter remains closed at rest and provides protection from the upward flow or reflux of stomach contents into the esophagus. The oral, pharyngeal, and laryngeal structures are in close proximity during the early months of life. Because their structures and functions are interrelated, structural defects or disorganized functional problems in one area may adversely affect other areas.

Muscles

More than 40 muscles participate in the complex process of coordinating the movement of food and air through the oral cavity. Muscles act in synchrony and function to affect lip movement, allow graded jaw movements, influence the shape and action of the tongue and cheeks, elevate the soft palate to seal the nasopharynx, protect the airway, and move and clear a bolus of food.

Neural Control

Just as the anatomical structures and functions of suck, swallow, and breathe overlap, so too do the nerves that innervate these structures and functions. Six cranial nerves overlap in neural function to allow the functions of suck, swallow, and breathe to occur (Table 3-1).

TABLE 3-1 Cranial Nerves Associated With Suck, Swallow, and Breathe

Cranial Nerve	Function
I Olfactory nerve (sensory)	Responsible for the sense of smell, which also affects the perception of taste.
V Trigeminal (sensory and motor functions)	Channels sensory information from the mouth
• Maxillary branch	• (suck), soft palate (swallow), nose (breathe)
• Mandibular branch	Gathers sensory input from the cheeks, nose, upper lip, teeth
• Ophthalmic branch (purely sensory and not involved with sucking, swallowing, or breathing)	• Gathers sensory input from the skin over the lower jaw, the lower lip, and lower teeth
	Motor aspect of the nerve innervates muscles that control chewing.
VII Facial (sensory and motor functions)	Sensory fibers on the anterior two-thirds of the tongue provide information on sweet, salty, and sour tastes. The motor fibers are involved with the muscles of facial expressions and the salivary glands.
IX Glossopharyngeal (sensory and motor functions)	Sensory fibers on the posterior third of the tongue for bitter taste. Motor fibers go to the muscles used in swallowing, to the salivary glands, and innervate the gag reflex.
X Vagus (sensory, somatic, and autonomic)	Sensory information from the palate, uvula, pharynx, larynx, esophagus, visceral organs. Motor connections to the pharynx, larynx, and heart. Autonomic nervous system functions are involved in heart rate, smooth muscle activity in the gut, glands that alter gastric motility, respiration, and blood pressure.
XII Hypoglossal (motor)	Contraction of the muscles of the tongue.
	Involved in the peristaltic action in bolus preparation, sucking, and swallowing.

Reflexes

Full-term infants come equipped with a number of well-developed reflexes that aid in securing food in a safe and efficient manner.

- Swallowing is seen in the fetus as early as 12 weeks of gestation. Infants are born with considerable experience in swallowing from the routine ingestion of amniotic fluid before birth.

- Sucking is present by 24 weeks of gestation with the fetus being capable of turning his or her head toward oral stimulation. Sucking is initiated by stimulation in the infant's mouth that causes the infant to extend his or her tongue over the lower gum, raise the mandible, draw the nipple–areola into his or her mouth, and initiate the sequence of sucking behaviors. Sucking is a reflex at birth, with the infant "obligated" to suck on anything placed in the mouth. By about 3 months, sucking changes from reflexive or automatic to voluntary. Some parents see this transition as a breastfeeding infant who refuses to suck on artificial nipples (even if they have been given in combination with breastfeeding since early after birth).

- The gag reflex is apparent at 26 weeks of gestation and is quite strong in a newborn. At first it can be stimulated when the posterior two-thirds of the tongue is touched. It gradually changes such that the gag reflex is elicited farther back on the posterior one-third of the tongue.

- The phasic bite and transverse tongue reflexes appear around 28 weeks of gestation. The phasic bite reflex is seen as the rhythmical opening and closing of the jaw when the gums are stimulated. The transverse tongue reflex is seen as the tongue gravitating toward a stimulus elicited by tracing the lower gum ridge and brushing the lateral edge of the tongue with the examiner's finger.

- The rooting reflex is seen at 32 weeks and occurs in response to stroking of the skin around the mouth. This mouth-orienting reflex is strongest around 40 weeks and fades after 3 months.

Sucking Mechanisms

Components of sucking, swallowing, and breathing along with the coordination between the three activities mature at different times and rates depending on the gestational age of the infant. For example, expression (positive pressure) matures before suction. They also need to occur sequentially from the oral phase, to the pharyngeal (swallowing) phase, to the pulmonary or breathing phase while ensuring that the swallow takes place during a safe phase of the respiratory cycle (Amaizu et al., 2008). Sucking at the breast involves a complex series of behaviors that have been studied for a number of years by various means. Changing research modalities have allowed researchers and clinicians to refine their understanding of how this process unfolds.

- Ardran and colleagues (1958) were some of the first researchers to visualize the breast inside the infant's mouth. In their study the breast was coated with a barium sulfate paste, and radiographic films were made while the infant nursed. Infants were positioned on a couch with the mother leaning over the baby, which may have prevented a deep latch and partially accounted for observations that have since been refined with newer imaging techniques. Notable was the confirmation that the nipple and areola were drawn into the mouth to the junction of the hard and soft palates and that the nipple widened and extended to about three times its resting length, forming the nipple–areolar complex or a teat. These authors also described the action of the infant forming the nipple–areola into a teat and drawing it far back into the mouth, with the tongue playing a major part in the sucking process and the breast being soft and pliable enough to allow this activity. According to these authors, "Any factor which causes edema or congestion [of the breast] will probably interfere with suckling." Their study was confined to the lateral plane and could not visualize other tongue actions. It also relied on x-rays, whose hazards halted the use of this type of research.

- The use of real-time ultrasound refined the interpretation of the sucking process at breast. Smith et al. (1985, 1988) noted the following points:

  1. Failure of the lips to form a complete seal is manifested on a scan by air leaking into the oral cavity.
  2. Tongue and jaw movements compress the nipple, which is highly elastic, elongating it along with 2 cm of areola to twice its resting length and to 70% of its original diameter.
  3. During the peristaltic action of the tongue, the teat is compressed 60% more in the vertical direction and widens by 20% in the lateral direction.
  4. The buccal mucosa and musculature (sucking pads, buccinator muscle) move inward as the tongue is depressed. This maintains a tight seal on the nipple–areola, conducts the milk toward the central depression in the

posterior portion of the tongue, and allows the milk to be propelled toward the oropharynx.

- Weber et al. (1986) described both feeding movements and the coordination of sucking, swallowing, and breathing:

  1. The action of the tongue in a breastfed infant was described as a rolling or peristaltic undulation in an anterior to posterior direction, whereas in bottle-fed infants the tongue worked in an up-and-down piston-type motion; when not sucking, the breastfed infants maintained their grasp on the nipple with the teat still moderately indented by the tongue.
  2. The lateral margins of the tongue cupped around the nipple, forming a central groove.
  3. One- to 3-day-old infants showed distinct interruptions of their breathing movements when a swallow occurred, whereas in infants 4 days and older, the breathing trace appeared as a smooth uninterrupted movement with swallows occurring at the natural boundary between expiration and inspiration.

Figure 3-2, a graphic rendering of ultrasound studies, summarizes the dynamics of a complete suck cycle that was postulated from this study (Woolridge, 1986).

Woolridge and Drewett (1986) also noted the importance of taking into account both positive and negative pressures. Fluid movement during breast-feeding occurs from an area of high pressure inside the breast—created by fluid volume and the milk ejection reflex—to an area of low pressure inside the infant's mouth, where suction or vacuum is created by sealing the oral cavity and enlarging it when the jaw and tongue drop. During bottle-feeding, either suction or compression can be the predominant determinant of efficient fluid flow depending on the type of nipple and opening in the nipple. Preterm infants are able to express milk from a bottle without applying vacuum (Lau et al., 1997), and although they may effectively feed from a bottle, they can demonstrate difficulty in removing milk from the breast. This suggests that the mechanics of milk removal from a bottle and the breast are different (Meier, 2003). Although infants can receive some milk by compressing an artificial nipple, in the absence of negative pressure (i.e., in infants who cannot develop sufficient suction), adequate amounts of milk may be reduced unless modifications are made to the nipple.

Figure 3-2 Complete Suck Cycle on Breast

a. The suck cycle is initiated by a welling up of the anterior tip of the tongue. Simultaneously, the lower jaw raises to constrict the base of the nipple, "pinching off" milk within the ducts of the teat.
b. The tongue moves along the underside of the nipple, pushing against the hard palate. This wavelike action squeezes milk from the nipple.
c. & d. This wave of compression passes beyond the tip of the nipple, pushing against the soft palate. The levatator muscles of the palate contract and raise to seal off the nasal cavity.
e. The cycle ends at the posterior base of the tongue. Tongue compression and negative pressure within the mouth maintain the tongue in close conformation to the nipple and the palate, drawing milk into the mouth. A lowering of the jaw allows milk back into the nipple.

Source: Reprinted with permission from Lauwers, *Counseling the Nursing Mother: A Lactation Consultant's Guide.* Sudbury, MA: Jones and Bartlett, 2000.

Current, more sensitive ultrasound studies describe the infant sucking dynamic (Figures 3-3 and 3-4) as follows (Geddes et al., 2008; Jacobs et al., 2007):

- Negative pressure draws the nipple–areola into the mouth, usually several millimeters anterior to the junction of the hard and soft palates, forms a teat, and holds it in place with a baseline vacuum of –60 mm Hg over the entire breastfeeding.

- The motion of the tongue during a suck cycle does not show a peristaltic action (as in bottle-feeding), but rather the tongue is up and in apposition with the hard palate with the anterior tongue not indenting the nipple.

- Vacuum is generated as the tongue and jaw move down, which allows milk flow from the nipple. Peak vacuum coincides with the tongue at its lowermost position.

- As the tongue moves back up, vacuum decreases and milk flow ceases. The tongue captures the milk that has flowed into the nipple, holding it in place until the tongue and jaw lower again with the milk subsequently flowing into the oral cavity. This mechanism ensures that milk is not

Figure 3-3

Ultrasound Images of Intra-oral Cavity During Breastfeeding

MD: milk ducts that are visible within the elongated nipple

MF: milk flow that is seen ejecting from the tip of the nipple

HSPJ: hard soft palate junction where the tip of the nipple rests just anterior to this spot

Source: Reprinted from *Early Human Development*, Donna T. Geddes, Jacqueline C. Kent, Leon R. Mitoulas and Peter E. Hartmann. Tongue movement and intra-oral vacuum in breastfeeding infants, 84:7, July 2008.

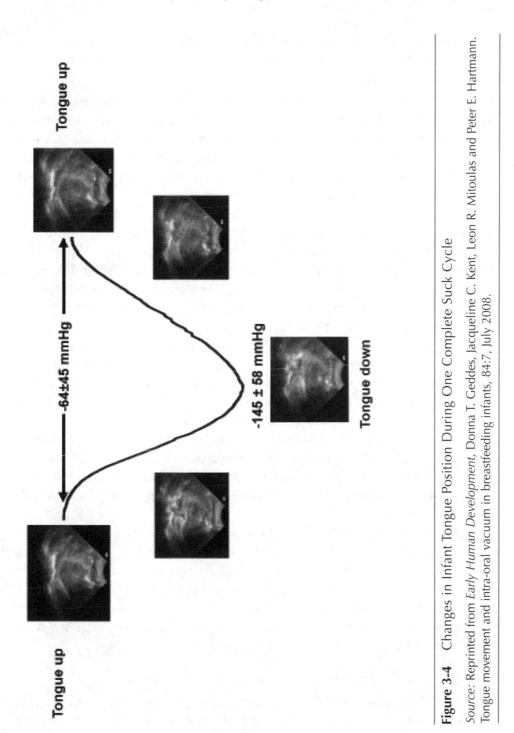

Figure 3-4 Changes in Infant Tongue Position During One Complete Suck Cycle

Source: Reprinted from *Early Human Development*, Donna T. Geddes, Jacqueline C. Kent, Leon R. Mitoulas and Peter E. Hartmann. Tongue movement and intra-oral vacuum in breastfeeding infants, 84:7, July 2008.

constantly flowing into the oral cavity but is apportioned into manageable boluses so that excessive swallowing does not interfere with breathing and oxygenation.

Mothers can remove milk by positive pressure only, as with manual expression and the milk ejection reflex, or by negative pressure, as with a breast pump. However, unless milk ejection occurs (positive pressure) when using a pump, mothers may not express very much milk. Vacuum seems to be the driving force working in concert with an intact milk ejection reflex to ensure appropriate milk transfer to the infant or maximum milk expression when using a breast pump. When mothers use a breast pump, they experience maximum milk yield in the shortest time when using the highest comfortable vacuum. Most of the milk is collected during the first two milk ejections occurring on average within the first 8 minutes after the start of the first milk ejection (Kent et al., 2008). Whereas too little vacuum may be problematic in removing milk from the breast, too much vacuum has also been shown to present potential problems. McClellan et al. (2008) studied two groups of mothers: those experiencing nipple pain during or after feedings and a control group with no complaints of pain. In spite of ongoing professional help by International Board Certified lactation consultants, infants of mothers with persistent nipple pain applied significantly stronger vacuums and transferred less milk than infants not causing pain. All components of the suck cycle were stronger, with the baseline vacuum or seal on the breast 61% stronger and the peak vacuum being 31% stronger in the infants causing the persistent nipple pain. These infants also applied more vacuum than an electric breast pump at the mothers' maximum comfort vacuum values. Mothers maintained their milk supply through expressing breastmilk if their nipples were too painful for direct breastfeeding.

Surface electromyography has shown differences in facial muscle activity between breastfeeding and bottle-feeding (Gomes et al., 2006). Cup feeding is closer to breastfeeding than is bottle-feeding, relative to the use of facial muscles during feeding. The masseter muscle is important in infant feeding, especially because its movements govern the growth and positioning of the jaw. Bottle-feeding reduces masseter muscle activity, increases buccinator activity, reduces jaw movements, and causes the tongue to retract.

Quantifying the Sucking Episode

A number of infant sucking and breast functioning parameters have been measured that are of interest in the understanding of sucking as well as in the assessment of what is in the range of normal and what may constitute a deviation or alteration from the norm (Table 3-2).

Sucking patterns change over the course of a feed. The typical 1:1 ratio of sucking to swallowing changes by the end of a feed to a ratio of 2:1 or 3:1 sucks per swallow (Weber, Woolridge, & Braum, 1986). The amount of milk transferred tends be higher from the first breast suckled and lower from the second breast. Prieto et al. (1996) showed a 58% decrease in amount of milk transferred from the second breast compared with the first: 63 ± 9 g from the first breast and 27 ± 8 g from the second breast in infants aged 21–240 days. Drewett and Woolridge (1981) measured 38.5 g from the first breast and 21.8 g from the second breast in 5- to 7-day-old infants. The volume of milk per suck also changes, with more than a 50% reduction from peak volume seen at the end of the feed on the second breast. The intake of the infants in these studies was not limited by the milk supply available but rather by the behavior of the infant in regulating his or her own intake.

Infants suck in bursts separated by rests, typically defined as a sequence of sucks with intersuck intervals of less than 2 seconds (Woolridge & Drewett, 1986). The sucking rate on the breast varies as a function of milk flow rate (Bowen-Jones et al., 1982); the higher the milk flow rate, the slower the sucking rate. The intersuck intervals (within bursts) range from 0.5 to 1.3 seconds depending on milk flow rates, leading these researchers to conclude that there was not a distinct separation of nutritive and non-nutritive sucking at breast (as with bottle-feeding) but rather a graded distribution between the two. Ramsay and Gisel (1996) measured a higher sucking rate in breastfed infants compared with bottle-fed infants and showed that infants spent 50% more time sucking when they were alert than when they were asleep. Also noted was that infants identified in this study as having feeding difficulties demonstrated shorter continuous sucking bursts and shorter sucking times than infants who had no problems feeding. Infants who later showed some feeding difficulties were already exhibiting poorer feeding ability shortly after birth.

Bromiker et al. (2006) demonstrated that full-term infants of insulin-managed mothers with diabetes had poorer sucking patterns. These infants averaged 5.2 fewer sucking bursts and 42 fewer sucks per 5-minute interval. This is consistent with descriptions by Pressler et al. (1999) of significantly poorer performance for motor processes and reflex functioning in infants of insulin-managed mothers with diabetes. These infants may be less neurologically mature, which would help explain the decrease seen in the number of sucks and number of bursts per 5-minute intervals.

TABLE 3-2   Infant Sucking and Breast Functioning Parameters

Parameter	Value	Reference
Infant negative pressure ranges		
Mean pressure	−50 ± 0.7 mm Hg	Prieto et al., 1996
Average range of pressure	−50 to −155 mm Hg	
Maximum pressure range	−197 ± 1 to −241 mm Hg	
Basal resting pressure to keep nipple in mouth	−70 to −200 mm Hg	
Infant positive pressure ranges		
Baby's tongue	73–3.6 mm Hg	
Baby's jaw	200–300 g	Kron & Litt, 1971
Full breast	28 mm Hg	Egnell, 1956
Additional pressure of milk ejection reflex	10 to 20 mm Hg	
Infant mechanics		
Cycles (sucks)	36–126 (mean 74) per minute	Bowen-Jones, Thompson, & Drewett, 1982
Duration of a suck	0.77 s	Chetwynd et al., 1998
Duration of rest	0.7 s	
Sucks per second	1.28	Ramsay & Gisel, 1996
Intersuck interval	0.5–0.6 s with no milk flow	Woolridge et al., 1982;
	0.9–1.0 s at a flow rate of 0.5 g/suck	Bowen-Jones,
Volume of milk per suck	0.14 mL to 0.21 mL at beginning of a feed	Thompson, & Drewett, 1982
	0.01 to 0.04 mL at the end of a feed	
Number of sucks per burst at beginning of feed	11 (with considerable variation)	Chetwynd et al., 1998
Number of sucks per burst at end of feed	5 (with considerable variation)	Chetwynd et al., 1998
Velocity of peristaltic wave motion of the tongue	15 cm/second	Shawker et al., 1983
Breast function parameters		
Mean diameter of lactiferous ducts before milk ejection	2.83 mm (range 1.1–5.9 mm)	Kent et al., 2003
Increase in cross-sectional area of ducts following milk ejection	6.45 mm ± 0.98 mm	Kent et al., 2003
Length of time ducts remain dilated per each milk ejection	86 seconds	Ramsay et al., 2001
Average yield for each milk ejection	35 g	Ramsay et al., 2001
Milk flow rate from breast	24.4 g/minute	Ramsay et al., 2001
Time from beginning of sucking to milk ejection	56 s	Kent et al., 2003
Time to milk ejection with pump	121 ± 11 s to 149 ± 12 s	Kent et al., 2003

Ramsay et al. (2001) found that milk intake was related to the number of milk ejections experienced by the mother rather than the total time an infant spent at the breast. Each milk ejection makes a certain amount of milk available to the infant, whereas the vacuum applied by the infant affects how fast this milk is removed.

Swallowing

More than two dozen muscles are involved in the process of swallowing. The pharyngeal swallow is thought to achieve rhythmic stability as early as 32–34 weeks gestation (Gewolb et al., 2001). To enable them to work in tandem, swallowing, sucking, and esophageal motility are linked together within a control center originating in a central pattern generator in the brainstem (Jean, 2001). Swallowing in the infant is initiated when the milk bolus accumulates either in the space between the soft palate and the tongue or in the space between the soft palate and the epiglottis. There are differences between an infant's and an adult's anatomy relative to the act of swallowing. As the infant grows and matures, the hyoid and larynx migrate downward, the epiglottis and soft palate are no longer in direct approximation after 3 to 4 months of age, and more mature protection of the airway allows the infant to cease relying on specialized anatomical structures and configurations to support sucking, swallowing, and breathing.

Swallowing can and should be assessed. Both the healthcare provider and the mother are encouraged to assess swallowing at each feeding in the early days to ensure milk transfer has occurred. Although an infant's jaw may move up and down, mimicking breastfeeding, jaw movement is not indicative of milk transfer. Signs of swallowing include the following:

- Deep jaw excursion (as opposed to shallow, biting, or chewing-like movements)
- Audible sound of swallowing
- Visualization of the throat during a swallow
- Vibration on the occipital region of the infant (a hand placed on the back of the baby's head may feel the swallow as a vibration)
- Movement of the throat felt by a finger over the trachea
- A small sound made by a puff of air from the nose
- A "ca" sound from the throat

Clinicians can assess swallow sounds by cervical auscultation with a stethoscope if they are uncertain that swallowing of milk is taking place.

- Placement of a small stethoscope adjacent to the lateral aspect of the larynx provides access to the sounds of the pharyngeal swallow (Vice et al., 1990).

- In the absence of definitive evidence of swallowing, pre- and postfeed weights could be taken to validate whether milk transfer took place if necessary.

Breathing

Breathing must also be coordinated while feeding. The airway is protected during sucking and swallowing and must remain stable (resist collapse) during feeding, because sucking and swallowing occur in a rapid sequence. The patency of the airway can be affected by the sleep state, structural abnormalities, position of the neck, rate of milk flow, maturation (preterm vs. full term), illness, or central nervous system involvement. Increasing neck flexion causes the airway to become more prone to collapse; conversely, increasing neck extension helps increase the resistance to collapse. Some infants who suffer respiratory distress or who are premature may adopt an extended head and neck position because this posture makes it easier for them to breathe.

Breathing always takes precedence over feeding. Feeding difficulties can sometimes be an indicator of breathing problems, either from faulty positioning or an anatomical or physiological aberration in the infant. Positioning such infants at the breast may include subtle adjustments in the position of the head and proper shoulder girdle support to allow infants to remain well ventilated while they feed. Although infants prefer to breathe through their noses, they are not obligate nose breathers. Infants can breathe through their mouths for short periods of time, but it is accomplished at the expense of respiratory efficiency (Miller et al., 1985).

The bulk of research looking at suck, swallow, breathe synchrony has been conducted during bottle-feeding (Mathew, 1991a; Mathew & Bhatia, 1989; Meier, 1988, 1996). Repeated airway closure during swallowing has been shown to interrupt breathing. The more rapid milk flow from soft artificial nipples with large holes results in more frequent swallowing, less frequent opportunities for breathing, and significantly increased interruption in ventilation (Duara, 1989; Mathew, 1991b). These breathing alterations are more pronounced in preterm infants but also occur in full-term infants (Mathew, 1988; Mathew & Bhatia,

1989). Sucking during bottle-feeding interrupts breathing more frequently and for more sustained durations than sucking during breastfeeding (Meier et al., 1990). During bottle-feedings, infants alternate clusters of sucks and breaths. During breastfeeding, breathing is integrated into the sucking bursts. The suck–breathe pattern during breastfeeding suggests that infants may manipulate sucking parameters to control milk flow and accommodate breathing in such a way that apnea, bradycardia, and fatigue do not occur (Meier, 2001).

Differing bottle systems can affect oxygenation and how swallows are distributed during feedings. Goldfield et al. (2006) demonstrated that swallowing during breastfeeding was distributed nonrandomly and occurred at the peaks of intraoral sucking pressures. The group of infants in this study that used a Playtex bottle system promoted a pattern of sucking, swallowing, and breathing that was more similar to the physiological norm of breastfeeding compared with the group who used an Avent bottle system. If infants need to be supplemented and a bottle is chosen to provide extra milk, clinicians may wish to choose those bottles that disrupt breastfeeding the least.

Clinical Implications

Alterations in an infant's functional anatomy and physiology related to feeding may affect milk intake to a greater or lesser extent. During breastfeeding evaluations and especially if an infant presents with feeding problems, it is important to include an assessment of the infant's anatomical structures related to breastfeeding and their functioning.

Assessment of the Lips

The lips should

- Appear soft at rest, remain closed when awake and asleep, have a bow-shaped upper lip, and have a well-defined philtrum (the median groove between the upper lip and the nose).
- Flange or flare outward when covering the areola.
- Be parted at a wide angle when measured from the corner of the mouth for proper latch. Aizawa et al. (2009) measured oral angles of breastfeeding and bottle-feeding infants, showing that the angle of the opened mouth of breastfed infants while nursing was approximately double that of infants sucking on standard artificial nipples. The angle at the corner of the mouth of infants feeding at the breast ranged from 112 degrees to 152 degrees, while infants

sucking on a standard artificial nipple had an oral angle ranging from 55 degrees to 72 degrees.

- Exert slight pressure to maintain a seal.

Alterations may include the following:

- Cleft lip: There is a great variation in cleft lip presentation, ranging from a small notch in the upper lip, either unilateral or bilateral, to a complete cleft through the lip into the nostril and through the upper alveolar ridge. A cleft in the lip compromises the seal needed to create negative pressure in the oral cavity. Many mothers fill the gap in the lip by manipulating the areola, their thumb, and the breast tissue to cover the defect. Infants with clefts of the lip are capable of generating suction, especially if the cleft is small (Reid et al., 2007). "Kissing" sounds heard during the feeding indicate that the anterior seal is being broken intermittently, which may compromise milk intake with each suck (Glass & Wolf, 1999).

- Loose, floppy, or asymmetrical lips: This problem can be associated with generalized hypotonia, partial paralysis or underdevelopment of the facial nerve (cranial nerve VII), facial asymmetry, mouth droop or immobility, with resulting failure to form a seal for the oral cavity, causing periodic breaks in suction, inability to generate suction, smacking sounds, and/ or milk leaking from the corners of the mouth. Asymmetrical lips may be seen if there is nerve damage or muscle weakness on either side of the face, causing one side of the mouth to droop and become slack on the weaker side.

- Retracted (forming a tight horizontal line over the mouth), pursed, or hypertonic lips: Increased tone may impair latch-on and active suckling, damage the nipple, and result in poor milk transfer. Pursed lips may result from feeding with artificial nipples that encourage mouth and lip closure. Lip retraction may also result from poor positioning where the neck or shoulder girdle is in extension.

- Tight (or short, inelastic) upper labial frenulum: This may impede the flanging of the upper lip over the areola. This could result in nipple abrasion, painful or improper sucking, difficulty achieving a proper latch, or awkward positioning attempts by the infant (Wiessinger & Miller, 1995).

- Lips and cheeks working together: Deviations or alterations in function in one affect the efficiency and functioning in the other.

Assessment of the Cheeks

The cheeks should appear soft, be symmetrical, have well-defined sucking pads, and maintain good tone during sucking. Cheeks with low tone or that are unstable may be pulled inward during the generation of vacuum, appearing as dimpled cheeks. In addition, they may contribute to reduced suction overall. Damage to cranial nerves VII (facial) and V (trigeminal) (either prenatally or from mechanical forces during delivery) could produce weakness or low tone in the cheeks, rendering them less able to sustain sucking during feeding. A tongue that is retracted or that lodges behind the lower gum line during sucking also produces dimpled cheeks. Dimpled cheeks indicate incorrect latch and/or suckling. Preterm infants have diminished sucking pads, such that the buccal surfaces of the cheeks may not come in contact with the mother's nipple–areola. This contributes to reduced stability and weaker structural support during feedings. Preterm infants may have difficulty both in opening their mouths wide enough and in closing their mouths over the areola.

Assessment of the Jaw

The lower jaw or mandible is typically in a neutral position at rest, with the lips touching. It moves in a smooth manner, correctly graded to engage in coordinated small excursions with a rhythmic quality. Several alterations in the structure of the jaw are possible.

- In recessed or retracted jaw structure (not caused by muscle tension or the normal slight recess of the newborn's jaw), the lower gum ridge is posterior to the upper gum ridge. The tongue is usually of normal size but is positioned farther back in the mouth. In utero, micrognathia can interfere with the normal positioning of the tongue, contributing to lack of fusion of the palatal shelves, and potentially lead to a cleft palate. Because of its posterior positioning, the tongue may be unable to move forward enough to engage in normal movements. The infant may also have difficulty opening the mouth wide enough to latch to the breast. Micrognathia frequently appears as part of various syndromes such as the following:
  - Pierre Robin syndrome, which also includes a small tongue and usually a wide, U-shaped cleft palate. Infants have a great deal of difficulty breastfeeding, usually because of the cleft. They also need to be placed in a prone position for feeding due to the tendency of the tongue to fall back into the throat, obstructing the airway.

- Hemifacial microsomia is a condition in which one side of the child's face is underdeveloped, affecting mainly the ear, mouth, and jaw. It is the second most common congenital facial anomaly after cleft lip/palate, occurring in 1 in every 3,000–5,600 live births. Involvement may range from mild, with just minor jaw asymmetry, to severe, with additional eye, vertebral, and cardiac involvement, which is known as Goldenhar syndrome. Underdevelopment of the jaw necessitates careful and creative positioning and close monitoring of milk transfer and weight gain.

- Asymmetrical jaw or deviations to one side may be the result of asymmetrical muscle tone, a structural defect, positioning in utero, or torticollis. Torticollis may be caused by fibrosis (replacement with connective tissue) of the sternocleidomastoid (SCM) muscle, resulting in rotation of the head to the opposite side. The typical right-sided head position preference when supine, cranial flattening, and long periods in the supine position with the head turned to the right may contribute to a shortening of the SCM. Infants with localized head flattening (plagiocephaly) at birth have an increased risk for other deformational anomalies, such as mandibular hypoplasia (underdeveloped lower jaw) (Peitsch et al., 2002). Boere-Boonekamp et al. (2001) examined 7,609 infants from a general population and found that 10% of infants less than 2 months of age had a preference for holding the head to one side and typically breastfeed better on one side. The infant with torticollis has spent many weeks in utero with the head turned to one side while pushing on the opposite shoulder. Breastfed infants may have difficulty achieving a comfortable breastfeeding position with the shortened SCM muscle (Stellwagen et al., 2004). Other physical features of infants with torticollis include misalignment of the eyes, asymmetry of the ears, upward tilting of the lower jaw and gum line, and limited neck movement. The mandible is tilted and not parallel with the upper jaw. Wall and Glass (2006) reported that mothers of infants with mandibular asymmetry may experience sore nipples, difficult latch, and reduced milk transfer. Chin support and use of a nipple shield may be helpful. The most expeditious intervention during the early days when an infant demonstrates torticollis/asymmetrical jaw is to position the infant at the breast with the head turned to the preferred side. Rather than switching positions to feed on the second breast, the infant is slid over in the same position to feed from the other breast. Stretching exercises may be prescribed or referral to an occupational or physical therapist may be necessary to improve the condition.

- Alterations in jaw functioning may show up as exaggerated jaw movements, jaw clenching, wide jaw excursions, clamping or biting down to achieve stability and hold onto the nipple, and low tone or poor control of the temporomandibular joint (TMJ). The TMJ may be affected by birth forces or instrument deliveries and may have an altered or limited range of movement. This joint moves in rather intricate ways: up and down like a hinge and gliding forward and down. A limited opening of the mouth caused by the inability of the TMJ to move in a full cycle of opening and closing may contribute to incremental latch-on in which an infant bites or nibbles his or her way onto the nipple rather than opening to a more optimal 160-degree angle. Wide jaw excursions beyond a 150- to 160-degree angle may be heard as smacking sounds as the tongue loses contact with the nipple–areola. Jaw instability is common in preterm infants and those with low orofacial tone, resulting in an unstable base for tongue movements. Sucking can be inefficient, and if the lips are unable to close, milk will leak from the corners of the mouth.

Assessment of the Tongue

The tongue should appear soft at rest, lying in the bottom of the mouth with a well-defined bowl shape, thin, flat, with a rounded tip and cupped sides. The tongue should neither protrude over the lips nor be seen when the mouth is closed. It should have sufficient tone and mobility to lift, extend, groove, and lateralize in a smooth and symmetrical manner. When a finger is placed in the infant's mouth, the tongue should cup around the finger, forming a distinct groove, and move in a rhythmical manner either in and out or up and down. Sucking pressure should be felt equally over the entire surface of the inserted finger. Besides playing a major role in sucking and swallowing, the tongue is an important oral structure that affects the shape of the palate, is involved in speech, contributes to the position of the teeth, and affects the development of the face.

Alterations of the tongue may include the following conditions:

- In tongue-tip elevation, the tip of the tongue is in opposition to the upper gum ridge, making it difficult for an infant to latch to the breast.

- Bunched (compressed in a lateral direction), retracted, or humped (in an anterior-posterior direction) tongue may be part of an infant's high tone. The tongue is unable to form a central groove in any of these positions.

- A tongue with low tone may demonstrate little to no shape, may feel excessively soft, may protrude over the lower gum ridge, or may appear excessively wide or large for the mouth.

- Tongue thrust (an in-and-out pattern of movement with a strong protrusion or push out of the mouth) during active sucking may be associated with high tone and result in difficulty generating negative pressure.

- Tongue alterations may be a sign of oral defensiveness or, with tongue protrusion, may be a result of respiratory problems where the infant positions the tongue forward to increase respiratory capacity.

- Tongue movement anomalies may be seen in cesarean-born infants from traction forces placed on the cranial base during delivery. The hypoglossal canal, through which the hypoglossal nerve passes, can be disrupted as the head is lifted through the cesarean incision (Smith, 2004).

- The action of the tongue can be altered by the use of artificial nipples: Whereas the shape of the human nipple–areola conforms to the inner boundaries of the infant's mouth, the infant's tongue and oral cavity are obligated to conform to the parameters presented to them by the shape and rigidity of an artificial nipple. The artificial nipple positions the tongue behind the lower gum (Figure 3-5). If a breastfed infant were to do this at

Figure 3-5 The artificial nipple does not extend to the junction of the hard and soft palates.

the breast, both the upper and lower gum would be in opposition to each other and the infant would actually bite the nipple. Such a scenario could result in extreme pain for the mother along with nipple damage and little milk transfer. High-flow artificial nipples may result in decreased oxygen levels due to rapid swallowing and limited intervals for breathing (Figure 3-6).The artificial nipple (Figure 3-7a) does not fill the oral cavity, alters the labial seal, may obliterate the central grooving of the tongue, and may result in forces that impinge on the alveolar ridges and press them inward. Even so-called orthodontic improvements made to artificial nipples still force the normal shape and physiological action of the tongue to change (Figure 3-7b).

Tongue-tie or ankyloglossia is one of the most common tongue alterations and can affect infant milk intake and the integrity of the mother's nipples. The exact incidence of tongue-tie is unknown, but studies report a 4.2–4.8% incidence in general populations of newborns (Ballard et al., 2002; Messner et al., 2000). Definitions and descriptions vary. Fernando (1998) described the condition based on both visual and functional aspects of the frenum: "Tongue-tie is a congenital condition, recognized by an unusually thickened, tightened, or shortened frenum [frenulum], which limits movement of the tongue in activities connected with feeding and which has an adverse impact on both dental health and speech." Hazelbaker (1993) defined tongue-tie as "impaired tongue function resulting from a tight and/or short lingual frenulum which may or may not involve fibers of the genioglossus muscle. Complete ankyloglossia can be defined as a 'fusing' of the tongue to the floor of the mouth."

Ankyloglossia limits the range of motion of the tongue and affects not only sucking but also speech, the position of the teeth, periodontal tissue (the tongue cannot clear residual fluid and food from the buccal cavities), jaw development, and swallowing. It has been associated with deviation of the epiglottis and larynx, harsh breath sounds, and mild oxygen desaturation during sucking (Mukai et al., 1991).

Tongue-tie is sometimes visualized during the newborn exam before hospital discharge. Mothers may complain of nipple pain and sore nipples, difficult latch, unsustained sucking, or the infant "popping" on and off the breast. Inability to transfer milk because of a mechanical difficulty can also lead to and present with insufficient milk, slow weight gain, engorgement, and plugged ducts. Observations of the breastfeeding may reveal milk leaking from the sides of the mouth, slow feeding, a clicking or smacking sound as the tongue loses

Figure 3-6   Throat Conformation for Swallowing Within the Bottle Suck Cycle

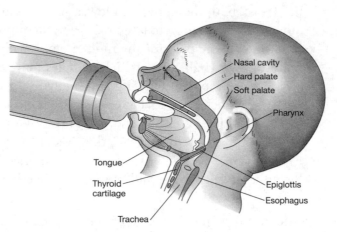

Figure 3-7
a. Traditional artificial nipple does not fill the oral cavity.
b. Altered "orthodontic" artificial nipple alters tongue position, compromising physiologic tongue action.

a.

b.

contact with the nipple–areolar complex, sucking blisters on the infant's lips, and distorted appearance of the nipple when released from the infant's mouth. Tongue-tie has been described and assessed by the appearance of the tongue, the functioning of the tongue, or a combination of both parameters. The affected tongue has variously been described as heart shaped (Figure 3-8), notched, unable to protrude beyond the lower gum or elevate to the roof of the mouth, unable to cup and form a central groove, having a short and/or tight frenulum, having a thick or thin frenulum, having a frenulum attached anywhere along the underside of the tongue, and anchored in various places from the lower alveolar ridge or farther back along the floor of the mouth. A tight or short frenulum may be less than 1 cm in length and feel tight when a finger is placed under the midline of the tongue (Notestine, 1990). During a digital assessment of the tongue, it may be felt to snap back to the mandibular floor because it may be unable to elevate or maintain extension for very long (Marmet et al., 1990).

Consistent definitions and assessment tools are scarce. Some mothers present with excoriated nipples caused by the infant's tongue being unable to engage in the peristaltic anterior-to-posterior movement used to extract milk. The compression between the gums and the up-and-down movements of the tongue may result in abrasions on the upper aspect of the nipple as it rubs against the upper gum ridge or rugae of the hard palate or on the underside of the nipple as it experiences friction over the uncovered lower gum. If the frenulum is attached at the very tip of the tongue, it can actually curl under. Tongue-tie restricts the tongue to a limited range of movements (Figure 3-9), making it problematic if the tongue tip remains unable to elevate as the jaw drops and/or interferes with the posterior tongue's movements in swallowing. Infants often engage in a

Figure 3-8
Heart-shaped Tongue

Heart-shaped tongue

Figure 3-9 Tight frenum causes problems elevating tongue.

Frenum

number of compensatory movements to facilitate milk intake, such as reliance on negative pressure to obtain milk, fluttering action of the tongue as it seeks the nipple, chewing motions, biting actions to hold onto the nipple, and head movements to help with swallowing.

Tongue-tie is usually an isolated condition, but it can also be seen as part of congenital syndromes, is more often seen in boys than in girls, and is often familial. If the mother has a small breast, if the breast is highly elastic, and if the infant can draw in enough of the areola, breastfeeding may not become compromised. However, failure to correct the tongue-tie may simply postpone problems with eating, dentition, and speech to an older age.

Assessment of the Hard Palate

The hard palate should be intact, smoothly contoured, and appear as if the tongue would comfortably fit within its contours. Several alterations of the hard palate have been noted.

- Cleft lip and cleft palate constitute the fourth most common congenital disability, affecting 1 in 700 children in the United States. A cleft of the palate can include the hard and/or soft palate, with or without involvement of the lip; can be unilateral or bilateral; and may exhibit varying degrees of severity and involvement. Clefting may occur as an isolated event or may be part of a syndrome such as Pierre Robin syndrome or Turner syndrome. A submucous cleft of the hard palate can sometimes be felt as a notch or depression in the bony palate when palpated with a finger. Although tongue movements during sucking may be normal, compression can be generated only if there is adequate hard palate surface to compress against; sealing of the oral cavity is always compromised with both hard and soft palate clefts (Glass & Wolf, 1999). Feedings are long, and if signs of aspiration, such as frequent coughing, choking, sputtering, or color change are observed, position changes may be required or assistive devices may be needed to ensure adequate intake (Edmondson & Reinhartsen, 1998). Usually, no airway obstruction or swallowing abnormalities are present, but with clefts of the palate, air is vented through the cleft, making it difficult to impossible to achieve vacuum depending on how much of the palate is involved. Infants born with a cleft lip only usually have fewer problems breastfeeding than those with palatal defects.

- Breastfeeding infants with clefts (or supplying pumped breastmilk) provides the same disease protection as for any other infant. Indeed, breastmilk is especially important in reducing the otitis media that cleft palate infants are so prone to develop. Breastfeeding encourages the proper use of the oral and facial musculature, promotes better speech development, and, when the infant is at breast, helps normalize maternal–infant interactions.

- Infants with cleft lip/palate are at an increased risk for insufficient milk intake. Weight gain, number of feedings, intake at each feeding, and diaper counts must be monitored to determine the need for supplemental breastmilk or other foods (Dowling, Danner, & Coffey, 1997).

- Poor feeding skills are common in newborns with cleft palate and cleft lip/cleft palate. Feeding efficiency is predictive of poor feeding in young infants. Neonates transferring less than 2.2 mL/min of milk and infants transferring less than 3.3 mL/min of milk are highly predictive of poor feeding skills (Reid et al., 2006).

- If the infant is unable to withdraw sufficient milk from the breast, expressed breastmilk can be provided through a supplemental tube feeding device at breast or through a special bottle feeder. Mothers will need an electric breast pump and a pumping plan to provide breastmilk and maintain an adequate supply. They may use alternate massage when the infant is at breast or hand express milk directly into the infant's mouth, but the infant may be unable to adequately drain the mother's breasts, increasing the risk of insufficient milk supply, engorgement, plugged ducts, and mastitis unless the breasts are more thoroughly drained at each feeding (Biancuzzo, 1998).

- Some infants may be fitted with a palatal obturator (a prosthesis molded to fill the cleft and provide an "artificial" palate). This device is designed to provide a solid surface against which to compress the nipple and seal the oral cavity to facilitate achieving negative pressure for milk withdrawal. It may also help to decrease the amount of time it takes for each feeding, reducing the fatigue for both infant and parents.

- Managing the infant with a cleft defect is typically accomplished by a team of healthcare professionals with surgeries, treatment, and therapy that can continue for many years. Because most oral-facial clefts are immediately apparent after birth, it is important that healthcare providers experienced with feeding cleft-involved infants be readily available to parents. Parents are especially concerned about feeding issues, and nurses caring for mothers of newborns with oral-facial clefts should quickly refer mothers to lactation specialists/consultants experienced with the associated feeding complications (Byrnes et al., 2003).

- Other palatal variations such as a bubble palate (Figure 3-10) may also impede breastfeeding. A bubble palate is defined as a "concavity in the hard palate, usually about ⅜ to ¾ in (1–2 cm) in diameter and ¼ in (½ cm) deep" (Marmet & Shell, 1993). Because of the position of the mother's nipple relative to the bubble, the nipples can become abraded, inflamed, and sore if the nipple is pulled into the bubble rather than maximally elongated to the juncture of the hard and soft palates. Weight gain problems may also ensue if the infant is unable to transfer sufficient milk (Snyder, 1997).

Figure 3-10   Bubble Palate

Assessment of the Soft Palate

The soft palate generally has thinner mucosa than the hard palate and may be somewhat darker in color. It is firm but spongy, the uvula should be in the midline and intact, and the soft palate should not sag to either side. Alterations include the following conditions:

- Cleft of the soft palate and uvula is always midline. A submucous cleft has intact mucosa lining the roof of the mouth that can make it difficult to see when looking into the mouth. The underlying muscle and bone are at least partially divided. A submucous cleft may be identified by the presence of a bifid uvula, a very thin translucent strip of mucosa in the middle of the roof of the mouth, and a notch at the back edge of the hard palate that can be felt with the fingertip. Infants may experience swallowing difficulties and persistent middle-ear disease. Damage to the glossopharyngeal nerve (cranial nerve IX) and the vagus nerve (cranial nerve X) may cause a paralysis of the soft palates, which will sag on the affected side.

- A congenital short palate can result in velopharyngeal insufficiency, as can insufficient tissue repair of a cleft palate (Morris & Klein, 2000).

- The soft palate is typically involved when the hard palate has a cleft. This can result in an open nasopharynx during swallowing and reflux of milk into the nasal cavity, swallowing of air into the stomach, and, if ear tubes are present, milk sometimes leaking through these out the ear.

Assessment of the Nasal Cavity, Pharynx, Larynx, and Trachea

These structures can be assessed with varying tests and instruments when significant deviations from normal are suspected. Alterations in swallowing and breathing or problems with the coordination of suck, swallow, breathe may alert the clinician to an anatomical or structural defect, such as the following:

- Choanal atresia—occlusion of the passage between the nose and pharynx by a bony or membranous structure.
- Vocal cord anomalies or paralysis.
- Edema from trauma such as intubation, extubation, or suctioning.
- Structural narrowing such as subglottic stenosis.
- Instability of a structure, such as tracheomalacia (softening of the tracheal cartilage) or laryngomalacia (softening of the tissues of the larynx, typically when the epiglottis bends over and partially obstructs the opening to the

larynx). Infants with tracheomalacia, laryngomalacia, and laryngotracheomalacia also have a higher incidence of gastroesophageal reflux (Bibi et al., 2001).

- Spasms of a structure such as laryngospasm.

Because these structures are not readily visible, the clinical presentation, feeding and health history, and behavioral observation of a feeding are necessary to gather data for a feeding plan and/or referral. Infants may present with one or a combination of signs and symptoms. The underlying cause of the problems may be unclear because similar signs and symptoms may reflect different etiologies. Complex medical diseases and conditions (e.g., bronchopulmonary dysplasia, cardiac problems, cerebral palsy, genetic syndromes) may also produce some of the following signs and symptoms even if they are not related to structural or anatomical defects. Infants presenting with these symptoms should be checked by their primary care provider and may be referred to a specialist or undergo testing (Arvedson & Lefton-Greif, 1998) to determine the primary problem:

- Noisy breathing
- Chronic congestion
- Inadequate weight gain
- Refusal to feed
- Apnea/bradycardia
- Coughing, choking, or gagging during a feeding
- Cyanosis, pallor, or sweating
- Wheezing, stridor, or suprasternal retractions
- Excessive drooling

Depending on the type and extent of interference with feeding at the breast, modifications may be warranted in such things as total body positioning, flexion or extension of the head, use of a nipple shield, expressing milk, and use of alternate feeding devices.

Assessment of the Esophagus

The most common disorder related to the esophagus in an infant is gastroesophageal reflux (GER), although other esophageal disorders can interfere with swallowing (e.g., upper or lower esophageal sphincter dysfunction, esophageal dysmotility, extrinsic compression, or mechanical obstruction) (Arvedson & Lefton-Greif, 1998). GER entails the passive backflow of stomach contents into the esophagus and implies a functional or physiological process in a healthy infant with no underlying systematic abnormalities. This disorder is associated with a transient relaxation of the lower esophageal sphincter, which allows gastric contents to wash back into the lower esophagus and often be regurgitated. GER (spitting up) generally peaks between 1 and 4 months of age and is seen in 40–65% of healthy infants. The supine position and the slumped seated position can exacerbate reflux during the times that the lower esophageal sphincter relaxes (Jung, 2001). Some infants with frequent GER have an inflamed throat and a hoarse cry.

Gastroesophageal reflux disease (GERD) is a pathological process characterized by clinical features such as regurgitation with poor weight gain, irritability, pain in the lower chest, possible apnea and cyanosis, wheezing, laryngospasm, and possibly aspiration, chronic cough, and stridor. In infants with more severe GERD, an abnormal hyperextension of the neck with torticollis (Sandifer syndrome) may be seen.

Infants with GER or GERD may demonstrate feeding resistance, arching at the breast, limited feeding time at the breasts, and discomfort when fed in the cradle position. These infants feed better when breastfed in an elevated position of 45 degrees or more (Boekel, 2000; Wolf & Glass, 1992). After each feeding infants should be kept upright, as in a front pack carrier, rather than slumped down in an infant seat or immediately put in a supine position. Care must be taken when using a sling so as not to increase intra-abdominal pressure.

Putting It All Together

The infant's feeding anatomy and associated physiology come together at feeding times in a complex series of actions that must occur in synchrony to ensure transfer of sufficient milk from the mother's breast into the infant. Guidelines for assessing the breastfeeding mother and infant have emphasized the importance of the visual assessment conducted in a coordinated manner (Walker, 1989). Assessment is the foundation of professional practice. Breastfeeding assessment is part of the community standard of care for hospital maternity units. The Committee on Fetus and Newborn of the American Academy of Pediatrics (2004) recommends that a number of criteria be met before any newborn discharge, including two items specific to breastfeeding:

1. The infant has completed at least two successful feedings, with documentation that the infant is able to coordinate sucking, swallowing, and breathing while feeding.

2. The mother's knowledge, ability, and confidence to provide adequate care for her baby are documented by the fact that she has received training and demonstrated competency regarding breastfeeding or bottle-feeding. The breastfeeding mother and baby should be assessed by trained staff regarding breastfeeding position, latch-on, and adequacy of swallowing.

Tools

Tools have been developed to predict future problems or to help identify mothers who are at risk for early weaning. Assessing breastfeeding activities using a systematic approach can be undertaken in a number of ways. Some clinicians either use or adapt one of a number of short clinical assessment tools that have been developed for the following purposes:

- Organize the breastfeeding assessment
- Identify both normal and abnormal patterns at the breast
- Determine whether milk transfer has occurred
- Document and chart breastfeeding behaviors
- Direct professional intervention and patient education to areas where it is needed
- Serve as a communication vehicle among professional caregivers
- Establish evaluation and teaching standards
- Reduce inappropriate supplementation
- Predict which infants are at risk for early weaning
- Recognize mother–baby pairs in need of referrals and follow-up

The use of such a tool or the modification of a tool helps objectively document feedings and may be expedient in the hospital or clinic setting. Some of the tools assign a score with cut-off points that serve as a basis for making referrals. Several have been shown to be predictive of risk for early weaning and are also used to justify the need for more intensive breastfeeding assistance. Not all tools have been shown to be valid (the tool measures what it states it measures) and/or clinically reliable (it consistently measures the intended behavior). However, the tools that assess feedings at the breast depend on the clinician's observation of a feeding and do not rely on subjective descriptions of "good–fair–poor" or number of minutes at each breast, descriptions that are inappropriate, inaccurate, and of little clinical relevance.

Infant Breastfeeding Assessment Tool

Matthews (1988) noted that Infant Breastfeeding Assessment Tool (IBFAT) scores (Table 3-3) were not predictive of abandonment of breastfeeding but rather illustrated that sucking behaviors improved over time. There was a significant difference in breastfeeding competence between infants of first-time mothers, who took a mean of 35 hours to establish effective breastfeeding, compared with infants of multiparous mothers, who took a mean of 21.2 hours to establish effective breastfeeding. A longer period to establish effective breastfeeding was also associated with the timing of drug administration in labor, as 83.4% of primiparous mothers received alphaprodine (Nisentil) within 1–4 hours before delivery compared with 45% of multiparous mothers.

The IBFAT does not assess swallowing, which can be a drawback in its use unless swallowing is included in the "sucking pattern" measurement score. Matthews (1991) also observed that mothers can use the IBFAT to assess their infants' feeding progress, with infants who score the highest having mothers who are more pleased with the feeding. Primiparous mothers had a significantly higher

TABLE 3-3   Infant Breastfeeding Assessment Tool

Component	3	2	1	0
Readiness to feed	started to feed readily without effort	needed mild stimulation to start feeding	needed vigorous stimulation to feed	cannot be roused
Rooting	rooted effectively at once	needed coaxing to root	rooted poorly, even with coaxing	did not try to root
Fixing (latch-on)	started to feed at once	took 3–10 minutes to start feeding	took >10 minutes to start feeding	did not feed
Sucking pattern	sucked well on one or both breasts	sucked off and on, but needed encouragement	some sucking efforts for short periods	did not suck

Maximum score: 12
Score of 10–12 = effective vigorous feeding
Score of 7–9 = moderately effective feeders
Score 0–6 = effective sucking rhythm not established

Source: Adapted from Matthews MK. Developing an instrument to assess infant breastfeeding behaviour in the early neonatal period. *Midwifery.* 1988;4:154–165.

percentage of feedings at which they were dissatisfied, with low scores tending to occur predominantly during the first 48 hours after birth. Mothers' satisfaction or positive feedback is important in the maternal decision to continue breastfeeding and persevere during breastfeeding difficulties. Mothers who experience dissatisfaction during the early time after birth will need more intensive support to curtail the negative feedback generated when an infant struggles to breastfeed. An infant who does not achieve a score in the 10 to 12 range of the IBFAT upon discharge from the hospital should be referred for follow-up (Matthews, 1993).

Latch Assessment Documentation Tool

This latch assessment tool (Table 3-4) was developed to serve as a quick and easy method for documenting a mother's ability to attach her baby properly to the breast and to observe the infant's sucking. Each component was defined and a plus or minus used to indicate whether the behavior was present or absent, respectively. If any component of the latch assessment is charted as insufficient, the nurse writes a progress note to detail the deviation or variance as well as to chart what corrective action was taken. Use of this form served to visually remind nurses to follow-up with mothers who needed assistance to latch their infants successfully (Jenks, 1991). Swallowing was not evaluated as a separate component but was mentioned as part of the adequate suction measurement (e.g., "suck/swallow ratio is 1–2/second"). No numerical score is assigned to the feeding effort; however, this

---

TABLE 3-4   Latch Assessment Documentation Tool

Parameter	Code + (Normal and Sufficient) − (Insufficient)
Baby's gum line placed over mother's lactiferous sinuses	
Both lips are flanged	
Complete jawbone movement	
Tongue is positioned under the areola	
Adequate suction	

Source: Adapted from Jenks M. Latch assessment documentation in the hospital. *J Hum Lact.* 1991;7:19–20.

---

tool is designed to identify breastfeeding problems so that a plan of care can be initiated as early as possible.

Breastfeeding Assessment Tool

Inaccurate, inadequate, or subjective/qualitative descriptions of breastfeeding in the hospital perpetuate inconsistencies in care and sometimes the communication of useless information. In an effort to improve breastfeeding assessment, the Breastfeeding Assessment Tool was developed to improve documentation of objective observations of breastfeeding status (Bono, 1992). Although nurses resisted filling out another form, practices supportive of breastfeeding increased with the improved awareness of the necessity of such documentation. Tools such as the Breastfeeding Assessment Tool, which includes audible swallowing as a component to be assessed, help prevent hospital staff from minimizing the importance of ongoing assessment of the breastfeeding couple.

Systematic Assessment of the Infant at Breast (SAIB)

It is recommended that each component of the SAIB (Table 3-5) be evaluated as part of an initial breastfeeding assessment and completed at least once before the mother and baby are discharged home. The SAIB delineates the essential components of a breastfeeding episode that are central to effective breastfeeding and milk transfer. It emphasizes the importance of assessing for and documenting that swallowing has occurred. Without an assessment of swallowing, it cannot be assumed that the infant has received any milk. A continuing pattern of no audible swallowing signals the need for careful investigation into the cause (Shrago & Bocar, 1990).

Mother-Baby Assessment Tool

The Mother-Baby Assessment (MBA) tool (Table 3-6) focuses on the mother's and baby's efforts in learning to breastfeed and tracks the progress of both partners (Mulford, 1992). The total number of pluses yields a numerical score that indicates the effectiveness of the breastfeeding session:

- A score of 3 or lower indicates that one partner (mother or baby) tried to initiate breastfeeding but the other was not ready.
- A score of 4 or 5 indicates that the infant was put to the breast but did not latch.

TABLE 3-5   Systematic Assessment of the Infant at Breast

Alignment

- Infant is in flexed position, relaxed with no muscular rigidity.
- Infant's head and body are at breast level.
- Infant's head is aligned with trunk and is not turned laterally, hyperextended, or hyperflexed.
- Correct alignment of infant's body is confirmed by an imaginary line from ear to shoulder to iliac crest.
- Mother's breast is supported with cupped hand during first 2 weeks of breastfeeding.

Areolar Grasp

- Mouth is open widely; lips are not pursed.
- Lips are visible and flanged outward.
- Complete seal and strong vacuum are formed by infant's mouth.
- Approximately ½ inch of areolar tissue behind the nipple is centered in the infant's mouth.
- Tongue covers lower alveolar ridge.
- Tongue is troughed (curved) around and below areola.
- No clicking or smacking sounds are heard during sucking.
- No drawing in (dimpling) of cheek pad is observed during sucking.

Areolar Compression

- Mandible moves in a rhythmic motion.
- If indicated, a digital suck assessment reveals a wavelike motion of the tongue from the anterior mouth toward the oropharynx (a digital suck assessment is not routinely performed).

Audible Swallowing

- Quiet sound of swallowing is heard.
- Sound may be preceded by several sucking motions.
- Sound may increase in frequency and consistency after milk ejection reflex occurs.

Source: Adapted from Shrago L, Bocar D. The infant's contribution to breastfeeding. *JOGNN.* 1990;19:209–215.

TABLE 3-6   Mother-Baby Assessment Tool

Steps/Points	What to look for/criteria
#1 Signaling:	
1	Mother watches and listens for baby's cues. She may hold, stroke, rock, talk to baby. She stimulates baby if he is sleepy, calms baby if he is fussy.
1	Baby gives readiness cues; stirring, alertness, rooting, sucking, hand-to-mouth, vocal cues, cry.
#2 Positioning:	
1	Mother holds baby in good alignment within latch-on range of the nipple. Baby's body is slightly flexed, entire ventral surface facing mother's body. Baby's head and shoulders are supported.
1	Baby roots well at breast, opens mouth wide, tongue cupped and covering lower gum.
#3 Fixing:	
1	Mother holds her breast to assist baby as needed, brings baby in close when his mouth is wide open. She may express drops of milk.
1	Baby latches on, takes all of nipple and about 2 cm (1 in) of areola into mouth, then suckles, demonstrating a recurrent burst-pause sucking pattern.
#4 Milk transfer:	
1	Mother reports feeling any of the following: thirst, uterine cramps, increased lochia, breast ache or tingling, relaxation, sleepiness. Milk leaks from opposite breast.
1	Baby swallows audibly; milk is observed in baby's mouth; baby may spit up milk when burping. Rapid "call-up sucking" rate (two sucks/second) changes to "nutritive sucking" rate of about 1 suck/second.
#5 Ending:	
1	Mother's breasts are comfortable; she lets baby suckle until he is finished. After nursing, her breasts feel softer; she has no lumps, engorgement, or nipple soreness.
1	Baby releases breast spontaneously, appears satiated. Baby does not root when stimulated. Baby's face, arms, and hands are relaxed; baby may fall asleep.

The MBA is an assessment method for rating the progress of a mother and baby who are learning to breastfeed. For every step both mother and baby should receive a + before either one can be scored on the following step. If the observer does not observe any of the designated indicators, score 0 for that person on that step. If help is needed at any step for either the mother or the baby, check "Help" for that step. This notation will not change the total score for mothers and babies.

Source: Adapted from Mulford C. The mother-baby assessment (MBA): An "Apgar score" for breastfeeding. *J Hum Lact.* 1992;8:79–82.

- A score of 6 indicates possible milk transfer.

- A score of 7 or 8 gives clearer evidence of milk transfer.

- A score of 9 or 10 scored consistently over a number of feedings indicates the need for only minimal follow-up

The higher the MBA score, the more effective the breastfeeding episode. A low score indicates the need for assistance from a skilled lactation specialist or consultant.

Via Christi Breastfeeding Assessment Tool

The Via Christi Breastfeeding Assessment Tool (Riordan & Riordan, 2000) (Table 3-7) assigns a score of 0, 1, or 2 to five factors. Scores range from 0 to 10.

- Immediate high risk: All mothers who have had breast surgery; all infants who have lost more than 10% of their birth weight

- 0 to 2 = High risk: Close, immediate postdischarge follow-up needed; phone call and visit to healthcare provider within 24 hours

TABLE 3-7 Via Christi Breastfeeding Assessment Tool

Assessment Factors	0 Points	1 Point	2 Points	Score
Latch-on	No latch-on achieved	Latch-on after repeated attempts	Eagerly grasped breast to latch on	
Length of time before latch-on and suckle	Over 10 minutes	4–6 minutes	0–3 minutes	
Suckling	Did not suckle	Suckled but needed encouragement	Suckled rhythmically and lips flanged	
Audible swallowing	None	Only if stimulated	Under 48 hours, intermittent; over 48 hours, frequent	
Mom's evaluation	Not pleased	Somewhat pleased	Pleased	

Total Score:

Source: Adapted from Riordan J. Via Christi breastfeeding assessment tool, 1999. Unpublished.

- 3 to 6 = Medium risk: Postdischarge phone call within 2 days; visit to healthcare provider within 3 days
- 7 to 10 = Low risk: Information given to mother and routine phone call

This tool was developed as an expedient way to assess excessively sleepy infants whose mothers received high does of labor analgesia and are at risk for breastfeeding problems. This research-based assessment tool scores early breastfeedings to establish a risk category for assigning appropriate follow-up.

Latch-on Assessment Tool

The Lactation Assessment Tool (Table 3-8) is a guided assessment form emphasizing comprehensive assessment from prefeeding behaviors through latch-on and during the actual feeding process. When used to study the elements of the feeding process that are thought to be related to nipple pain and damage, positioning errors were found to be related to pain, but no one element was shown to be the sole cause of sore nipples. Rather, many aspects of the breastfeeding episode, especially the latching process, contribute in elevating or reducing the mother's level of pain (Blair et al., 2003).

LATCH Scoring System

Mothers who use the LATCH criteria after discharge have reported increased confidence in the assessment of their infants' breastfeeding and knowledge about when to seek help for breastfeeding problems (Hamelin & McLennan, 2000). Audible swallowing is an integral part of this tool, which evaluates the amount of help a mother needs to physically breastfeed. A composite score ranging from 0 to 10 is possible in the LATCH scoring system (Table 3-9), facilitating the identification of needed interventions and improving charting (Jensen et al., 1994). Breastfeeding behavioral changes can be followed over time, and the tool can also be used by mothers as a means of continuing assessment.

Breastfeeding Assessment Score

The Breastfeeding Assessment Score (Table 3-10) is designed to be administered before hospital discharge to identify infants at risk for breastfeeding cessation in the first 7–10 days of life (Hall et al., 2002). Hall et al. (2002) demonstrated that approximately 10.5% of mothers from the study sample of 1,075 women had completely weaned by 7–10 days postpartum. Scoring with the tool ranges from 0 to 2,

TABLE 3-8   Latch-on Assessment Tool/Lactation Assessment Tool

The latching process
- Rooting
- Gape
- Suck
- Seal

Angle of infant's mouth opening
- 160 degrees
- 100 degrees
- 90 degrees
- 60 degrees

Infant's lip position
- Top and bottom lips flanged
- Top lip turned in
- Bottom lip turned in
- Top and bottom lips turned in

Infant's head position
- Nose and chin
- Chin away
- Nose away
- Chin and nose away

Infant's cheekline
- Smooth
- Broken
- Dimpled

Height at the breast
- Nose opposite nipple
- Too high
- Too low

Body rotation
- Chest to mother's breast
- Head only turned to breast

Body relationship
- Horizontal
- Angle

Breastfeeding dynamic
- Bursts 2:1 or 1:1
- Occasional 8+:1
- Sucks, no swallows

Rhythm of mother's breast while breastfeeding
- Breast moves rhythmically
- Breast stays stationary

Source: Adapted from Healthy Children Project 2000. *Latch-on Assessment Tool (LAT)*. East Sandwich, MA: Healthy Children Project.

TABLE 3-9 LATCH Criteria

	0	1	2
L			
Latch	Too sleepy or reluctant No latch achieved	Repeated attempts Hold nipple in mouth Stimulate to suck	Grasps breast Tongue down Lips flanged Rhythmic sucking
A			
Audible swallowing	None	A few with stimulation	Spontaneous and intermittent <24 hours Spontaneous and frequent >24 hours
T			
Type of nipple	Inverted	Flat	Everted (after stimulation)
C			
Comfort (breast/nipple)	Engorged Cracked, bleeding, large blisters, or bruises Severe discomfort	Filling Reddened/small blisters or bruises Mild/moderate discomfort	Soft Tender
H			
Hold (positioning)	Full assist (staff holds infant at breast)	Minimal assist (i.e., elevate head of bed; place pillows for support Teach one side; mother does the other Staff holds and then mother takes over	No assist from staff Mother able to position/hold infant

Source: Adapted from Jensen D, Wallace S, Kelsay P. LATCH: A breastfeeding charting system and documentation tool. *JOGNN.* 1994;23:27–32.

representing low, moderate, or high risk of early weaning. The highest overall score is 10, with 2 points being subtracted for each of the three variables of previous breast surgery, maternal hypertension, and vacuum extraction at delivery, creating a score range of –6 to +10. Results from the study were as follows:

Score	No. of Mothers	Cessation Rate at 7–10 Days Postpartum
≥8	705 of 1,075	5% (37 of 705)
<8	370 of 1,075	21% (77 of 370)

TABLE 3-10   Breastfeeding Assessment Score

Variable	0	1	2
Maternal age (y)	<21	21–24	>24
Previous breastfeeding experience	Failure	None	Success
Latching difficulty	every feeding	half the feedings	<3 feedings
Breastfeeding interval (# of hours between feedings)	>6	3–6	<3
Number of bottles of formula before enrollment (Babies were enrolled into the study if they were at least 20 hours old.)	>2	1	0

Two points each should be subtracted for the presence of previous breast surgery, maternal hypertension during pregnancy, and/or vacuum vaginal delivery.

Source: Adapted from Hall RT, Mercer AM, Teasley SL, et al. A breastfeeding assessment score to evaluate the risk for cessation of breastfeeding by 7 to 10 days of age. *J Pediatr.* 2002;141:659–664.

The Breastfeeding Assessment Score identifies those mothers most in need of additional follow-up. The 370 women scoring lower than 8 on this screening tool represented about one-third of the study population, pointing out the significant need for continued professional lactation support (Nommensen-Rivers, 2003). The mean age of breastfeeding cessation was 5.4 days ($\pm$ 2.2), suggesting a strong association between events occurring during the first 3–5 days of life and the early abandonment of breastfeeding.

Maternal Breastfeeding Evaluation Scale (MBFES)

The MBFES (Leff et al., 1994) consists of 30 items divided into three categories identified as maternal perceptions of successful breastfeeding: (1) maternal enjoyment/ role attainment, (2) infant satisfaction/growth, and (3) lifestyle/body image. It is designed to measure the positive and negative aspects of breastfeeding that mothers deem important in defining successful breastfeeding.

Potential Early Breastfeeding Problem Tool (PEBPT)

The PEBPT was developed to determine which breastfeeding problems rated highest among breastfeeding mothers (Kearney et al., 1990). This tool uses 23 questions with a four-point Likert scale questionnaire, giving a possible total score of 88. Higher scores indicate more breastfeeding problems have occurred.

H & H Lactation Scale

The H & H Lactation Scale and its three subscales (maternal confidence/commitment to breastfeeding, perceived infant breastfeeding satiety, and maternal/infant breast-feeding satisfaction) are designed to measure a mother's perception of insufficient milk supply, a leading cause of premature weaning from the breast (Hill & Humenick, 1996). This tool can be used prospectively with both full-term and preterm mothers.

Breastfeeding Self-Efficacy Scale (BSES)

The BSES (Dennis & Faux, 1999) is a 33-item self-report tool that assesses breast-feeding self-efficacy expectancies in new mothers. Self-efficacy is the mother's perception regarding her ability to perform a specific behavior, in this case, breastfeeding. The scale is designed to identify mothers with low breastfeeding confidence and to provide assessment information so as to assist the healthcare provider in creating care plans specific to the items identified as problematic (Dennis, 1999). The BSES was modified to a shortened version (BSES-SF) that keeps 14 items and deletes 18 items that were shown to be redundant, making it easier and quicker to administer (Dennis, 2003).

Breastfeeding Attrition Prediction Tool (BAPT)

The BAPT (Janke, 1992) uses four subscales to measure the theory of planned behavior: positive breastfeeding sentiment (18 items), negative breastfeeding sentiment (9 items), social and professional support (10 items), and control (12 items). The original tool used 49 items to help predict breastfeeding status at 8 weeks postpartum.

Neonatal Oral-Motor Assessment Scale

This scale assesses 28 characteristics of sucking and is used to diagnose both disorganized and dysfunctional sucking (Palmer et al., 1993). This differentiation is often subtle, necessitating that users of the Neonatal Oral-Motor Assessment Scale be certified in the administration and scoring of the tool. Deviations in sucking include a disorganized suck that is defined as a lack of rhythm of the total sucking activity (Crook, 1979), with the infant demonstrating difficulty in coordinating sucking and swallowing with breathing. Clinical signs of disorganized sucking include labored breathing, color changes, apnea, bradycardia, and nasal flaring (Palmer, 1993), often seen with premature infants. Dysfunctional sucking is characterized by abnormality in orofacial tone that may present as minimal jaw excursions, excessively wide jaw excursions, tongue retraction, and/or flaccid tongue (Palmer, 2002). Such situations usually require specialized referrals and follow-up because dysfunctional sucking in the neonate has been correlated with developmental delay at 24 months of age (Hawdon et al., 2000; Palmer & Heyman, 1999).

Newborn Individualized Developmental Care and Assessment Program (NIDCAP)

The NIDCAP is an infant behavior assessment system (Als, 1995) originally developed for preterm infants that assesses behavior in the autonomic system (heart rate, respiration, skin color, startles, twitches, gastrointestinal signs), motor system (muscle tone, posture, active movements), state system (level of wakefulness, clarity of state, pattern of state transitions), and attention or interaction (availability, responsiveness). The observation is designed to provide data for descriptions of an infant's strengths and weaknesses, current developmental goals, and recommendations for caregiving, including feeding. NIDCAP observations have been used to guide modifications to the infant's environment and to provide recommendations to facilitate optimal breastfeeding experiences for compromised infants (Nyqvist et al., 1996a). Most users of the NIDCAP tool are certified in its administration and interpretation.

Preterm Infant Breastfeeding Behavior Scale

The Preterm Infant Breastfeeding Behavior Scale was developed to describe the maturational steps and developmental stages in preterm infant breastfeeding behavior through operational definitions ranging from immature to mature behavior (Nyqvist et al., 1999). It is also used to reduce the delays in going to breast that commonly occur with preterm infants by quantifying the appearance of parameters necessary for full breastfeeding (Nyqvist et al., 1996a, 1996b). Maturational steps in preterm infants' breastfeeding behavior are scored for rooting, areolar grasp, latching, sucking, longest sucking burst, and swallowing.

Mother-Infant Breastfeeding Progress Tool

This tool was developed in recognition that both the mother and infant contribute to the development and success of breastfeeding (Johnson et al., 2007). The Mother-Infant Breastfeeding Progress Tool is designed to evaluate the presence of maternal and infant behaviors that are necessary for the mother to independently latch her infant to the breast. The tool is used during breastfeeding and consists of eight items (Table 3-11). Rather than using a single score to identify or predict problems and guide interventions, the checklist is not scored but is used over time to assess whether progress toward effective breastfeeding is being made. It is unclear if swallowing is included under nutritive sucking. If swallowing does not happen, then no milk transfer occurs and the infant is left undernourished

TABLE 3-11 Mother-Infant Breastfeeding Progress Tool

Mother responds to infant feeding cues	Infant eagerly roots and latches
Mother goes no longer than 3 h between feeding attempts	Infant grasps areolar tissue with mouth open wide, lips visible and flanged outward
	Nutritive sucking bursts noted
Mother independently positions self for feeding	Does not require assistance, including position pillows
Mother able to independently latch infant onto breast	Does not require any assistance to position herself or infant for latch
No nipple trauma is present	Includes redness, blistering, bruising, bleeding, or scabbing
No negative comments about breastfeeding	No comments that reflect insecurity about ability to breastfeed or satisfy her infant

Source: Adapted from Johnson TS, Mulder PJ, Strube K. Mother-infant breastfeeding progress tool: a guide for education and support of the breastfeeding dyad. *JOGNN.* 2007;36:319–327.

even though he or she may be latched to the breast and the mother can independently breastfeed her infant.

Validity and Reliability

The validity and reliability of breastfeeding assessment tools vary depending on a number of issues, including the outcome criteria under study. Some tools were constructed for charting and descriptive purposes, not necessarily for their predictive value. Efforts have been made to scrutinize a number of breastfeeding assessment tools to discover their usefulness in the clinical setting as well as in areas of policy and research. Howe et al. (2008) reviewed seven clinical feeding assessment tools, five of which related to breastfed infants (IBFAT, LATCH, MBS, Preterm Infant Breastfeeding Behavior Scale, and SAIB) and reported that none was satisfactory in terms of being empirically validated. Mixed results of reliability and validity were noted for the LATCH and IBFAT, and limited evidence of psychometric properties was seen for the MBA and SAIB.

LATCH, IBFAT, and MBA

Riordan and Koehn (1997) assessed three tools, LATCH, IBFAT, and MBA, to ascertain whether any or all were accurate predictors of adequate infant intake, especially after discharge. Each tool uses different components to assess effective breastfeeding. Interrater agreement among the tools was low on some of the components. Agreement reached 0.90 (a number on which clinical decisions can be made) on two items in the LATCH tool (audible swallowing and type of nipple), two items in the MBA (readiness to feed and positioning), and no items in the IBFAT. The study concluded that none of these tools was reliable or valid in the clinical setting. No tools used any type of swallow count or weight measurements to determine actual intake at a feeding, nor did the study use these techniques to test validity of the tools. Raters were maternity nurses who viewed videotapes of feedings and were not present in the clinical setting where the feedings occurred.

Comparisons among existing tools as a way to test validity may be difficult because they measure feedings at the breast in different ways. Thus the results may not be highly correlated to one another (Riordan, 1998).

Hamelim and McLennan (2000) assessed the relationship between the use of the LATCH tool and breastfeeding outcomes, determining that even after the tool went into use in the hospital setting, breastfeeding outcomes did not improve. The authors concluded that the LATCH tool lacked predictive ability. This result could have been related to hospital practices that delayed the first breastfeed for an average of 2 hours and to the fact that 30% of all infants in the study were supplemented with formula during their hospital stay. Individual LATCH scores of breastfeeding sessions in the hospital setting were not collected.

Adams and Hewell (1997) compared maternally derived LATCH scores and professional LATCH scores to see whether relationships existed between these measures and maternal reports of satisfaction with breastfeeding. Their results showed moderate correlations overall but significant discrepancies in specific areas. The weakest correlations between mother and professional assessments were in the areas of audible swallowing and positioning, where the maternal assessments were less accurate. These areas involve assessing the infant's contribution to breastfeeding rather than the mother's contribution. As the maternal scores increased on the LATCH, mothers ranked themselves as being more satisfied with breastfeeding. The interrater agreement between the researcher and the clinic lactation consultants for total LATCH scores was 94.4%. The interrater agreement was greater than 85% (range, 85.7–100%) for each of the five LATCH components, supporting the reliability of the LATCH as an effective tool for professional assessment of breastfeeding and for the communication of those findings. This conclusion contradicts the findings of Riordan and Koehn, possibly because the Riordan study used maternity nurses who evaluated videotaped breastfeeding sessions, whereas this study used lactation consultants who were physically present to evaluate each feeding.

LATCH/IBFAT and MBFES/PEBPT

The LATCH and IBFAT tools and the MBFES and PEBPT tools were assessed to see whether a relationship existed between scores on the LATCH/IBFAT breastfeeding assessment and maternal satisfaction (MBFES) and breastfeeding problems (PEBPT) experienced at 1 week postpartum (Schlomer et al., 1999). A moderate association was seen: As the scores on both the LATCH and IBFAT increased, maternal satisfaction scores increased and breastfeeding problem scores tended to decrease.

The LATCH tool was assessed for its validity in predicting breastfeeding status at 6 weeks postpartum. Mothers who scored lower on the comfort domain (engorged, cracked, or bleeding nipples) were less likely to be breastfeeding at 6 weeks, despite their intention to feed at least that long (Riordan et al., 2001). The LATCH tool proved useful in identifying the need for follow-up with breastfeeding mothers at risk for early weaning because of sore nipples. The authors recommend that mothers who score 2 or lower on the comfort measure be closely followed after discharge.

Riordan and coworkers (1994) tested the validity and reliability of the MBFES as a way to directly measure maternal satisfaction with breastfeeding. The MBFES scale and subscales were positively correlated with the length of time the mother intended to breastfeed as well as the length of time she actually breastfed. Maternal satisfaction with breastfeeding was also positively linked to the length of time mothers intended to breastfeed. The MBFES was found to be a valid and reliable tool and was useful for measuring outcomes of interventions such as breastfeeding classes or breastfeeding rounds.

Low breastfeeding satisfaction as measured by the MBFES appeared to be the most important predictor of weaning at survey ages of 6 weeks and 3 months, even after adjusting for other breastfeeding experiences (Cooke et al., 2003). Most breastfeeding problems were not predictive of weaning. Mothers with low breastfeeding satisfaction scores were 3–15 times more likely to wean during the 2-week, 6-week, and 3-month survey periods in the Cooke study.

H & H Lactation Scale

The H & H Lactation Scale and its three subscales were found to have a high degree of reliability as well as concurrent and predictive validity when used prospectively with breastfeeding mothers of both full-term and preterm infants (Hill & Humenick, 1996). The tool's predictive ability suggested that a mother's perception of insufficient milk supply was most closely tied to her perception of infant satiety.

BSES

Predictive validity for the BSES was demonstrated with positive correlations between BSES scores and infant feeding patterns at 6 weeks postpartum. The BSES was found to be valid and reliable in predicting which women would still be breastfeeding at 6 weeks (Dennis & Faux, 1999). In other words, the higher the BSES score, the more likely the mother would be exclusively breastfeeding at 6 weeks postpartum. The BSES was also shown to be significantly related to breastfeeding duration and intensity (exclusivity).

Low antenatal breastfeeding self-efficacy scores were positively related to bottle-feeding at 1 week postpartum. High self-efficacy scores at 1 week postpartum were related to mothers being more likely to continue to breastfeed until 4 months postpartum and to do so exclusively (Blyth et al., 2002). The BSES has been translated into Spanish and replicated in a sample of 100 Puerto Rican women. It was found to be a valid and reliable measure of breastfeeding confidence among Puerto Rican mothers (Torres et al., 2003). This tool has also been translated into Mandarin Chinese and shown to be a reliable and valid instrument when administered to 186 Chinese mothers (Dai & Dennis, 2003). The short form, BSES-SF, proved both valid and reliable in identifying mothers who needed additional interventions as well as pointing out that cesarean-delivered mothers had lower self-efficacy in breastfeeding than vaginally delivered mothers (Dennis, 2003).

BAPT

Janke (1994) established construct validity of the BAPT by factor analysis. The original BAPT was able to predict breastfeeding status at 8 weeks in 73% of the mother studies (Janke, 1994). Shortening the instrument increased its reliability scores while maintaining adequate prediction of early attrition. The modified BAPT was an effective predictor of 78% of women who stopped breastfeeding before 8 weeks and 68% of those who were still breastfeeding at that time (Dick et al., 2002). These results were consistent with Wambach's results that showed a mother's attitude and sense of control were the strongest predictors of breast-feeding behavior (Wambach, 1997). Evans et al. (2004) determined that the BAPT was not an effective predictor of early breastfeeding attrition at either the prenatal or postpartum administration of the tool.

Summary: The Design in Nature

The human infant, although born immature in many regards, is uniquely adapted to secure food and nurturance from the maternal breast right from the start. Alterations in the infant's anatomy and physiology may temporarily (or rarely permanently) affect his or her ability to feed at the breast, but breastmilk can almost always be fed to the infant. Prompt recognition of deviations and appropriate referrals and follow-up often permit breastfeeding or the provision of breastmilk in even the most extreme situations. All infants benefit from human milk, especially in the presence of anatomical or physiological compromise.

References

Adams, D., Hewell, S. (1997). Maternal and professional assessment of breastfeeding. *J Hum Lact.* 13: 279–283.

Aizawa, M., Mizuno, K., Tamura, M. (2009). Neonatal sucking behavior -comparison of perioral movement during breastfeeding and bottle feeding. *Pediatr Int.* Accepted article [ePub ahead of print]

Als, H. (1995). Manual for the Naturalistic Observation of Newborn Behavior. Newborn Individualized Developmental Care and Assessment Program (NIDCAP). Boston: Harvard Medical School.

Amaizu, N., Shulman, R. J., Schanler, R. J., Lau, C. (2008). Maturation of oral feeding skills in preterm infants. *Acta Paediatr.* 97:61–67.

American Academy of Pediatrics, Committee on Fetus and Newborn. (2004). Hospital stay for healthy term newborns. *Pediatrics.* 113:1434–1436.

Ardran, G. M., Kemp, F. H., Lind, J. (1958). A cineradiographic study of breast feeding. *Br J Radiol.* 31: 156–162.

Arvedson, J. C., Lefton-Greif, M, A. (1998). Pediatric Videofluoroscopic Swallow Studies. San Antonio, TX: Communication Skill Builders.

Ballard, J. L., Auer, C. E., Khoury, J. C. (2002). Ankyloglossia: Assessment, incidence, and effect of frenuloplasty on the breastfeeding dyad. *Pediatrics.* 110:e63. Retrieved August 23, 2005 from www.pediatrics. org/cgi/content/full/110/5/e63

Biancuzzo, M. (1998). Yes! Infants with clefts can breastfeed. *AWHONN Lifelines.* 2:45–49.

Bibi, H., Khvolis, E., Shoseyov, D., et al. (2001). The prevalence of gastroesophageal reflux in children with tracheomalacia and laryngomalacia. *Chest.* 119:409–413.

Blair, A., Cadwell, K., Turner-Maffei, C., Brimdyr, K. (2003). The relationship between positioning, the breastfeeding dynamic, the latching process and pain in breastfeeding mothers with sore nipples. *Breastfeeding Rev.* 11:5–10.

Blyth, R., Creedy, D. K., Dennis, C.-L., et al. (2002). Effect of maternal confidence on breastfeeding duration: an application of breastfeeding self-efficacy theory. *Birth.* 29:278–284.

Boekel, S. (2000). Gastroesophageal Reflux Disease (GERD) and the Breastfeeding Baby. Independent Study Module. Raleigh, NC: International Lactation Consultant Association.

Boere-Boonekamp, M., van der Linden-Kuiper, L. (2001). Positional preference: prevalence in infants and follow-up after two years. *Pediatrics.* 107:339–343.

Bono, B. J. (1992). Assessment and documentation of the breastfeeding couple by health care professionals. *J Hum Lact.* 8:17–22.

Bosma, J. F., Hepburn, L. G., Josell, S. D., Baker, K. (1990). Ultrasound demonstration of tongue motions during suckle feeding. *Dev Med Child Neurol.* 32:223–229.

Bowen-Jones, A., Thompson, C., Drewett, R. F. (1982). Milk flow and sucking rate during breastfeeding. *Devel Med Child Neurol.* 24:626–633.

Bromiker, R., Rachamim, A., Hammerman, C., Schimmel, M., Kaplan, M., Medoff-Cooper, B. (2006). Immature sucking patterns in infants of mothers with diabetes. *J Pediatr.* 149:640–643.

Byrnes, A. L., Berk, N. W., Cooper, M. E., Marazita, M. L. (2003). Parental evaluation of informing interviews for cleft lip and/or palate. *Pediatrics.* 112:308–313.

Chetwynd, A. G., Diggle, P. J., Drewett, R. F., Young, B. (1998). A mixture model for sucking patterns of breastfed infants. *Stats Med.* 17:395–405.

Cooke, M., Sheehan, A., Schmied, V. (2003). A description of the relationship between breastfeeding experiences, breastfeeding satisfaction, and weaning in the first 3 months after birth. *J Hum Lact.* 19:145–156.

Crook, C. K. (1979). The organization and control of infant sucking. *Adv Child Dev Behav.* 14:209–252.

Dai, X., Dennis, C. L. (2003). Translation and validation of the Breastfeeding Self-Efficacy Scale into Chinese. *J Midwifery Womens Health.* 48:350–356.

Dennis, C.-L. (2003). The Breastfeeding Self-Efficacy Scale: psychometric assessment of the short form. *JOGNN.* 32:734–744.

Dennis, C.-L. (1999). Theoretical underpinnings of breastfeeding confidence: A self-efficacy framework [Commentary]. *J Hum Lact.* 15:195–201.

Dennis, C.-L., Faux, S. (1999). Development and psychometric testing of the Breastfeeding Self-Efficacy Scale. *Res Nurs Health.* 22:399–409.

Dick, M. J., Evans, M. L., Arthurs, J. B., et al. (2002). Predicting early breastfeeding attrition. *J Hum Lact.* 18: 21–28.

Dowling, D., Danner, S., Coffey, P. (1997). Breastfeeding the Infant with Special Needs. White Plains, NY: March of Dimes.

Drewett, R. F., Woolridge, M. (1981). Milk taken by human babies from the first and second breast. *Physiol Behav.* 26:327–329.

Duara, S. (1989). Oral feeding containers and their influence on intake and ventilation in preterm infants. *Biol Neonate.* 56:270–276.

Edmondson, R., Reinhartsen, D. (1998). The young child with cleft lip and palate: intervention needs in the first three years. *Inf Young Children.* 11:12–20.

Egnell, E. (1956). The mechanism of different methods of emptying the female breast. *J Swed Med Assoc.* 40:1–8.

Evans, M. L., Dick, M. J., Lewallen, L. P., Jeffrey, C. (2004). Modified breastfeeding attrition prediction tool: prenatal and postpartum tests. *J Perinatal Educ.* 13:1–8.

Fernando, C. (1998). Tongue Tie: From Confusion to Clarity. Sydney, Australia: Tandem Publications.

Geddes, D. T., Kent, J. C., Mitoulas, L. R., Hartmann, P. E. (2008). Tongue movement and intra-oral vacuum in breastfeeding infants. *Early Hum Dev.* 84:471–477.

Gewolb, I. H., Vice, F. L., Schweitzer-Kenney, E. L., et al. (2001). Developmental patterns of rhythmic suckle and swallow in preterm infants. *Dev Med Child Neurol.* 43:22–27.

Glass, R. P., Wolf, L. S. (1999). Feeding management of infants with cleft lip and palate and micrognathia. *Inf Young Children.* 12:70–81.

Goldfield, E. C., Richardson, M. J., Lee, K. G., Margetts, S. (2006). Coordination of sucking, swallowing, and breathing and oxygen saturation during early infant breastfeeding and bottle-feeding. *Pediatr Res.* 59:1–7.

Gomes, C. F., Trezza, E. M. C., Murade, E. C. M., Padovani, C. R. (2006). Surface electromyography of facial muscles during natural and artificial feeding of infants. *J Pediatr (Rio J).* 82:103–109.

Hall, R. T., Mercer, A. M., Teasley, S. L., et al. (2002). A breastfeeding assessment score to evaluate the risk for cessation of breastfeeding by 7 to 10 days of age. *J Pediatr.* 141:659–664.

Hamelin, K., McLennan, J. (2000). Examination of the use of an in-hospital breastfeeding assessment tool. *Mother Baby J.* 5:29–37.

Hawdon, J. M., Beauregard, N., Kennedy, G. (2000). Identification of neonates at risk of developing feeding problems in infancy. *Dev Med Child Neurol.* 42:235–239.

Hazelbaker, A. K. (1993). The Assessment Tool for Lingual Frenulum Function (ATLFF): use in a lactation consultant private practice. Thesis. Pasadena, CA: Pacific Oaks College.

Hill, P., Humenick, S. Development of the H & H Lactation Scale. *Nurs Res.* 45:136–140.

Howe, T.-H., Lin, K.-C., Fu, C.-P., Su, C.-T., Hsieh, C.-L.(2008). A review of psychometric properties of feeding assessment tools used in neonates. *JOGNN.* 37:338–349.

Iskander, A., Sanders, I. (2003). Morphological comparison between neonatal and adult human tongues. *Ann Otol Rhinol Laryngol.* 112:768–776.

Jacobs, L. A., Dickinson, J. E., Hart, P. D., Doherty, D. A., Faulkner, S. J. (2007). Normal nipple position in term infants measured on breastfeeding ultrasound. *J Hum Lact.* 23:52–59.

Janke, J. R. (1994). Development of the Breastfeeding Attrition Prediction Tool. *Nurs Res.* 43:100–104.

Janke, J. R. (1992). Prediction of breastfeeding attrition: Instrument development. *Appl Nurs Res.* 5:48–53.

Jean, A. (2001). Brain stem control of swallowing: Neuronal network and cellular mechanisms. *Physiol Rev.* 81:929–969.

Jenks, M. (1991). Latch assessment documentation in the hospital nursery. *J Hum Lact.* 7:19–20.

Jensen, D., Wallace, S., Kelsay, P. (1994). LATCH: a breastfeeding charting system and documentation tool. *JOGNN.* 23:27–32.

Johnson, T. S., Mulder, P. J., Strube, K. (2007). Mother-infant breastfeeding progress tool: a guide for education and support of the breastfeeding dyad. *JOGNN.* 36:319–327.

Jung, A. D. (2001). Gastroesophageal reflux in infants and children. *Am Fam Physician*. 64:1853–1860.

Kearney, M., Cronenwett, L., Barrett, J. (1990). Breastfeeding problems in the first week postpartum. *Nurs Res*. 39:90–95.

Kent, J. C., Mitoulas, L. R., Cregan, M. D., et al. (2008). Importance of vacuum for breastmilk expression. *Breastfeeding Med*. 3:11–19.

Kent, J. C., Ramsay, D. T., Doherty, D., et al. (2003). Response of breasts to different stimulation patterns of an electric breast pump. *J Hum Lact*. 19:179–186.

Kron, R. E., Litt, M. (1971). Fluid mechanics of nutritive sucking behaviour: the suckling infant's oral apparatus analysed as a hydraulic pump. *Med Biol Eng*. 9:45–60.

Lau, C., Sheena, H. R., Shulman, R. J., Schanler, R. J. (1997). Oral feeding in low birth weight infants. *J Pediatr*. 130:561–569.

Leff, E., Jeffries, S., Gagne, M. (1994). The development of the Maternal Breastfeeding Evaluation Scale. *J Hum Lact*. 10:105–111.

Marmet, C., Shell, E. (1993). Lactation Forms: A Guide to Lactation Consultant Charting. Encino, CA: Lactation Institute and Breastfeeding Clinic; pp. 4–7.

Marmet, C., Shell, E., Marmet, R. (1990). Neonatal frenotomy may be necessary to correct breastfeeding problems. *J Hum Lact*. 6:117–121.

Mathew, O. P. (1988). Respiratory control during nipple feeding in preterm infants. *Pediatr Pulmonol*. 5:220–224.

Mathew, O. P. (1991a). Science of bottle feeding. *J Pediatr*. 119:511–519.

Mathew, O. P. (1991b). Breathing patterns of preterm infants during bottle feeding: Role of milk flow. *J Pediatr*. 119:960–965.

Mathew, O. P., Bhatia, J. (1989). Sucking and breathing patterns during breast- and bottle-feeding in term neonates. *Am J Dis Child*. 143:588–592.

Matthews, M. K. (1988). Developing an instrument to assess infant breastfeeding behaviour in the early neonatal period. *Midwifery*. 4:154–165.

Matthews, M. K. (1991). Mothers' satisfaction with their neonates' breastfeeding behaviors. *JOGNN*. 20:49–55.

Matthews, M. K. (1993). Assessments and suggested interventions to assist newborn breastfeeding behavior. *J Hum Lact*. 9:243–248.

McClellan, H. L., Geddes, D. T., Kent, J. C., Garbin, C. P., Mitoulas, L. R., Hartmann, P. E. (2008). Infants of mothers with persistent nipple pain exert strong sucking vacuums. Acta *Paediatr*. 97:1205–1209.

Meier, P. P. (1988). Bottle and breastfeeding: effects on transcutaneous oxygen pressure and temperature in preterm infants. *Nurs Res*. 37:36–41.

Meier, P. P. (1996). Suck-breathe patterning during bottle and breastfeeding for preterm infants. In: David TJ, ed. Major Controversies in Infant Nutrition. International Congress and Symposium Series 215. London: Royal Society of Medicine Press; pp. 9–20.

Meier, P. P. (2001). Breastfeeding in the special care nursery: Prematures and infants with medical problems. *Pediatr Clin North Am*. 48:425–442.

Meier, P. P. (2003). Supporting lactation in mothers with very low birth weight infants. *Pediatr Ann*. 32:317–325.

Meier, P. P., Lysakowski, T. Y., Engstrom, J. L., et al. (1990). The accuracy of test-weighing for preterm infants. *J Pediatr Gastroenterol Nutr*. 10:62–65.

Messner, A. H., Lalakea, L., Aby, J., et al. (2000). Ankyloglossia: incidence and associated feeding difficulties. *Arch Otolaryngol Head Neck Surg*. 126:36–39.

Miller, M. J., Martin, R. J., Carlo, W. A., et al. (1985). Oral breathing in newborn infants. *J Pediatr*. 107:465–469.

Morris, S. E., Klein, M. D. (2000). Pre-Feeding Skills: A Comprehensive Resource for Mealtime Development. 2nd ed. San Antonio, TX: Therapy Skill Builders.

Mukai, S., Mukai, C., Asaoka, K. (1991). Ankyloglossia with deviation of the epiglottis and larynx. *Ann Otol Rhinol Laryngol.* 100:3–20.

Mulford, C. (1992). The Mother-Baby Assessment (MBA): An "Apgar score" for breastfeeding. *J Hum Lact.* 8:79–82.

Nommsen-Rivers, L. (2003). Research Spotlight. Identifying mothers at risk for early abandonment of breastfeeding. *J Hum Lact.* 19:217–218.

Notestine, G. E. (1990). The importance of the identification of ankyloglossia (short lingual frenulum) as a cause of breastfeeding problems. *J Hum Lact.* 6:113–115.

Nyqvist, K. H., Ewald, U., Sjoden, P.-O. (1996a). Supporting a preterm infant's behaviour during breast-feeding: A case report. *J Hum Lact.* 12:221–228.

Nyqvist, K. H., Rubertsson, C., Ewald, U., Sjoden, P.-O. (1996b). Development of the Preterm Infant Breastfeeding Behavior Scale (PIBBS): a study of nurse–mother agreement. *J Hum Lact.* 12:207–219.

Nyqvist, K. H., Sjoden, P.-O., Ewald, U. (1999). The development of preterm infants' breastfeeding behavior. *Early Hum Dev.* 55:247–264.

Page, D. C. (2001). Breastfeeding and early functional jaw orthopedics (an introduction). *Funct Orthod.* 18:24–27.

Palmer, B. (1998). The influence of breastfeeding on the development of the oral cavity: A commentary. *J Hum Lact.* 14:93–98.

Palmer, M. M. (1993). Identification and management of the transitional suck pattern in premature infants. *J Perinat Neonat Nurs.* 7:66–75.

Palmer, M. M. (2002). Recognizing and resolving infant suck difficulties. *J Hum Lact.* 18:166–167.

Palmer, M. M., Crawley, K., Blanco, I. (1993). The Neonatal Oral-Motor Assessment Scale: a reliability study. *J Perinatol.* 13:28–35.

Palmer, M. M., Heyman, M. B. (1999). Developmental outcome for neonates with dysfunctional and dis-organized sucking patterns: preliminary findings. Infant-Toddler Intervention: *Transdisc J.* 9:299–308.

Peitsch, W. K., Keefer, C. H., LaBrie, R. A., Mulliken, J. B. (2002). Incidence of cranial asymmetry in healthy newborns. *Pediatrics.* 110(6). Retrieved February 3, 2005 from www.pediatrics.org/cgi/content/full/110/6/e72

Pressler, J. L., Hepworth, J. T., LaMontagne, L. L., Sevcik, R. H., Hesselink, L. F. (1999). Behavioral responses of newborns of insulin-dependent and nondiabetic healthy mothers. *Clin Nurs Res.* 8:103–118.

Prieto, C. R., Cardenas, H., Salvatierra, A. M., et al. (1996). Sucking pressure and its relationship to milk transfer during breastfeeding in humans. *J Reprod Fertil.* 108:69–74.

Ramsay, D. T., Kent, J. C., Owens, R. A., Hartmann, P. E. (2001). Ultrasound imaging of milk ejection in the human lactating breast. Society for Reproductive Biology, Proceedings of the Thirty-Second Annual Conference, Gold Coast, Queensland, September 2001, Abstract 30.

Ramsay, M., Gisel, E. G. (1996). Neonatal sucking and maternal feeding practices. *Dev Med Child Neurol.* 38:34–47.

Reid, J., Reilly, S., Kilpatrick, N. (2007). Sucking performance of babies with cleft conditions. *Cleft Palate Craniofac J.* 44:312–320.

Reid, J., Kilpatrick, N., Reilly, S. (2006). A prospective, longitudinal study of feeding skills in a cohort of babies with cleft conditions. *Cleft Palate-Craniofac J.* 43:702–709.

Riordan, J. (1998). Predicting breastfeeding problems. *AWHONN Lifelines.* 2:31–33.

Riordan, J., Bibb, D., Miller, M., Rawlins, T. (2001). Predicting breastfeeding duration using the LATCH breastfeeding assessment tool. *J Hum Lact.* 17:20–23.

Riordan, J. M., Koehn, M. (1997). Reliability and validity testing of three breastfeeding assessment tools. *JOGNN.* 26:181–187.

Riordan, J., Riordan, S. (2000). The Effect of Labor Epidurals on Breastfeeding. Unit 4/Lactation Consultant Series Two. Schaumburg, IL: La Leche League International.

Riordan, J. M., Woodley, G., Heaton, K. (1994). Testing validity and reliability of an instrument which measures maternal evaluation of breastfeeding. *J Hum Lact*. 10:231–235.

Schlomer, J. A., Kemmerer, J., Twiss, J. J. (1999). Evaluating the association of two breastfeeding assessment tools with breastfeeding problems and breastfeeding satisfaction. *J Hum Lact*. 15:35–39.

Shawker, T. H., Sonies, B., Stone, M., Baum, B. J. (1983). Real-time ultrasound visualization of tongue movement during swallowing. *J Clin Ultrasound*. 11:485–490.

Shrago, L., Bocar, D. (1990). The infant's contribution to breastfeeding. *JOGNN*. 19:209–215.

Smith, L. J. (2004). Physics, forces, and mechanical effects of birth on breastfeeding. In: Kroeger M, ed. Impact of Birthing Practices on Breastfeeding. Sudbury, MA: Jones and Bartlett, pp. 119–145.

Smith, W. L., Erenberg, A., Nowak, A. (1988). Imaging evaluation of the human nipple during breastfeeding. *Am J Dis Child*. 142:76–78.

Smith, W. L., Erenberg, A., Nowak, A., et al. (1985). Physiology of sucking in the normal term infant using real-time US. *Radiology*. 156:379–381.

Snyder, J. B. (1995). Variation in infant palatal structure and breastfeeding. A project submitted in partial fulfillment of the requirements for the degree master of arts in human development specialization in lactation. Encino, CA: Lactation Institute.

Snyder, J. B. (1997). Bubble palate and failure to thrive: A case report. *J Hum Lact*. 13:139–143.

Stellwagen, L., Hubbard, E., Vaux, K. (2004). Look for the "stuck baby" to identify congenital torticollis. *Contemp Pediatr*. 21–55.

Tamura, Y., Horikawa, Y., Yoshida, S. (1996). Coordination of tongue movements and peri-oral muscle activities during nutritive sucking. *Dev Med Child Neurol*. 38:503–510.

Torres, M. M., Torres, R. R. D., Rodriguez, A. M. P., Dennis, C.-L. (2003). Translation and validation of the Breastfeeding Self-Efficacy Scale into Spanish: data from a Puerto Rican population. *J Hum Lact*. 19:35–42.

Vice, F. L., Heinz, J. M., Giuriati, G., et al. (1990). Cervical auscultation of suckle feeding in newborn infants. *Dev Med Child Neurol*. 32:760–768.

Walker, M. (1989). Functional assessment of infant breastfeeding patterns. *Birth*. 16:140–147.

Wall, V., Glass, R. (2006). Mandibular asymmetry and breastfeeding problems: experience from 11 cases. *J Hum Lact*. 22:328–334.

Wambach, K. A. (1997). Breastfeeding intention and outcome: a test of the theory of planned behavior. *Res Nurs Health*. 20:51–59.

Weber, F., Woolridge, M. W., Baum, J. D. (1986). An ultrasonographic study of the organisation of sucking and swallowing by newborn infants. *Dev Med Child Neurol*. 28:19–24.

Wiessinger, D., Miller, M. (1995). Breastfeeding difficulties as a result of tight lingual and labial frena: a case report. *J Hum Lact*. 11:313–316.

Wilson-Clay, B., Hoover, K. (2002). The Breastfeeding Atlas. 2nd ed. Austin, TX: LactNews Press.

Wolf, L. S., Glass, R. P. (1992). Feeding and Swallowing Disorders in Infancy: Assessment and Management. Tucson, AZ: Therapy Skill Builders.

Woolridge, M., Drewett, R. (1986). Sucking rates of human babies on the breast: a study using direct observation and intraoral pressure measurements. *J Reprod Infant Psychol*. 4:69–75.

Woolridge, M. W. (1986). The "anatomy" of infant sucking. *Midwifery*. 2:164–171.

Woolridge, M. W., How, T. V., Drewett, R. F., et al. (1982). The continuous measurement of milk intake at a feed in breastfed babies. *Early Hum Dev*. 6:365–373.

Chapter 4

Influence of Peripartum Factors, Birthing Practices, and Early Caretaking Behaviors

Introduction

The environment in which an infant lives before, during, and immediately after birth can affect breastfeeding through a number of mechanisms. Early sucking behaviors can be affected by medications that a mother receives during her pregnancy and during her delivery. Instrument-assisted deliveries can affect the mechanics of breastfeeding. Separation, supplementation, crying, and tight wrapping diminish breastfeeding efforts. This chapter delineates a number of factors in the early environment that can influence the initiation of breastfeeding.

Birth Interventions and Breastfeeding

"Natural childbirth" is fast becoming an extinct practice. In a 2002 landmark U.S. survey of 1,583 mothers conducted by the Maternity Center Association, no births occurred without some form of medical intervention (Declercq et al., 2002). Birth interventions and their side effects have the potential to significantly disrupt early breastfeeding behaviors, especially if more than one intervention is experienced. The Maternity Center Association's Listening to Mothers survey outlined the extent to which childbirth has been transformed into a technologically choreographed event. Similar outcomes were seen in the 1,573 women who participated in the 2006 Listening to Mothers Survey II (Box 4-1) conducted by Childbirth Connection (formerly the Maternity Center Association) (Declercq et al., 2006). What was once a "normal" progression of labor and delivery has been tinkered with to the point that the absence of birth interventions is rare (Kroeger, 2004).

BOX 4-1   Selected Birth Interventions From Listening to Mothers Survey II

- 41% of women had their labor induced
- 86% of mothers used one or more types of medication for pain relief
- 76% of women used epidural or spinal analgesia; 22% were given narcotics such as Demerol or Stadol
- 80% received intravenous fluids
- 59% had their membranes broken; 55% received Pitocin to augment the labor
- 25% had an episiotomy
- 5% experienced vacuum extraction, and 2% experienced the use of forceps
- 32% experienced a cesarean delivery
- 34% of newborn infants were not kept in the mothers' arms
- 69% of mothers with a vaginal birth experienced rooming-in compared with 49% of cesarean mothers
- 61% of mothers hoped to breastfeed exclusively; 19% planned to use a combination of breastfeeding and formula; 20% planned to use formula only
- 34% of mothers perceived that hospital staff expressed no infant feeding preference; 3% encouraged formula feeding
- Of those mothers intending to breastfeed only, 66% were given free formula samples or offers; 44% of their infants were given pacifiers by staff; 38% were given formula or water supplements
- One week after giving birth, 51% of the mothers were exclusively breastfeeding; 75% of the mothers intending to breastfeed exclusively were doing so by the end of the first week

Source: Declercq, ER, Sakala, C, Corry MP, et al. Listening to mothers: Report of the first national US survey of women's childbearing experiences. New York: Maternity Center Association; October 2002.

Abundant physical contact and frequent breastfeeding have been replaced with artificial feeding, minimal contact, early separation, medication, and misinformation. Lozoff et al. (1977) explained that perinatal medical management practices (such as routine postpartum separation) approach the limits beyond which breastfeeding may fail: "the limits of adaptability." For the mother and baby with a problem, breastfeeding success is even more tenuous. Variations in practice abound, with many perinatal interventions claiming to be scientifically based but with large gaps existing between common practices and what the research actually says (Goer, 1995). Interference with the natural process of childbirth should proceed from a sound base of evidence and do more good than harm. Maternity care practices in hospitals and birth centers throughout the intrapartum period, such as ensuring mother–newborn skin-to-skin contact, keeping mother and newborn together, and not giving supplemental feedings to breastfed newborns unless medically indicated, can positively influence breastfeeding behaviors during a period critical to the successful establishment of lactation (Chien et al., 2007; Dewey et al., 2003; DiGirolamo et al., 2001; Murray et al., 2007; Rosenberg et al., 2008a; World Health Organization/United Nations Children's Fund, 1989).

Certain maternity care practices experienced by mothers during their hospital stay have been shown to promote breastfeeding (Cadwell & Turner-Maffei, 2009). Specifically, the Baby-Friendly Hospital Initiative (BFHI), an international initiative introduced in 1991 by the World Health Organization and the United Nations Children's Fund (1989), has been shown to contribute to positive breastfeeding outcomes. Ten evidence-based best practices form BFHI's core of breastfeeding support in the hospital (Table 4-1). The Ten Steps address a major factor in the erosion of exclusive and sustained breastfeeding—maternity care practices that interfere with or are ineffective in supporting breastfeeding. Achievement of the components of all 10 steps earns a birthing facility the designation of Baby-Friendly and the assurance to patients that breastfeeding support services engaged in by the hospital are deemed as best practices. During the implementation of the BFHI in one inner city hospital, breastfeeding rates rose from 58% to 87%. Of note was the increase among U.S.-born African-American mothers, whose breastfeeding rates rose from 34% to 74% (Philipp et al., 2001).

DiGirolamo et al. (2001) surveyed 1,085 new mothers in the Infant Feeding Practices Study I regarding the breastfeeding support they received during the hospital stay after the birth of their baby. They studied the presence or absence of 5 of the 10 steps (i.e., initiation of breastfeeding within 1 hour of birth, 24-hour rooming-in, infant receipt of supplements, feeding on cue, and use of pacifiers). All five steps were experienced by only 7% of the mothers surveyed. Mothers experiencing none of the steps were eight times more likely to have stopped breastfeeding before 6 weeks postpartum. A dose-response relationship was seen, as the more steps a mother experienced, the more likely she was to continue breastfeeding to 6 weeks and beyond. The major risk factors for early abandonment of breastfeeding were late initiation of breastfeeding and supplementation

---

TABLE 4-1   Ten Steps to Successful Breastfeeding

---

1. Maintain and routinely communicate a written breastfeeding policy to all staff.
2. Train all healthcare staff in skills necessary to implement this policy.
3. Inform all pregnant women about the benefits and management of breastfeeding.
4. Help mothers initiate breastfeeding within 1 hour of birth.
5. Show mothers how to breastfeed and how to maintain lactation, even if they are separated from their infants.
6. Give infants no food or drink other than breastmilk, unless medically indicated.
7. Practice rooming-in, which allows mothers and infants to remain together 24 hours a day.
8. Encourage unrestricted breastfeeding.
9. Give no pacifiers or artificial nipples to breastfeeding infants.
10. Foster the establishment of breastfeeding support groups and refer mothers to them on discharge from the hospital or clinic.

Source: World Health Organization/United Nations Children's Fund. *Protecting, promoting and supporting breastfeeding: the special role of maternity services.* Geneva, Switzerland: World Health Organization, 1989.

---

of the infant. A dose-response relationship between the number of steps experienced and the time of breastfeeding discontinuation was replicated in the Infant Feeding Practices Study II (DiGirolamo et al., 2008). Only 8% of the mothers experienced all six of the steps studied. A consistent association of breastfeeding beyond 6 weeks was seen with initiation of breastfeeding within 1 hour of birth, giving only breastmilk, and avoiding pacifier use. Mothers who experienced none of the practices were 13 times more likely to stop breastfeeding early.

These studies suggest a cumulative effect of the practices with no one practice in isolation contributing to enhanced outcomes, but the combination of practices as the important goal (Forster & McLachlan, 2007). Hospitals designated as Baby-Friendly have elevated rates of breastfeeding initiation and exclusivity compared with national and state levels, demonstrating the effectiveness of institutional investments in breastfeeding (Merewood et al., 2005).

One of the most important practices contained in the Ten Steps is that of having a written breastfeeding policy that is routinely communicated to all healthcare staff. Rosenberg et al. (2008b) found that this step was associated with continued breastfeeding at 2 weeks and that if a hospital had to prioritize the Ten

Steps, that breastfeeding policy development and implementation was an effective place to start. Although there may be concerns or misinformation regarding implementation of the BFHI (Walker, 2007), institutional changes in hospital practices are effective in increasing both initiation and duration of breastfeeding (Fairbank et al., 2000). Kruse et al. (2005) reported that hospital practices are extremely important to breastfeeding outcomes. Although sociodemographic variables predicted about 60% of the variation in hospital-specific rates of exclusive breastfeeding at discharge, other contributions, including hospital practices, predicted the remaining 40%.

In 2007 the Centers for Disease Control and Prevention (CDC) conducted the first national Maternity Practices in Infant Nutrition and Care (mPINC) survey to characterize intrapartum practices in hospitals and birth centers in the United States. Questions regarding maternity practices were grouped into seven categories that served as subscales in the analyses:

1. Labor and delivery
2. Breastfeeding assistance
3. Mother–newborn contact
4. Newborn feeding practices
5. Breastfeeding support after discharge
6. Nurse/birth attendant breastfeeding training and education
7. Structural and organizational factors related to breastfeeding

The findings from the 2,690 hospitals that responded to the survey indicated widespread use of maternity practices that are not evidence-based and that are known to interfere with breastfeeding. For example, 24% of birth facilities reported supplementing more than half of healthy, full-term, breastfed newborns with something other than breastmilk during the postpartum stay, a practice shown to be unnecessary and detrimental to breastfeeding. In addition, 70% of facilities reported giving breastfeeding mothers gift bags containing infant formula samples. Scores on the seven items will help facilities identify specific maternity practices that might be changed to better support breastfeeding (CDC, 2008).

Because the mPINC survey questions draw heavily from the Ten Steps to Successful Breastfeeding, the BFHI remains an important goal for hospitals to achieve. At the very least, hospitals should strive to implement the Ten Steps to provide optimal evidence-based breastfeeding support to new mothers. Sample policies and more information on the BFHI are listed in the Additional Reading/Resources at the end of this chapter.

Maternity Care Practices and Breastfeeding

Prenatal Maternal Medications

Although the possibility always exists that recreational drugs (i.e., maternal prenatal smoking and its association with infantile colic) (Sondergaard et al., 2001) or drugs of abuse can affect an infant's feeding behaviors, some prescribed medications taken by the mother during the third trimester also have the potential to influence such behaviors. For example, selective serotonin reuptake inhibitors are a group of antidepressants used to treat mild to moderate depression. When taken by a mother during the second or third trimester, withdrawal symptoms may be evident in infants during the early days after birth. These symptoms may include irritability, constant crying, shivering, increased tone, feeding and sleeping difficulties, and convulsions, all described as part of the neonatal withdrawal syndrome by Nordeng et al. (2001). Conversely, Laine et al. (2003) suggest that the cluster of symptoms that includes tremor, restlessness, and rigidity, although seen four times more frequently in exposed newborns, is due to central nervous system serotogenic overstimulation (serotonin-using pathways) rather than an actual withdrawal syndrome.

Some evidence suggests that symptoms are not always due to toxic or withdrawal actions but that selective serotonin reuptake inhibitors may interfere with the physiology of the infant's respiratory system and parasympathetic activity (Gentile, 2007). Symptoms may occur during the early hours after birth and/or may appear after discharge and further include respiratory distress, transient tachypnea, hypoglycemia, bradycardia, and sucking problems depending on the particular drug and dosage. Some of these symptoms are suggestive of other conditions, such as dehydration or intracranial hemorrhage.

Paroxetine (Paxil) and fluoxetine (Prozac) are most commonly reported as being associated with neonatal side effects (Moses-Kolko et al., 2005). When mothers receive a combination of paroxetine and clonazepam (Klonopin), infants may be at a higher risk of experiencing poor neonatal adaptation (Oberlander et al., 2004). The clinician may need to check the mother's records or ask whether she has taken any of these medications. Education of the parents is important and should include that these symptoms are short-lived (2–4 weeks) and may disrupt feeding, motor tone, sleeping, and consolability of the infant. Although the symptoms may subside during the first 4–7 days or so, extra vigilance and assistance with breastfeeding may be necessary during the hospital stay and the first week home. Suggested interventions include the provision of a dim, quiet environment (visitors should be minimized), frequent small feedings to address increased caloric requirements and feeding difficulties, skin-to-skin contact to improve breastfeeding, behavioral states and breathing regularity, swaddling, and cue-based feedings. Extra vigilance is also called for with mothers who have received mood-stabilizing drugs for treating bipolar disorders because a number of undesirable effects have been described in neonates whose mothers received antimanic or maintenance drugs for mood disorders (Iqbal et al., 2001).

Labor Medications

Pharmacological relief of the pain from labor has a long history. Various drugs, combinations of drugs, and routes of delivery have fallen in and out of favor through the years.

Systemic Agents

Drugs such as opioids provide some pain relief during labor but carry a number of potential side effects. More than 40 years ago, Brazelton (1961) described the central nervous system depressant effects that occurred in newborns of heavily medicated mothers (i.e., those who received scopolamine, barbiturates, spinal block, pudendal block, saddle block, ether, trichloroethylene, Nisentil, or nitrous oxide). Behavioral disorganization, difficulty in the modulation of state control, and difficulties with breastfeeding that included a sleepy, unresponsive infant who was challenging to wake and keep alert were common. Bricker and Lavender (2002) summarized the association of opioid use during labor with neonatal respiratory depression, decreased alertness, inhibition of sucking, lower neurobehavioral scores, and delay in effective feeding. Other side effects in infants exposed to narcotics include a shorter duration of wakefulness, less efficient suckling, depressed visual and auditory attention, longer time to habituate to noise, and decreased social responsiveness. This behavior can be evident for as long as 4 days (Weiner et al., 1977). The drug-to-delivery interval is the time from when the drug was administered to the mother to the time of the infant's birth. It is an important consideration regarding the extent to which the newborn is affected by medications administered to the mother. Effects on newborns are minimized when narcotics have been given within an hour of birth (Rooth et al., 1983). Maximal accumulation of a drug and its metabolites in fetal tissues occurs when the agent is given more than 3 hours before delivery (Brice et al., 1979) or given repeatedly over a longer period of time.

Although older medications may no longer be used during childbirth, drugs used today still exert a number of undesirable effects on the newborn. Demerol (meperidine) replaced morphine as a popular labor medication for many years. It is now being phased out in many institutions due to its unpleasant side effects on laboring mothers, its depressive effects on newborns, its long half-life in neonates (13 hours), and the extremely long half-life of its potent metabolite normeperidine (62 hours in the neonate). Side effects of concern include depressed suckling (Righard & Alade, 1990), decreased tone and reflexes (Coalson & Glosten, 1991), respiratory depression (Hamza et al., 1992), delayed rooting reflex (Nissen et al., 1995a), and delayed neonatal sucking behavior (Nissen et al., 1997).

Nisentil (alphaprodine) is a rapid-acting narcotic analgesic with a short duration of action. Matthews (1989) compared infants from nonmedicated mothers and mothers medicated with Nisentil in terms of time to effective breastfeeding. Also studied was the effect of the drug-to-delivery interval on mean time to effective breastfeeding. Ninety-three percent of the infants of mothers from the nonmedicated group and from a group whose mothers received Nisentil within an hour of delivery were effectively breastfeeding by 24 hours of age. Mean time to effective breastfeeding for this group was 11.86 hours. By comparison, infants of mothers who received Nisentil 1–3 hours before birth experienced a mean time to effective breastfeeding of 21.2 hours. Only 66% of these infants had established effective breastfeeding by 24 hours.

Crowell and coworkers (1994) studied Stadol (butorphanol) and Nubain (nalbuphine), comparing the effects on breastfeeding relative to the drug-to-delivery interval and when the first breastfeeding occurred (Table 4-2). Their data also identified a subgroup of mothers and infants who were especially at risk of suboptimal breastfeeding, namely primiparous mothers of boys.

In 2005 the U.S. Food and Drug Administration (FDA) approved safety labeling revisions for nalbuphine (Nubain) injection, warning of the risk for serious fetal and neonatal adverse events associated with its use during labor and delivery. Reports to the FDA of fetal and neonatal adverse events have included fetal bradycardia, respiratory depression at birth, apnea, cyanosis, and hypotonia. Some of these events have been life threatening. Although maternal administration of naloxone during labor has sometimes counteracted these effects, severe prolonged

TABLE 4-2 Comparative Effects on Breastfeeding of DDI* and First Breastfeed

IBFAT scoring system was used to determine the establishment of effective breastfeeding	No analgesia or analgesia administered less than 1 hour prior to delivery	Analgesia administered more than 1 hour prior to delivery
Early initiator: Breastfeeding started less than 1 hour after delivery	Mean time to effective breastfeeding: 6.4 hours	Mean time to effective breastfeeding: 50.3 hours
Late initiator: Breastfeeding started more than 1 hour after delivery	Mean time to effective breastfeeding: 49.7 hours	Mean time to effective breastfeeding: 62.5 hours

*Drug to Delivery Interval

fetal bradycardia has occurred and, in some cases, resulted in permanent neurological damage. The FDA advised that nalbuphine be used during labor and delivery only if clearly indicated and the potential benefit outweighed the risk to the infant. The FDA recommended that newborns exposed to maternal nalbuphine should be monitored for respiratory depression, apnea, bradycardia, and arrhythmias.

Systemic analgesics can be highly lipid soluble. They rapidly cross the placenta and are quickly absorbed into fetal circulation. Immaturity of the fetal liver and renal system can delay detoxification and clearance of the drug, which prolongs its action, sometimes well past discharge from the hospital. Peak fetal depressant effects can be seen approximately 1.5–2 hours after administration. To reduce the possibility of newborn depression from opioid analgesia, birth should occur within 1 hour of or 4 hours after its administration (Poole, 2003), something over which clinicians have little control.

Concerns have surfaced regarding the concept of genetic imprinting at birth for self-destructive behavior and opiate or amphetamine addiction later in life as possible long-term consequences to an infant whose mother received narcotics during labor (Jacobson et al., 1987, 1988, 1990). The potential for adult drug abuse may be programmed early in life with obstetric narcotics exposure serving as an early risk factor (Nyberg et al., 2000). Animal models have demonstrated that the course of behavioral maturation during certain periods of infancy is influenced by both meperidine and bupivacaine administration at birth, possibly by interfering with the programming of brain development or the alteration of early experiences (Golub, 1996).

Regional Analgesia/Anesthesia

These methods include spinal, epidural, intrathecal, and combined spinal-epidural techniques. They use various types and amounts of drugs and drug combinations and may be administered over short or long periods of time, before or after the cervix is 3–4 cm dilated, or after laboring women have already been dosed with systemic analgesics. The relationship between epidural use and breast-feeding has yielded conflicting data, with difficulties experienced in comparing studies whose methodologies vary widely and which may not take into account the influence of cointerventions (Camann, 2007). In an analysis of the Infant Feeding Practices Study II that looked at 1,907 mothers who intended to breast-feed for greater than 2 months, mothers who did not receive any pain medication during labor and delivery were more likely to continue breastfeeding beyond 6 weeks. This association remained after controlling for demographic, behavioral, and attitudinal variables (DiGirolamo et al., 2008). Torvaldsen and colleagues (2006) studied 1,295 women to determine any association between epidural analgesia and breastfeeding in the first week postpartum and breastfeeding cessation during the first 6 months. Epidurals were significantly associated with partial breastfeeding during the first week due to difficulty breastfeeding. Women who used no pain medication had the lowest rates of breastfeeding cessation at 6 months compared with mothers who experienced epidurals having the highest rates of abandoning breastfeeding. Although epidural use may not have been causal, breastfeeding difficulties were more frequent during the first week post-partum, formula supplementation occurred early, and breastfeeding cessation was more common in mothers who had been given epidural analgesia. Infants whose mothers received epidural analgesia appear to be at an increased risk for difficulty initiating breastfeeding, being supplemented with formula, and not being breastfed until 6 months of age. These mother–baby pairs will benefit from tar-geted interventions (Jordan, 2006), and clinicians may wish to place such pairs in a higher risk category for breastfeeding problems and premature weaning.

Early studies failed to examine breastfeeding as an outcome of epidural use and may not have used nonmedicated control groups (Walker, 1997). Nevertheless, epidural analgesia has been associated with neonatal respiratory depression (Kumar & Paes, 2003), a lower rate of spontaneous vaginal delivery, fetal mal-positioning, a higher rate of instrumental vaginal delivery, an increased cesarean section rate, longer labors, increased incidence of oxytocin-augmented labor, increased incidence of intrapartum fever (with the infants more likely to be evalu-ated and treated for suspected sepsis as well as experiencing unexplained neonatal seizures), infant hypotonia, decreased performance on the Neonatal Behavioral Assessment Scale, and increased occurrence of neonatal jaundice (Lieberman & O'Donoghue, 2002).

Cointerventions designed to reduce the common side effects of epidurals have their own side effects (Mayberry et al., 2002). Epidural drugs and their side effects on the laboring woman, their effects on the labor and delivery, the consequences to the fetus and newborn plus the cointerventions administered to reduce side effects and their own side effects all make it difficult to pinpoint which intervention affects breastfeeding, how they influence breastfeeding, and how varying combinations of interventions may act synergistically (Riordan & Riordan, 2000). Some studies claim that epidural use does not affect breastfeeding initiation or duration (Halpern et al., 1999) or that epidurals actually promote breastfeeding (Leighton & Halpern, 2002a). Halpern et al. (1999) studied the duration of breastfeeding as a means to evaluate the effect of labor pain medication on successful breastfeeding outcomes. Of the 189 women enrolled in the study, 171 were interviewed at 6–8 weeks postpartum. These mothers had received intravenous (IV) narcotics, epidural analgesia, or no medications for labor pain relief. Although 59% had received epidural anesthesia, there was no discrimination between breastfeeding outcomes among the various labor experiences. Seventy-two percent of the entire sample was breastfeeding exclusively at 6 weeks, 20% were partially breastfeeding, and the rest had weaned. Thirty-six percent reported difficulty in initiating breastfeeding in the hospital, 55 of the mothers visited a free lactation clinic at least once, and intensive breastfeeding support was used during and after the hospital stay.

The study did not say whether these problems were associated with analgesia use during labor but concluded that epidurals do not affect breastfeeding. Perhaps breastfeeding succeeded despite the medications, due to the rigorous amount of lactation care and services provided to all the mothers in this study. Not all mothers who receive epidural analgesia will be fortunate enough to have access to the sometimes extensive services of lactation professionals that may be needed to overcome this impediment to breastfeeding. Henderson et al. (2003) found that nulliparous women who chose epidural analgesia were significantly more likely to breastfeed for shorter durations.

Epidural Drugs

All drugs used in epidurals reach the fetus in greater or lesser amounts, including bupivacaine (Kuhnert et al., 1982), an anesthetic that is measurable in the fetus within 10 minutes of maternal administration (Rosenblatt et al., 1981), and any of the narcotics combined in the epidural, such as fentanyl and sufentanil (Loftus et al., 1995). The effects on breastfeeding may be either direct or indirect and can vary from agent to agent. Fentanyl has a half-life of 2–4 hours in an adult but 3–13 hours in neonates (Hale, 2006). If it takes approximately five half-lives to eliminate the drug from the body, a neonate with a sluggish liver could take as long as 65 hours to eliminate the fentanyl that accumulated during the birthing process. The concentration of fentanyl increases as infant pH decreases, placing crying infants and cesarean-delivered infants at an elevated risk for much higher concentrations of fentanyl (Jordan et al., 2005). This point is well after discharge from the hospital and may signal the need for closer follow-up in infants whose mothers received fentanyl during labor.

Spontaneous breast-seeking and suckling behaviors soon after delivery are reduced in newborns whose mothers receive analgesics and epidurals (Righard & Alade, 1992; Widstrom et al., 1987). Developing and early discreet breastfeeding movements are also altered or blunted by maternal labor medications. Administration of analgesia and epidurals disturbs the behavioral sequence of prefeeding behaviors immediately after delivery such as hand-to-mouth movements, touching of the areola, suckling movements, and the sucking pattern itself (Ransjo-Arvidson et al., 2001).

Using the Infant Breastfeeding Assessment Tool, Riordan et al. (2000) compared four groups of infants whose mothers received (1) no labor pain medication, (2) only epidural analgesia, (3) only intravenous narcotics, or (4) both epidural and IV analgesia. On a scale where 12 represented the highest suckling score, infants whose mothers had no labor pain analgesia scored 11.1 ± 0.9. Infants whose mothers had IV analgesia scored 8.5 ± 3.2, whereas infants whose mothers had an epidural scored 8.5 ± 3.4. Infants whose mothers had both IV analgesia and an epidural had significantly lower suckling scores of 6.4 ± 3.0. Infants with scores less than 10 are in need of significant follow-up, because both IV medications and epidurals diminish neonatal sucking.

Baumgarder et al. (2003) also found that epidural anesthesia had a negative impact on breastfeeding in the first 24 hours of life. The primary outcome of interest in their study was the ability of the infant to accomplish two successful breastfeedings by 24 hours as defined by the LATCH breastfeeding assessment tool (see Table 3-10). This outcome was achieved by 81% of infants whose mothers did not have an epidural compared with 69.6% of infants whose mothers received epidural analgesia. Another disturbing outcome of this study was the finding that infants exposed to epidural anesthesia were significantly more likely to receive a bottle supplement during hospitalization. Mothers who received an epidural and did not breastfeed within 1 hour of delivery were at extremely high risk for their infants to receive bottle supplementation.

Formula supplementation was reported to be more common among infants of mothers who received epidural analgesia containing a bupivacaine concentration of 0.25% (Volmanen et al., 2004). Wiklund et al. (2009) reported that compared with infants of mothers not receiving an epidural, fewer infants of mothers with epidurals suckled the breast within the first 4 hours of birth, that they were given formula more often during their hospital stay, and fewer were exclusively breastfed upon discharge.

In an attempt to reduce the negative effects of epidurals on laboring mothers and their newborns, some obstetric services use an ultra-low dose of drugs in the epidural mixture (0.125% bupivacaine, 50 μg fentanyl, and 1:600,000 epinephrine as the loading dose and a continuing infusion of 0.044% bupivacaine, 0.000125% fentanyl, and 1:800,000 epinephrine). Radzyminski (2003) concluded that there were no measurable differences between the breastfeeding behaviors of infants of 28 mothers who received this type of epidural and 28 infants whose mothers received no labor medication. However, it is interesting to note that 72% of the medicated mothers received oxytocin to induce or augment their labor compared with 32% of the mothers in the unmedicated group. The subgroup of infants who experienced difficulty in initiating breastfeeding had mothers who experienced more maternal fatigue, anxiety, lack of previous breastfeeding experience, induction of labor, and extremes of the labor curve. One difference between the two groups was the greater amount of swallowing in the unmedicated group, although it was not statistically significant. Bupivacaine in the epidural affected the newborn's passive and active tone and total score on the Neurologic and Adaptive Capacity Score instrument used to measure neurobehavior in this study (Amiel-Tison et al., 1982). This could possibly impede early suckling movements. It remains unknown whether any of these drugs become sequestered in the neonatal central nervous system during the early days after discharge.

In animals, epidural anesthesia can interfere with maternal attachment and the onset of mothering behavior by blocking sensory stimuli for the release of oxytocin (Krehbiel et al., 1987). In human mothers a spontaneous peak of oxytocin release is usually observed about 15 minutes postdelivery, with several more peaks of oxytocin occurring up to 60 minutes postpartum (Nissen et al., 1995b). Epidural use is associated with a decrease or deficiency in plasma oxytocin levels in mothers after delivery (Goodfellow et al., 1983; Rahm et al., 2002). Sepkoski et al. (1992) showed that mothers with bupivacaine (0.5%) epidurals spent less time with their infants while in the hospital (9.7 vs. 13.7 hours) than did a nonmedicated group of mothers. The medicated infants showed clear depression in motor abilities and exhibited poor state control.

Intrapartum fever is associated with epidural use. Whereas maternal fever is a marker for potential infection, most intrapartum fevers originate as a side effect of epidural use (Lieberman et al., 1997). Lieberman et al. (1997) analyzed 1,047 laboring women, 63% of whom received epidurals and 37% of whom did not. Of the women who received an epidural, 14.5% developed a fever of more than 100.4°F (38°C) during labor compared with only 1% of women not receiving an epidural. Ninety-six percent of the intrapartum fevers occurred within the group receiving an epidural, resulting in 85.6% of neonatal sepsis workups occurring in the group of infants whose mothers received an epidural. These infants were also four times more likely to be treated with antibiotics.

Gross et al. (2002) evaluated the records of 1,233 mothers whose labor analgesia was managed with no medication, epidural medication only, nalbuphine alone, or both epidural and nalbuphine. The incidence of fever was 17% for mothers receiving only epidurals and 1% for the no-medication group.

Intrapartum maternal fever is associated with an increased risk of cesarean section and operative vaginal delivery (Lieberman et al., 1999) as well as a number of transient adverse effects in the newborn such as low Apgar score, hypotonia, bag and mask resuscitation, and oxygen therapy in the nursery (Lieberman et al., 2000b). High maternal fever increases the risk of neurological injury to the fetus independent of infection. It is associated with a 3.4-fold increase in the risk of unexplained neonatal seizures and is a strong predictor of later morbidity and mortality in term infants (Lieberman et al., 2000a). Even in afebrile mothers, those who receive epidural analgesia have infants who are more likely to be evaluated for sepsis compared with mothers who do not receive such medications (20.4% vs. 8.9%) (Goetzl et al., 2001). Sepsis workups usually result in separation, invasive procedures, expressing milk rather than having an infant at the breast, and maternal anxiety that contributes to a slow start to breastfeeding.

Delivery and immediate postpartum care practices can affect breastfeeding in mothers who have received an epidural, possibly exacerbating problems that could have been minimized with early frequent contact such as skin to skin (Anderson et al., 2003), minimal to no separation (Leighton & Halpern, 2002b), opportunities for self-attachment to the breast, and frequent feedings. It is possible that with intense lactation care and services both during the hospital stay and after discharge, many of the side effects of epidurals on breastfeeding may be overcome. However, if mothers do not have these services available or lack access to them, then breastfeeding is placed in jeopardy with mixed feeding and early weaning distinct possibilities.

When an epidural is administered, it is usually accompanied by a cascade of interventions that either individually or in combination can significantly affect breastfeeding:

- IV infusion of regional anesthesia/analgesia can cause hypotension. To reduce the risks of this side effect, a preepidural IV infusion of 500–1,000 mL of non–glucose-balanced sodium chloride solution (isotonic saline or lactated Ringer's) is usually administered 15–30 minutes before the procedure. Glucose solutions are contraindicated due to the risk for fetal hyperglycemia and rebound hypoglycemia in the newborn. Large amounts of fluid can be administered over the course of a long labor or if maternal IV medications are used during and after the labor and delivery (1–6 L of fluid are possible). A healthy pregnant woman at term already has approximately 2 L of fluid stored in her extravascular space (Lind, 1983). One adverse outcome of a delay in the expected postpartum fluid shift and diuresis of excess fluid has been observed as areolar edema (Cotterman, 2004). An edematous areola envelops the nipple and increases subareolar tissue resistance, resulting in a difficult, painful latch or an areola that cannot be drawn into the infant's mouth. Fluid retention is further exacerbated by the normally increased vasopressin (antidiuretic hormone) production during childbirth. Hypotension is also managed with intravenous vasopressor agents, such as ephedrine and phenylephrine (Camann, 2003), adding yet more drugs (which also contribute to fluid retention) into the laboring woman. Omitting the fluid preload before epidural administration has been studied, with findings of similar rates of maternal hypotension between no preload and a 1 L preload in low-dose epidurals but with a higher rate of deterioration in fetal heart rates seen where no fluid preload was administered (Kinsella et al., 2000).

- Oxytocin administration for inducing or augmenting labor can further contribute to edema (as well as dilutional hyponatremia or water intoxication), because it has an antidiuretic effect similar to vasopressin. If oxytocin is administered in a glucose solution, this formulation further potentiates the antidiuretic effects of oxytocin. A few hospitals still use a dextrose solution for the mainline IV (Ruchala et al., 2002). Water overload, dilutional hyponatremia (Omigbodun et al., 1991), hyperbilirubinemia (Omigbodun et al., 1993), respiratory distress, and feeding difficulties can be seen in newborns whose mothers are the recipients of excessive or inappropriate fluids during labor (Borcherding & Ruchala, 2002–2003).

- Fetal malposition is strongly and consistently associated with epidural analgesia (Ponkey et al., 2003). Lieberman et al. (2005) found that epidurals were associated with a fourfold increase in the risk of occiput posterior birth. Persistent occiput posterior is associated with increased rates of operative vaginal and cesarean deliveries and other peripartum complications such as prolonged first and second stages of labor, oxytocin augmentation, excessive blood loss, third- and fourth-degree perineal lacerations, and chorioamnionitis (Cheng et al., 2006). Infants of mothers who experienced a cesarean delivery compared with those delivered vaginally were shown to demonstrate poorer scores on the LATCH scoring system at each of their first three feedings (Cakmak & Kuguoglu, 2007), creating the need for more intensive lactation support.

- Instrument delivery by forceps, vacuum extraction, or both is commonly associated with epidural use (Walker & O'Brien, 1999), often due to fetal malposition. Thorp et al. (1993) found a fourfold increase in the rate of malposition (19% vs. 4%) in a group of mothers who received epidural analgesia. Epidural analgesia increases the risk for labor dystocia and has been identified as an independent risk factor for vacuum extraction (O'Hana et al., 2008). Vacuum extraction has the potential to disrupt the autonomic balance in infants, increasing their vulnerability to stress (Moehler et al., 2007; Porges, 1992). Intracranial hemorrhage is higher among infants delivered by forceps or vacuum extraction. Towner et al. (1999) identified one-third of a sample of 583,340 live-born singleton infants as being born by operative techniques. Intracranial hemorrhage occurred in 1 of 860 infants delivered by vacuum extraction, 1 of 664 infants delivered by forceps, and 1 of 1,900 infants delivered spontaneously. Vacuum extraction causes less maternal trauma but increases the risk of certain types of intracranial hemorrhage such as subarachnoid hemorrhage (Wen et al., 2001). Compared with spontaneous vaginal deliveries, deliveries by sequential use of vacuum and forceps had even higher rates of injuries, with almost four times the rate of intracranial hemorrhage and increased risk of brachial plexus, facial nerve injury, seizures, depressed 5-minute

Apgar scores, and maternal perineal lacerations. The relative risk of sequential vacuum and forceps use was greater than the sum of the individual relative risks of each instrument for intracranial hemorrhage, facial nerve injury, seizure, hematoma, and perineal and vaginal lacerations (Gardella et al., 2001).

The FDA became sufficiently concerned about the serious injuries and deaths related to the use of vacuum extraction devices that it issued a public health advisory to healthcare professionals on May 21, 1998 (FDA, 1998). The FDA warned that these devices could cause serious or fatal injuries and noted that those who care for these infants after delivery might not be aware that the devices could produce life-threatening complications. The FDA was also concerned that if healthcare providers were not alerted to an infant who had been vacuum extracted, they might not adequately monitor for signs and symptoms of device-related injuries.

- Infants exposed to vacuum-assisted delivery devices usually have a caput succedaneum; that is, an extracranial hemorrhage producing edema of the soft tissues of the scalp that resolves spontaneously within the first week of life. The FDA, however, warned of two major life-threatening complications of vacuum extraction:

  1. Subgaleal hematoma (subaponeurotic hematoma) (Cavlovich, 1994) is an extracranial hemorrhage that represents a significant blood loss to the infant. It occurs when emissary veins are damaged and blood accumulates in the potential space between the galea aponeurotica and the periosteum of the skull. Because this space has no boundaries, blood may accumulate from the orbital ridges above the eyes to the nape of the neck. The signs may be present at delivery or may not become apparent until several hours or days after delivery. Signs include diffuse swelling of the head, pallor, hypotension, tachycardia, lethargy, and increased respiration rate. Significant blood loss can occur with subsequent brain compression, disseminated intravascular coagulation, and shock (Amar et al., 2003; Uchil & Arulkumaran, 2003).

  2. Intracranial hemorrhage may include subdural, subarachnoid, intraventricular, and/or intraparenchymal hemorrhage. Signs are not visible from the outside and may include seizure activity, lethargy, apnea, bulging fontanel, poor feeding, increased irritability, bradycardia, and shock. Clinical evidence of neurologic damage may develop over time and not become apparent until 4 weeks to 6 months of age (Steinbach, 1999).

The FDA estimated that almost 6% of all deliveries in 1998 used vacuum extraction devices. The rate of delivery by vacuum extraction, which had increased by 59% between 1990 (3.9%) and 1996–1997 (6.2%), has since decreased to 3.7% for 2006. This is due primarily to the large increase in cesarean deliveries (Martin et al., 2009).

Infants delivered by vacuum extraction often start suckling later, are given formula more often, and are breastfed less at night, and their mothers may experience a delay in lactogenesis II (Vestermark et al., 1991). Hall et al. (2002) demonstrated that vacuum extraction was a significant contributor to poor scores on the Breastfeeding Assessment Score that was predictive of increased risk of breastfeeding cessation during the first 7–10 days after birth.

Separation

When the predominant location for birth moved to the hospital setting in the early 20th century, caretaking routines developed that are still in use today. It remains common to see mothers and their babies separated at birth, infants cared for in a nursery, mothers and babies together only during the day, infant interventions performed not at the bedside but in the nursery, and the expectation that continuous contact between mother and baby will somehow lead to the baby becoming "dependent" on the mother. Although there are medical reasons for separation, most occur due to non–evidence-based views; for example, nursery care allows better supervision of the infant, routine monitoring or physician evaluations must be done where better light is available, interventions such as phototherapy must occur in the nursery, or mothers are told that they should allow the nurses to care for the infant (especially at night) so that they can get more rest. Separating mothers and infants reduces the interaction between mother and baby, hinders a mother's opportunity to learn her baby's feeding cues, decreases access to the breast resulting in fewer breastfeeds (Yamauchi & Yamanouchi, 1990a), may increase the occurrence of complementary or supplementary feedings of water or formula, delays lactogenesis II, and produces undesirable physiological side effects in newborns (Anderson, 1989).

Separation and Sleep

Separation does not result in more sleep for mothers at night if infants are returned to the nursery. Keefe (1988) demonstrated that mothers slept an average of 5.35 hours during an 8-hour night period when their infants were returned to the nursery, whereas mothers who roomed-in with their babies slept an average of 5.55 hours. The American Academy of Pediatrics (AAP, 2005) recommends that mothers sleep in close proximity to their infants to facilitate breastfeeding.

Infants cared for in a nursery at night are exposed to greater light and sound levels than those cared for in the mother's room, receive less contact with a caregiver, experience less quiet sleep, and cry more than infants who remain with their mothers. Keefe (1987) reported illumination levels in a nursery as 35 footcandles compared with 3 footcandles in the mother's room. Infants kept in the nursery at night were exposed to noise levels equal to or greater than 80 decibels for approximately one-third of the night. The most persistent and striking noise in the nursery was the sound of infants crying. Infants kept in their mothers' rooms also engaged in more quiet sleep and less crying. The presence of the newborn in the mother's room did not significantly alter maternal sleep but did improve infant sleep.

Infants separated from their mothers cry more, frequently startle, have lower body and skin temperatures, and have lower blood glucose levels than do infants who remain with their mothers after birth. In a study following 50 infants for the first 90 minutes after birth, Christensson et al. (1992) found that the maternal body was an efficient heat source for the newborn because the skin-to-skin infants remained warmer. Blood glucose levels in the separated infants at 90 minutes after birth averaged 46.6 mg/dL compared with the skin-to-skin infants whose blood glucose averaged 57.6 mg/dL. The latter infants also cried significantly less, preserving high blood glucose levels and glycogen stores and contributing to a more rapid metabolic adaptation to extrauterine life.

Separating mothers and babies during their hospital stay has been associated with a reduced length of breastfeeding (Murray et al., 2007). Rooming-in for 60% or more of the hospital stay is significantly associated with the continuation of full breastfeeding at 4 months of age (Wright et al., 1996). Rooming-in results in higher milk yields during the first 4 days after birth, most likely due to the high intensity of nonsupplemented breastfeeding (Bystrova et al., 2007). Staff attitudes and support for rooming-in have a significant effect on the practice. Svensson et al. (2005) demonstrated that mothers who had not roomed-in with their infants were more likely to perceive that the staff believed their babies should stay in the nursery at night compared with those mothers who roomed in with their babies. Negative staff attitudes toward night rooming-in may implicitly suggest to mothers that closeness and contact at this time are not important.

Crying

Adaptation to extrauterine life can be physiologically demanding for an infant. Misconceptions about newborn crying persist, such as the belief that newborns need to cry to expand or exercise their lungs. A full-term newborn's lungs carry an adequate functional reserve after the first breath (Karlberg, 1960) and are as fully expanded at 30 minutes after birth as they are at 24 hours after birth (Klaus et al., 1963). Crying results in a surprising number of undesirable side effects (Ludington-Hoe et al., 2002), which can render an infant less capable of breastfeeding.

Crying raises the heart rate by at least 19 beats per minute, varying with the intensity and duration of crying from 170 beats per minute with slight crying to more than 200 beats per minute with hard crying, resulting in tachycardia. Crying causes both systolic and diastolic pressures to increase by 135%, and the all-important pulse pressure is reduced to values less than 1% at rest, impairing circulation to the brain (Dinwiddie et al., 1979a). Unoxygenated blood is shunted to the body, reducing arterial oxygen levels by 16.8 mm Hg and resulting in desaturation (Dinwiddie et al., 1979b). Decreased oxygen levels and excessive right-sided heart pressures may cause the foramen ovale to open, shunting blood into the left atrium and reestablishing fetal circulation (Brazy, 1988); fluctuations in cerebral blood flow and pressure plus immature vascularization (Figure 4-1) can contribute to intraventricular hemorrhage in preterm infants and, if severe, result in developmental delays (Brazy, 1988; Hiraishi et al., 1991).

Full-term infants are also vulnerable to intracranial hemorrhage during this transitional time. In a study conducted on 505 asymptomatic, normal, full-term

Figure 4-1   Stressor: Crying

Source: © Gene Cranston Anderson, PhD, RN, FAAN, Emeritus Professor of Nursing, Case Western Reserve University, Cleveland, Ohio. Used with permission.

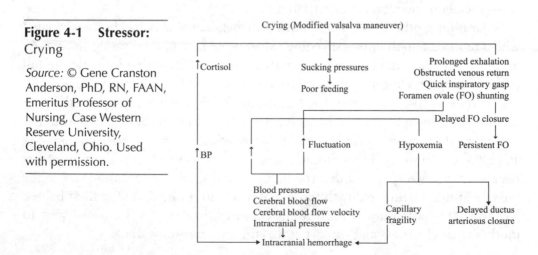

infants in a general nursery, such hemorrhages were documented at 72 hours after birth in 3% of these apparently healthy infants (Hayden et al., 1985). Salivary cortisol levels increase as the length of crying increases, signaling stress. High levels of cortisol act as an immunosuppressant, weakening the infant's ability to fight infection. Infants can swallow a large amount of air when crying. In a study of 2- to 3-week-old infants, a mean of 360 mL of air was swallowed during crying (Shaker et al., 1973). Distention of the stomach contributes to discomfort, reduced intake of milk, and the possibility of further crying, spitting up, and disruption in the normal feeding and digestive processes. Gastric rupture has been reported with prolonged (30 minutes) hard crying associated with circumcision (Connelly et al., 1992); as crying progresses, infant behavior becomes more disorganized (Anderson, 1976) and the exhausted infant may be unable to make eye contact or breastfeed effectively.

Newborns cared for in hospital nurseries rather than in close contact with the mother have often begun crying before they are taken to their mothers. One-hour-old infants were observed displaying many oral cues and signs of stress over a time period of 30 minutes before reaching a sustained cry (Gill et al., 1984). In busy hospital nurseries the sustained cry typically prompts the nurse (or the mother) to determine it is time to feed the infant. A better approach is to take advantage of the infant's feeding readiness cues such as mouthing or hand-to-mouth movements and to feed him or her at that point rather than after crying has begun and the infant experiences stress (Figure 4-2).

A crying infant is also stressful to the mother, raising a woman's systolic blood pressure by 8–10 mm Hg when she first hears her baby cry (Zeskind, 1980). The

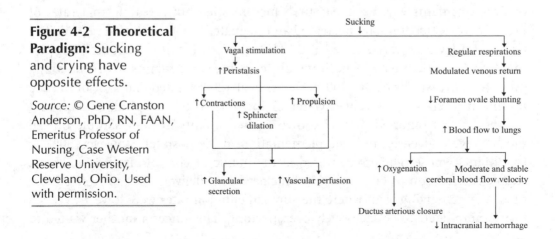

Figure 4-2   Theoretical Paradigm: Sucking and crying have opposite effects.

Source: © Gene Cranston Anderson, PhD, RN, FAAN, Emeritus Professor of Nursing, Case Western Reserve University, Cleveland, Ohio. Used with permission.

cry represents a distress signal and is designed to cause a caregiving response that will meet the needs of the infant at that time (Ludington-Hoe et al., 2002); energy reserves are depleted as a result of vigorous motor movements during crying (Ludington, 1990). When crying is reduced (such as when keeping the mother and baby in close contact), blood glucose levels remain high due to decreased metabolic demand for circulating or stored glucose (Christensson et al., 1992).

Supplementation

Supplementing or complementing breastmilk with other fluids and foods from an early age has been described since antiquity (Fildes, 1986). Supplementary and complementary feedings have been defined in many ways, and these terms are often used interchangeably in the literature and in clinical practice. Supplementation can refer to a feeding given in place of a breastfeed or as an extra feeding, whereas complementation often describes topping off a breastfeed with formula, water, or expressed breastmilk. Both mothers and healthcare providers may request or advise that a breastfed infant receive something other than breast-milk for a number of reasons, some of which may not be medically indicated or evidence based. Supplementing breastfed infants both in the hospital and after discharge is a common practice (Kovach, 1997). Abbott Nutritionals (formerly Ross Laboratories and Ross Products Division), an infant formula manufacturer, has collected breastfeeding data through the Mothers Survey since 1955. Data from recent years show a disturbing trend of decreasing exclusive breastfeeding in hospital and increasing amounts of supplementation (Table 4-3).

The CDC currently monitors breastfeeding statistics, showing an all time high of 77% of infants who were at some time breastfed but revealing that rates of exclusive breastfeeding have decreased and stagnated (McDowell et al., 2008). The CDC's mPINC survey revealed that 24% of birth facilities reported supple-menting more than 50% of healthy, full-term, breastfed infants with something other than breastmilk (CDC, 2007). Dewey et al. (2003) noted that 21% of the 280 infants in their study received water or formula in the hospital. Kurinij and Shiono (1991) reported that 37% of breastfed infants in their sample of 726 mothers were given formula supplementation in the hospital. However, 50% of the infants whose mothers delivered at the public or community hospital were supplemented, compared with 15% of the newborns delivered at a university hos-pital. Women giving birth where the supplementation rates were lowest were 3.5 times more likely to be exclusively breastfeeding. The longer a mother waited to

---

TABLE 4-3 Hospital Formula Supplementation Trends

1971

- 21% exclusive breastfeeding in hospital
- 3% additionally supplemented

1982

- 55% exclusive breastfeeding in hospital
- 6.9% additionally supplemented

2001

- 46.3% exclusive breastfeeding in hospital
- 23% additionally supplemented

2003

- 44.0% exclusively breastfeeding in hospital
- 22% additionally supplemented

2006

- 38.4% exclusively breastfeeding in hospital
- 25.2% additionally supplemented

Source: From: Ryan et al. *Pediatrics* 2002; 110:1103–1109; Mothers Survey, Ross Products, Breastfeeding Trends—2003, 2006..

---

initiate breastfeeding, the more likely she was to use formula. Seventeen reasons were cited in the Kurinij and Shiono study for supplementing breastfed infants, with the top three being (1) to give the mother some rest, (2) because the mother was ill, or (3) because the mother did not have enough breastmilk.

Tender et al. (2009) reported that 78% of breastfed infants in their study received formula supplementation while hospitalized. Only 13% of these infants received supplementation based on the supplementation guidelines from the Academy of Breastfeeding Medicine (2002). Reasons for supplementation included the mother's perception of not enough milk and that milk was not in at birth and providers' reasons that infant was lactose intolerant, to help simplify weaning, mother was taking medications, and to allow the mother to sleep. Over 20% of mothers did not know why their infant was supplemented. Within the cohort of women receiving WIC benefits, 80% of breastfed infants were given supplements in the hospital, 87% of which was medically unnecessary. Infants of mothers who did not attend a prenatal breastfeeding class were 4.7 times more likely to receive formula supplementation in hospital. This study demonstrated the importance of improving medical providers' knowledge about breastfeeding and medical indications for supplementation as well as the necessity of correcting misinformation on the part of the mother.

Gagnon et al. (2005) discovered that the highest risk time of day for an infant to receive supplementation was between 7 pm and 9 am, regardless of the time of birth. Nurses in this study revealed that "insufficient milk" was a common reason for supplementing. Infant behaviors such as fussiness, sleepiness, or latching difficulties often triggered supplementation even though there are numerous breastfeeding interventions that can address these issues and do not involve supplementation. Highly anxious mothers were a subgroup of women who needed extra support and special interventions to avoid unnecessary supplementation.

Other common reasons for supplementation include a fussy unsettled infant, a sleepy infant, a certain number of hours have passed without a feeding at the breast, the mother (or nurse) believes she does not have enough milk, and non–evidenced-based assumptions or opinions that supplementation will prevent hypoglycemia, weight loss, dehydration, or hyperbilirubinemia in the breastfed infant. A preponderance of data supports the opposite conclusion (WHO, 1998). Inappropriate supplementation can also negatively affect the immediate and long-term intensity (exclusivity) and duration of breastfeeding (Semenic et al., 2008) and serve as a potential environmental trigger for some acute and chronic diseases and conditions later in life.

Intensity and Duration of Breastfeeding

Research from as early as the 1970s has shown that the introduction of breastmilk substitutes (water or formula), whether in the hospital or in the first month of life, has a consistently negative effect on the duration of breastfeeding. Blomquist et al. (1994) found that breastfed infants who had been given supplements in the hospital were almost four times more likely to have weaned by 3 months of age and were seven times less likely to be breastfed at 3 months if they experienced in-hospital supplementation and experienced a loss of 10% birth weight or more. However, among infants receiving supplements for the specific indications of maternal insulin-dependent diabetes mellitus or gestational diabetes, the duration of breastfeeding was similar to that in the nonsupplemented group. Supplementation without medical reasons significantly reduces the duration of both exclusive and partial breastfeeding; conversely, supplementation for medical reasons does not have this type of dramatic effect on intensity or duration of breastfeeding (Ekstrom et al., 2003). Even one bottle of formula can affect the duration of breastfeeding. Chezem et al. (1998) looked at the patterns of human milk replacement during hospitalization. In a small sample of 53 mothers, 28% of their infants received at least one oral replacement while in the hospital. Duration of breastfeeding was significantly shorter in women whose infants received any formula during hospitalization (9 weeks) compared with women whose infants were not fed formula (20 weeks). Only 40% of the infants fed formula in the hospital were still breastfeeding at 6 weeks compared with 88% of those not fed formula.

In a population of low-income women, Bolton et al. (2009) reported that formula introduction on day 1 postpartum was associated with a significantly shorter breastfeeding duration and that the most dramatic predictor of breastfeeding duration was introduction of formula on day 1. Because early weaning is associated with the early introduction of formula (Hornell et al., 2001), delaying formula introduction may be highly effective in lengthening the duration of breastfeeding. Breastfeeding support interventions must address methods to reduce excessive formula supplementation in-hospital.

One such intervention that reduces formula supplementation in-hospital is to ensure that mothers breastfeed in the labor, delivery, and recovery room (Komara et al., 2007). Newborn medications can be stocked in the labor, delivery, and recovery room so staff can administer the required medications while avoiding the separation of mothers and infants during the early time after birth. Because staff members may perceive infant formula to be free, it is used and given away liberally. Not only is infant formula frequently seen as a fix for breastfeeding problems, but some hospital staff give large quantities of formula to breastfeeding mothers at discharge from the hospital. One way hospitals have helped restrict formula use in breastfed infants to actual medical indications is to lock up the formula and require staff to log out the formula, noting the formula batch number in case there is a recall, date and time of formula use, patient and staff member's names, and reason for use. Some hospitals manage formula use by placing it in a medication distribution system such as Pyxis. This helps provide information on where additional staff education may be needed and helps reduce unnecessary formula supplementation (Cadwell & Turner-Maffei, 2009).

Distribution of discharge bags from formula companies is another form of supplementation with commercial overtones. These bags represent a marketing tactic (not a gift) designed to cause breastfeeding mothers to supplement and purchase more of the product, thus creating a market where none existed before (Walker 2001, 2007). Women who received these packs were more likely to exclusively breastfeed for fewer than 10 weeks than were women who had not received the packs (Rosenberg et al., 2008a). The distribution of these bags to new mothers by hospitals is part of a long-standing marketing campaign by infant formula manufacturers and implies hospital and staff endorsement of infant formula. Many hospitals have recognized the ethical problems created by commercial relationships with infant formula manufacturers and have eliminated the distribution of formula company bags. They have created their own bags, marketing their birthing services rather than allowing formula company access to their patients. Over 300 U.S. hospitals have eliminated these bags, often with help from the Ban the Bags campaign (www.banthebags.org), which provides materials and assistance with formula company bag elimination.

Use of daily human milk replacements is also negatively correlated with breastfeeding duration, regardless of the mother's prenatal intentions to exclusively or partially breastfeed (Chezem et al., 2003). Bottles of formula can be the cause of breastfeeding problems or a symptom of breastfeeding difficulties. Infants who are given nonbreastmilk fluids in the first 48 hours or offered pacifiers have been shown to be two to three times more likely to have suboptimal breastfeeding behaviors on days 3 and 7 (Infant Breastfeeding Assessment Tool score < 10), interfering with the establishment of effective breastfeeding (Dewey et al., 2003). Sievers et al. (2003) studied peripartum indicators for mothers and infants who were most at risk for early lactation failure. Partial feeding of infant formula or an intake of less than 150 g of human milk per day 24–48 hours after lactogenesis II was linked to weaning within 4 weeks.

Supplementation has a marked effect on lactogenesis III, or the calibration and maintenance of a sufficient milk supply (Daly et al., 1993). This interference with the body's ability to accomplish and sustain the production of copious amounts of milk can result in reduced amounts of breastmilk transferred to the infant (Drewett et al., 1989) and a repeating cycle of more formula supplementation until the body receives the signal for breast involution. Breastfeeding frequency and duration decline quickly after the start of regular formula supplementation (one or more bottles of formula per day). Indeed, the younger infants are at the start of regular formula supplementation, the younger they are when they stop breastfeeding (Hornell et al., 2001). The most frequent reason for supplementing young infants is the mother's impression that she does not have enough milk to satisfy the infant. Whether this shortage is real or merely perceived, intervention is needed to prevent the downward spiral toward weaning.

Breastfeeding intensity or degree of exclusivity has been shown to be predictive of duration of breastfeeding up to 1 year of age. Hill et al. (1997) followed 343 mothers for 20 weeks or until weaning, observing the supplementation patterns and subsequent rate of breastfeeding at 5 months postpartum. The breastfeeding rate at 20 weeks was significantly greater for mothers who reported feeding breastmilk exclusively at 2 weeks postpartum ($\approx$61%) compared with mothers who supplemented with formula ($\approx$26%). Using data from the 1988 National Maternal-Infant Health Survey, Piper and Parks (1996) reported that exclusive breastfeeding during the first month postpartum was associated with a breastfeeding duration of longer than 6 months. The strongest association with breastfeeding duration of 1 year was a higher breastfeeding intensity during months 4–6 postpartum (Piper & Parks, 2001).

Weight Loss

Concern about the potential for excessive weight loss in an exclusively breastfed infant has been used to justify the prophylactic and "therapeutic" feeding of water, glucose water, and formula. Lack of understanding regarding the amount of colostrum available and required by newborns has led both parents and health-care providers to urge breastfed infants to consume sterile water, 5% dextrose water, 10% dextrose water, or formula in an attempt to compensate for "insufficient milk," feed the infant "until the milk comes in," or because the infant is "too big" or "too small." Research shows that breastfed infants on the average lose about 5–7% of their birth weight in the first few days of life, peaking on day 3 after birth and recovering by day 8 (Macdonald et al., 2003; Rodriguez et al., 2000). Clinicians become watchful and may intervene when this weight loss reaches 7–10%. Weight loss exceeding 10% of birth weight must be addressed.

Supplementing breastfed infants in the hospital with water or formula, however, does not prevent weight loss (Herrera, 1984; Shrago, 1987). Bertini et al. (2001) also confirmed the relationship between supplementation of breastfed infants with formula and weight loss. Breastfed infants supplemented with formula lost significantly more weight than exclusively breastfed infants or exclusively bottle-fed infants (Table 4-4). In a chart audit of 74 mothers, breastfed infants who received glucose water demonstrated a larger percentage of birth weight loss (2.43–15.87%) compared with unsupplemented breastfed newborns

TABLE 4-4 Weight Loss After Birth and Neonatal Hyperbilirubinemia

	Weight Loss After 72 h of life (g)	*p* Value
All infants studied	214.63 ± 146	< 0.001
Infants with TSB ≥ 12.9 mg/dL	264.49 ± 74	< 0.001
Supplement-fed infants	266 ± 150	< 0.01
Breastfed infants	200.33 ± 145	< 0.01
Formula-fed infants	207.2 ± 70	< 0.01

p Values were < 0.001 among infants with TSB (total serum bilirubin) ≥12.9 mg/dL and all infants studied, <0.01 among supplement- and breastfed infants, and <0.01 among supplement- and formula-fed infants.
Source: Reproduced with permission. *Pediatrics,* Vol 107, ppe41, Table 3, Copyright 2001.

(2.97–7.48%) (Glover, 1990). Weight loss in infants supplemented with sterile water or 5% glucose water is consistent with the lower caloric density of these fluids compared with colostrum, transitional, and mature milk. One ounce of 5% dextrose water contains 5 calories, 1 ounce of 10% dextrose water contains 10 calories, and 1 ounce of colostrum contains 18–20 calories. For each ounce of 5% dextrose water consumed by a breastfed infant, his or her caloric intake is reduced by approximately two-thirds. The risk of excess infant weight loss has been shown to be 7.1 times greater if the mother has delayed onset of milk production (Dewey et al., 2003). Neifert (1998, 1999) recommended that weight loss of 8% or more from birth weight, failure to surpass birth weight by 2 weeks of age, or failure to commence weight gain of approximately 28 g per day by 5 days of age warrant further investigation.

Healthy full-term newborns have an abundance of extracellular and extravascular water. Caution therefore is necessary in the use of water supplementation of newborns. Water intoxication with seizures has been reported in a breastfed infant who was given 675 mL (22.5 oz) of supplementary glucose water during the 24 hours before transfer from the maternity unit to the neonatal intensive care unit (Ruth-Sanchez & Greene, 1997). Supplementation should not be used in place of skilled assessment and prompt and correct lactation care and services. Neonates born to mothers who have received dextrose-containing IV fluids during labor can experience enough of a fluid shift to skew weight loss calculations toward the appearance of a clinical problem of excessive loss of birth weight, when what is really taking place is a diuresis of excess fluid (Keppler, 1988).

Dahlenburg et al. (1980) examined the serum sodium levels in newborns whose mothers received IV fluids containing 5% dextrose and oxytocin. The mean sodium levels were significantly lower in the infants whose mothers had IV fluids compared with those who did not. Percentage of weight loss in infants whose mothers received IV fluids was 6.17% ± 3.36% compared with 4.07% ± 2.20% weight loss in infants whose mothers did not receive IV fluids during labor. Both maternal and neonatal serum sodium concentrations are significantly decreased even when dextrose is used only as the diluent (rather than normal saline) for oxytocin infusion in induction or augmentation of labor (Higgins et al., 1996; Stratton et al., 1995).

Breastfed infants whose mothers received epidurals have been shown to lose more weight in the first 24 hours than infants whose mothers did not have an epidural. Merry and Montgomery (2000) reported that the average weight loss in the first day for infants whose mothers had an epidural was 226 g (8 oz) compared with 142 g (5 oz) in a nonepidural group. It is possible that administration of IV fluids during labor, which is more common in women receiving analgesia or anesthesia, could initially increase the hydration status of the newborn, with a subsequent rapid weight loss mimicking underfeeding. Once started, water supplementation remains prevalent in the first month of life, even in exclusively breastfed infants (Scariati et al., 1997).

Martens and Romphf (2007) demonstrated that factors significantly increasing the percentage of weight loss in newborn infants included birth weight, female sex, epidural use, and a longer hospital stay. In this study, supplemented breastfed infants lost more weight than exclusively breastfed newborns, as did those whose mothers had epidurals during labor and delivery. Formula-fed infants lost approximately 3% of birth weight, substantially less than a breastfed infant who represents the norm. The authors speculated that formula-fed infants (who were 111 g heavier than breastfed infants during the first 3 days postpartum) may be at risk for overfeeding in the early days, a time when early feeding experiences could be critical to metabolic imprinting and future overweight or obesity (Lucas, 1998; de Moura et al., 2008). Unnecessary or unphysiological amounts of formula supplement may predispose infants to later weight problems. Stettler et al. (2005) found a 28% increased risk of obesity in adults for every 100 g of weight an infant gained in his or her first week of life.

Caglar et al. (2006) reported that infants with a weight loss of more than 10% were more likely to be from primiparous mothers, to experience a delay in receiving their first breastfeeding, to pass less than four stools per day, and to have uric acid crystals in their diaper. This alerts the clinician to the need by first-time mothers for extra vigilance, ensuring that the infant is swallowing milk and that the mother knows how to tell when the infant is swallowing.

Assessment of effective or ineffective breastfeeding and supplementation interventions must rely on more than just weight loss. Often, the underlying assumption is that weight loss is due to insufficient milk supply or ineffective milk transfer, but other confounding factors may also be present. Birthing practices, hospital routines, and birth experiences are also associated with weight loss. Seldom is the amount of stooling and voiding entered into the equation of neonatal weight loss. Weight change patterns help clinicians identify situations of concern, but interventions such as supplementing breastfed infants with formula should not be solely based on maintaining an infant's weight within preestablished norms (Noel-Weiss et al., 2008).

Dehydration

Prophylactic or routine administration of water or formula to breastfed infants to prevent dehydration has not been shown to be necessary. Dehydration is unlikely to occur in full-term healthy newborns who are able to successfully transfer colostrum and milk from the breast and who are given ample opportunities to do so when they demonstrate feeding readiness cues. Rodriguez et al. (2000) calculated the loss of total body water and body solids during the first 3 days of life. The percentage of total body water actually increased, indicating adequate hydration, whereas the weight of the infant decreased due to the greater loss of body solids (stool), not the loss of total body water. Infants who pass several large meconium stools during the first 24–48 hours may give the appearance of not being adequately fed or hydrated but do not require intervention unless other feeding parameters are not acceptable.

Renal function in the newborn differs from that in older children and adults. The normal neonate has 6–44 mL of urine in the bladder at birth. Approximately 17% of newborns void directly after delivery, 92% by 24 hours, and 99% by 48 hours. Newborns tend to be oliguric (low urinary output) for the first day because of high circulating levels of antidiuretic hormone after birth. If the infant voided at delivery, urine output in the first 24 hours may be misleading (Black, 2001) because another void may not become apparent until many hours later. The full-term infant typically creates a urine volume of 15–60 mL per 24 hours. Voiding size is 19.3 mL, with urine formation ranging from 0.5 to 5.0 mg/kg/h at all gestational ages. Normal neonates void 2–6 times per day during the first 48 hours of life and 5–25 times daily thereafter. Voiding during the first 2–3 days reflects the depletion of the infant's extravascular and extracellular reserve and may be reflected in diaper counts of one to two diapers, with amounts increasing as lactogenesis II occurs on days 3–4. Urine output increases rapidly after this time (Table 4-5).

Hypernatremic dehydration, however, can represent the extreme spectrum of a deteriorating clinical situation (Neifert, 2001). An infant who is unable to transfer milk and a mother who has a depleted milk supply, delayed lactogenesis II, under-production, or any number of other risk factors (Tables 4-6 and 4-7) should be evaluated promptly to avoid true infant dehydration. Fever and hypernatremia are often found in neonates with excessive weight loss. In low-risk, full-term infants, fever with no other symptoms during the first days is frequently related to dehydration and problems with breastfeeding. Jaundice and poor sucking may be the major presenting symptoms (Unal et al., 2008). Hypernatremia can cause disruption in the blood–brain barrier, facilitating the diffusion of bilirubin into the brain. This can lead to a worsening cycle of dehydration, jaundice, and hyper-natremia. Often, jaundice is the presenting complaint along with a weight loss of greater than 7% (Uras et al., 2007). Hypernatremic dehydration may be difficult to recognize clinically, but weight loss and inadequate stooling are sensitive indi-cators of dehydration (Moritz et al., 2005). Scant bowel output during the first 5 days after delivery or delayed transition of bowel movements to a yellow color are markers for immediate follow-up (Shrago et al., 2006). Konetzny et al. (2009) found that infants born by cesarean section had a 3.4 times higher risk for hyper-natremia than those born vaginally, reminding clinicians that these babies may need closer follow-up both during the hospital stay and post discharge. Weighing infants at 72–96 hours after birth helps in the early recognition of hypernatremic dehydration and reduces the extent of the dehydration and hypernatremia while preserving breastfeeding (Iyer et al., 2008). Mothers should be provided with information (Figure 4-3) that addresses feeding adequacy and alerts them to when they should consult a healthcare provider (Livingstone et al., 2000).

TABLE 4-5 Urine Volume mL/24 h

Full term	2 Weeks	8 Weeks	1 Year
15–60	250–400	250–400	500–600

Source: Ingelfinger JR. Renal conditions in the newborn period. In: Cloherty JP, Stark AR, eds. *Manual of Neonatal Care.* 3rd ed. Boston: Little, Brown and Company; 1991, pp. 477–495.

TABLE 4-6   Maternal Risk Factors for Infant Dehydration

- Previous insufficient milk or underweight, breastfed infant
- Flat or inverted nipples affecting infant latch or milk removal
- Breast anomalies such as markedly asymmetrical, tubular, or hypoplastic breasts
- Excessive, prolonged, or unrelieved breast engorgement
- Previous breast surgery (periareolar incisions, abscess)
- Cracked, bleeding nipples or persistent nipple pain
- Perinatal complications (hemorrhage, hypertension, infection)
- Preexisting maternal conditions (overweight, obesity, diabetes, endocrine disorders)
- Lack of previous breastfeeding experience
- Maternal age older than 37 years
- Labor and delivery variations (vacuum extraction, labor medications, prolonged labor)

TABLE 4-7   Early Infant Breastfeeding Risk Factors for Dehydration

---

- Gestation age (preterm and near-term 36–37 weeks)
- Small for gestation age, intrauterine growth retardation, low birth weight
- Separation from mother for more than 24 h
- Oral anatomical defects (cleft lip/palate, micrognathia, macroglossia, ankyloglossia, bubble palate)
- Neurological or neuromotor problems (Down syndrome, dysfunctional sucking)
- Sucking variations (nonsustained, non-nutritive, disorganized, weak)
- Hyperbilirubinemia, especially if using phototherapy
- Multiple births
- Systemic illness (increased oxygen requirement, cardiac defect, infection)
- Difficulty latching correctly to one or both breasts
- Sleepy infant with poor or subtle feeding cues
- Irritability, fretfulness, apparent hunger after feeds
- Excessive pacifier use
- Weight loss of more than 7% of birth weight
- Not passing yellow, breastmilk stools by 4 days of age; fewer than four sizable stools per day between 4 days and 4 weeks of age
- Fewer than six clear voids per day by 4 days of age
- Appearance of urate crystals in the diaper after 3 days of age
- Failure to exceed birth weight by 10–14 days of age
- Failure to begin weight gain of approximately 28 g/day after day 4 or 5

Sources: Adapted from Neifert MR. Prevention of breastfeeding tragedies. *Ped Clin North Am.* 2001;48: 273–297; Walker M. Functional assessment of infant breastfeeding patterns. *Birth.* 1989;16:140–147.

Breastfeeding Checklist for Newborns

Post on your refrigerator or on the back of your bathroom door.

Baby's birth date and time: _____

Your baby will be 4 days old on _____

Baby's birth weight: _____

Baby's discharge weight: _____
(*It's normal to lose up to 7% from birth.*)

Baby's weight at check-up 2 days after discharge: _____

Baby's second week weight: _____
(*Baby should have regained his birth weight by 14 days.*)

Important Numbers:

Pediatrician: _____

OB-GYN Doctor: _____

Lactation Consultant: _____

Find more support near you at Zipmilk.org – just enter your zip code.

Some signs that breastfeeding is going well:

❑ Your baby is breastfeeding at least 8 times every 24 hours.

❑ Your baby has at least 4 yellow bowel movements every 24 hours by day 4.

❑ You can hear your baby gulping or swallowing at feedings.

❑ Once your baby latches on, your nipples do not hurt when your baby nurses.

❑ Your baby is receiving only breastmilk.

Check in with your pediatrician's office or lactation consultant if:

❑ Your baby is having fewer than 4 poopy diapers per 24 hours by day 4.

❑ There are any red stains in the diaper after day 3. (It can be normal in the first 3 days.)

❑ Your baby is still having black tarry bowel movements on day 4.

❑ Your baby is not breastfeeding at least 8 times every 24 hours.

❑ You can't hear your baby gulping or swallowing, or you can't tell.

❑ Your nipples hurt during feeding, even after the baby is first latched on.

❑ Your baby does not seem satisfied after most feedings.

It is your responsibility to contact your baby's doctor
to schedule visits, including a visit 2 days after going home.

**Do not wait to call your baby's doctor or the
lactation consultant if *you* think breastfeeding
is not going well.**

Figure 4-3   Breastfeeding Checklist for Newborns

Source: Massachusetts Breastfeeding Coalition (www.massbfc.org). Used with permission.

Hyperbilirubinemia

Prevention of hyperbilirubinemia is a frequently cited reason for recommending supplementation, as is the misconception that bilirubin can be flushed out of the system by increasing water intake. At birth normal, healthy, full-term infants have a cord total serum bilirubin concentration of about 1.5 mg/dL (25.5 μmol/L). This increases in the early days to a mean peak of approximately 5.5 mg/dL (93.5 μmol/L) by the third day in black and white infants and 10 mg/dL (170 μmol/L) in infants of Asian origin (Halamek & Stevenson, 1996). Breastfed infants of Asian origin (Japanese, Korean, and Chinese) as well as breastfed Navajo Indian and Alaska Native newborns appear to have exaggerated physiological jaundice independent of feeding method (Saland et al., 1974).

Breastfed and formula-fed infants have been shown to have differing bilirubin patterns, with breastfed infants experiencing a more gradual decline in bilirubin levels or with bilirubin concentration reaching a second peak around the 10th day of life (Gartner & Herschel, 2001). Breastfed infants have had a persistent reputation of demonstrating higher serum bilirubin concentrations than do formula-fed infants (Adams et al., 1985; Schneider, 1986). This perception may be a holdover perhaps from early studies or an artifact of restrictive policies on the frequency and duration of breastfeeding and the practice of routinely or liberally supplementing breastfed newborns with water or formula.

- Feeding frequency and bilirubin levels are inversely associated in the first 3 days of life. Infants fed eight times or less per 24 hours had significantly higher bilirubin levels on day 3 (9.3 mg/dL) than did infants fed more than eight times per 24 hours (6.5 mg/dL) (De Carvalho et al., 1982). As the frequency of breastfeeding decreases, the incidence and levels of bilirubin increase over the first week of life. Yamauchi and Yamanouchi (1990) looked at the frequency of breastfeeding during the first 24 hours and the incidence of bilirubin levels exceeding 15 mg/dL at 6 days. Infants who fed 9–11 times per day had a 0% rate, those feeding 7–8 times per 24 hours had a rate of 11.8%, those feeding 5–6 times per 24 hours yielded a 15.2% rate, 3–4 times showed a 24.5% rate, and infants fed less frequently than that showed a 28.1% rate of significant jaundice.

- Water supplementation has an inverse relationship with bilirubin levels. The more water given to breastfed infants, the higher their bilirubin levels (Nicoll et al., 1982). Supplementary water does not prophylactically prevent or lower bilirubin levels (De Carvalho et al., 1981).

- Meconium passage is also related to bilirubin levels. As stooling volume increases, serum bilirubin levels decrease. Early initiation and more frequent breastfeeding avoid delayed fecal bilirubin clearance (De Carvalho et al., 1985).

Bertini et al. (2001) reported a significant correlation between breastfed infants with significant jaundice (bilirubin levels > 12.9 mg/dL; 221 mmol/L) and supplementary feeding. Breastfed infants did not have higher bilirubin levels in the first days of life, except for a subpopulation that showed a greater weight loss than the mean. Jaundice was not associated with breastfeeding per se but rather with an increased weight loss after birth subsequent to fasting, suggesting the important role of caloric intake in the regulation of serum bilirubin. Thus breastfed infants who receive low-calorie supplements in place of colostrum and breastfed infants who are unable to transfer colostrum and subsequently receive supplementation show much higher levels of bilirubin. Among the other conditions favoring jaundice (ABO blood incompatibility, supplementary feeding, weight loss, and Asian ethnicity) was the finding that infants born by vacuum extraction were at a high risk for exaggerated jaundice. Seventeen percent of vacuum-extracted infants had total serum bilirubin values exceeding 12.9 mg/dL. This finding is consistent with the development of scalp or brain bleeding and has been reported in the past (Rubaltelli, 1968).

Once formed, bilirubin cannot be diluted or flushed out by giving additional water. This substance is conjugated by the liver, and almost all of it is excreted via the bile into the stools. Water is not a limiting or facilitating factor in bilirubin metabolism. Giving additional water decreases breastmilk and caloric intake, reduces breast stimulation, increases the risk for insufficient milk, increases bilirubin levels, and is counterproductive to establishing breastfeeding and adequate lactation. Water supplements may result in adequate hydration but create simultaneous caloric deprivation, contributing to the very situation the supplements were supposed to avoid. As Gartner (1994) reminds clinicians, "In the great majority of cases of breastfeeding jaundice, the evidence points to inappropriate or thoughtless policies and procedures regarding breastfeeding advice and management." The AAP (2004) recommends against routine supplementation of non-dehydrated breastfed infants with water or dextrose water. In spite of the data and recommendations to the contrary, the mPINC survey found that 30% of facilities gave feedings of glucose water and 15% gave water to breastfed infants, practices known to be detrimental to breastfeeding (CDC, 2008). Dextrose/water supplements may prevent clinical interventions necessary to prevent excessive bilirubin levels from developing pre and post discharge. Rather than water supplements, clinicians should use a preventive approach to hyperbilirubinemia (Bhutani & Johnson, 2009) that includes optimal breastfeeding support (making sure that mothers know when their infant is swallowing milk), risk assessment for hyper-bilirubinemia in the hospital through use of a bilirubin nomogram, more intense monitoring of infants at increased risk (such as late preterm infants), and a follow-up appointment with the infant's physician within 48 hours of discharge.

Hypoglycemia

Hypoglycemia (or the potential for hypoglycemia) represents a frequent reason for supplementing the breastfed newborn. A major physiological challenge for newborns is to establish and regulate their own metabolic processes, including the self-regulation of glucose metabolism when this function is no longer performed by the maternal placental unit. A quarter of a century ago newborns were routinely fed nothing by mouth for 6–12 hours after birth, reflecting a number of non–evidence-based assumptions. Inappropriate supplementation trends persist today due to a lack of consensus on what constitutes hypoglycemia, misunderstanding of neonatal glucose metabolism, and uncertainty about when to intervene. After delivery, the maternal glucose supply is abruptly withdrawn, causing a self-limiting decline in the infant's blood sugar for about the first 3 hours of life (Srinivasan et al., 1986). The infant must then initiate counterregulatory compensation through three processes, plus the formation of alternative fuels (Williams, 1997):

1. Glycolysis, the conversion of glucose to lactate and pyruvate
2. Glycogenolysis, the release of glycogen from body stores to form glucose
3. Gluconeogenesis, the production of glucose by the liver and kidneys from substrates such as fatty acids and amino acids

Additional sources of fuel for the brain include ketone bodies derived from a brisk ketogenic response to low blood glucose levels through fatty acid mobilization. Especially at low blood glucose levels, breastfed infants show high concentrations of ketone bodies, a response that is blunted by supplementation with formula (De Rooy & Hawdon, 2002). Early feeding of human milk/colostrum enhances the process of gluconeogenesis by providing amino acid precursors, presents fatty acids that facilitate the formation of an enzyme critical to ketogenesis, and provides lactose that minimizes insulin secretion. Feeding either 5% or 10% glucose water in the immediate period after birth increases insulin secretion (which suppresses gluconeogenesis), decreases secretion of glucagon (a hormone that stimulates the liver to change stored glycogen to glucose and encourages the use of fats and amino acids for energy production), and delays the natural gluconeogenesis and ketogenic processes (Eidelman, 2001). The breastfed term infants who lose the most weight have the highest ketone body concentrations (Hawdon et al., 1992; Swenne et al., 1994), suggesting that ketogenesis is an adaptive response to temporarily low nutrient intake during the time it takes for the infant to successfully establish feeding at the breast (Cornblath et al., 2000).

Formula- and breastfed infants demonstrate different patterns of serum glucose concentrations. Hawdon and coworkers (1992) reported a mean of 3.6 mmol/L (58 mg/dL) with a range of 1.5–5.3 mmol/L (27–95 mg/dL) in breastfed infants and a mean of 4.0 mmol/L (72 mg/dL) with a range of 2.5–6.2 mmol/L (45–111 mg/dL) in formula-fed infants. None of the breastfed infants became symptomatic, and all responded with significant increases in ketone bodies. Only the interval between feedings was correlated with glucose concentrations, reinforcing the recommendation for frequent breastfeeding. Considerable controversy exists regarding the actual definition of hypoglycemia, with some current definitions not being applicable to breastfed infants because these infants can tolerate lower plasma glucose levels (Cornblath et al., 1990). Statistical rather than functional blood glucose levels have been described for hypoglycemia cut-off points that are the lower limits of normal (Table 4-8). These distinctions are based on serum or plasma glucose concentrations, which are 10–15% higher than in whole blood and do not distinguish between breastfed and formula-fed infants.

Symptomatic hypoglycemia is the association of clinical signs (which can be vague and nonspecific) and blood glucose concentrations of less than arbitrary

TABLE 4-8 Statistical Definition of Hypoglycemia

Author	Age (h)	Serum or Plasma Glucose Concentration
Srinivasan et al. (1986)	0–3 hours	<35 mg/dL (2.0 mmol/L)
	3–24 hours	<40 mg/dL (2.2 mmol/L)
	24–48 hours	<45 mg/dL (2.5 mmol/L)
Heck & Erenberg (1987)	0–24 hours	<30 mg/dL (1.7 mmol/L)
	24–48 hours	<40 mg/dL (2.2 mmol/L)

level. Healthy, normal, full-term infants do not develop symptomatic hypoglycemia simply as a result of underfeeding (Williams, 1997) and do not require routine monitoring of blood glucose levels (Eidelman, 2001). The use of bedside screening tests using reagent strips can have as high as a 20% rate of false positives (i.e., normoglycemic infants labeled erroneously as hypoglycemic) (Holtrop et al., 1990; Reynolds & Davies, 1993). Laboratory determinations should confirm the results before supplementing a breastfed infant. Hypoglycemia is minimized in breastfed infants who are fed early, often, and exclusively and who are actually and adequately transferring milk (colostrum) that is confirmed by documenting swallowing. Early breastfeeding is not precluded simply because an infant meets the criteria for glucose monitoring (Academy of Breastfeeding Medicine, 2006). Some maternity units supplement normal, healthy, full-term infants as if they were high risk, using specific glucose levels that may inappropriately call for supplementing infants who have no medical need. Maternity units should not use glucose measurements adapted for sick infants, such as in the S.T.A.B.L.E. program (http://www.stableprogram.org/index.php), a program for postresuscitation/pretransport stabilization care of sick infants. Gross overfeeding of breastfed infants with infant formula to prevent or ameliorate low blood sugar levels may unintentionally result in long-term problems. Screening should be restricted to at-risk and symptomatic infants, with symptomatic infants receiving intravenous glucose therapy, not forced feedings (Wight, 2006).

"Just One Bottle Won't Hurt" (Or Will It?)

Early supplementation of the breastfed infant with infant formula has significant effects on the recipient infant's gut flora (Brown & Bosworth, 1922; Bullen et al., 1977), can provoke sensitivity and allergy to cow's milk protein (Host, 1991), and has been identified as an environmental triggering event in the development of diabetes in susceptible families (Karjalainen et al., 1992). Gimeno and deSouza (1997) demonstrated that the introduction to cow's milk products before 8 days of age is a risk factor for insulin-dependent diabetes mellitus. Careful consideration should be undertaken before supplementing a breastfed infant, including establishing the presence of a history of allergy or diabetes in the infant's family. Liberal or cavalier supplementing of a breastfed infant with standard cow's milk–based formula can have long-lasting negative effects. Exposure of an exclusively breastfed infant to the cow's milk in infant formula during the hospital stay can sensitize the infant to cow's milk protein (Juvonen et al., 1999), setting up an allergic response when challenged with cow's milk later in the first year of life (Saarinen et al., 1999; Saarinen & Savilahti, 2000). IgA antibodies in colostrum and mature human milk prevent antigen entry at the intestinal surface of a breastfed infant. Infants whose mothers have a low IgA content in their milk may experience defective exclusion of food antigens and be predisposed to the development of food allergies (Jarvinen et al., 2000). Only tiny amounts of an allergen are necessary to sensitize a susceptible infant. Just 1 ng of bovine beta-lactalbumin is sufficient to set the stage for an undesired outcome (Businco et al., 1999). Cantani and Micera (2005) demonstrated that small doses of allergens are more sensitizing than larger ones. Isolated supplementary cow's milk–based formula feedings of breastfed infants should be avoided during the early days. If a formula is needed, a hydrolyzed formula should be used (AAP, 1994). The Nutritional Committees from the AAP and jointly the European Society for Pediatric Allergology and Clinical Immunology and the European Society for Pediatric Gastroenterology, Hepatology, and Nutrition recommend exclusive breastfeeding as the most critical measure for food allergy prevention (Zeiger, 2003).

Indications for Supplementation

According to the World Health Organization, there are a few medical indications in a maternity facility that may require individual infants be given fluids or food in addition to, or in place of, breastmilk (Box 4-2). If supplementation is being considered, a thorough breastfeeding assessment and evaluation of the mother and infant should take place and should include a direct observation of a feeding at breast; an evaluation of the maternal milk supply; a labor, delivery, and feeding history; evaluation of the infant's positioning, latch, suck, and swallow; and assessment of the infant's overall condition (Walker, 1989). A number of indications or conditions present in the mother (Table 4-9) or the infant (Table 4-10) would alert the clinician to the possibility of the need for either temporary or ongoing supplementation—the infant must always be fed.

What to Supplement

If it is determined that supplementation is necessary, what should be used? A hierarchy of supplemental feedings (Table 4-11) in descending order of preference can be used as a guide. Fresh expressed mother's own milk is always preferable (AAP, 2005) unless very rare conditions or situations temporarily or permanently

BOX 4-2 Acceptable Medical Reasons for Supplementing Breastfed Infants

It is assumed that severely ill infants, infants in need of surgery, and very-low-birth-weight infants will be in a special care unit. Their feeding will be individually decided, given their particular nutritional requirements and functional capabilities, although breastmilk is recommended whenever possible. These infants in special care are likely to include the following groups:

- Infants with very low birth weight (less than 1,500 g) or who are born before 32 weeks gestational age
- Infants with severe dysmaturity with potentially severe hypoglycemia or who require therapy for hypoglycemia and who do not improve through increased breastfeeding or by being given breastmilk

For infants who are well enough to be with their mothers on the maternity unit, there are very few indications for supplements. To assess whether a facility is inappropriately using fluids or artificial feeds, any infants receiving supplements must have been diagnosed as

- Infants whose mothers are severely ill (e.g., with psychosis, sepsis, eclampsia, or shock) or with HIV infection, herpes simplex virus type 1 if lesions are on the breast
- Infants with inborn errors of metabolism (e.g., galactosemia, phenylketonuria, maple syrup urine disease)
- Infants with acute water loss (e.g., during phototherapy for jaundice), if increased breastfeeding cannot provide adequate hydration
- Infants whose mothers are taking medication that is contraindicated when breastfeeding (e.g., cytotoxic drugs, certain radioactive drugs such as iodine-131, and antithyroid drugs other than propylthiouracil) or mothers engaged in substance abuse
- Newborn infants at risk of hypoglycemia due to impaired metabolic adaptation or increased glucose demand (small for gestational age, late preterm, experienced hypoxic/ischemic stress, those who are ill, and those whose mothers are diabetic) if their blood sugar fails to respond to breastfeeding or breastmilk feeding

When breastfeeding has to be temporarily delayed or interrupted, mothers should be helped to establish or maintain lactation; for example, through manual or hand-pumped expression of milk in preparation for the moment when breastfeeding may be begun or resumed.

Source: World Health Organization/United Nations Children's Fund. *Baby-Friendly Hospital Initiative. Part II: Hospital Level Implementation.* Geneva: World Health Organization; 1992; World Health Organization/United Nations Children's Fund. *Acceptable medical reasons for use of breast-milk substitutes.* Geneva: World Health Organization; 2009.

TABLE 4-9   Possible Maternal Indications for Supplementing the Breastfed Infant

---

- Maternal illness or condition (psychosis, eclampsia, herpes simplex lesion on the breast until healed, postpartum hemorrhage/Sheehan syndrome, varicella-zoster [chickenpox] until the mother is noninfectious, active tuberculosis until 2 or more weeks of treatment have occurred, Lyme disease until mother has initiated treatment, retained placenta)
- Geographic separation (mother and baby at different hospitals, mother or baby remaining in the hospital, custody or visitation issues)
- Maternal medications or recreational drugs (certain diagnostic radiopharmaceuticals until cleared from maternal plasma, most street or recreational drugs except cigarettes and small amounts of alcohol, and a very small number of medications)
- Delayed lactogenesis II (after day 5 with signs of inadequate infant intake)
- Intolerable pain and/or extensive damage to the nipples
- Breast anomalies, surgery, insufficient glandular tissue

Sources: Adapted from Lawrence RA. *A review of the medical benefits and contraindications to breastfeeding in the United States.* (Maternal and Child Health Technical Information Bulletin). Arlington, VA: National Center for Education in Maternal and Child Health; 1997; Powers NG, Slusser W. Breastfeeding update 2: Clinical lactation management. *Pediatr Rev.* 1997;18:147–161; Wight NE. *Supplements and the breastfed infant: When are they needed and how should they be supplied?* Independent Study Module. Schaumburg, IL: La Leche League International; 2001.

TABLE 4-10   Possible Infant Indications for Supplementing the Breastfed Infant

---

- Hypoglycemia validated with laboratory measurements, after the infant has been shown to unsuccessfully transfer colostrum during suckling opportunities
- Impending or significant dehydration (usually picked up after hospital discharge)
- Weight loss of 7–10% after days 3–5 with evidence of delayed lactogenesis II
- Meconium stools at day 5
- Inability of infant to transfer sufficient milk in the presence of an adequate milk supply
- Hyperbilirubinemia when the infant cannot sustain feedings at the breast
- Preterm, low birth weight, late preterm, congenital anomalies, illness, or other conditions that preclude the infant from either feeding directly at breast or feeding at breast but being unable to transfer sufficient quantities of milk

Sources: Adapted from Powers NG, Slusser W. Breastfeeding update 2: Clinical lactation management. *Pediatr Rev.* 1997;18:147–161; Wight NE. *Supplements and the breastfed infant: When are they needed and how should they be supplied?* Independent Study Module. Schaumburg, IL: La Leche League International; 2001.

TABLE 4-11 Hierarchy of Supplements

- Fresh mother's own milk/colostrum
- Refrigerated mother's own milk
- Frozen and thawed mother's own milk
- Fortified (if necessary) mother's own milk for preterm infants
- Pasteurized donor banked human milk
- Hypoallergenic infant formula
- Elemental infant formula
- Cow's milk–based infant formula
- Soy infant formula
- Water or glucose water

---

preclude its use. Diabetic mothers may wish to express colostrum prenatally, freeze it, and bring it to the hospital in case their infant requires supplementation (Cox, 2006). Mothers can begin expressing colostrum by drawing it into a 1-mL or 3-mL syringe at 34 weeks for 3–5 minutes on each breast as long as they experience no uterine cramping.

The potential risks and benefits of supplementation must be considered within the overall goal of preserving breastfeeding (Academy of Breastfeeding Medicine, 2002). Each type of supplement (Table 4-12) should be considered in terms of its potential to provide appropriate nutrition, protect the maternal milk supply, and avoid feeding-related morbidities (Wight, 2001).

The amount of supplement to be provided also depends on the situation. Wight (2006) recommended 3–5 mL/kg of expressed breastmilk or breastmilk substitute. This volume is based on normal volumes of colostrum, the average size of the infant's stomach, and average volumes of milk typically ingested by newborns. If an infant needed an entire feeding supplemented, this amount may vary based on the infant's health status, weight, and feeding goals. For late preterm infants, Stellwagen et al. (2007) recommend feeding volumes of 5–10 mL every 2–3 hours on day 1, 10–20 mL on day 2, and 20–30 mL on day 3.

How to Supplement

There are a number of different ways to supplement a breastfed infant. Healthcare providers often recommend that the supplement be delivered by bottle, because it

TABLE 4-12 Comparison of Supplements on Selected Parameters

Supplement	Calories/oz/28 cc	Allergic potential	Effect on milk production	Effect on bilirubin levels	Effect on blood sugar
Expressed mother's milk	18 colostrum 20 or more mature	None	Increases	Normal	Stabilizes and increases
Cow's milk–based formula	20	High	Decreases	Lowers	Increases
Soy formula	20	Medium to high	Decreases	Lowers	Increases
Hydrolyzed formula	20	Low	Decreases	Lowers	Increases
Sterile water	0	None	Decreases	Increases	None
D5W	6	None	Decreases	Increases	Bounces

presents a rapid and easy way to feed an infant. However, sucking on an artificial nipple is not the same as suckling from the breast. Perioral muscle function differs between bottle-feeding and breastfeeding (Inoue et al., 1995). Artificial nipples that require mostly suction rather than mostly compression can contribute to reduced masseter muscle activity as the muscle adjusts to bottle-feeding (Sakashita, Kamegai, & Inoue, 1996). Buccinator muscles are recruited to compensate for altered tongue function during bottle-feeding. Changes in tongue function alter and weaken other muscles, such as the styloglossus and palatoglossus, used during sucking and swallowing. This change in oral muscle function may contribute to an infant experiencing difficulty in transitioning to the breast after being bottle-fed (Ferrante et al., 2006). There can be significant differences between bottle-feeding and breastfeeding in terms of swallowing and the stability of the suck-swallow-breathe cycle (Goldfield et al., 2006). Mizuno and Ueda (2006) reported that sucking pressures for nutritive and non-nutritive sucking are exactly the opposite when comparing breastfeeding and sucking on an artificial nipple. Random, frequent, and uncoordinated swallowing seen with some bottle-feeding systems can contribute to desaturation, poor intake, and a delay in breastfeeding skill acquisition.

If supplementation is done by bottle, choice of an artificial nipple can be problematic. Nipple flow rates are not standardized, many nipples are too stiff for an infant with a weak suck, some have rapid flow rates that compromise ventilation, and none fits the anatomical shape of an infant's oral structures. The mechanics of sucking on specific artificial nipples have been sparsely studied (Fadavi et al., 1997; Goldfield et al., 2006), and care must be taken in interpreting the results because nipple parameters (material, deflection, and extension capabilities) are changed frequently by manufacturers. Aizawa et al. (2009) demonstrated that the angle of mouth opening on the breast was double that of infants feeding from a standard size artificial nipple. A partially closed mouth configuration on the breast may result in nipple pain and damage and reduced milk intake.

When choosing an artificial nipple for a breastfed infant, consider the following. The artificial nipple should have a soft nipple (silicone rather than latex) that can be slightly elongated and deflected upward, mimicking the shape changes of the human nipple–areola. The human nipple is not stationary during breast-feeding and has a mean movement of 4.0 ± 1.3 mm during infant sucking (Jacobs et al., 2007). If the strength required to alter the artificial nipple shape is beyond the infant's capacity, the tongue may be forced down, reinforcing an incorrect swallow pattern (Ferrante et al., 2006).

The length of the artificial nipple is also important. Jacobs et al. (2007) found on ultrasound scans that the nipple tip of the human nipple was usually not drawn into the mouth to a point where it rested directly under the junction of the hard and soft palates but was positioned approximately 5 mm in front of this spot. The artificial nipple should not be so long that it causes the infant to gag. Shorter, softer, more mobile nipples may result in a supplementation experience that does not compromise the transition to feeding at the breast.

Artificial nipples are typically less elastic than the human nipple, may elongate only minimally (Nowak et al., 1994), may have varying flow rates (Mathew, 1988a, 1990) (which may or may not be appropriate for an individual infant), and may deliver milk using only vacuum or only compression rather than both. The "orthodontic" type of nipple may eliminate the central grooving of the tongue (Wolf & Glass, 1992). The tongue motion on an artificial nipple, especially a firm one, is more squeezing or piston-like (Weber et al., 1986). Artificial nipples also increase the amount of air that an infant swallows (Ardran et al., 1958). Random, frequent, and uncoordinated swallowing seen with some bottle systems can provoke oxygen desaturation, poor intake, and a delay in breastfeeding skill acquisition, especially in a compromised infant. If a bottle is used, paced feedings may avoid fatigue and desaturation in less mature infants.

Because of these differences, which can sometimes be quite subtle, questions may arise about an infant's ability to correctly suckle at breast if he or she has been exposed to an artificial nipple that requires different sucking dynamics. This phenomenon has been referred to as nipple confusion or nipple preference. Neifert et al. (1995) defined nipple confusion as "an infant's difficulty in achieving the correct oral configuration, latching technique, and suckling pattern necessary for successful breastfeeding after bottle feeding or other exposure to an artificial nipple." The fact that nipple confusion occurs is probably best illustrated by infants who have difficulty changing between bottle nipples of varying designs. Although the term "confusion" may be inaccurate, it may be that it is the tactile and proprioceptive qualities of an object that influence or alter the infant's oral movements and acceptance (Wolf & Glass, 1992). These qualities may act as a "super-stimulus" and simply overwhelm an infant's sensitive mouth.

Some infants have no difficulty alternating between the breast and an artificial nipple. Others may experience difficulty in rapidly adapting to a change or may take time to learn a different behavior. A subset of infants may be unable to differentiate between the sucking movements required to extract milk relative to the differing types of nipples presented to them. According to Sakashita et al. (1996), "Bottle feeding is a non-physiological condition and the physiological behavior is replaced by an adaptive change, the sucking action." There are a number of other variables whose interaction with one another and effect on any given infant require the clinician's attention (Box 4-3).

There is currently no way to predict which infants will have difficulty and which ones will transition between breast and bottle effortlessly. In an effort to prevent or reduce latch, suck, and numerous other problems attributed to artificial nipples, alternatives to bottles may be recommended. These devices can be used temporarily to deliver nutrition, may be selected to assist with latch-on, or may be necessary for longer periods of time to deliver nutrients while an infant learns to feed at breast. Common devices include tube feeding setups, cups, spoons, droppers, syringes, and paladai. (For more information on devices, please refer to Additional Readings/Resources at the end of this chapter.)

Tube feeding devices include commercial versions such as the Supplemental Nursing System and the Starter Supplemental Nursing System by Medela, Inc., and the Lact-Aid Nursing Trainer System by Lactaid International. Similarly acting devices can be created from gavage tubing, from a length of butterfly tubing (with the needle removed) attached to a 20-cc or 30-cc syringe (Edgehouse & Radzyminski, 1990), or a 36-inch length of 5 French tubing threaded through an artificial nipple on a feeding bottle (Newman, 1990). Finger feeding with any of these tubing devices utilizes the tubing attached to a caregiver's finger in the infant's mouth (Bull & Barger, 1987).

Use of these devices is usually temporary because the mother uses them to establish the infant at breast and/or supplement the infant at breast (Figure 4-4).

> **BOX 4-3   Other Possible Effects of Feeding Bottles and Artificial Nipples on Selected Infant Parameters**
>
> - Muscles of mastication along with jaw development may be affected temporarily with short-term supplementation or permanently with long-term bottle use.
> - Respiratory patterns and ventilation in both term and preterm (Shivpuri et al., 1983) infants are affected during bottle-feeding (Mathew, 1988b, 1991a).
>   - As swallowing frequency increases, the time between swallows available for breathing decreases, and obstructed breathing can occur (Koenig et al., 1990).
>   - Apnea and bradycardia can occur in both preterm (Mathew, 1991b) and term infants (Mathew et al., 1985).
> - Transcutaneous oxygen pressure declines in preterm infants, resulting in desaturation with the use of fast-flow nipples (Meier, 1988; Meier & Anderson, 1987).
> - Cardiac parameters can be adversely affected by bottle-feeding (Butte et al., 1991; Zeskind et al., 1992).
>   - Bottle-fed neonates exhibit differences in physiological organization compared with breastfed infants; higher heart rates, lesser heart period variability, and lowered vagal tone are seen in bottle-fed infants (DiPietro et al., 1987). Higher vagal tone as seen in breastfed infants is a reflection of better physiological status and enhanced nervous system organization, and it results in a subsequent improved behavioral repertoire (Porges, 1983).

However, some mothers use tube feeding devices for longer-term breastfeeding such as for adoptive nursing, if the mother has had a breast reduction or other surgery on the breasts, if she is experiencing insufficient breastmilk, or if the infant is not capable of feeding directly at the breast without assistance because of oral anomalies, genetic or anatomical problems, or neurological compromise. When using these devices, small boluses can be effective if needed to help the infant initiate and sustain sucking, as flow regulates suck. Flow rate can be adjusted to either augment or reduce the flow. If the infant is looking distressed, sputtering, coughing, or choking, then the flow needs to be reduced such that a

Figure 4-4 Infant Feeding with Assistance from a Supplemental Nutrition System

Source: Courtesy of Marsha Walker, RN, IBCLC.

comfortable ratio of sucking to swallowing is seen and the infant inhibits breathing only when swallowing (Wolf & Glass, 2008). Although some mothers may find these devices awkward or inconvenient, they have been shown to be an effective tool in addressing selected breastfeeding problems and extending the duration of breastfeeding (Borucki, 2005; Guoth-Gumberger, 2006).

Commercial infant feeding cups are available in hard and soft plastic in varying shapes and sizes from Medela, Inc., Ameda, Maternal Concepts, and Foley. Some clinicians use a 28-mL medicine cup or a small party-favor-size Dixie cup with a rounded rim. Cup feeding allows the participation of the masseter and temporalis muscles, similar to the functioning of these muscles during breastfeeding (Gomes et al., 2006). Cup feeding of supplements to breastfed infants has been shown to be safe, resulting in a lower incidence of desaturation episodes (especially in preterm infants) and helping to prolong breastfeeding, particularly if multiple supplements are required (Rocha et al., 2002; Howard et al., 1999, 2003). Huang et al (2009) demonstrated that full term infants supplemented with bottles displayed more negative sucking behavior during attempts to latch to the breast and that mothers who used bottles to supplement breastfeeding had a lower perception of milk supply up to 4 weeks postpartum. Abouelfettoh, et al. (2008) showed that preterm infants who were supplemented by cup demonstrated more mature breastfeeding behaviors when compared to bottle-fed infants over 6 weeks and had a significantly higher proportion of breastfeedings one week after discharge. Cup feeding, however, can be slow and involve spillage, which must be accounted for when feeding fragile preterm infants. Cup feeding has the potential to delay discharge from the hospital for some preterm infants (Collins et al., 2008).

Small plastic spoons can be used to hand express colostrum into and spoon-feed a newborn unable to latch onto the breast (Hoover, 1998). The Medela Soft Feeder has a spoon-shaped spout at the end of a milk reservoir.

Glass or plastic medicine droppers or soft plastic clinical droppers are useful to provide milk incentives at the breast for teaching latch-on (Figure 4-5). TB (tuberculin) syringes can be used for this purpose, or periodontal syringes may be selected to deliver larger quantities of milk on a temporary basis. A curved tip or periodontal syringe allows for a very precise control of milk flow. A paladai resembles a small gravy boat with a spout that is similar to cup feeding but reduces the spillage common with cup feeding (Malhotra et al., 1999). Use of a paladai has more spillage than the use of a bottle and increases feeding time in preterm infants (Aloysius & Hickson, 2007).

All alternative feeding methods have strengths and weaknesses (Table 4-13). Therefore they must be selected with the goals of establishing or returning the infant to feedings at the breast while preserving the milk supply.

Supplementation should be undertaken with specific therapeutic goals in mind. Documentation when supplementing should include the indication, route of delivery, type of supplement, and amount ingested by the infant. When a mother requests that her infant be supplemented, the clinician will need to ask

Figure 4-5 Assisting Latch On with a Small Clinic Dropper

Source: Courtesy of Marsha Walker, RN, IBCLC.

TABLE 4-13 Strengths and Limitations of Selected Alternative Feeding Methods

Tube Feeding Devices

Strengths	Limitations
All feeding experience is at the breast	May be cumbersome and unappealing
Less opportunity for faulty imprinting	Needs continuing expert follow-up and teaching
Consistent practice and reinforcement for appropriate sucking at breast	Improper tube placement
Frequent breast stimulation for enhanced milk production	May exacerbate problem with baby's sucking action and mouth conformation
Establishes milk flow to regulate sucking	May suck on the tube like on a straw
	Parts can break, may be expensive for some parents

Finger Feeding

Strengths	Limitations
May reduce improper mouth conformation for sucking at breast	Finger is firm and does not change shape with sucking
Must open mouth wide	Baby may become reliant on firm nature of finger
Keeps tongue down, forward, and cupped	Baby may not learn to draw nipple into mouth if finger is simply inserted through closed lips
Delivers milk only with correct sucking action	No breast stimulation
Can be used to train sucking	

Syringe/Dropper

Strengths	Limitations
Can be used to assist baby to breast	Often needs a second person to help
Can reinforce proper sucking	Is a foreign object in the mouth
Can create milk flow to establish and regulate sucking	Milk can be improperly injected into mouth causing the baby to choke
Rewards sucking attempts	Is a slow way to feed baby
Avoids nipple confusion	

Bottle-Feeding

Strengths	Limitations
Faster and easier for baby to obtain milk	Ease of use may decrease mother's desire to continue breastfeeding
Does not require large time expenditure to teach mothers how to use a bottle	Artificial nipple may weaken baby's suck, suppress central grooving of the tongue, and decrease masseter muscle activity and development
May need to be considered if long-term supplementation is necessary	May reinforce improper oral configuration
	May induce bradycardia, apnea, and oxygen desaturation
	Can contribute to oral cavity alterations and malocclusions

(continues)

TABLE 4-13   Strengths and Limitations of Selected Alternative Feeding Methods
(continued)

Cup Feeding

Strengths	Limitations
Quick way to supplement a baby that does not contribute to nipple confusion (Lang, Lawrence, & Orme, 1994)	Does not teach sucking at breast
	Does not increase milk supply
Allows baby to pace his or her feeding (Lang, 1994)	Term babies can easily become so accustomed to the cup that they will not go to breast
Decreases amount of time gavage tubes are used	Caregivers can become so accustomed to the cup that breastfeeding is not encouraged
Is less invasive than gavage tubes	Significant loss of fluid from the cup as spillage or dribbling may cause difficulty in quantifying the actual amount of milk consumed by the baby (Dowling et al., 2002)
Decreases oral defensiveness	
Decreases risk of misplaced tube or esophageal perforation (Vandenplas et al., 1989)	
Helps tongue move down and forward	Pouring milk into the mouth can contribute to aspiration and loss of feeding skills (Thorley, 1997)
Does not cause breathing problems, oxygen desaturation (Rocha, Martinez, & Jorge, 2002), or physiologic instability (Howard et al., 1999)	
Provides positive feeding experiences	
Can be used with an already nipple-confused baby	

why the mother is requesting this action, dispel any misconceptions, advise of potential risks and consequences, and educate other family members if they are the cause of the request. Mothers or staff may feel the need to supplement infants in the evening or at night, because many infants are unsettled at these times. Mothers may state they are "feeding all the time," that the infant does not appear to be getting enough, and that the infant does not fall asleep after feeding. Rather than giving the infant a bottle of formula, clinicians should first directly assess a feeding at breast, recommend techniques to improve milk transfer, and recognize that they may be observing a normal diurnal feeding pattern that is common during the hospital stay and beyond. Benson (2001) demonstrated that the frequency of feeding in infants during the first 60 hours after birth was lowest between 3:00 am and 9:00 am and then gradually increased throughout the day to the highest frequency between 9:00 pm and 3:00 am. This is the precise time that staffing levels are at their lowest, lactation consultants are unavailable, and family members have either gone home or are as tired as the mother. Evening and night staffing that includes lactation consultants, staff nurses with additional breast-feeding management expertise, and staffing ratios that allow for more time per patient might alleviate unnecessary supplementation and its resulting side effects.

Summary: The Design in Nature

Although circumstances and the environment surrounding the birth of an infant vary considerably, the process of lactation and the needs of an infant remain constant. Even after the umbilical cord is cut, the mother and newborn demonstrate a physiological attachment to each other. The mutual release of hormones when they touch each other, the explorations of each other's face, and the need to be with each other should be honored within the birthing environment. Minimizing birth interventions and constructing caretaking behaviors that facilitate and enhance close contact, promote early and frequent breastfeeding, and provide correct and consistent support chart the course for a successful breastfeeding experience See Appendix 4-1.

References

Abouelfettoh, A. M., Dowling, D. A., Dabash, S. A., Elguindy, S. R., & Seoud, I. A. (2008). Cup versus bottle feeding for hospitalized late preterm infants in Egypt: a quasi-experimental study. *Intl Breastfeed J.*, *3*, 27.

Academy of Breastfeeding Medicine. (2002).*Hospital guidelines for the use of supplementary feedings in the healthy term breastfed neonate* Clinical Protocol #3. Retrieved February 19, 2009, from www.bfmed.org

Academy of Breastfeeding Medicine. (2006) *Guidelines for glucose monitoring and treatment of hypoglycemia in term breastfed neonates.* Clinical Protocol #1. Retrieved February 19, 2009, from www.bfmed.org

Adams, J. A., et al. (1985). Incidence of hyperbilirubinemia in breast- vs. formula-fed infants. *Clin Pediatr.*, *24*, 69–73.

Aizawa, M., Mizuno, K., & Tamura, M. (2009). Neonatal sucking behavior-comparison of perioral movement during breastfeeding and bottle-feeding. *Pediatr Intl.* Accepted article ahead of print

Aloysius, A., Hickson, M. (2007). Evaluation of paladai cup feeding in breast-fed preterm infants compared with bottle feeding. *Early Hum Dev.* 83, 619–621.

Amar, A. P., Aryan, H. E., Meltzer, H. S., Levy, M. L. (2003). Neonatal subgaleal hematoma causing brain compression: report of two cases and review of the literature. *Neurosurgery.* 52, 1470–1474.

American Academy of Pediatrics [AAP], Section on Breastfeeding. (2005). Breastfeeding and the use of human milk. *Pediatrics.* 115, 496–506.

American Academy of Pediatrics [AAP], Subcommittee on Hyperbilirubinemia. (2004). Management of hyperbilirubinemia in the newborn infant 35 or more weeks of gestation. *Pediatrics.* 114:297–316. Retrieved February 16, 2009, from http://aappolicy.aappublications.org/cgi/reprint/pediatrics;114/1/297.pdf

American Academy of Pediatrics [AAP], Work Group on Cow's Milk Protein and Diabetes Mellitus. (1994). Infant feeding practices and their possible relationship to the etiology of diabetes mellitus. *Pediatrics.* 94, 752–754.

Amiel-Tison, C., Barrier, G., & Shnider, S. (1982). A new neurologic adaptive capacity scoring system for evaluating obstetric medication in full term infants. *Anesthesiology.* 56, 340–347.

Anderson, G. C. (1976). *The Transitional Newborn* [videotape]. Chicago: Aldine

Anderson, G. C. (1989). Risk in mother-infant separation postbirth. *IMAGE: J Nurs Scholarship.*, *21*, 196–199.

Anderson, G.C., Moore, E., Hepworth, J., Bergman, N. (2003). *Early skin-to-skin contact for mothers and their healthy newborn infants (Cochrane Review).* In: The Cochrane Library, Issue 2, 2003. Oxford: Update Software.

Ardran, G. M., Kemp, F. H., & Lind, J. (1958). A cineradiographic study of bottle feeding. *Br J Radiol.* 31, 11–22.

Baumgarder, D., Muehl, P., Fischer, M., & Pribbenow, B. (2003). Effect of labor epidural anesthesia on breastfeeding of healthy full-term newborns delivered vaginally. *J Am Board Fam Pract.*, 16, 7–13.

Benson, S. (2001). What is normal? A study of normal breastfeeding dyads during the first sixty hours of life. *Breastfeeding Rev.*, 9, 27–32.

Bertini, G., Dani, C., Tronchin, M., & Rubaltelli, F. F. (2001). Is breastfeeding really favoring early neonatal jaundice? *Pediatrics.*, *107*(3). Retrieved March 7, 2009, from www.pediatrics.org/cgi/content/full/107/3/e41

Bhutani, V. K., & Johnson, L. (2009). A proposal to prevent severe neonatal hyperbilirubinemia and kernicterus. *J Perinatol.*, *29*, S61–S67.

Black, L. S. (2001). Incorporating breastfeeding care into daily newborn rounds and pediatric office practice. *Pediatr Clin North Am.*, 48, 299–319.

Blomquist, H. K., Jonsbo, F., Serenius, F., & Persson, L. A. (1994). Supplementary feeding in the maternity ward shortens the duration of breastfeeding. *Acta Paediatr Scand.*, *83*, 1122–1126.

Bolton, T. A., Chow, T., Benton, P. A., & Olson, B. H. (2009). Characteristics associated with longer breastfeeding duration: an analysis of a peer counseling support program. *J Hum Lact.*, *25*, 18–27.

Borcherding, K. E., & Ruchala, P. L. (2002). Maternal hyponatremia. *AWHONN Lifelines.*, 514–519.

Borucki, L. C. (2005). Breastfeeding mothers' experience using a supplemental feeding tube device: finding an alternative. *J Hum Lact.*, *21*, 429–438.

Brazelton, T. B. (1961). Psychophysiologic reactions in the neonate. II. Effect of maternal medication on the neonate and his behavior. *J Pediatr.*, *58*, 513–518.

Brazy, J. E. (1988). Effects of crying on cerebral blood volume and cytochrome aa3. *J Pediatr.*, *112*, 457–461.

Brice, J. E., Moreland, T. A., & Walker, C. H. (1979). Effects of pethidine and its antagonists on the newborn. *Arch Dis Child.*, *54*, 356–361.

Bricker, L., & Lavender, T. (2002). Parenteral opioids for labor pain relief: A systematic review. *Am J Obstet Gynecol.*, *186*, S94–S109.

Brown, E. W., & Bosworth, A. W. (1922). Studies of infant feeding. VI. A bacteriological study of the feces and the food of normal babies receiving breast milk. *Am J Dis Child.*, *23*, 243.

Bull, P., & Barger, J. Fingerfeeding with the SNS. (1987). *Rental Roundup.*, 25–34.

Bullen, C. L., Tearle, P.V., & Stewart, M. G. (1977). The effect of humanized milks and supplemented breast feeding on the faecal flora of infants. *J Med Microbiol.*, *10*, 403–413.

Businco, L., Bruno, G., & Giampietro, P. G. (1999). Prevention and management of food allergy. *Acta Paediatr.*, *88*(Suppl. 430), 104–109.

Butte, N. F., Smith, E., & Garza, C. (1991). Heart rates of breast-fed and formula-fed infants. *J Pediatr Gastroenterol Nutr.*, *13*, 391–396.

Bystrova, K., Widstrom, A. M., Matthiesen, A. S., et al. (2007). Early lactation performance in primiparous and multiparous women in relation to different maternity home practices. A randomized trial in St. Petersburg. *Int Breastfeed J.*, *8*, 2–9.

Cadwell, K., & Turner-Maffei, C. (2009). *Continuity of Care in Breastfeeding*. Sudbury, MA: Jones and Bartlett.

Caglar, M. K., Ozer, I., & Altugan F. S. (2006). Risk factors for excess weight loss and hypernatremia in exclusively breastfed infants. *Braz J Med Biol Res., 39*, 539–544.

Cakmak, H., & Kuguoglu, S. (2007). Comparison of the breastfeeding patterns of mothers who delivered their babies per vagina and via cesarean section: an observational study using the LATCH breast-feeding charting system. *Int J Nurs Stud., 44*, 1128–1137.

Camann, W. (2007). Labor analgesia and breastfeeding: avoid parenteral narcotics and provide lactation support. *Int J Obstet Anesth., 16*, 199–201.

Camann, W. (2003). *Spinal anesthesia in obstetrics—new concepts and developments*. Medscape Ob/Gyn Women's Health. *8*(2). Retrieved September 4, 2005, from www.medscape.com/viewarticle/464413

Cantani, A., & Micera, M. (2005). Neonatal cow milk sensitization in 143 case-reports: role of early expo-sure to cow's milk formula. *Eur Rev Med Pharmacol Sci., 9*, 227–230.

Cavlovich, F. E. (1994). Subgaleal hemorrhage in the neonate. *JOGNN., 24*, 397–404.

Centers for Disease Control and Prevention [CDC]. (2008). *Breastfeeding-related maternity practices at hospitals and birth centers*—United States, 2007. MMWR., *57*, 621–625. Retrieved January 27, 2009, from http://www.cdc.gov/mmwr/preview/mmwrhtml/mm5723a1.htm

Cheng, Y. W., Shaffer, B. L., & Caughey, A. B. (2006). Associated factors and outcomes of persistent occiput posterior position: a retrospective cohort study from 1976 to 2001. *J Matern Fetal Neonat Med., 19*, 563–568.

Chezem, J. C., Friesen, C., & Boettcher, J. (2003). Breastfeeding knowledge, breastfeeding confidence, and infant feeding plans: effects on actual feeding practices. *JOGNN., 32*, 40–47.

Chezem, J. C., Friesen, C., Montgomery, P., et al. (1998). Lactation duration: influences of human milk replacements and formula samples on women planning postpartum employment. *JOGNN., 27*, 646–651.

Chien, L. Y., Tai, C. J., Chu, K. H., Ko, Y. L., & Chiu YC. (2007). The number of baby friendly hospital practices experienced by mothers is positively associated with breastfeeding: a questionnaire survey. *Int J Nurs Stud., 44*, 1138–1146.

Christensson, K., Siles, C., Moreno, L., et al. (1992). Temperature, metabolic adaptation and crying in healthy full-term newborns cared for skin-to-skin or in a cot. *Acta Paediatr., 81*, 488–493.

Coalson, D. W., & Glosten, B. (1991). Alternatives to epidural analgesia. *Semin Perinatol., 15*, 375–385.

Collins, C. T., Makrides, M., Gillis, J., & McPhee, A. J. (2008). Avoidance of bottles during the establish-ment of breast feeds in preterm infants. *Cochrane Database Syst Rev., 8*(4), CD005252.

Connelly, K. P., Shropshire, L. C, & Salzberg, A. (1992). Gastric rupture associated with prolonged crying in a newborn undergoing circumcision. *Clin Pediatr., 31*, 560–561.

Cornblath, M., Hawdon, J.M., & Williams, A. F., et al. (2000). Controversies regarding definition of neonatal hypoglycemia: Suggested operational thresholds. *Pediatrics. 105*, 1141–1145.

Cornblath, M., Schwartz, R., & Aynsley-Green, A., et al. (1990). Hypoglycemia in infancy: the need for a rational definition. *Pediatrics., 85*, 834–837.

Cotterman, K. J. (2004). Reverse pressure softening: a simple tool to prepare areola for easier latching during engorgement. *J Hum Lact., 20*, 227–237.

Cox, S. G. (2006). Expressing and storing colostrum antenatally for use in the newborn period. *Breastfeeding Rev., 14*, 11–16.

Crowell, M. K., Hill, P. D., & Humenick, S. S. (1994). Relationship between obstetric analgesia and time of effective breastfeeding. *J Nurse Midwifery., 39*, 150–155.

Dahlenburg, G.W., Burnell, R.H., & Braybrook, R. (1980). The relation between cord serum sodium levels in newborn infants and maternal intravenous therapy during labor. *Br J Obstet Gynaecol., 87*, 519–522.

Daly, S. E. J., Owens, R. A., & Hartmann, P. E. (1993). The short-term synthesis and infant-regulated removal of milk in lactating women. *Exp Physiol., 78*, 209–220.

De Carvalho, M., Hall, M., & Harvey, D. (1981). Effects of water supplementation on physiological jaundice in breastfed babies. *Arch Dis Child., 56*, 568–569.

De Carvalho, M., Klaus, M. H., & Merkatz, R. B. (1982). Frequency of breastfeeding and serum bilirubin concentration. *Am J Dis Child., 136*, 737–738.

De Carvalho, M., Robertson, S., & Klaus, M. (1985). Fecal bilirubin excretion and serum bilirubin concentrations in breastfed and bottle-fed infants. *J Pediatr., 107*, 786–790.

de Moura, E. G., Lisboa, P. C., & Passos, M. C. (2008). Neonatal programming of neuroimmunomodulation—role of adipocytokines and neuropeptides. Neuroimmunomodulation. *15*, 176–188.

De Rooy, L., & Hawdon, J. (2002). Nutritional factors that affect the postnatal adaptation of full-term small- and large-for gestational-age infants. *Pediatrics., 109*(3). Retrieved February 15, 2009, from www.pediatrics.org/cgi/content/full/109/3/e42

Declercq, E.R., Sakala, C., Corry, M. P., et al. (2002). *Listening to Mothers: Report of the First National US Survey of Women's Childbearing Experiences.* New York: Maternity Center Association; Retrieved March 7, 2009, from www.maternitywise.org/listeningtomothers/

Declercq, E. R., Sakala, C., Corry, M. P., & Applebaum, S. (2006). *Listening to Mothers Survey II: Report of the Second National US Survey of Womens' Childbearing Experiences.* New York: Childbirth Connection. Retrieved January 23, 2009, from http://www.childbirthconnection.org/article.asp?ck=10396

Dewey, K. G., Nommsen-Rivers, L. A., Heinig, M. J., & Cohen, R. J. (2003). Risk factors for suboptimal infant breastfeeding behavior, delayed onset of lactation, and excess neonatal weight loss. *Pediatrics., 112*, 607–619.

DiGirolamo, A. M., Grummer-Strawn, L. M., & Fein, S. (2001). Maternity care practices: implications for breastfeeding. *Birth., 28*, 94–100.

DiGirolamo, A. M., Grummer-Strawn, L. M., & Fein, S. B. (2008). Effect of maternity-care practices on breastfeeding. *Pediatrics., 122*, S43–S49.

Dinwiddie, R., Patel, B. D., Kumar, S. P., & Fox, W. W. (1979a). The effects of crying on arterial oxygen tension in infants recovering from respiratory distress. *Critical Care Med., 7*, 50–53.

Dinwiddie, R., Pitcher-Wilmott, R., & Schwartz, J. G., et al. (1979b). Cardiopulmonary changes in the crying neonate. *Pediatr Res., 13*, 900–903.

DiPietro, J. A., Larson, S. K., & Porges, S. W. (1987). Behavioral and heart rate pattern differences between breast-fed and bottle-fed neonates. *Dev Psych., 23*, 467–474.

Dowling, D. A., Meier, P. P., & DiFiore, J. M., et al. (2002). Cup-feeding for preterm infants: mechanics and safety. *J Hum Lact., 18*, 13–20.

Drewett, R. F., Woolridge, M. W., Jackson, D. A., et al. (1989). Relationships between nursing patterns, supplementary food intake and breast milk intake in a rural Thai population. *Early Hum Dev., 20*, 13–23.

Edgehouse, L., & Radzyminski, S. G. (1990). A device for supplementing breastfeeding. *MCN., 15*, 34–35.

Eidelman, A. I. (2001). Hypoglycemia and the breastfed neonate. *Pediatr Clin North Am., 48*, 377–387.

Ekstrom, A., Widstrom, A.-M., & Nissen, E. (2003). Duration of breastfeeding in Swedish primiparous and multiparous women. *J Hum Lact., 19*, 172–178.

Fadavi, S., Punwani, I. C., Jain, L., & Vidyasagar, D. (1997). Mechanics and energetics of nutritive sucking: a functional comparison of commercially available nipples. *J Pediatr., 130*, 740–745.

Fairbank, L., O'Meara, S., Renfrew, M. J., Woolridge, M., Sowden, A. J., & Lister-Sharp, D. A. (2000). Systematic review to evaluate the effectiveness of interventions to promote the initiation of breastfeeding. *Health Technol Assess., 4*, 1-171

Ferrante, A., Silvestri, R., & Montinaro, C. (2006). The importance of choosing the right feeding aids to maintain breastfeeding after interruption. *Int J Orofac Myol., 32*, 58–67.

Fildes, V. A. (1986) *Breasts, Bottles and Babies: A History of Infant Feeding.* Edinburgh, Scotland: Edinburgh University Press

Forster, D. A., & McLachlan, H. L. (2007). Breastfeeding initiation and birth setting practices: a review of the literature. *J Midwifery Women's Health.*, *52*, 273–280.

Gagnon, A. J., Leduc, G., Waghorn, K., Yang, H., & Platt, R. W. (2005). In-hospital formula supplementation of health breastfeeding newborns. *J Hum Lact.*, *21*, 397–405.

Gardella, C., Taylor, M., & Benedetti, T., et al. (2001). The effect of sequential use of vacuum and forceps for assisted vaginal delivery on neonatal and maternal outcomes. *Am J Obstet Gynecol.*, *185*, 896–902.

Gartner, L. M. (1994). On the question of the relationship between breastfeeding and jaundice in the first 5 days of life. *Semin Perinatol.*, 18, 502, 508–509.

Gartner, L. M., Herschel, M. (2001). Jaundice and breastfeeding. *Pediatr Clin North Am.* 48, 389–399.

Gentile, S. (2007). Serotonin reuptake inhibitor-induced perinatal complications. *Paediatr Drugs.*, *9*, 97–106.

Gill, N. E., White, M. A., & Anderson, G. C. (1984). Transitional newborn infants in a hospital nursery: from first oral cue to first sustained cry. *Nurs Res.*, *33*, 213–217.

Gimeno, S.G., & deSouza, J. M. (1997). IDDM and milk consumption: a case-control study in Sao Paulo, Brazil. *Diabetes Care.*, *20*, 1256–1260.

Glover, J. (1990). Supplementation of breastfeeding infants and weight loss in hospital. *J Hum Lact.*, *6*, 163–166.

Goer, H. (1995).*Obstetric myths versus research realities: A guide to the medical literature.* Westport, CT: Bergin & Garvey.

Goetzl, L., Cohen, A., Frigoletto, F., et al. (2001). Maternal epidural use and neonatal sepsis evaluation in afebrile mothers. *Pediatrics.*, 108, 1099–1102.

Goldfield, E. C., Richardson, M. J., Lee, K. G., & Margetts, S. (2006). Coordination of sucking, swallowing, and breathing and oxygen saturation during early infant breastfeeding and bottle-feeding. *Pediatr Res.*, *60*, 450–455.

Golub, M. S. (1996). Labor analgesia and infant brain development. *Pharmacol Biochem Behav.*, *55*, 619–628.

Gomes, C. F., Trezza, E. M. C., Murade, E. C. M., & Padovani, C. R. (2006). Surface electromyography of facial muscles during natural and artificial feeding of infants. *J Pediatr (Rio J).*, *82*, 103–109.

Goodfellow, C. F., Hull, M. G. R., Swaab, D. F., et al. (1983). Oxytocin deficiency at delivery with epidural analgesia. *Br J Obstet Gynaecol.*, *90*, 214–219.

Gross, J. B., Cohen, A. P., Lang, J. M., et al. (2002). Differences in systemic opioid use do not explain fever incidence in parturients receiving epidural analgesia. *Anesthesiology.*, *97*, 157–161.

Guoth-Gumberger, M. (2006). *Breastfeeding with the supplementary nursing system.* Retrieved March 7, 2009, from www.breastfeeding-support.de/eng/sns-more.htm

Halamek, L. P., & Stevenson, D. K. (1996). Neonatal jaundice and liver disease. In: Fanarof A., Martin, R., eds. Neonatal-Perinatal Medicine: Diseases of the Fetus and Infant. Vol. 2, 6th ed. St. Louis, MO: Mosby-Year Book; pp. 1345–1389.

Hale, T. (2008). *Medications and mother's milk.* 13th ed. Amarillo, TX: Hale Publishing.

Hall, R. T., Mercer, A. M., Teasley, S. L., et al. (2002). A breastfeeding assessment score to evaluate the risk for cessation of breastfeeding by 7 to 10 days of age. *J Pediatr.*, *141*, 659–664.

Halpern, S.H., Levine, T., Wilson, D. B., et al. (1999). Effect of labor analgesia on breastfeeding success. *Birth.*, *26*, 83–88.

Hamza, J., Benlabed, M., Orhant, G., et al. (1992). Neonatal pattern of breathing during active and quiet sleep after maternal administration of meperidine. *Pediatr Res.*, *4*, 412–416.

Hawdon, J. M., Ward-Platt, M. P., & Aynsley-Green, A. (1992). Patterns of metabolic adaptation for term and preterm infants in the first neonatal week. *Arch Dis Child.*, *67*, 357–365.

Hayden, C. K., Shattuck, K. E., Richardson, C. V., et al. (1985). Subependymal germinal matrix hemorrhage in full-term neonates. *Pediatrics.*, *75*, 714–718.

Heck, L. J., & Erenberg, A. (1987). Serum glucose levels in term neonates during the first 48 hours of life. *J Pediatr.*, 110, 119–122.

Henderson, J. J., Dickinson, J. E., Evans, S. F., et al. (2003). Impact of intrapartum epidural analgesia on breastfeeding duration. *Aust NZ J Obstet Gynaecol.*, *43*, 372–377.

Herrera, A. J. (1984). Supplemented versus unsupplemented breastfeeding. *Perinatol/Neonatol.*, *8*, 70–71.

Higgins, J., Gleeson, R., Holohan, M., et al. (1996). Maternal and neonatal hyponatremia: a comparison of Hartmann's solution with 5% dextrose for the delivery of oxytocin in labour. *Eur J Obstet Gynaecol Reprod Biol.*, *68*, 47–48.

Hill, P. D., Humenick, S. S., Brennan, M. L., & Woolley, D. (1997).Does early supplementation affect long-term breastfeeding? *Clin Pediatr.*, *36*, 345–350.

Hiraishi, S., et al. (1991). Inter-atrial shunt flow profiles in newborn infants: a colour flow and pulsed Doppler echocardiographic study. *Br Heart J.*, *65*, 41–45.

Holtrop, P. C., Madison, K. A., Kiechle, F. L., et al. (1990). A comparison of chromogen test strip (Chemstrip bG) and serum glucose values in newborns. *Am J Dis Child.*, *144*, 183–185.

Hoover, K. (1998). Supplementation of the newborn by spoon in the first 24 hours. *J Hum Lact.*, *14*, 245.

Hornell, A., Hofvander, Y., & Kylberg, E. (2001). Solids and formula: association with pattern and duration of breastfeeding. *Pediatrics.*, *107*(3). Retrieved March 7, 2009, from www.pediatrics.org/cgi/content/full/107/3/e38

Host, A. (1991). Importance of the first meal on the development of cow's milk allergy and intolerance. *Allerg Proc.*, *10*, 227–232.

Howard, C. R., de Blieck, E. A., ten Hoopen, C. B., et al. (1999). Physiologic stability of newborns during cup- and bottle-feeding. *Pediatrics.*, *104*, 1204–1207.

Howard, C. R., Howard, F. M., Lanphear, B., et al. (2003). Randomized clinical trial of pacifier use and bottle-feeding or cupfeeding and their effect on breastfeeding. *Pediatrics.*, *111*, 511–518.

Huang, Y.-Y., Gau, M.-L., Huang, C.-M., & Lee, J.-T. (2009). Supplementation with cup-feeding as a substitute for bottle-feeding to promote breastfeeding. *Chang Gung Med J.*, *32*, 423–431.

Inoue, I., Sakashita, R., & Kamegai, T. (1995). Reduction of masseter muscle activity in bottle-fed babies. *Early Hum Dev.*, *42*, 185–193.

Iqbal, M. M., Gundlapalli, S.P., Ryan, W.G., et al. (2001). Effects of mood-stabilizing drugs on fetuses, neonates, and nursing infants. *South Med J.*, *94*, 305–322.

Iyer, N. P., Srinivasan, R., Evans, K., Ward, L., Cheung, W. Y., & Matthes, J. W. (2008). Impact of early weighing policy on neonatal hypernatraemic dehydration and breastfeeding. *Arch Dis Child.*, *93*, 297–299.

Jacobs, L. A., Dickinson, J. E., Hart, P. D., Doherty, D. A., & Faulkner, S. J. (2007). Normal nipple position in term infants measured on breastfeeding ultrasound. *J Hum Lact.*, *23*, 52–59.

Jacobson, B., Eklund, G., Hamberger, L., et al. (1987). Perinatal origin of adult self-destructive behavior. *Acta Psychiatr Scand.*, *76*, 364–371.

Jacobson, B., Nyberg, K., Eklund, G., et al. (1988). Obstetric pain medication and eventual adult amphetamine addiction in offspring. *Acta Obstet Gynaecol Scand.*, *67*, 677–682.

Jacobson, B., Nyberg, K., Gronbladh, L., et al. (1990). Opiate addiction in adult offspring through possible imprinting after obstetric treatment. *Br Med J.*, *301*, 1067–1070.

Jarvinen, K. M., Laine, S. T., Jarvenpaa, A. L., & Suomaiainen, H. K. (2000). Does low IgA in human milk predispose the infant to development of cow's milk allergy? *Pediatr Res. 48*, 457–462.

Jordan, S. (2006). Infant feeding and analgesia in labour: the evidence is accumulating. *Intl Breastfeeding J. 1*, 25. Retrieved February 11, 2009, from http://www.internationalbreastfeedingjournal.com/content/1/1/25

Jordan, S., Emery, S., Bradshaw, C., et al. (2005). The impact of intrapartum analgesia on infant feeding. BJOG: *Int J Obstet Gynaecol.*, *112*, 927–934.

Juvonen, P., Mansson, M., Kjellman, N. I., et al. (1999). Development of immunoglobulin G and immunoglobulin E antibodies to cow's milk proteins and ovalbumin after a temporary neonatal exposure to hydrolyzed and whole cow's milk proteins. *Pediatr Allerg Immunol.*, *10*, 191–198.

Karjalainen, J., Martin, J. M., Knip, M., et al. (1992). A bovine albumin peptide as a possible trigger of insulin-dependent diabetes mellitus. *N Engl J Med.*, *327*, 302–307.

Karlberg, P. (1960). The adaptive changes in the immediate postnatal period with particular reference to respiration. *J Pediatr.*, *56*, 585–604.

Keefe, M.R. (1987). Comparison of neonatal nighttime sleep-wake patterns in nursery versus rooming-in environments. *Nurs Res.*, *36*, 140–144.

Keefe, M. R. (1988). The impact of infant rooming-in on maternal sleep at night. *JOGNN.* *17*, 122–126.

Keppler, A. B. (1988). The use of intravenous fluids during labor. *Birth.*, *15*, 75–79.

Kinsella, S. M., Pirlet, M., & Mills, M. S., et al. (2000). Randomized study of intravenous fluid preload before epidural analgesia during labour. *Br J Anaesth.*, *85*, 311–313.

Klaus, M. H., Tooley, W. H., Weaver, K.H , & Clements, J. A. (1963). Lung volume in the newborn infant. *Pediatrics.*, *30*, 111–116.

Koenig, J. S., Davies, A. M., & Thach, B. T. (1990). Coordination of breathing, sucking, and swallowing during bottle feedings in human infants. *J Appl Physiol.*, *69*, 1623–1629.

Komara, C., Simpson, D., Teasdale, C., Whalen, G., Bell, S., & Giovanetto, L. (2007). Intervening to promote early initiation of breastfeeding in the LDR. *MCN.*, *32*, 117–121.

Konetzny, G., Bucher, H. U., & Arlettaz, R. (2009). Prevention of hypernatraemic dehydration in breastfed newborn infants by daily weighing. *Eur J Pediatr.*, *168*, 815-818.

Kostraba, J. N., Cruickshanks, K. J., Lawler-Heavner, J., et al. (1993). Early exposure to cow's milk and solid foods in infancy, genetic predisposition, and risk of IDDM. *Diabetes.*, *42*, 288–295.

Kovach, A. C. (1997). Hospital breastfeeding policies in the Philadelphia area: a comparison with the Ten Steps to Successful Breastfeeding. *Birth.*, *24*, 41–48.

Krehbiel, D., Pomdron, P., Levy, F., & Prud'Homme, M.J. (1987). Peridural anesthesia disturbs maternal behavior in primiparous and multiparous parturient ewes. *Physiol Behav.*, *40*, 463–467.

Kroeger, M. (2004). Impact of Birthing Practices on Breastfeeding: Protecting the Mother and Baby Continuum. Sudbury, MA: Jones and Bartlett.

Kruse, L., Denk, C.E., Feldman-Winter, L., & Rotondo, F. M. (2005). Comparing sociodemographic and hospital influences on breastfeeding initiation. *Birth.*, *32*, 81-85.

Kuhnert, B. R., Kuhnert, P.M., & Gross, T. L. (1982). The disposition of bupivacaine following epidural anesthesia for cesarean section. *Anesthesiology.*, *57*, 249–250.

Kumar, M., & Paes, B. (2003). Epidural opioid analgesia and neonatal respiratory depression. *J Perinatol.*, *23*, 425–427.

Kurinij, N., et al. (1984). Predicting duration of breastfeeding in a group of urban primiparae. *Ecol Food Nutr.*, *15*, 281–291.

Kurinij, N., Shiono, P. H. (1991). Early formula supplementation of breastfeeding. *Pediatrics.* 88, 745–750.

Laine, K., Heikkinen, T., Ekbald, U., & Kero, P. (2003). Effects of exposure to selective serotonin reuptake inhibitors during pregnancy on serotonergic symptoms in newborns and cord blood monoamine and prolactin concentrations. *Arch Gen Psychiatry.*, *60*, 720–726.

Lang, S. (1994). Cup-feeding: an alternative method. *Midwives Chron Nurs Notes.*, *107*, 171–176.

Lang, S., Lawrence, C. J., & L'E Orme, R. (1994). Cup feeding: An alternative method of infant feeding. *Arch Dis Child.*, *71*, 365–369.

Lawrence, R. A. (1997). A Review of the Medical Benefits and Contraindications to Breastfeeding in the United States. (Maternal and Child Health Technical Information Bulletin). Arlington, VA: National Center for Education in Maternal and Child Health.

Leighton, B., & Halpern, S. H. (2002a). Epidural analgesia: effects on labor progress and maternal and neonatal outcome. *Semin Perinatol.*, *26*, 122–135.

Leighton, B. L., & Halpern, S. H. (2002b). The effects of epidural analgesia on labor, maternal, and neonatal outcomes: a systematic review. *Am J Obstet Gynecol.*, *186*, S69–S77.

Lieberman, E., Cohen, A. P., & Lang, J. M., et al. (1999). Maternal intrapartum temperature elevation as a risk factor for cesarean section and assisted vaginal delivery. *Am J Pub Health.*, *89*, 506–510.

Lieberman, E., Davidson, K., Lee-Parritz, A., & Shearer, E. (2005).Changes in fetal position during labor and their association with epidural analgesia. *Obstet Gynecol.*, *105*, 974–982.

Lieberman, E., Eichenwald, E., & Mathur, G., et al. (2000a). Intrapartum fever and unexplained seizures in term infants. *Pediatrics.*, *106*, 983–988.

Lieberman, E., Lang, J. M., & Frigoletto, F., et al. (1997). Epidural analgesia, intrapartum fever, and neonatal sepsis evaluation. *Pediatrics.*, *99*, 415–419.

Lieberman, E., Lang, J., & Richardson, D. K., et al. (2000b). Intrapartum maternal fever and neonatal outcome. *Pediatrics.*, *105*, 8–13.

Lieberman, E., & O'Donoghue, C. (2002). Unintended effects of epidural analgesia during labor: a systematic review. *Am J Obstet Gynecol.*, *186*, S31–S68.

Lind, T. (1983). Fluid balance during labour: a review. *J R Soc Med.*, *76*, 870–875.

Livingstone, V. H., Willis, C. E., Abdel-Wareth, L., Thiessen, P., & Lockitch, G. (2000). Neonatal hypernatremic dehydration associated with breastfeeding malnutrition: retrospective survey. *CMAJ.*, *162*, 647–652.

Loftus, J. R., Hill, H., & Cohen, S. E. (1995). Placental transfer and neonatal effects of epidural sufentanil and fentanyl administered with bupivacaine during labor. *Anesthesiology.*, *83*, 300–308.

Lozoff, B., Brittenham, G. M., & Trause, M. A., et al. (1977). The mother-newborn relationship: limits of adaptability. *J Pediatr.*, *91*, 1–12.

Lucas, A.. (1998). Programming by early nutrition: an experimental approach. *J Nutr.* 128(2 Suppl), 401S–406S.

Ludington, S. M.. (1990). Energy conservation during skin-to-skin contact between premature infants and their mothers. *Heart Lung.* 19, 445–451.

Ludington-Hoe, S. M., Cong, X., & Hashemi, F. (2002). Infant crying: Nature, physiologic consequences, and select interventions. *Neonat Netw.*, *21*, 29–36.

Macdonald, P. D., Ross, S. R., Grant, L., & Young, D. (2003). Neonatal weight loss in breast and formula fed infants. *Arch Dis Child Fetal Neonat Ed.*, *88*, F472–F476.

Malhotra, N., Vishwambaran, L., Sundaram, K. R., & Narayanan, I. (1999). A controlled trial of alternative methods of oral feeding in neonates. *Early Hum Dev.*, *54*, 29–38.

Martens, P. J., & Romphf, L. (2007). Factors associated with newborn in-hospital weight loss: comparisons by feeding method, demographics, and birthing procedures. *J Hum Lact.*, *23*, 233–241.

Mathew, O. P. (1988a). Nipple units for newborn infants: a functional comparison. *Pediatrics.*, *81*, 688–691.

Mathew, O. P. (1988b). Respiratory control during nipple feeding in preterm infants. *Pediatr Pulmonol.*, *5*, 220–224.

Mathew, O. P. (1990). Determinants of milk flow through nipple units: role of hole size and nipple thickness. *Am J Dis Child.*, *144*, 222–224.

Mathew, O. P. (1991a). Breathing patterns of preterm infants during bottle feeding: role of milk flow. *J Pediatr.*, *119*, 960–965.

Mathew, O. P. (1991b). Science of bottle feeding. *J Pediatr.*, *119*, 511–519.

Mathew, O. P., Clark, M. L., & Pronske, M. H. (1985). Apnea, bradycardia, and cyanosis during oral feeding in term neonates Letter. *Pediatrics.*, *106*, 857.

Matthews, M. K. (1989). The relationship between maternal labour analgesia and delay in the initiation of breastfeeding in healthy neonates in the early neonatal period. *Midwifery.*, *5*, 3–10.

Mayberry, L. J., Clemmens, D., & De, A. (2002). Epidural analgesia side effects, co-interventions, and care of women during childbirth: a systematic review. *Am J Obstet Gynecol.*, *186*, S81–S93.

McDowell, M. A., Wang, C.-Y., & Kennedy-Stephenson, J. (1999). Breastfeeding in the United States: Findings from the National Health and Nutrition Examination Surveys –2006. NCHS data briefs, (2008). no. 5, Hyattsville, MD: National Center for Health Statistics. Retrieved August 22, 2009, from http://www.cdc.gov/nchs/data/databriefs/db05.htm

Meier, P. (1988). Bottle- and breast-feeding: effects on transcutaneous oxygen pressure and temperature in preterm infants. *Nurs Res.*, *37*, 36–41.

Meier, P., & Anderson, G. C. (1987). Responses of small preterm infants to bottle- and breast-feeding. *MCN.*, *12*, 97–105.

Merewood, A., Mehta, S. D., Chamberlain, L. B., Phillip, B. L., & Bauchner, H. (2005). Breastfeeding rates in US Baby-Friendly hospitals: results of a national survey. *Pediatrics.*, *116*, 628–634.

Merry, H., & Montgomery, A. (2000). Do breastfed babies whose mothers have had labor epidurals lose more weight in the first 24 hours of life? Annual Meeting Abstracts. Academy of Breastfeeding Medicine News and Views; *6*, 21.

Mizuno, K., & Ueda, A. (2006). Changes in sucking performance from nonnutritive sucking to nutritive sucking during breast and bottle-feeding. *Pediatr Res.*, *59*, 728–731.

Moehler, E., Poustka, L., & Resch, F. (2007). Vacuum extraction and autonomic balance in human infants. *J Perinatal Med.* 35, 347–349.

Moritz, M. L., Manole, M., Bogen, D. L., & Ayus, J. C. (2005). Breastfeeding-associated hypernatremia: are we missing the diagnosis? *Pediatrics.*, *116*, e343–e347.

Moses-Kolko, E. L., Bogen, D., & Perel, J., et al. (2005). Neonatal signs after late in utero exposure to serotonin reuptake inhibitors. *JAMA.*, *293*, 2372–2383.

Murray, E. K., Ricketts, S., & Dellaport, J. (2007). Hospital practices that increase breastfeeding duration: results from a population-based study. *Birth.*, *34*, 202–211.

Neifert, M. R. (1999). Clinical aspects of lactation: promoting breastfeeding success. *Clin Perinatol.*, *26*, 281–306.

Neifert, M. R. (2001). Prevention of breastfeeding tragedies. *Pediatr Clin North Am.*, *48*, 273–297.

Neifert, M. R. (1998). The optimization of breastfeeding in the perinatal period. *Clin Perinatol.*, *25*, 303–326.

Neifert, M. R., Lawrence R., & Seacat, J. (1995). Nipple confusion: toward a formal definition. *J Pediatr.*, *126*, S125–S129.

Newman, J. (1990). Breastfeeding problems associated with the early introduction of bottles and pacifiers. *J Hum Lact.*, *6*, 59–63.

Nicoll, A., Ginsburg, R., & Tripp, J. H. (1982). Supplementary feeding and jaundice in newborns. *Acta Paediatr Scand.*, *71*, 759–761.

Nissen, E., Lilja, G., & Matthiesen, A.-S., et al. (1995a). Effects of maternal pethidine on infants' developing breastfeeding behavior. *Acta Paediatr.*, *84*, 140–145.

Nissen, E., Lilja, G., Winstrom, A.-M., & Uvnas-Moberg, K. (1995b). Elevation of oxytocin levels early post partum in women. *Acta Obstet Gynaecol Scand.*, *74*, 530–533.

Nissen , E., Widstrom, A. M., & Lilja, G., et al. (1997).Effects of routinely given pethidine during labour on infants' developing breastfeeding behavior. Effects of dose-delivery time interval and various concentrations of pethidine/norpethidine in cord plasma. *Acta Paediatr.*, *86*, 201–208.

Noel-Weiss, J., Courant, G., & Woodend, A. K. (2008). Physiological weight loss in the breastfed neonate: a systematic review. *Open Med.*, *2*, 11–22.

Nordeng, H., Lindemann, R., Perminov, K. V., & Reikvam, A. (2001). Neonatal withdrawal syndrome after in utero exposure to selective serotonin reuptake inhibitors. *Acta Paediatr.*, *90*, 288–291.

Nowak, A. J., Smith, W. L., & Erenberg, A. (1994). Imaging evaluation of artificial nipples during bottle feeding. *Arch Pediatr Adolesc Med.*, *148*, 40–42.

Nyberg, K., Buka, S. L., & Lipsitt, L. P. (2000). Perinatal medication as a potential risk factor for adult drug abuse in a North American cohort. *Epidemiology.*, *11*, 715–716.

Oberlander, T. F., Misri, S., Fitzgerald, C. E., Kostaras, X., Rurak, D., & Riggs, W. (2004). Pharmacologic factors associated with transient neonatal symptoms following prenatal psychotropic medication exposure. *J Clin Psychiatry.*, *65*, 230–237.

O'Hana, H. P., Levy, A., Rozen, A., Greemberg, L., Shapira, Y., & Sheiner, E. (2008). The effect of epidural analgesia on labor progress and outcome in nulliparous women. *J Matern Fetal Neonat Med.*, *21*, 517–521.

Omigbodun, A. O., Akindele, J. A., & Osotimehin, B. O., et al. (1993). Effect of saline and glucose infusions of oxytocin on neonatal bilirubin levels. *Int J Gynaecol Obstet.*, *40*, 235–239.

Omigbodun, A. O., Fajimi, J. L., & Adeleye, J. A. (1991). Effects of using either saline or glucose as a vehicle for infusion in labour. *East Afr Med J.*, *68*, 88–92.

Philipp, B. L., Merewood, A., & Miller, L. W., et al. (2001). Baby-Friendly Hospital Initiative improves breastfeeding initiation rates in a US hospital Setting. *Pediatrics.*, *108*, 677–681.

Piper, S., & Parks, P. L. (1996). Predicting the duration of lactation: evidence from a national survey. *Birth.*, *23*, 7–12.

Piper, S., & Parks, P. L. (2001). Use of an intensity ratio to describe breastfeeding exclusivity in a national sample. *J Hum Lact.*, *17*, 227–232.

Ponkey, S. E., Cohen, A. P., Heffner, L. J., & Lieberman, E. (2003). Persistent fetal occiput posterior position: obstetric outcomes. *Obstet Gynecol.*, *101*, 915–920.

Poole, J. H. (2003). Analgesia and anesthesia during labor and birth: Implications for mother and fetus. *JOGNN.*, *32*, 780–793.

Porges, S. W. (1983). Heart rate patterns in neonates: a potential diagnostic window to the brain. In: Field T, Sostek A, eds. Infants Born at Risk: Physiological, Perceptual, and Cognitive Processes. New York: Grune and Stratton; pp. 3–22.

Porges, S. W. (1992). Vagal tone: a physiologic marker of stress vulnerability. *Pediatrics.*, *90*, 498–504.

Powers, N. G., & Slusser, W. (1997). Breastfeeding update 2: clinical lactation management. *Pediatr Rev.*, *18*, 147–161.

Radzyminski, S. (2003). The effect of ultra low dose epidural analgesia on newborn breastfeeding behaviors. *JOGNN.*, *32*, 322–331.

Rahm, V.-A., Hallgren, A., & Hogberg, H., et al. (2002). Plasma oxytocin levels in women during labor with or without epidural analgesia: a prospective study. *Acta Obstet Gynaecol Scand.*, *81*, 1033–1039.

Ransjo-Arvidson, A.-B., Matthiesen, A.-S., & Lilja, G., et al. (2001). Maternal analgesia during labor disturbs newborn behavior: effects on breastfeeding, temperature, and crying. *Birth.*, *28*, 5–12.

Reynolds, G. J., & Davies, S. (1993). A clinical audit of cotside blood glucose measurement in the detection of neonatal hypoglycemia. *J Pediatr Child Health.*, *29*, 289–291.

Righard, L., & Alade, M. (1990). Effect of delivery room routines on success of first breastfeed. *Lancet.*, *336*, 1105–1107.

Righard, L., & Alade, M. O. (1992). Sucking technique and its effects on success of breastfeeding. *Birth.*, *19*, 185–189.

Riordan, J., Gross, A., & Angeron, J., et al. (2000). The effect of labor pain relief medication on neonatal suckling and breastfeeding duration. *J Hum Lact.*, *16*, 7–12.

Riordan, J., & Riordan, S. (2000). *The effect of labor epidurals on breastfeeding.* Unit 4/Lactation Consultant Series Two. Schaumburg, IL: La Leche League International.

Rocha, N. M. N., Martinez, F. E., & Jorge, S. M. (2002). Cup or bottle for preterm infants: effects on oxygen saturation, weight gain, and breastfeeding. *J Hum Lact., 18*, 132–138.

Rodriguez ,G., Ventura, P., Samper, M. P., et al. (2000). Changes in body composition during the initial hours of life in breastfed healthy term newborns. *Biol Neonate., 77*, 12–16.

Rooth, G., Lysikiewicz, Huch, R., & Huch, A. (1983). Some effects of maternal pethidine administration on the newborn. *Br J Obstet Gynaecol., 90*, 28–33.

Rosenberg, K. D., Eastham, C. A., & Kasehagen, L. J., (2008a). Sandoval AP. Marketing infant formula through hospitals: the impact of commercial hospital discharge packs on breastfeeding. *Am J Public Health., 98*, 290–295.

Rosenberg, K. D., Stull, J. D., Adler, M. R., Kasehagen, L. J., & Crivelli-Kovach, A. (2008b). Impact of hospital policies on breastfeeding outcomes. *Breastfeeding Med., 3*, 110–116.

Rosenblatt, D. B., Belsy, E. M., Redshaw, M., et al. (1981). The influence of maternal analgesia on neonatal behavior: II. Epidural bupivacaine. *Br J Obstet Gynaecol., 88*, 407–413.

Rubaltelli, F. F. (1968). The frequency of neonatal hyperbilirubinemia in newborns with vacuum extractor. *Attual Ostet Ginecol., 14*, 1–4.

Ruchala, P. L., Metheny, N., Essenpreis, H., & Borcherding, K. (2002). Current practice in oxytocin dilution and fluid administration for induction of labor. *JOGNN., 31*, 545–550.

Ruth-Sanchez, V., Greene, C. V. (1997). Water intoxication in a three day old: a case presentation. *Mother Baby J., 2*, 5–11.

Saarinen, K. M., Juntunen-Backman, K., Jarvenpaa, A. L., et al. (1999). Supplementary feeding in maternity hospitals and the risk of cow's milk allergy: a prospective study of 6209 infants. *J Allerg Clin Immunol.* 104, 457–461.

Saarinen, K. M., & Savilahti, E. (2000). Infant feeding patterns affect the subsequent immunological features in cow's milk allergy. *Clin Exp Allerg., 30*, 400–406.

Sakashita, R., Kamegai, T., & Inoue, N. (1996). Masseter muscle activity in bottle feeding with the chewing type bottle teat: evidence from electromyographs. *Early Hum Dev., 45*, 83–92.

Saland, J., McNamara, H., & Cohen, M. I. (1974). Navajo jaundice: a variant of neonatal hyperbilirubinemia associated with breastfeeding. *J Pediatr., 85*, 271–275.

Savilahti, E., Tuomilehto, J., Saukkonen, T. T., et al. (1993). Increased levels of cow's milk and b-lactoglobulin antibodies in young children with newly diagnosed IDDM. *Diabetes Care., 16*, 984–989.

Scariati, P. D., Grummer-Strawn, L. M., & Fein, S. B. (1997). Water supplementation of infants in the first month of life. *Arch Pediatr Adolesc Med., 151*, 830–832.

Schneider, A. P. (1986). Breast milk jaundice in the newborn: a real entity. JAMA., 255, 3270–3274.

Semenic, S., Loiselle, C., & Gottlieb, L. (2008). Predictors of the duration of exclusive breastfeeding among first-time mothers. *Res Nurs Health., 31*, 428–441.

Sepkoski, C. M., Lester, B. M., Ostheimer, G. W., & Brazelton, T. B. (1992). The effects of maternal epidural anesthesia on neonatal behavior during the first month. *Dev Med Child Neurol., 34*, 1072–1080.

Shaker, I. J., Schaefer, J. A., James, A. E. Jr, & White, J. J. (1973). Aerophagia, a mechanism for spontaneous rupture of the stomach in the newborn. *Ann Surg., 39*, 619–623.

Shrago, L. (1987). Glucose water supplementation of the breastfed infant during the first three days of life. *J Hum Lact., 3*, 82–86.

Shrago, L. C., Reifsnider, E., & Insel, K. (2006). The neonatal bowel output study: indicators of adequate breast milk intake in neonates. *Pediatr Nurs., 32*, 195–201.

Shivpuri, C. R., Martin, R. J., Carlo, W. A., & Fanaroff, A. A. (1983). Decreased ventilation in preterm infants during oral feeding. *J Pediatr., 103*, 285–289.

Sievers, E., Haase, S., Oldigs, H.-D., & Schaub, J. (2003). The impact of peripartum factors on the onset and duration of lactation. *Biol Neonate.*, *83*, 246–252.

Sondergaard, C., Henriksen, T. B., Obel, C., & Wisborg, K. (2001). Smoking during pregnancy and infantile colic. *Pediatrics.*, *108*, 342–346.

Srinivasan, G., Pildes, R. S., & Cattamanchi, G., et al. (1986). Plasma glucose values in normal neonates: A new look. *J Pediatr.*, *109*, 114–117.

Steinbach, M. T. (1999). Traumatic birth injury-intracranial hemorrhage. *Mother Baby J.*, *4*, 5–14.

Stellwagen, L. M., Hubbard, E. T., & Wolf, A. (2007). The late preterm infant: A little baby with big needs. *Contemporary Pediatr.*, Retrieved February 17, 2009, from http://www.modernmedicine.com/modernmedicine/CME+Showcase/The-late-preterm-infant-A-little-baby-with-big-nee/CME/Article/detail/522990

Stettler, N., Stallings, V. A., Troxel, A. B., Zhao, J., Schinnar, R., Nelson, S. E., Ziegler, E. E., & Strom, B.L. (2005). Weight gain in the first week of life and overweight in adulthood: a cohort study of European American subjects fed infant formula. *Circulation.*, *111*, 1897-1903.

Stratton, J. F., Stronge, J., & Boylan, P. C. (1995). Hyponatremia and non-electrolyte solutions in labouring primigravida. *Eur J Obstet Gynaecol Reprod Biol.*, *59*, 149–151.

Svensson, K., Matthiesen, A.S., & Widstrom, A. M. (2005). Night rooming-in: who decides? An example of staff influence on mother's attitude. *Birth.*, *32*, 99–106.

Swenne, I., et al. (1994). Inter-relationship between serum concentrations of glucose, glucagon, and insulin during the first two days of life in healthy newborns. *Acta Pediatr.*, *83*, 915–919.

Tender, J. A. F., Janakiram, J., Arce, E., et al. (2009). Reasons for in-hospital formula supplementation of breastfed infants from low-income families. *J Hum Lact.*, *25*, 11–17.

Thorley, V. (1997), Cup feeding: problems created by incorrect use. *J Hum Lact.*, *13*, 54–55.

Thorp, J. A., Hu, D. H., Albin, R. M., et al. (1993). The effect of intrapartum epidural analgesia on nulliparous labor: A randomized, controlled, prospective trial. *Am J Obstet Gynecol.*, *169*, 851–858.

Torvaldsen, S., Roberts, C. L., Simpson, J. M., Thompson, J. F., & Ellwood, D. A. (2006). Intrapartum epidural analgesia and breastfeeding: A prospective cohort study. *Int Breastfeeding J.*, *1*, 24. Retrieved February 11, 2009, from www.internationalbreastfeedingjournal.com/content/1/1/24

Towner, D., Castro, M. A., Eby-Wilkens, E., & Hilbert, W. M. (1999). Effect of mode of delivery in nulliparous women on neonatal intracranial injury. *N Engl J Med.*, *341*, 1709–1714.

Uchil, D., & Arulkumaran, S. (2003). Neonatal subgaleal hemorrhage and its relationship to delivery by vacuum extraction. *Obstet Gynecol Surv.*, *58*, 687–693.

Unal, S., Arhan, E., Kara, N., Uncu, N., & Alliefendioglu, D. (2008). Breastfeeding-associated hypernatremia: retrospective analysis of 169 term newborns. *Pediatr Int.*, *50*, 29–34.

Uras, N., Karadag, A., Dogan, G., Tonbul, A., & Tatli, M. M. (2007). Moderate hypernatremic dehydration in newborn infants: retrospective evaluation of 64 cases. *J Matern Fetal Neonat Med.*, *20*, 449–452.

U.S. Food and Drug Administration [FDA]. (1998). FDA public health advisory: Need for CAUTION when using vacuum assisted delivery devices. Retrieved March 7, 2009, from www.fda.gov/cdrh/safety.html

Vandenplas, Y., Delree, M., Bougatef, A., & Sacre, L. (1989). Cervical esophageal perforation diagnosed by endoscopy in a premature infant: Review of recent literature. *J Pediatr Gastroenterol Nutr.*, *8*, 390–393.

Vestermark, V., Hogdall, C. K., Birch, M., et al. (1991). Influence of the mode of delivery on initiation of breastfeeding. *Eur J Obstet Gynaecol Reprod Biol.*, *38*, 33–38.

Volmanen, P., Valanne, J., & Alahuhta, S. (2004). Breastfeeding problems after epidural analgesia for labour: a retrospective cohort study of pain, obstetrical procedures and breastfeeding practices. *Int J Obstet Anesth.*, *13*, 25–29.

Walker, M. (1997). Do labor medications affect breastfeeding? *J Hum Lact.*, *13*, 131–137.

Walker, M. (1989). Functional assessment of infant breastfeeding patterns. *Birth.*, *16*, 140–147.

Walker, M. (2007). *Still selling out mothers and babies: Marketing of breastmilk substitutes in the USA.* Weston, MA: National Alliance for Breastfeeding Advocacy.

Walker, N. C., & O'Brien, B. (1999). The relationship between method of pain management during labor and birth outcomes. *Clin Nurs Res.*, *8*, 119–134.

Weber, F., Woolridge, M. W., & Baum, J. D. (1986). An ultrasonographic study of the organization of sucking and swallowing by newborn infants. *Dev Med Child Neurol.*, *28*, 19–24.

Weiner, P. C., Hogg, M. I. J., & Rosen, M. (1977). Effects of naloxone on pethidine-induced neonatal depression. *Br Med J.*, *2*, 228–231.

Wen, S. W., Liu, S., Kramer, M. S., et al. (2001). Comparison of maternal and infant outcomes between vacuum extraction and forceps deliveries. *Am J Epidemiol.*, *153*, 103–107.

Widstrom, A. M., Ransjo-Arvidsson, A.-B., Christensson, K., et al. (1987). Gastric suction in healthy newborn infants. *Acta Paediatr Scand.*, *76*, 566–572.

Wight, N. E. (2001). *Supplements and the breastfed infant: When Are they needed and how should they be supplied?* Independent Study Module. Schaumburg, IL: La Leche League International.

Wight, N. E. (2006). Hypoglycemia in breastfed neonates. *Breastfeeding Med.*, *1*, 253–262.

Wiklund, I., Norman, M., Uvnas-Moberg, K., Ranjo-Arvidson, A. B., & Andolf, E. (2009). Epidural analgesia: breastfeeding success and related factors. *Midwifery.*, *25*, e31-e38.

Williams, A. F. (1997). *Hypoglycemia of the newborn: Review of the literature.* Geneva: World Health Organization; Retrieved September 4, 2005, from www.who.int/chd/pub/imic/bf/hypoglyc/hypoglyc.htm

Wolf, L. S., & Glass, R. P. (1992). *Feeding and swallowing disorders in infancy.* Tucson, AZ: Therapy Skill Builders.

Wolf, L. S., & Glass, R. P. (2008). The Goldilocks problem: milk flow that is not too fast, not too slow, but just right. In: Genna CW, ed. *Supporting Sucking Skills in Breastfeeding Infants.* Sudbury, MA: Jones and Bartlett; pp. 131–152.

World Health Organization. (1998). Evidence for the Ten Steps to Successful Breastfeeding. Geneva: World Health Organization.

World Health Organization/United Nations Children's Fund. (1989). Protecting, Promoting and Supporting Breastfeeding: The Special Role of Maternity Services. Geneva: World Health Organization.

Wright, A., Rice, S., & Wells, S. (1996). Changing hospital practices to increase the duration of breastfeeding. *Pediatrics.*, *97*, 669–675.

Yamauchi, Y., & Yamanouchi, I. (1990a). The relationship between rooming-in/not rooming-in and breastfeeding variables. *Acta Paediatr (Oslo).*, *79*, 1017–1022.

Yamauchi, Y., & Yamanouchi, I. (1990b). Breastfeeding frequency during the first 24 hours after birth in full term neonates. *Pediatrics.*, *86*, 171–175.

Zeiger, R. S. (2003). Food allergen avoidance in the prevention of food allergy in infants and children. *Pediatrics.*, *111*(Suppl.), 1662–1671.

Zeskind, P. S. (1980). Adult responses to the cries of low-risk and high-risk infants. *Infant Behav Dev.* 3, 167–177.

Zeskind, P. S., Marshall, T. R., & Goff, D. M. (1992). Rhythmic organization of heart rate in breast-fed and bottle-fed newborn infants. *Early Dev Parent.*, *1*, 79–87.

Additional Reading/Resources

Sources for Improving Hospital Care of the Breastfeeding Mother and Infant

Baby-Friendly USA (administers the Baby Friendly certifying process for hospitals)
327 Quaker Meeting House Rd.
E. Sandwich, MA 02537
508-888-8092
www.babyfriendlyusa.org

"Breastfeeding Best Practice Guidelines for Nurses" includes evidence-based nursing practice guidelines for providing lactation care and services. It is available from the Registered Nurses of Ontario at www.rnao.org/bestpractices

"Providing Breastfeeding Support: Model Hospital Policy Recommendations" (June 2005, 3rd ed.) is available from http://www.cdph.ca.gov/programs/breastfeeding/Documents/MO05ModelHospitalPolicyRecommend.pdf

On-line toolkit for the Model Hospital Policy Recommendations http://www.cdph.ca.gov/HealthInfo/healthyliving/childfamily/Pages/MainPageofBreastfeedingToolkit.aspx

Sample Hospital Breastfeeding Policy for Newborns from the American Academy of Pediatrics Section on Breastfeeding http://www.aap.org/breastfeeding/samplehospitalpolicy.pdf

Academy of Breastfeeding Medicine. Protocol #7: Model Breastfeeding Policy. Retrieved www.bfmed.org/protocol/mhpolicy_ABM.pdf

International Lactation Consultant Association. Clinical Guidelines for the Establishment of Exclusive Breastfeeding. ILCA in cooperation with the United States Health Resources and Services Administration's Maternal and Child Health Bureau, Department of Health and Human Services. Raleigh, NC, 2005. Retrieved from www.ilca.org

Shealy, K. R., Benton-Davis, S., Grummer-Strawn, L. M. *The CDC Guide to Breastfeeding Interventions.* U.S. Department of Health and Human Services, Centers for Disease Control and Prevention; 2005. Retrieved from www.cdc.gov/breastfeeding/resources/guide.htm

Alternative Devices for Supplementing the Breastfed Infant

Books

Genna CW. *Selecting and using breastfeeding tools.* Amarillo, TX: Hale Publishing, 2009.
Wolf LS, Glass RP. *Feeding and swallowing disorders in infancy.* Tucson, AZ: Therapy Skill Builders, 1992.

Cups

Foley cup
Foley Development, Inc.
PO Box 50
Conway, MI 49722
888-463-2688
www.FOLEYCUP.com

Suckle cup
Maternal Concepts
130 North Public St.
Elmwood, WI 54740
800-310-5817
www.maternalconcepts.com

Ameda baby cup
Ameda
475 Half Day Rd.
Lincolnshire, IL 60069
1-866-99-AMEDA
www.ameda.com

Soft Feeder
Medela, Inc.
1101 Corporate Dr.
McHenry, IL 60050
800-435-8316 or 1-815-363-1166
www.medela.com

Flexi-Cut cup (uses a cutout design to prevent neck extension)
New Visions
1124 Roberts Mountain Rd.
Faber, VA 22938
800-606-7112
www.new-vis.com

Tube-feeding devices
Lact-Aid International, Inc. (Lact-Aid nursing training device)
PO Box 1066
Athens, TN 37371
423-744-9090
www.lact-aid.com

Supplemental Nursing System
Starter Supplemental Nursing System
Medela, Inc.
1101 Corporate Dr.
McHenry, IL 60050
800-435-8316 or 1-815-363-1166
www.medela.com

Summary Interventions Based on Peripartum Factors, Birthing Practices, and Early Caretaking Behaviors

1. Encourage mothers to attend prenatal childbirth preparation classes.

2. Discuss potential effects on breastfeeding of common birth interventions and what actions parents may take to reduce adverse effects on breastfeeding.

3. After delivery, facilitate the breast-seeking behaviors of the infant; encourage the first breastfeeding within 60–80 minutes of birth. Avoid forcing the infant to the breast during this time by not pushing the infant's head into the breast or placing pressure on the occipital region of the head.

4. Keep mothers and babies together after delivery and around the clock unless the mother's or infant's condition does not permit or special circumstances arise.

5. Supplementation should occur for medical reasons, using the method least likely to cause disruption of feeding at the breast and with the lowest potential to provoke allergy or diabetes in a susceptible family. Mothers should be asked if there is a family history of allergy or diabetes.

6. If breastfeeding is delayed or interrupted, mothers should be helped to initiate and maintain their milk supply.

7. Alternative feeding methods, equipment, techniques, and instructions should be selected with the goals of establishing or returning the infant to feeding at the breast while preserving the maternal milk supply.

8. When a mother requests that her baby be supplemented, clinicians should ascertain why the mother wishes this, learn what infant behaviors she interprets

as indicating insufficient milk production or inadequate intake, and perform an assessment of a feeding at breast before supplementing the infant.

9. Clinicians should be aware of the possible side effects that many birth interventions can produce in the breastfeeding dyad. See Boxes 4-4 through 4-6.

BOX 4-4   Possible Labor Medication Side Effects

Infant behavioral disorganization

Difficulty modulating state control

Sleepy baby

Respiratory depression

Decreased alertness

Inhibition of sucking

Less efficient sucking

Lower neurobehavioral scores

Increased incidence of sepsis workups

Delay in effective breastfeeding

Shorter duration of wakefulness

Depressed visual and auditory attention

Longer time to habituate to noise

Decreased social responsiveness

Decreased tone and reflexes

Delayed rooting reflex

Higher rates of instrument delivery

Maternal and infant edema/water overload

Increased use of oxytocin

Increased incidence of intrapartum fever

Unexplained neonatal seizures

Increased incidence of jaundice

Decreased spontaneous breast-seeking behaviors

Disturbance of prefeeding sequence of behavior

Altered sucking patterns

Less time spent with baby during hospital stay

Increased incidence of intracranial hemorrhage

BOX 4-5   Possible Side Effects of Separation

Reduced interaction between mother and baby

Reduced opportunity to learn infant feeding cues

Decreased access to the breast/fewer breastfeeds

Increased use of supplementary feedings

Can delay lactogenesis II

Babies cry more

Infants experience less quiet sleep

Infants startle more

Infants may have lower body and skin temperatures

Infants can have lower blood glucose levels

Is associated with reduced length of breastfeeding

Care in nursery exposes infants to bright lights and loud noise

Babies receive less contact with caregiver

BOX 4-6 Possible Side Effects of Supplementation

Decreases incidence of exclusive breastfeeding (in hospital and long term)

Can delay lactogenesis II

Contributes to insufficient milk supply

Water supplements can

- Contribute to weight loss
- Increase hyperbilirubinemia
- Exacerbate hypoglycemia
- Result in caloric deprivation

Infant formula supplements can

- Alter gut flora
- Provoke sensitivity and allergy to cow's milk protein in susceptible families
- Act as the environmental triggering event in the development of diabetes in susceptible families

Infant-Related Challenges to Breastfeeding

Chapter 5

First 24–48 Hours: Common Challenges

Introduction

Proper positioning of the mother and infant and a correct latch of the infant to the breast form the foundation of each breastfeeding encounter. Many problems stem from improper positioning, incorrect latch, and subsequent failure to transfer milk. Some problems innate to the infant or the mother require modification of positioning and latching techniques. This chapter explores positioning, latch, and other infant-related problems encountered during the first few days after birth.

Clinician Influence

Mothers benefit most when a nurse or lactation consultant remains with her for early feedings, ensuring that the infant is latched correctly and transferring milk. Nurses need to demonstrate appropriate positioning and latch, while allowing the mother to perform the task (Gill, 2001). Mothers find it helpful when clinicians offer prenatal information of the realities of breastfeeding, deliver practical help with positioning and latch-on, perform effective interventions for early problems, and offer enlightenment on questions such as how long and how often to breastfeed, when to switch breasts, and whether nipple shields and supplementing with bottles of formula will undermine breastfeeding (Graffy & Taylor, 2005). Inadequate, insensitive, or apathetic approaches to breastfeeding often culminate in a downward spiral of fatigue, frustration, and weaning by 2 weeks postpartum. Neutrality of clinicians regarding infant feeding negatively affects breastfeeding initiation and duration. Mothers reporting that hospital staff expressed no preference regarding infant feeding were more likely to be bottle-feeding at 6 weeks, especially if the mothers had intended to breastfeed for less than 2 months (DiGirolamo et al., 2003).

Mothers are especially frustrated by inconsistent advice about breastfeeding techniques and the tendency of some clinicians to quickly support the use of a bottle when feeding difficulties are present, sometimes even offering a bottle before the infant goes to breast (Mozingo et al., 2000). Inconsistent advice, rushed encounters with mothers, lack of skilled nurses, unavailability of lactation consultants, and the promotion of unhelpful practices sabotage breastfeeding right from the start (McInnes & Chambers, 2008). Failure to offer assistance with latch-on, failure to follow up after a feeding, inadequate assessment of breastfeeding technique, anecdotal descriptions of personal experience that differs from other professional information, and failure to provide information regarding community resources have been further identified by mothers as behaviors by clinicians that are nonsupportive of learning to breastfeed (Hong et al., 2003).

Clinicians must be mindful of interventions perceived by the mother as being unhelpful, discouraging, or ineffective (Ebersold et al., 2007). Staff shortages and increasing demands on nurses can contribute to the inability of staff to provide the type of assistance and care that new mothers require. When mothers deem nurses to be too busy or rushed, they may feel disinclined to ask for the help they need (Hong et al., 2003). Mothers with low confidence levels are particularly vulnerable to insufficient and inadequate lactation care and services (Mantha et al., 2008). Short postpartum hospital stays, inadequate staffing, and busy maternity units decrease contact between nurses and mothers, limiting teaching time and resulting in many mothers being discharged with unmet learning needs.

On busy maternity units nurses can teach content that mothers and families are most in need of knowing (Ruchala, 2000), which may be different from or in addition to unit checklists. Some nurses find it helpful to teach mothers basic breastfeeding information and observe infant feeding with small groups of two or three mother–baby pairs to ensure that each mother has a core knowledge of breastfeeding and each infant has been assessed for successful milk transfer. Clinicians must also refrain from telling mothers what to do rather than acknowledging the mothers' feelings and helping them develop their own solutions. Karl et al. (2006) described a compelling role for the nurse during the newborn period as an "attacher." Facilitating physical closeness and regular contact with her baby strengthens the attachment system between mother and infant, providing an oxytocin-rich environment that has a physiological and psychological positive effect on both of them.

It is especially important that mothers who anticipate or who are having difficulty with breastfeeding have access to a consultant with the International Board Certified Lactation Consultant credential. Castrucci et al. (2006) showed a positive association between delivering an infant at a hospital using certified lactation consultants and breastfeeding at hospital discharge. Optimal lactation consultant (staff with the International Board Certified Lactation Consultant credential) staffing has been calculated to require 1 full-time equivalent lactation consultant per 783 breastfeeding couplets in the in-patient unit (Mannel & Mannel, 2006).

Positioning of the Mother

When the mother is first learning to breastfeed, she needs to be positioned comfortably herself before putting the infant to breast. Typically, she may be in a sitting position on a bed, chair, or couch. She also may be reclining in a bed or lying on her side. Her back and arms can be supported with pillows when necessary so that her posture is relaxed. Some mothers appreciate a footstool when sitting in a chair, which tilts the mother's pelvis back, prevents her from feeling the need to lean forward, and elevates the infant so that the mother is not compelled to lean down or over her infant. Some mothers use commercial pillows designed to provide an inclined and/or firmer support surface than bed pillows, finding that they reduce back strain and facilitate an easier latch (Humenick et al., 1998) (Figure 5-1). For other mothers pillows simply get in the way.

A mother who experiences a cesarean birth may wish to breastfeed in a side-lying position, sitting upright with a pillow in her lap, or placing the infant to her side in a clutch or football hold (Frantz & Kalmen, 1979). A pillow under her knees or elevation of the knee gatch in a hospital bed may also be helpful. If an intrathecal or epidural catheter remains in place for continued pain relief after birth, care must be taken in positioning the mother and placing pillows behind her back such that the catheter is not dislodged. Mothers may have a number of areas of postpartum pain, including the perineum, back, cesarean incision site, intravenous (IV) line site, muscle aches and strains, or headache. Positioning options should also take these considerations into account so that pain is not exacerbated in these areas, the mother is medicated if needed, and she is able to remain comfortable during the time it takes to feed the infant.

Figure 5-1
Commercial Pillow for Firm Surface Support

Source: Courtesy of Marsha Walker, RN, IBCLC.

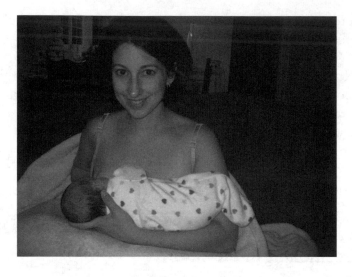

Assistance with positioning and latch is usually necessary during the early days of learning for both primiparous and multiparous mothers because each infant and each situation are different. Under normal circumstances, once the mother and baby have mastered the art of positioning and latch, positioning techniques and latch approaches become integrated into daily life, mothers and babies work out a mutually comfortable arrangement, and special or intricate positioning and latch techniques are no longer needed.

Hand Positions

Most mothers and many babies find it helpful if the breast is supported during the early learning period. There are two common ways to hold the breast, scissors and C-hold, with a number of variations also available for special situations. The way in which a mother is positioned and how she holds her breast can affect the angle at which the infant approaches the breast and can distort and firm the shape of both the breast and the areola (Minchin, 1998).

1. Scissors or V-hold. The breast is held by the index and middle fingers separated over the top and bottom of the areola. Some mothers and babies thrive with this hand position. Others find that although this is not "wrong," it has some potential drawbacks.
    - The fingers may exert enough pressure over milk ducts to partially obstruct the milk flow.

- If the areola is large and/or the mother's hands are small, the fingers may cover parts of the areola that should be in the infant's mouth, causing an incorrect latch-on to only the nipple.
- Too much pressure from one or the other finger could distort the nipple shape in the infant's mouth by tipping it up or down.
- Pressure toward the chest wall from either or both fingers could exert enough traction on the nipple–areola to keep the infant from drawing sufficient tissue far enough into the mouth or pull the nipple out of the infant's mouth such that the infant applies vacuum to just the tip of the nipple.

2. C-hold. The breast is supported by four fingers underneath the breast and the thumb rests on top (Figure 5-2). This position helps keep the infant's jaw from having to support the weight of the breast. Women with large breasts may find that they cannot comfortably hold the breast in this manner and may benefit from folded towels or a rolled receiving blanket tucked under the breast for support. The support from the C-hold often helps to firm a very soft breast, stabilizing it during the latch, and controlling the angle of the nipple–areola as it is presented to the infant (Chute, 1992).

- U-hold or Dancer hand position. This is a C-hold rotated 90 degrees such that the thumb is placed on the lateral margin of the breast and the four fingers rest on the medial aspect of the breast or vice versa (Figure 5-3). This hand position is often recommended for preterm infants, infants with a weak suck, or infants with muscular or neurological problems that prevent them from executing normal jaw movements (Danner & Cerutti, 1984). The entire jaw is supported simultaneously with the breast. The thumb and index finger are in a position to be placed on both cheeks of the infant and can be gently pressed inward to cause contact between the buccal surfaces of the

Figure 5-2   The C-hold

Figure 5-3   The Dancer Hand Position
This position supports the baby's mouth while gently compressing the cheeks.

Source: Photo Courtesy of Childbirth Graphics, copyright 1984 Sarah Coulter Daniel.

mouth and the nipple. This action fills the gap in a preterm infant's mouth between the buccal surface inside the mouth and the nipple, causing all parts of the infant's mouth to come in contact with the breast.

- A modified C-hold with index finger slipped under infant's chin provides support for jaw instability when an infant's mandible exhibits excessive jaw excursion to the point where contact is lost with the nipple. In this situation, smacking sounds may be heard, indicating that the infant's jaw movement is excessive. A finger that is moved slightly back from the chin can also be gently placed under where the base of the tongue attaches to provide external support for the tongue.

There is a great variety of shapes, sizes, and tissue elasticity of breasts, as well as numerous variations in the anatomical structure and function of infants' mouths. Although most of these combinations eventually accommodate to each other, some mismatches require more attention to positioning and alterations of standard positioning and latch techniques (Escott, 1989). In particular, the breast can be shaped (Figure 5-4) and adjusted to present a better match to the long axis of the infant's mouth depending on how the infant is positioned (Wiessinger, 1998).

- The breast can be shaped into a horizontal or vertical oval by the use of a U-hold or scissors hold modified to a more vertical position.
- Sometimes presenting "less" breast tissue (as with large or very soft breasts) for the latch results in more tissue being drawn into the infant's mouth.
- In very small infants, an elastic areola can be shaped with the index finger and thumb to present tissue in a manner more easily grasped by a tiny mouth.

Figure 5-4 Shaping
the Breast

Positioning of the Infant

Poor positioning can compromise an infant's ability to feed effectively. Proper head, neck, and trunk alignment are important to smooth feeding performance (Shrago & Bocar, 1990). The head and neck are typically in neutral alignment, with the overall body position being one of slight flexion, including the hips (Wolf & Glass, 1992). There is a strong interaction between head and neck position and feeding function. Proper positioning during feeding affects respiratory mechanisms, oral-motor control, swallowing, and the development of head and neck postural responses (Bosma, 1988). Blair et al. (2003) found that no one attribute of positioning (head flexion, body alignment, etc.) was more important than others in relation to the degree of nipple pain experienced by the mother. It appears that all attributes work together to achieve a position that is compatible for good milk transfer in each individual mother–baby pair.

Four common positions for breastfeeding exist, with many variations available to suit special circumstances. A mother does not need to know all these positions but can be assisted to find which position or positions work best for her and her infant. Before her discharge from the hospital, the mother should be able to demonstrate at least one position in which she is comfortable and in which she can position the baby by herself on both sides or with minimal help.

1. Cradle hold. The infant is held completely facing the mother, typically on a slight angle with the head and shoulders a little higher than the hips (Figure 5-5).

Figure 5-5 The Cradle Position

The infant lays on his or her side in direct contact with the mother's midriff. The infant's head rests on the upper forearm. The breast should not be pushed sideways to the infant. The infant is well supported by the mother's arm across his or her back, tucking the hips into flexion and molding or wrapping the infant's body around her waist. This positioning should place the infant's nose at about the level of the nipple and the lower lip and chin below the nipple. The infant's head and neck should be straightly aligned with the shoulders and hips. Some mothers find this position awkward at first, with the infant's head difficult to control and position and the breast difficult to embrace in a C-hold without disrupting the contact between the infant's mouth and the breast.

2. Cross-cradle hold. The infant is in the same position as in the cradle hold but is held with the mother's opposite arm (Figure 5-6). The neck and shoulders of the infant are supported with the mother's hand, her fingers rest back behind the ears, there is no pressure on the occipital region of the head, and the mother's forearm supports the infant's back. This gives the mother more control over positioning the infant's head and may be easier to learn at first. The breast is accessed by the mother's hand without having to be inserted between the infant and the breast tissue, and the nipple–areola is more visible to the mother. Some mothers start the feeding with the cross-cradle hold and, once the infant is positioned, change to the cradle hold. This position is frequently used as a learning position for a full-term infant or to position a small or preterm infant who tends to "roll" up when placed in a cradle hold.

Figure 5-6 The Cross-Cradle Hold

3. Clutch or football hold. The infant is positioned on a pillow to the side of the mother turned slightly sideways or sitting partially upright (Figure 5-7). The mother's hand and wrist support the infant's back and shoulders, and her fingers rest behind the infant's ears. This position may be much easier for some mothers, giving them the most control over the infant's head and allowing the best visualization of the nipple–areola. Care should be taken that the weight of the breast is not placed on the infant's chest, that the infant is not placed so low that he or she pulls down on the nipple, or that the mother leans down over the infant. This position is also good for learning and for small or preterm infants.

Figure 5-7 The Football Hold

4. Lying down. Many mothers find this position an especially restful way to feed their infant, although some mothers may find it difficult to learn at first. The mother lies on her side with the infant's body on his or her side and completely facing and in contact with her (Figure 5-8). The infant's head may be resting on the bed or on the mother's forearm that supports the infant's back and hips. Some mothers place a rolled towel or blanket behind the infant to keep the infant on his or her side and place a pillow behind her own back for support. Mothers can offer the top breast by adjusting their position such that they are turned further prone, thus avoiding having to move the infant and themselves to the other side.

Marmet and Shell (2008) described a number of therapeutic positions that function to compensate for sucking problems or for use in infants with anatomical variations, neurological deficits, respiratory issues, state control problems, young gestational age, or sensory integration variations:

- *Infant and mother sitting.* Useful in infants older than 6 weeks to help bring down an elevated tongue, for infants with a cleft palate, to help improve alertness in a sleepy infant, for velopharyngeal inadequacy, or repeated ear infections. The infant sits facing the mother's breast with legs straddled over the mother's leg.

- *Mother supine and infant prone.* The prone position is frequently used for positioning sick or preterm infants because it improves oxygenation and has been shown to increase sucking pressures when bottle-feeding (Mizuno et

Figure 5-8 The Side-Lying Position

al., 2000). With the mother supine and the infant prone, infants who need to bring their tongue forward, such as with tongue-tie or infants who have difficulty handling a fast flow of milk, may feed better.

- *Mother semireclining, infant semiprone.* This position may be helpful for infants with upper respiratory problems such as tracheomalacia or laryngomalacia (Figure 5-9). It is also helpful for infants with a receding chin or for a mother who has had a cesarean delivery. This position is also referred to within the biological nurturing concept.

Biological Nurturing

Biological nurturing is a concept that involves how certain feeding positions and behaviors are associated with the release of primitive neonatal reflexes necessary to establish successful breastfeeding (Colson et al., 2003, 2008). It is any mother–baby behavior at the breast where the infant is in close chest contact with the mother's body contours.

- For the infant, biological nurturing means
  - Mouthing, licking, smelling, nuzzling, and nestling at the breast
  - Sleeping at the breast
  - Groping and rooting at the breast
  - Latching onto the breast
  - Sucking and swallowing breastmilk through active feeding

Figure 5-9 Semi-Reclining Position of Mother and Semi-Prone Position of Infant

- For the mother, biological nurturing means
  - Holding the infant in close contact with a maternal body contour
  - Offering unrestricted access to the breast with as much skin-to-skin contact as the mother desires

Extended holding in postures where the mother leans back and the infant lies prone in close frontal apposition with maternal body contours (ventral positioning) is thought to aid in the release of primitive neonatal reflex–like movements, necessary for successful breastfeeding.

Primitive neonatal reflexes is a collective name given to more than 50 unconditioned reflex responses and spontaneous behaviors to environmental stimuli such as rooting, sucking, swallowing; head, cheek, tongue and lip reflexes; hand-to-mouth; stepping; and crawling. A greater number of primitive neonatal reflexes and a reduction in feeding problems at the breast were observed when mothers were in full biological nurturing postures (Colson et al., 2008). Biological nurturing positions also work well for the late preterm infant. Colson et al. (2003) noticed that although infants appeared to be asleep in the biological nurturing position, they were often actively feeding with strong sucking and swallowing. Thus an infant may not need to be fully awake to engage in nutritive sucking and swallowing.

The maternal semireclined position with the infant in a prone position adhering to her body contours may also be an effective intervention for the infant who "fights" at the breast. Clinicians have seen infants who arch away from the breast, bob their heads, and engage in erratic and jerky movements at the breast, preventing latch-on. Placing the mother and infant into a biological nurturing position may use gravity to assist in moving the infant's chin and tongue forward and stop the movements that are preventing the infant from latching on. Biological nurturing during the first 72 hours may also trigger higher peak concentrations of oxytocin at an earlier time, helping to offset oxytocin aberrations caused by oxytocin infusion during labor epidurals. The higher the dose of oxytocin infusion during labor epidurals, the lower the oxytocin levels in mothers during breastfeeding on day 2 (Jonas et al., 2009).

Latch

Latch has been described as possibly the single most important moment and movement in breastfeeding (Brandt et al., 1998). Once the infant is positioned correctly, the infant's lips can be brushed gently against the areola if his or her mouth is not already opening in anticipation. When it is opened like a yawn, the infant's mouth is moved to the breast, with the chin and lower lip making contact first, followed by the upper lip and tip of the nose. The infant's mouth must open wide, ranging up to approximately 160 degrees. Only the lower jaw can move to achieve this type of opening, so the infant's head must tilt back far enough to accommodate the dropping of the jaw (Cadwell, 2007). Some mothers and infants find an easier latch when the mother shapes the breast to offer the areola under the nipple as the first contact point, making that area more accessible. The lower lip and chin can be planted well down on the areola with the infant's mouth rolled the rest of the way on as the upper lip makes contact just above the nipple. An infant who is crying or who has an elevated tongue tip will need to be calmed, and the tongue can be stroked down and forward before latching.

In an effort to aid or hasten latch-on, some mothers, helpers, or healthcare providers push on the back of the infant's head as the infant is brought to the breast. Pushing on the occiput may cause the infant to compensate by extending the head, biting the nipple, or detaching from the breast. Increasing neck flexion causes the airway to become more prone to collapse, interfering with breathing. Anatomical structures change their relative positions when pressure is exerted on the occiput. The hyoid bone should move up and forward, which happens with slight extension of the head to facilitate swallowing. Excessive flexion with distortion of the cervical vertebrae can impinge on the proper movement of the hyoid bone, which has six other connections involved in sucking, swallowing, and breathing. Forcing the infant's head onto the breast may disturb placement of the tongue, encouraging it to elevate rather than cupping and moving down and forward (Widstrom & Thringstrom-Paulsson, 1993). Too much flexion of the neck, nose-first attachment to the breast, and continued pressure on the occiput create a scenario for nipple pain and poor milk transfer.

Blair et al. (2003) looked at positioning and latching behaviors of infants whose mothers reported varying degrees of nipple pain. Several factors of the latch and positioning of the infant combined to contribute to the soreness experienced by the mothers in the study, including the observations that only 18% of 92 infants had the optimal angle of mouth opening of 160 degrees (Figure 5-10), just 36.6% had both their nose and chin on or in close proximity of the breast, and merely 34.4% had their nose opposite the mother's nipple at latch. Poor attachment to the breast that leaves the nipple in the anterior portion of the mouth can contribute to sore nipples as well as obstructed milk flow (Morton, 1992), resulting in weight loss, hyperbilirubinemia, and low milk supply.

A deep latch or attachment to the breast is important to ensure uniform drainage of all the mammary lobes. Mizuno et al. (2008) found on examination of milk from three milk ducts in each breast that each duct contained milk with differing compositions. They measured the degree of emptying in three milk ducts from each breast of 37 breastfeeding mothers. Findings confirmed that the changes in the degree of emptying of each mammary lobe differed by the depth of attachment of the infant at the breast as measured by the creamatocrit of milk obtained before and after breastfeeding. A deep attachment was defined as the nipple and approximately 0.7–1.3 cm of the areola in the infant's mouth and the angle of the open mouth greater than 130 degrees. If the depth of attachment was shallow, milk was excreted unevenly from different mammary lobes.

Milk retention in a lobe can predispose a breast to plugged ducts and mastitis. If the depth of attachment is deep, the lobes drain uniformly, leaving a reduced risk of plugged ducts and mastitis. If a lobe is poorly drained over an extended period of time, less milk will be made in that lobe, reducing the amount of milk that the breast produces. Thus achieving a deep latch is important in preventing breast problems and milk supply issues.

Problems with Latch

A number of indicators of poor positioning or latch should be checked before hospital discharge, if the mother reports nipple pain or damage, if there is a low milk supply, or if weight gain problems arise. A mother and infant who are experiencing difficulties with latch should be checked for the following:

- Body position of the infant
  - Misalignment of the head, trunk, and hips
  - Infant not tucked close and facing the mother, hips extended or back arched, neck flexed, or nose buried in the breast tissue

Figure 5-10   Optimal Angle of Mouth Opening

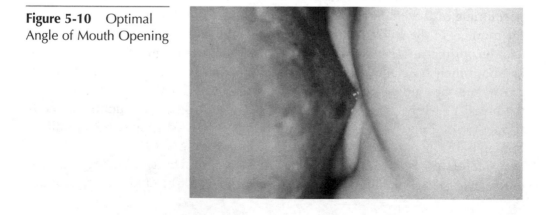

- Head too high over the breast
- Nose or chin not touching the breast
- Mouth and tongue
  - Angle of the infant's mouth opening less than 160 degrees (Figure 5-11)
  - Upper (tight labial frenulum) or lower lip not flanged
  - Tongue not down, cupped, and forward
    - Humped (anterior to posterior direction)
    - Bunched (compressed in a lateral direction)
    - Retracted (tip behind alveolar ridges)
    - Elevated
    - Flat (Figure 5-12)
    - Short or tight lingual frenulum
    - Large tongue, protruding tongue, short tongue
- Palate
  - High or arched
  - Bubble
  - Cleft (hard, soft)
- Cheeks
  - Drawn in, dimpled, or hollowed with each suck
  - Cheekline not a smooth arc (Figure 5-13)
- Jaw
  - Retrognathia or receding jaw (Figure 5-14) (can position the tongue posteriorly where it leads to obstruction of the airway; can contribute to sore nipples unless chin is brought very close to the breast)

Figure 5-11 Mouth Angle Less Than 160 Degrees

Figure 5-12
Flat Tongue

Figure 5-13   Cheekline
Not in a Smooth Arc

Figure 5-14
Receding Jaw

- Large jaw excursions (cannot close over the areola)
- Small jaw excursions (cannot open over the areola)
- Lack of graded jaw excursions heard as clicking or smacking sounds
- Jaw asymmetry or tilted jaws (may include torticollis) (Wall & Glass, 2006)

- Lips
  - Poor occlusion of lips around the areola (milk leaking from the sides of the mouth)
  - Lips do not form a seal, preventing the creation of a pressure gradient between breast and mouth

- Nipple
  - Slides back and forth within the infant's mouth during the feeding
  - Pops in and out of mouth (may indicate tongue-tie)
  - Creased in a horizontal, vertical, or oblique plane
  - Distorted shape or flattened
  - Blanched or in spasm after the infant releases the nipple
  - Pain, blisters, maceration, fissures, cracks, bleeding, craters
  - Flat, dimpled, retracted
  - Edematous areola that envelopes the nipple
  - Engorged breast that flattens the nipple

- Rhythmicity or coordination of suck, swallow, breathe
  - Diminished suck-to-swallow ratio less than 1–3:1
  - High respiratory rate, stridor
  - Coughing or choking

Other situations may occur that cause problems with latch. These are described below.

State and Feeding Readiness

Many breastfeeding recommendations from the past and, to some extent, those used currently tend to lead to insufficient breastmilk and a hungry infant. Feeding schedules that are determined by the clock rather than infant feeding readiness cues can result in an over-hungry crying infant (Millard, 1990), or one who remains underfed because scheduled feeds coincide with deep sleep states. An infant in a deep sleep state cannot feed, nor can a vigorously crying infant organize his or her behavior to latch and feed effectively. Infants can breastfeed in the other four states: light sleep, drowsy, quiet alert, and active alert. Infants feed best in a quiet alert state but should be put to breast whenever feeding cues are demonstrated. The quiet alert state may be difficult for some newborns to achieve and may require organizational maturation before they develop competency in alerting themselves to feed from a sleeping state. Other infants may experience state control problems as a result of maternal labor medications, becoming more competent at state control as the drugs clear their body and the effects of the medications diminish.

Some newborns require help in achieving a state that is optimal for latch, whereas other infants demonstrate state organization and sucking competency with a minimum of effort on the part of the mother. The ability of infants to suck appropriately, demonstrate alertness and stamina, and possess the ability to self-regulate and respond to maternal soothing behaviors are major influences on the initial pattern and the ultimate duration of breastfeeding (Lothian, 1995). Sucking behavior in the early neonatal period affects the breastfeeding duration at 3 and 6 months. Vigorously feeding infants are much more likely to be fully breastfed and to breastfeed longer than infants described by their mothers as "procrastinators," who are at a higher risk for short-term breastfeeding (Mizuno et al., 2004). Karl (2004) used an arousal model (Als, 1995) to describe behavioral breastfeeding difficulties on a continuum, with the quiet alert state as a neutral arousal reference and newborns unable to manage their state well enough to latch being viewed as either under-aroused (the sleepy infant) or over-aroused (the fussy or reluctant nurser).

Infants experiencing state overload appear to be sleeping but may be shut down or closed down in an attempt to block out negative stimuli that have raised their arousal levels beyond that which they can manage. A shut-down infant may appear to be asleep, and parents may have difficulty differentiating between these two states (Table 5-1). Increasing stimulation to an infant who is shut down further exacerbates the problem. Parents need to become knowledgeable regarding infant states and how best to assist their infant in achieving a latchable state. One of the most effective interventions for modulating infant arousal levels in over-aroused, under-aroused, and shut-down infants is the use of a combination of vestibular (upright rocking) and skin-to-skin tactile stimulation that affect state organization itself (Anderson, 1991). In an effort to encourage infant self-regulation and to positively modulate infant state, skin-to-skin care can be initiated directly after birth, which is the normal mammalian postnatal condition (Ferber & Makhoul, 2004).

Previous or Concurrent Use of Artificial Nipples and Pacifiers

Milk transfer from the breast to the infant is contingent upon the smooth functioning of a group of interrelated behaviors, intact anatomical structures, and

TABLE 5-1 Differentiation Between Sleeping Infants and Over-Aroused, Shut-Down Infants

Sleeping Infant Descriptors	Shut-Down Infant Descriptors
Relaxed muscle tone	Tense muscle tone (not relaxed)
Peaceful facial expression	May reflect internal tension with furrowed eyebrows
Normal skin color	Color flushed or pale
Eyelids fluttering in light sleep	Eyes held tightly closed

Source: Adapted from Karl DJ. Using principles of newborn behavioral state organization to facilitate breastfeeding. *MCN.* 2004;29:292–298.

coordinated physiological actions. Some infants have been observed to have difficulty in latching and sucking from the breast if artificial nipples and/or pacifiers have been introduced before breastfeeding is well established (Neifert et al., 1995). Pacifier use is associated with a reduced length of breastfeeding (DiGirolamo et al., 2008). This may be due to interference with proper sucking or may be an indicator of breastfeeding problems where a pacifier is used to soothe an infant who is not adequately transferring milk.

Pacifier shape, length, and material, just as with other artificial nipples, can have an impact on the mechanics of sucking (Nowak et al., 1995). Characteristics of the nipple can impact tongue and lip position as well as their movements during sucking. Orthodontic-shaped nipples may interfere with the central grooving of the tongue, whereas pacifiers with a ball-shaped tip may result in reduced functional sucking activity (Wolf & Glass, 1992). Levrini et al. (2007) evaluated the distribution of stress on the palate using three different types of pacifiers, showing that pacifiers with different geometrical shapes caused a different stress distribution on the palate. Orthodontic-shaped pacifiers distributed the stress on the palate during sucking over a wider area than pacifiers that were narrow or that had a bulblike tip. The latter two types of pacifiers concentrate stress on the central part of the palate that could lead to a narrowing of the palatal arch. Not only could sucking be affected, but the eventual position of the child's dentition and speech may also be involved.

The concept of human imprinting has been advanced to help explain the observation of nipple preference. Mobbs (1989) discusses imprinting as an aspect of learning that takes place early in life. It is known that nonhuman mammals imprint or demonstrate a one-nipple preference; for example, the piglet and kitten establish their preferred teat and drive away others who would use it. The human infant is thought to be programmed to seek and attach to a suitable object on which to imprint using its most powerful sense organs at birth—the nose and mouth. Olfaction is one of the guides to the nipple directly after birth (Varendi & Porter, 2001). Within minutes of birth, maternal breast odors elicit preferential head orientation of the infant, contributing to successful nipple localization. The chemical profile of breast secretions overlaps somewhat with that of amniotic fluid. Lactating women emit odor cues that release activity in newborns. Such cues may be carried in various substrates, including milk or areolar secretions.

A study by Doucet and colleagues (2007) examined the responses of infants facing their mother's breast with the goal of sorting out the source(s) of active volatile compounds emitted by the lactating breast. Infants (aged 3–4 days) were presented their mother's breast in two consecutive trials of 90 seconds each: a scentless condition (breast entirely covered with a transparent film) paired with one of four odorous conditions (fully exposed breast, n = 15; nipple only exposed, n = 15; areola only exposed, n = 13; and milk exposed, n = 12). The infants were more orally activated when facing any of the odorous breast conditions than when facing the scentless breast. They cried earlier and longer and opened their eyes less,when facing the scentless breast. Nipple, areola, and milk odors appeared to be equivalent to the whole breast odor in stimulating oral activity and in delaying crying onset. This study showed that volatile compounds originating in areolar secretions or milk release mouthing, stimulate eye opening, and delay and reduce crying in newborns.

The early attraction to the breast may also be a reflection of prenatal exposure and the recognition of a familiar scent (Mizuno & Ueda, 2004; Porter & Winberg, 1999). Infants are able to discriminate between their mother's scent on a breast pad and that of an unfamiliar woman (Macfarlane, 1975). Olfactory breast-associated cues are so important that both 3- to 4-day-old breastfeeding and bottle-feeding infants orient toward a pad worn on a breast rather than an unused or clean pad (Makin & Porter, 1989). Preferences to mother's milk odor lasts as long as 2 weeks, with 14-day-old bottle-fed infants responding preferentially to a breast pad from an unfamiliar lactating woman rather than a pad treated with their own familiar formula (Porter et al., 1991). Washing the breast or separating the infant from the mother before the infant becomes oriented to the biologically relevant chemical signal from the breast could be one precursor that inhibits correct latch (Varendi et al., 1994). This reason is also why the use of scented pacifiers should be avoided in breastfed infants. One of the first ways an infant recognizes his or her mother is through the distinctive features of her nipple. As with birds, who are known to be preferentially selective to supernormal size stimuli, a human infant may experience a mishap in attaching to the mother's nipple by fixating on an artificial nipple whose large, rigid features predominate when there is a choice between sizes (Mobbs, 1989).

Tongue placement and the sequential movements of the tongue are crucial to the infant latching to the breast, drawing the nipple–areola into the mouth by forming a teat, and covering the lower gum to prevent nipple damage. The extrusion reflex has been defined as the forward movement of the cupped tongue over the lower gum so as to grasp the breast at the start of the formation of a teat (Stephens & Kotowski, 1994). With an artificial nipple, the teat is already formed and is inserted into a fully or partially closed mouth. This can lead to the extrusion reflex being diminished or extinguished from lack of use. If the extrusion reflex does not occur in the latch sequence of events at the breast, a teat cannot be formed. Consequently, the infant will apply the gums to the breast first rather than the tongue, resulting in nipple pain and poor milk transfer. One of the prime motoric differences between sucking on an artificial nipple and sucking at the breast may be in the initiation of sucking (Wolf & Glass, 1992).

The muscles involved with breastfeeding are also affected by the use of artificial nipples. Masseter muscle activity is significantly weakened by the use of artificial nipples. Muscles involved with breastfeeding are either immobilized (masseter, orbicularis oris), overactive (chin muscle), or malpositioned (tongue is pushed backward) during artificial nipple use (Inoue et al., 1995).

Gestational Age

Developmental maturity and feeding behaviors may vary depending on the gestational age of the infant, postnatal age of the infant (days since birth), and any growth rate abnormalities. Sucking patterns vary, change, and mature along a continuum of gestational age, postnatal age, and health status. In measurements taken on an artificial nipple, preterm infants compared with full-term infants generally demonstrate lower sucking pressures, less fluid consumption per suck, fewer sucks per feeding, and an inability to maintain the suction for long periods of time (Medoff-Cooper et al., 1989). As gestational age increases, feeding behavioral organization improves, with more reliable maximum sucking pressures starting an upward trend at 34 weeks (Medoff-Cooper, 1991). Preterm breastfed infants who are encouraged to feed at breast can catch up and exhibit similar milk consumption to those born after a longer gestation (Nyqvist, 2001). Gestational age and birth weight classifications (Hankins et al., 2006) and their effects on breastfeeding typically include the following categories:

- Preterm: less than 34 weeks. Latch may be complicated by poor initiation of sucking with excessive rooting, inability to close the mouth/wide jaw excursions, lapping at the nipple, oral defensiveness, elevated tongue tip, oral/facial hypotonia, a closed mouth, weak suck (suboptimal or immature sucking pressure), and jaw instability. If the infant cannot form a teat and draw it into his or her mouth, the infant's gums may contact the breast at the base of the nipple rather than farther back on the areola, interfering with efficient milk removal (Meier et al., 2000).

- Late preterm: 34 0/7 to 36 6/7 weeks. Latch may be complicated by respiratory instability in some breastfeeding positions, little energy reserve or stamina, immature state regulation, sleepiness, low tone, depressed sucking vacuum, or uncoordinated sucking (Wight, 2003).

- Early term: 37 0/7 to 38 6/7 weeks. Latch may be compromised by the increased risk from severe respiratory distress syndrome.

- Term: 39 0/7 to 41 6/7 weeks. Latch may be compromised by maternal labor medications, an overstimulating environment, high ambient temperature (Elder, 1970), or artificial nipple use.

- Postterm: 42 weeks or more. The infant may be lethargic; may have trouble sustaining sucking; may have experienced hypoxia (with depressed suck), birth injury, or trauma; and is prone to hypoglycemia.

- Macrosomia or large for gestational age: 4,000 g or more (8 lb, 14 oz). The infant may have experienced birth trauma and be susceptible to hypoglycemia.

- Normal birth weight: 2,500–3,999 g (5 lb, 9 oz to 8 lb, 13 oz)

- Low birth weight: less than 2,500 g (<5 lb, 9 oz)

- Very low birth weight: less than 1,500 g (<3 lb, 5 oz)

- Small for gestation age: can occur in term, near-term, and preterm infants; mostly defined as two standard deviations below the mean for gestational age or as below the 10th percentile; sometimes referred to as intrauterine growth retardation. One may see poorer reflex performance with rooting and sucking, poor tone, difficulty coming to an alert state, stress when handled, and an easily fatigued infant (Als et al., 1976).

Birth Trauma, Medications, Conditions, and Events

Events or conditions experienced during birth, such as hypoxia, brachial plexus injuries, fractured clavicle, vacuum extraction, facial muscle trauma, or deep or aggressive suctioning, can impinge on achieving a correct latch. Congenital conditions not discovered prenatally may first become apparent when an infant experiences feeding difficulties. Epidural analgesia (0.25% bupivacaine) is associated with insufficient milk and early formula supplementation, because infants may have difficulty in executing correct and effective suckling that results in diminishing maternal milk production (Volmanen et al., 2004).

Widstrom et al. (1987) observed that organized breastfeeding behaviors in full-term infants develop in a predictable way during the first hours of life. These behaviors are initially expressed as spontaneous sucking (low at 15 minutes after birth, maximal at 45 minutes postdelivery, and absent by 2–2½ hours after birth when asleep) and rooting movements (low at 15 minutes and maximal at 60 minutes after birth) when placed on the mother's chest immediately at birth. They progress to hand-to-mouth movements (observed at a mean time of 34 ± 2 minutes), more intense rooting and sucking activity, and breast-seeking behaviors, and they culminate in attachment to the breast. Unmedicated infants found the breast unassisted and started vigorous suckling at 55 ± 4 minutes after delivery.

Although newborn human infants and other mammals both crawl to the breast soon after birth to feed, this "instinctive" behavior is easily disturbed. Separation of the infant from the mother before the first attachment to the breast has occurred can disrupt subsequent correct latch to the breast (Righard & Alade, 1990). Infants separated from their mothers before they have suckled from the breast may have more difficulty in latching and exhibit an incorrect latch and suck at the subsequent feeding. Combinations of these factors may cause difficulties in latching and staying attached to the breast.

A young infant who is reluctant to feed at breast may be unable to do so because of residual conditions still present from the delivery. The normal overlap or overriding of the cranial bone plates generally self-corrects within a couple of days after birth. Traction on the head during either a vaginal or a cesarean delivery, and the possible resulting hyperextension of the neck, may displace the occipital bone forward, potentially compromising the jugular foramen and/or the foramen magnum (Smith, 2004). The jugular foramina provide passage out of the skull for three nerves:

1. The glossopharyngeal (IX) cranial nerve works with the vagus nerve to help control swallowing and airway function along with function of the tongue. It also works with the hypoglossal (XII) nerve to control the tongue. The hypoglossal nerve exits the skull through the hypoglossal canals located beside and beneath the joint surfaces of the occiput.

2. The vagus (X) nerve also helps maintain a normal heart rate.

3. The spinal accessory (XI) nerve innervates major neck muscles such as the sternocleidomastoid and a portion of the trapezius.

Pressure on these nerves is thought to contribute to some feeding problems. Abnormal presentations such as face, mentum (chin), arm, footling breech, or breech may also set the stage for compressive forces on nerves that are responsible for normal feeding activities.

An infant whose head is misshapen (one side of the head higher than the other) or whose bones are out of alignment may signal the need for closer inspection of the infant's feeding capacity. Fascia or connective tissue surrounds, supports, and connects one type of tissue to another and affects the normal range of motion for structures. Observations of infants and their limiting movements have led to a number of forms of bodywork for infants to correct these limitations. Craniosacral therapy (CST) is a gentle form of massage that focuses on the bones, connective tissues, and fluid that surround the brain and spinal cord to relieve constrictions that may be impinging on the functioning of these structures (Upledger, 2003a, 2003b). About 5 g of pressure is used to evaluate and correct mobility restrictions or misalignments along the cranial sutures (Brussel, 2001). Practitioners of CST may be chiropractors, massage therapists, physical therapists, physicians, dentists, or allied healthcare providers who have taken courses in CST.

Myofascial release is another therapy intended to produce and improve changes in tissue mobility. Most evidence on the usefulness or outcomes of CST is anecdotal or consists of case studies (Hewitt, 1999; Turney, 2002). Holtrop (2000) described resolution by cranial adjusting of sucking dysfunction in a 6-month-old infant with an inward dishing at the occipitoparietal junction and upper cervical (C1–C2) asymmetry and fixation. Although the available health outcome research consists mainly of low-grade evidence (Green et al., 1999), Vallone (2004) suggested that biomechanical dysfunction based on articular or muscular integrity may influence the ability of an infant to suckle successfully and that intervention via soft tissue work, cranial therapy, and spinal adjustments may have a direct result in improving the infant's ability to suckle efficiently. Wescott (2004) believed that cranial osteopathy is a useful treatment when dealing with instances of breastfeeding problems resulting from birth trauma. If parents are interested in these forms of therapy, the practitioners of these treatment modalities should be qualified to provide them safely.

Some infants experience troublesome breastfeeding due to a nervous system that does not respond appropriately to sensory stimuli. Sensory-processing difficulties were first described in the 1960s by A. Jean Ayers, who was working with neurologically involved children (Ayers, 1977). Sensory integration has evolved over time and is now defined as the ability of the nervous system to accept sensory information, process it, and respond with motor and behavioral responses that are appropriate to the context (Weiss-Salinas & Williams, 2001). The nervous system is designed to modulate environmental stimuli and provide graded responses. However, with sensory-processing difficulties, there may be poor coordination, sensory defensiveness (extreme reactions to ordinary sensations), or sensory modulation difficulties (extremes in activity, emotional levels, and arousal levels) (Reisman, 2002). An infant can be hypersensitive to some stimuli and hyposensitive to others (Genna, 2001). Indications of sensory integration disturbance may first be manifested in the newborn as feeding difficulties and should be followed and remedied (Table 5-2). Infants with poor tactile processing who fail to root, attach to the breast, or ignore the breast may benefit from use of a nipple shield. The shield may present a stronger tactile signal to such an infant helping to trigger rooting and mouth opening (Genna, 2008).

Some infants may simply become overwhelmed by multiple people handling them, loud noise, bright lights, radio, television, and ringing telephones. As a result, they may basically shut down until the environment becomes quieter.

Oral aversion or oral-tactile hypersensitivity may be another manifestation of sensory integration difficulties but can often have iatrogenic origins. These conditions and the ensuing aversive responses can be caused by prematurity, immaturity, illness, delayed oral feeding, and unpleasant oral-tactile experiences (Wolf & Glass, 1992). The possibility of oral aversion resulting in maladaptive imprinting, faulty sucking techniques, and dysphagia (difficulty in swallowing) should be taken into account when an infant is reluctant to breastfeed (Healow & Hugh, 2000). Suctioning, intubation, and gavage feeding are all invasive to the oral cavity. Petechiae and bruises on the posterior palates of infants who were suctioned with

---

TABLE 5-2   Possible Indicators of Sensory Integration Difficulties

---

Hyperactive gag reflex

Shallow latch (breast not drawn deeply into mouth)

Low oral muscle tone

Poor sucking rhythmicity

Excessive jaw compression

Malpositioning of the tongue

Unusual posturing

Avoidance of certain positions (arching of the back)

Increased tone, withdrawal responses from the breast

Latch refusal, tonic bite

Passive at breast

Mother's belief that the infant does not like to breastfeed or does not like her

---

a standard bulb syringe after a vaginal delivery have been reported (Black, 1993). Conditioned dysphagia from aggressive suctioning and procedures can be acquired and learned when a negative stimulus is associated with swallowing (Di Scipio et al., 1978). Other intrusions into a newborn's mouth that may contribute to oral-aversive behaviors include gastric lavage, use of artificial nipples or pacifiers, digital assessment of the mouth, finger feeding, use of latex gloves or finger cots, unpleasant-tasting fluids, and repeated suctioning with a bulb syringe.

Latch difficulties may be an early marker of a congenital condition previously called benign congenital hypotonia. Although not identifying a disease, this general descriptive term refers to an infant with low muscle tone at birth and a generalized floppiness. Diagnostic advances have been able to identify specific neurological disorders and myopathies such as central core disease, congenital muscular dystrophy, and spinal muscle atrophy, resulting in this term being phased out in favor of the more accurate diagnoses (Prasad & Prasad, 2003). An accurate diagnosis is important, because some neuromuscular disorders carry the risk of malignant hyperthermia (Thompson, 2002). The "floppy baby" referred to here represents a neuromuscular disorder of unknown origin that is nonprogressive and tends to improve over time. The infant feels like a rag doll with general weakness and flaccidity of the muscles. The infant may be unable to lift his or her head, has a weak cry, displays poor reflexes, shows poor suckling, has hypermobile joints, demonstrates an underactive gag reflex, has a high arched palate, demonstrates fasciculations of the tongue, and has an open mouth. Mothers may describe decreased fetal movements during the pregnancy. Some infants are born with joint contractures (arthrogryposis) of the ankles, knees, elbows, or wrists. An affected infant may also have congenitally dislocated hips and weakness in the anterior neck muscles, causing the head to lag when lifted. Sucking difficulties may be found with inactive lip, cheek, and tongue muscles as well as lack of sensory input from hand-to-mouth movements (Cohen, 1998). Such hypotonia may originate from an insult to the central nervous system that was not severe enough to cause permanent damage. It can also result from perinatal asphyxia, intraventricular hemorrhage, and prematurity. Clinicians may wish to look at the labor and delivery records to check for hypoxia, difficult delivery, or vacuum extraction in such cases.

Drug-exposed infants experiencing neonatal abstinence syndrome (NAS) present an almost completely opposite picture; that is, they may be hypertonic, be irritable, demonstrate abnormal movements, be hypersensitive, thrash at the breast, clamp down on the nipple, be unable to modulate their state to feed well, be difficult to position at breast, and pull back from the breast if experiencing nasal stuffiness (Jansson et al., 2004). Intrauterine drug exposure may temporarily impact the development of brainstem respiratory and swallow centers, transiently altering the suck-swallow-breathe cycle. During the early days after birth, some of these infants may ingest less volume of milk per sucking burst and/or demonstrate less rhythmical swallowing, especially if they have been opiate exposed in utero (Gewolb et al., 2004).

The substance abuse rate in pregnant women in the United States has been estimated to be approximately 10% (King, 1997), though this rate probably underestimates the actual extent of chemical dependency among pregnant women. Mothers on methadone maintenance who are receiving proper care and counseling through substance abuse treatment programs may be candidates for breastfeeding with close follow-up. Often, their infants must be medicated as the infants withdraw from opioids, because 60–90% of opiate-exposed infants develop NAS (Kandall, 1995) and the amount of methadone in breastmilk is low and not therapeutic to the infant (Begg et al., 2001; Jansson et al., 2008). However, Dryden et al. (2009) demonstrated that breastfeeding was associated with reduced odds of the infant requiring treatment for NAS. Abdel-Latif et al. (2006) documented that breastfeeding has a significant positive impact on the neonate that included reduced NAS severity, delayed onset of NAS, and decreased need for pharmacological treatment regardless of gestational age and the type of drug exposure. Thus breastfeeding is to be encouraged and supported because these infants are extremely vulnerable and can benefit greatly by not only the receipt of breastmilk but by the act of breastfeeding itself. Jansson and coworkers (2004) identified eight potential challenges to breastfeeding presented by methadone-exposed infants and suggestions for handling them (Table 5-3).

Infants who are exposed to other drugs during pregnancy may also exhibit stress or abstinence behaviors. Prenatal use of less potent opiates, some nonopiate central nervous system depressants, alcohol, marijuana, and tobacco can all generate side effects in the newborn (Lester et al., 2002).

Women who smoke are less likely to breastfeed than those who do not smoke and are more likely to wean earlier than nonsmoking mothers (Liu et al., 2006). There may be a number of explanations for this:

- Smoking ≥ 10 cigarettes daily was reported to decrease milk production and alter milk composition (Hopkinson et al., 1992).

- Mothers who smoke may perceive that their milk supply is inadequate (Hill & Aldag, 1996).

- The milk of smoking breastfeeding mothers has a lower fat content than the milk of mothers who do not smoke (Powers, 1999).

- Mothers who smoked five or more cigarettes daily had infants who exhibited behaviors such as colic and crying that may contribute to early weaning (Matheson & Rivrud, 1989).

- Smoking mothers perceived a strong risk of harming the infant by smoking and weaned earlier due to concerns regarding the toxic effects of nicotine on the composition and quantity of their milk. Mothers did not receive a strong message from healthcare providers that the benefits of breastfeeding superseded the harm of smoking, as many smoking mothers remain unaware that the benefits of breastfeeding outweigh the potential harm posed to their infants by nicotine in their breastmilk (Goldade et al., 2008).

Tobacco-exposed infants have been shown to demonstrate neurotoxic effects such as greater excitability, greater hypertonia, the need for more handling, and signs of withdrawal or abstinence (Law et al., 2003). Smoking-exposed infants may demonstrate poor self-regulation with all side effects persisting up to a month after birth (Stroud et al., 2009). Postnatal exposure to the nicotine in breastmilk can alter autonomic cardiovascular control in infants. Heart rate variability has

TABLE 5-3   Challenges to Breastfeeding in Methadone-Exposed Infants

Challenge	Intervention
1. Irritability/crying	Feed when in a drowsy state or before full crying appears Swaddle Vertical rocking Hold baby's hand Gentle cupping of head if tolerated "Tame" the environment by dimming lights and minimizing noise

2. State lability
  • Rapid fluctuation between states
  • Not achieving quiet alert state
	Minimize stimulation
	Bring infant from sleep to quiet alert state slowly
	Watch for signs of stress

3. Hypertonicity
  • Generalized, often with asymmetries
  • Clenched jaw and poor gape (mouth opening)
  • Easily overstimulated
    ▪ Neck arching
    ▪ Side-to-side head thrashing
  • Arched posture
	Gradual oral stimulation
	Respond to overstimulation cues (irritability, hiccups, tremors, excessive gas, gaze aversion, tachypnea [rapid breathing], mottling)
	Head support
	Wrap baby in a soft blanket to restrain thrashing movements
	Avoid the clutch hold and have baby facing the mother
	Use ventral positioning

4. Suck-and-swallow incoordination • Poor or disorganized suck patterns	Feeding therapy referral to occupational therapist, physical therapist, or speech/language pathologist Mothers may need to pump their milk Alternative feeding devices may be required until baby can feed at breast
5. Hypersensitivity	Feed in a dim, quiet room with comfortable, constant temperature Gentle and minimal handling Swaddling Have mother breastfeed in a side-lying position Artificial nipples may not be well tolerated and should be avoided Shape the breast to fit the long axis of the baby's mouth if he or she does not open wide enough to latch Wrap a soft blanket around baby's arms, upper body, and back of head to minimize thrashing
6. Nasal stuffiness (may cause detaching from the nipple, pulling back of baby's head, arching, and stiffening)	May require gentle nasal suctioning with saline drops

(continues)

TABLE 5-3 Challenges to Breastfeeding in Methadone-Exposed Infants *(continued)*

Challenge	Intervention
7. Vomiting	Small, frequent feeds and frequent burping
8. Pull-down (may appear to be sedated or asleep in an effort to avoid stimuli and create a tolerable environment)	Baby may actually be in an awake or hypersensitive state; vigorous stimulation should be avoided in an attempt to wake baby Soft handling, gentle talking, and skin-to-skin contact

Source: Adapted from Jansson LM, Velez M, Harrow C. Methadone maintenance and lactation: a review of the literature and current management guidelines. *J Hum Lact.* 2004;20:62–71.

been shown to decrease as the amount of nicotine in breastmilk increases (Dahlstrom et al., 2008). Shorter times between the mother smoking a cigarette and the onset of breastfeeding increase the concentration of nicotine in breastmilk (Dahlstrom et al., 2004). Mothers who smoke can be advised to smoke immediately after a breastfeeding to prolong the interval between nicotine intake and breastfeeding. Nicotine is not stored in breastmilk, and levels peak in breastmilk 30 to 60 minutes after cessation of smoking (Mennella & Beauchamp, 1998). Even passive smoke in the household increases the nicotine levels in breastmilk. Although mothers who smoke should be encouraged to breastfeed, they should also be helped to eliminate smoking from their homes. The following may provide potential motivations to stop smoking:

- Infants spend significantly less time sleeping during the hours immediately after breastfeeding when their mothers have recently smoked (Mennella et al., 2007).

- Smoking is a leading risk factor for sudden infant death syndrome (Anderson et al., 2005).

- Nicotine-induced disruptions in sleep may contribute to long-term behavioral and learning deficits (DiFranza et al., 2004), because sleep promotes learning in infants (Gomez et al., 2006) and deprivation of active sleep impairs learning and the formation of new memories in animal models (McDermott et al., 2003).

Infants born to mothers who were treated prenatally for depression with selective serotonin reuptake inhibitors, such as the commonly prescribed paroxetine (Paxil), fluoxetine (Prozac), citalopram (Celexa), and sertraline (Zoloft), can demonstrate a wide range of neurobehavioral alterations (Lattimore et al., 2005), including increased tremulousness and difficulty achieving more alert states (Zeskind & Stephens, 2004). As many as 35% of women use psychotropic medications during pregnancy (Goldberg & Nissim, 1994). A neonatal behavioral syndrome has been described in infants whose mothers have been treated with selective serotonin reuptake inhibitors that includes tremors, shaking, agitation, spasms, hyper- or hypotonia, irritability, and sleep disturbances. Respiratory system involvement includes indrawing, apnea/bradycardia, and tachypnea (Jordan et al., 2008). These signs appear during the first day of life and resolve within 3 to 5 days (Ferreira et al., 2007). Other differences observed in the exposed group were higher rates of vomiting, tachycardia, and jaundice. Any or all of these signs may disturb early breastfeeding behaviors, necessitating close observation and a potential need for intense breastfeeding support. Some of the signs and symptoms of withdrawal are seen in healthy non-drug-exposed infants or are indicative of other types of underlying problems. A withdrawal scoring sheet may be helpful to identify the drug-withdrawing infant from a collection of symptoms that persist over time (http://newborns.stanford.edu/ScoringSheet.html). The Neonatal Intensive Care Unit Network Neurobehavioral Scale was developed to provide a comprehensive assessment of neurological integrity and behavioral function in drug-exposed infants and to identify the types and ranges of withdrawal and stress behaviors likely to be seen in these infants (Lester & Tronick, 2004). Use of this scale is intended to ensure a home environment sensitive to infant tolerance for stimulation and handling and to provide insight to the clinician regarding positioning, handling, and environmental conditions that are most beneficial in caring for these infants during hospitalization (Boukydis et al., 2004).

Early feeding resistance in some infants may have an organic basis. Abadie et al. (2001) described a set of feeding behaviors in bottle-fed infants that they attributed to poor organic perinatal control of oroesophageal motility: early onset of poor sucking and swallowing skills, refusal to feed, excessive regurgitation, and occasional cough or pallor attacks during bottle-feeding. Some infants also displayed minor facial dysmorphism (retrognathia and arched palate) and mild hypotonia of the tongue base or larynx. The congenital nature of these behaviors combined with manometric findings in the esophagus led to the suspicion that these feeding behaviors were the result of prenatal factors, because central control of the coordinated peristalsis of esophageal motility, sucking, and swallowing originates in a central pattern generator in the brainstem (Jean, 2001). Also, retrognathia and arched palate are anatomical variations that have been observed in children with poor fetal sucking movements (Sherer et al., 1995).

Persistent and unresolved difficulties with latching may result in an infant who never achieves latch, early weaning from the breast, or a mother who pumps her milk and provides it to her baby in a bottle. Clinicians have the option of using a nipple shield to achieve latch. Although early shield design and use often yielded unwanted and detrimental outcomes to breastfeeding (Desmarais & Browne, 1990), more recent data have described beneficial outcomes. Central to such outcomes are the use of ultrathin silicone shields, critical assessment by a skilled lactation consultant, and continuous follow-up, both in the hospital and postdischarge. Many infants who otherwise may have been unable to breastfeed can and have benefited from the judicious use of this tool.

Nipple Shields

The use of nipple shields can be quite helpful as an intervention in certain breastfeeding situations (Brigham, 1996; Wilson-Clay, 2003). An understanding of what shields can and cannot accomplish is essential in the clinical decision-making process. Shields can

- Therapeutically supply oral stimulation that an infant cannot obtain from the mother's nipples due to inability to latch or transfer milk
- Create a nipple shape in the infant's mouth
- Allow extraction of milk by expression with minimal suction, with negative pressure inside the shield tip keeping milk available
- Compensate for weak infant suction
- Present a stable nipple shape that remains during pauses in sucking bursts
- Maintain the nipple in a protruded position
- Affect the rate of milk flow

Shields cannot

- Correct milk transfer problems or weight gain if the mother has inadequate milk volume
- Fix damaged nipples if the cause is not discovered and remedied
- Replace skilled intervention and close follow-up

Shield use permits learning to feed at breast, allows supplementation to occur at breast (i.e., thread tubing under or alongside of the shield), encourages nipple protractility, does not overwhelm the mother with gadgets, and avoids the infant fighting the breast. Shield use may prevent premature termination of breastfeeding. Use of shields does not affect maternal prolactin levels, and infants are able to gain weight appropriately while using a nipple shield (Chertok et al., 2006).

The clinician must also consider some of the disadvantages of nipple shield use. It is sometimes used as a substitute for skilled care or as a quick fix but may not correct the underlying problem; may exacerbate the original problem; may lead to insufficient milk volume, inadequate weight gain, or weaning; can be problematic without follow-up; may prevent proper extension of the nipple back into the infant's mouth (Minchin, 1998); could pinch the nipple and areola, causing abrasion, pain, skin breakdown, and internal trauma to the breast if not applied properly; could create nipple shield addiction (DeNicola, 1986), after which the infant will not feed at breast without the shield in place; might predispose the nipple to damage when the infant is put to breast without the shield, because the infant may chew rather than suckle; and could be discarded as a useful intervention in selected situations.

Use of a nipple shield should be considered in situations involving latch difficulty, oral cavity problems, upper airway problems, prematurity (Clum & Primomo, 1996), and damaged nipples when other avenues to achieve latch have been attempted and failed to produce the desired outcome and when discharge or weaning is imminent. (A complete list of such situational examples can be found in Appendix 5-1.)

Shield Composition and Dimensions

Shields composed of all rubber are no longer seen today, and standard bottle nipples placed over the mother's nipple or attached to a glass or plastic base are not appropriate interventions (Figure 5-15a). Latex and silicone shields are extremely thin and flexible, with a firmer nipple portion. Because the silicone is so thin, more stimulation reaches the areola and milk volume is not as seriously depleted as with the other designs (Auerbach, 1990). With the increasing reports of latex allergy in the general population, latex-containing shields should be avoided. Silicone shields (Figure 5-15b) are available in a number of sizes (Table 5-4).

Few data exist in the literature regarding shield selection and instructions for their use. The height of the nipple portion of the shield should not exceed the

(a)   (b)

Figure 5-15 **(a)** Old Style Nipple Shields; **(b)** Modern Silicone Nipple Shields

length of the infant's mouth from the juncture of the hard and soft palates to lip closure (Wilson-Clay & Hoover, 2002). If the height of the teat of a shield is greater than this length, the infant's jaw closure and tongue compression will fall on the shaft of the teat, and not over the breast. The teat must be large enough to allow for the expansion of the nipple during sucking. If the height of the teat is too short for the nipple, it may abrade against the inside of the teat or extrude through the teat holes. The base diameter should fit the mother's nipple and better results occur with the shortest teat height and smallest base diameter. (A summary of shield-use instructions is presented in Appendix 5-1.)

TABLE 5-4 Dimensions of Silicone Nipple Shields

Product	Diameter	Height of Nipple	Width of Nipple	Number of Holes
Avent	2⅝″	⅞″	⅝″ at tip, 1″ at base	3
Medela				
Standard	2⅝″	⅞″	⅝″ at tip, 1″ at base	4
Extra Small	2⅝″	⅝″	⅜″ at tip, ⅝″ at base	3
Ameda	2⅝″	⅞″	⅘″ at tip, ⅞″ at base	5

Source: Walker M. Breast pumps and other technologies. In: Riordan J, ed. *Breastfeeding and Human Lactation.* 3rd ed. Sudbury, MA: Jones and Bartlett Publishers; 2005:352.

Weaning From the Shield

There is no set time to wean an infant (or mother) from shield use. Extended use of the ultrathin silicone shield has not been shown to be detrimental (Bodley & Powers, 1996). Mothers start the shield-weaning process by just encouraging skin-to-skin contact next to the nipple, starting the feed with the shield and then removing it, and gradually trying feeds without the shield. The tip of the shield should not be cut off in an attempt to present less and less of the device to the infant. Rough edges may scrape the infant's mouth, and the altered shape and consistency of the shield may not be appropriate to the desired outcome. Clinicians should document all encounters and instructions and communicate these to the primary health provider.

Consent and Follow-Up

Some hospital units use informed consent before using a shield (Kutner, 1986). A consent form is signed by the mother, the father (if available), and the provider who is recommending the shield. This approach ensures that everyone knows the downside of using a shield as well as how to use it so that it maximizes the chances of achieving an optimal outcome. A consent form used in this manner also serves as a teaching aid to professionals who are unaware of potential long-range problems. A copy should be given to the mother, another copy is retained in the medical record, and a third copy is sent to the pediatrician.

Clinicians should provide proper written instructions for the mother and referrals if a shield is recommended as an interim measure to assist with breastfeeding. If a mother is discharged from the hospital using a shield, a community referral must be made to a lactation consultant or the nurse practitioner at the pediatrician's office for daily follow-up. Weight checks may need to be obtained twice a week. The pediatrician should be alerted to the problem that required use of the shield in the first place and should be aware of suggestions for discontinuing its use.

Reluctant Nurser

The mother is likely to experience frustration and anxiety over an infant who cannot feed at her breast. If breastfeeding attempts are internalized as failure, the mother may experience disappointment and disconnection with her infant rather than the beginnings of connection and competence (Driscoll, 1992). The mother's perception of the neonate's competence at breast serves as a primary reinforcer in her persistence with breastfeeding. An infant who does not latch to the breast generally presents a reality clash with a mother's expectation of breastfeeding as automatic and pleasing (Mozingo et al., 2000). It acts as a stressor that can lead directly to weaning if sensitive, consistent, and evidence-based interventions are not received. Mothers whose infants experience difficulty latching or sucking are significantly less likely to be breastfeeding at all at 12 weeks (Taveras et al., 2004). Positive feedback in the form of an infant who breastfeeds well reinforces the mother's decision to breastfeed and increases maternal self-esteem (Matthews, 1991). Problems related to latch include the infant who is reluctant to or unable to latch to the breast, with interventions for the reluctant nurser varying depending on what is contributing to the problem (Box 5-1).

Sleepy Infant

An infant who is "unavailable" to feed can be especially worrisome to both the mother and the clinician. With hospital stays of 48 hours or less being the norm for full-term healthy infants, many infants can be discharged without ever having actually fed at the breast. Sleep architecture in newborns during the first days after birth shows both ultradian (biological rhythms that occur less frequently than every 24 hours) and circadian (biological rhythms that occur every 24 hours) cyclicity (Freudigman & Thoman, 1994) that is responsive to a number of variables, including mode of delivery (Freudigman & Thoman, 1998), maternal labor medications, gestational age, and the surrounding environment. The earliest postnatal sleep patterns differ between vaginally and cesarean-born infants. The diurnal sleep pattern of infants is disrupted by a cesarean delivery such that infants born by cesarean section have shown significantly less active sleep. During the first 2 days, vaginally born infants show significant day/night differences with more wakefulness, shorter mean sleep periods, and shorter longest-sleep periods during the daytime on both days (Freudigman & Thoman, 1998). This presents as a vaginally born infant having more opportunities to breastfeed, whereas a cesarean-born infant may not demonstrate breastfeeding cues as frequently. Heavier infants of diabetic mothers have been shown to have higher amounts of quiet and motionless sleep (Sadeh et al., 1996), which may limit optimal breastfeeding opportunities. Jaundiced newborns tend to sleep more than nonjaundiced infants, which may have origins in increased carbon monoxide production. Carbon monoxide is formed from the breakdown of heme to bilirubin and is produced at a rate equal to the rate

BOX 5-1 Problem of the Reluctant Nurser

Problem Description

- Baby may latch to the breast only after many attempts.
- Baby may be unable to latch.
- Baby may completely refuse to latch to breast, either falling asleep or aggressively pushing away with an arched body.
- Baby may exhibit rapid side-to-side head movements and may or may not latch to breast.
- Baby may have a one-sided preference.

Contributing Factors

- poor positioning at breast
- hypertonia (jaw clenching, pursed lips, neck and back hyperextension, tongue retraction or elevation)
- interruption in the organized sequence of prefeeding behaviors immediately after birth
- infrequent feeds leading to an overhungry baby and excessive or prolonged crying resulting in behavioral disorganization
- drug-induced interference that prolongs the period of state disorganization in the newborn (epidural, Stadol, Nubain, Demerol)
- interference with imprinting on the breast from separation, artificial nipples, or pacifiers
- fetal history of breech presentation, extension in utero, protracted labor, cervical spine pain or damage, precipitous delivery, dislocated hip, fractured clavicle, or asymmetrical positioning in utero with right-sided preference
- excessive pressure on the occipital region of baby's head from pushing the head forward into the breast
- vigorous or deep suctioning or intubation that causes swelling or discomfort in the mouth or throat with resulting clenched mouth, tongue thrusting, neck extension, or pushing away from the breast
- oral aversion or other sensory integration problems
- vacuum extraction, forceps, shoulder dystocia with misalignment of head, neck, and shoulders
- cephalohematoma
- short or tight lingual frenulum
- flat or inverted nipples
- upper airway disorders

(continues)

Management	Rationale
Check the positioning of baby at breast: • baby completely facing mother with head, neck, and spine aligned • mouth in front of and slightly below where nipple points • baby brought to breast and held close • mother does not lean forward or maneuver the breast sideways	Poor positioning increases the number of latch attempts needed before obtaining milk, which can frustrate both mother and baby. Improper positioning increases the chances that the baby will not attach to the breast, leading to sore nipples, engorgement, insufficient milk production, and slow weight gain.
Positioning may vary depending on the symmetry of the baby. Babies with a right-sided preference may need to be held in a football hold for the right breast and in a cradle or prone position for the left breast. Some babies do better when the mother is in a sidelying position. Breech babies may feed better sitting upright in a clutch hold (Figure 5-16). Babies with delivery trauma such as a cephalohematoma may be more comfortable and feed better when held with the affected side up. Babies with a fractured clavicle may feed better in a clutch hold if the weight of the breast is kept off the chest or in a cradle hold with the affected side up.	Positioning in utero and delivery events influence breastfeeding patterns. Several different positions may need to be explored to find one that is satisfactory.

Figure 5-16   Upright Hold

Allow the baby time on the mother's breast immediately after delivery. Let baby seek and find the nipple before removal from the mother's chest.	This provides the opportunity for the prefeeding sequence of behaviors to occur, which increases the likelihood of proper attachment to the breast.

Management

Keep the mother and baby together. Place the baby skin-to-skin on the mother's chest (Meyer & Anderson, 1999). Instruct the mother to feed her baby on cue: when he stirs at breast, when she sees rapid eye movements under the eyelids, when she sees movements of the tongue and mouth, when baby exhibits hand-to-mouth movements, or when baby makes small sounds.

An alternative technique is to place mother and baby in a bath allowing baby to repattern in the warm water. To keep baby warm and soothed, a helper can gently pour warm water over the baby's back as he creeps to the breast and attaches (Harris, 1994).

Place a warm towel over baby's neck; massage the shoulders and arms. This is helpful after a precipitous delivery, forceps, or vacuum extraction. It is also soothing to a high-tone baby.

For rapid side-to-side head movements, touch the midline of baby's upper lip with a dropper of colostrum or D_5 (Figure 5-17). Move baby onto the breast as he follows the dropper to the nipple. When his mouth is wide open, place a few drops of water or colostrum on his tongue to elicit sucking and swallowing.

Rationale

This reestablishes and/or repatterns the initial sucking sequence that may not have occurred immediately postdelivery. With the baby in close, the mother can feel the infant's feeding cues and place him to breast before he becomes over-hungry and when he is most likely to latch on.

Baby may be in pain from overriding cervical vertebrae. This helps relax the cervical structures and decrease tone in a high-tone baby.

The dropper acts to provide external control and food incentives for attachment and sucking at breast.

Figure 5-17 Use of Dropper to Orient Infant to Breast

(continues)

Management	Rationale
An arching baby can be placed either in the football hold or with the mother lying on her side. The mother can also use a sling to help position the baby in flexion. If this does not calm the baby, place him on a receiving blanket, have two adults pick up the corners of the blanket and rock the baby from side-to-side like a hammock. Then put the baby to breast.	These techniques help to flex the back and hips to avoid arching and jaw clenching.
Provide latch and sucking incentives to the baby, which can include:	This helps prevent the baby from pulling away from the breast before he latches on or swallows.

- A periodontal syringe placed in the side of the baby's mouth that delivers a small amount of colostrum or sugar water with each suck until the baby demonstrates rhythmic suck and swallow at breast.

- A syringe or soft clinic dropper can be used to elicit sucking (Figure 5-18).

- Butterfly tubing attached to a 10 cc syringe and taped to the breast can provide these incentives as well as a supplement if needed.

Figure 5-18   Use of Soft Clinic Dropper to Elicit Sucking

Management	Rationale
A baby who is crying hard or has been crying for a period of time may not be able to organize himself to feed. Allow this baby to suck on a finger or place the tubing on a finger and allow baby to suck (Figure 5-19) a little colostrum or sugar water by finger feeding him before putting him to breast. Avoid pacifiers and bottles. If the baby will not suck on a finger, place some colostrum in a 28 cc medicine cup and have the baby sip from the cup until he calms down and has a little food in his stomach.	

Figure 5-19 Tubing Taped to the Finger to Elicit Sucking

Management	Rationale
If the baby will not open his mouth wide enough for painless latch-on or clenches his jaw, hold the baby's jaw between your thumb and index finger and move the jaw a small amount from side to side. If the lower lip is rolled under, keeping the mouth from achieving a large enough gape, or the mouth is not open to >130 degrees, **gently** pull down on the chin to evert the lower lip and encourage a more open mouth (Figure 5-20).	This helps inhibit jaw clenching. Pulling down on the chin too hard may dislodge the baby from the breast or cause him to bite down to stay attached.

(continues)

Management	Rationale

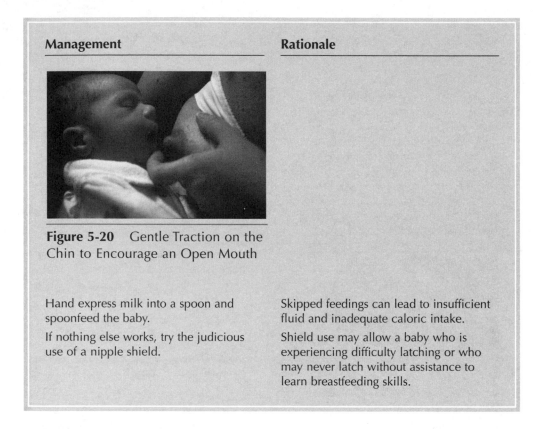

Figure 5-20   Gentle Traction on the Chin to Encourage an Open Mouth

Management	Rationale
Hand express milk into a spoon and spoonfeed the baby.	Skipped feedings can lead to insufficient fluid and inadequate caloric intake.
If nothing else works, try the judicious use of a nipple shield.	Shield use may allow a baby who is experiencing difficulty latching or who may never latch without assistance to learn breastfeeding skills.

of bilirubin synthesis. Increased carbon monoxide production in jaundiced infants may likely play a role in increased sleep states due to the regulatory effects on sleep circadian rhythm and rapid-eye-movement sleep via the cholinergic system activation (Ozkan et al., 2008). The first 2 hours after delivery offer the earliest opportunity for imprinting and latch to take place. However, infants do not fall into a deep sleep state for the next 24 hours after that point. Infants experience sleep cycles during this time, which makes it important that infants be kept with their mothers to take advantage of feeding opportunities during sleep–wake transition times.

Many mothers may be under the impression that crying indicates when it is time to feed an infant. In reality, crying is a late sign of hunger, and a sleepy infant may not come to a full arousal state and cry. Feeding cues in some infants can be very subtle and easily overlooked. Maternal labor medications can interfere with state control in infants, making it difficult to feed a sleepy infant. When such an infant arouses, he or she may go from sound sleep to hard crying, bypassing the graded levels of arousal in between. Sleeping is not an indication that an infant is receiving sufficient amounts of milk. Some parents have been told to never wake a sleeping infant, believe that sleeping is an indication that the infant is content, work toward causing the infant to sleep as much as possible, and have unrealistic expectations regarding the nature of newborn sleep.

The sleep organization of breastfed and formula-fed infants is different (Butte et al., 1992), changes over time, and is influenced by maturation, development, nutrition, and caretaking patterns. Over the first 4 months of life, non–rapid-eye-movement sleep (light sleep) increases to about 60% and rapid-eye-movement sleep (deep sleep) decreases to approximately 40% of total sleep (Roffwarg et al., 1966). Breastfed infants typically show more spontaneous arousals from sleep (McKenna et al., 1990), especially in the early morning, spend more time in non–rapid-eye-movement sleep, and demonstrate accelerated maturation of the central nervous system compared with formula-fed infants.

Many infant training programs (Pinilla & Birch, 1993) exist to cause young infants to lengthen their nighttime sleep bouts, especially during the early months of life, when they are also at higher risk for sudden infant death syndrome (Schechtman et al., 1992). Parents should be aware that sleep training books and programs may not be in the best interest of a young infant. Arousal from sleep is a survival mechanism that can be impaired by the major risk factors for sudden infant death syndrome such as prone sleeping and maternal smoking. Horne et al. (2004) found that 2- to 3-month-old formula-fed infants are less arousable in active sleep than breastfed 2- to 3-month-old infants. They also state that breastfeeding during the critical risk period for sudden infant death syndrome (2–4 months) remains very important, because reduced arousability in active sleep could impair the ability of an infant to respond to a life-threatening situation.

Some infants whose breastfeeding needs are not met at night, when it is "not" all right to breastfeed, may be unable to differentiate when it is permissible or not permissible to breastfeed and refuse to breastfeed during the day. Young breastfed infants during the early weeks of life need to feed at night. This ensures adequate weight gain and an abundant milk supply. Feeding very young infants cereal at night to make them sleep longer is a misconception, does not cause longer sleep (Macknin et al., 1989), and displaces breastmilk from the diet. An infant who is very sleepy in the early days of life is a challenge to the breastfeeding mother (Walker, 1997). She needs to know when the infant is actually swallowing milk (Table 5-5) and how to know that the infant is getting enough milk (Table 5-6).

These data assume that infants have not experienced breastfeeding difficulties or any interventions that might disrupt the normal acquisition of early breastfeeding

---

TABLE 5-5   Signs of Swallowing

- Hearing a puff of air from the nose
- Hearing a "ca" sound
- Hearing a swallow in the throat
- Feeling the areola drawn farther into the infant's mouth
- Seeing the areola move toward the infant's lips
- Observing the infant's jaw drop lower than during non-nutritive sucking
- Feeling the swallow by placing fingers on the infant's throat
- Hearing swallowing by listening with a stethoscope on the infant's throat

---

skills. The length of time for meconium to transition to the typical breastfed stool varies with gestational age, pattern of feedings, amount of intake, and supplementation with other fluids. Transitioning stool color serves as one of a number of indicators of sufficient breastmilk intake and infant well-being (Salariya & Robertson, 1993). Parents and clinicians often find it easier and more accurate to use a handout that illustrates stool color and consistency changes (Figure 5-21), as well as a diaper log, which ensures adequate intake or signals a need for clinical intervention.

TABLE 5-6   Signs of Sufficient Breast Milk Intake

Age	Wet Diapers	Color	Urates	Stools	Color	Volume	Consistency	Weight Gain
Day 1	1	pale	possible	1	black	≥15 gm	tarry/ sticky	<5% loss
Day 2	2–3	pale	possible	1–2	greenish/ black	≥15 gm	changing	<5% loss
Day 3	3–4	pale	possible	3–4	greenish/ yellow	≥15 gm	soft	≤8–10% loss
Day 4	≥4–6 disposable	pale	none	4 large	yellow/ seedy	≥15 gm	soft/ liquidy	15–30 gm/day
	≥6–8 cloth			10 small				

Sources: Adapted from Powers NG, Slusser W. Breastfeeding update 2: clinical lactation management. *Pediatr Rev.* 1997;18:147–161; Black LS. Incorporating breastfeeding care into daily newborn rounds and pediatric office practice. *Ped Clin N Am.* 2001;48:299–319; Neifert MR. Prevention of breastfeeding tragedies. *Ped Clin N Am.* 2001;48:273–297.

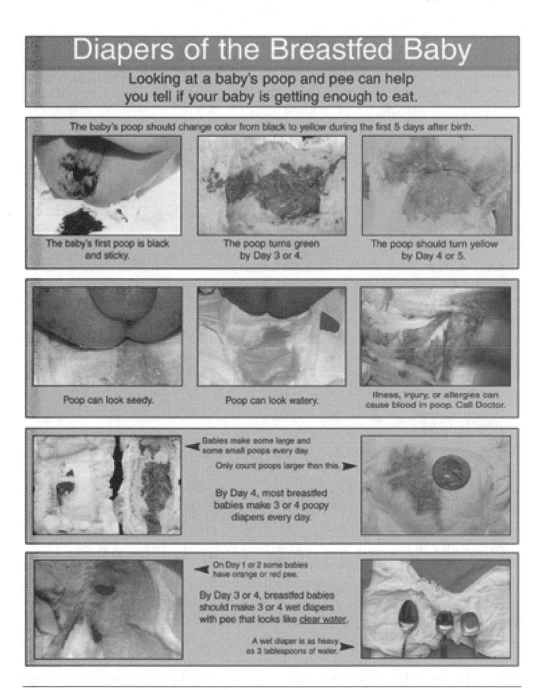

Babies make some large and some small poops every day.

Only count poops larger than this.

By Day 4, most breastfed babies make 3 or 4 poopy diapers every day.

On Day 1 or 2 some babies have orange or red pee.

By Day 3 or 4, breastfed babies should make 3 or 4 wet diapers with pee that looks like clear water.

A wet diaper is as heavy as 3 tablespoons of water.

Figure 5-21   Diapers of the Breastfed Baby

Source: © 2002 Kay Hoover, M Ed, IBCLC, and Barbara Wilson-Clay, BS, IBCLC.

Drowsiness at breast may also be related to the normal release of metabolic hormones that occurs when an infant breastfeeds. One such hormone, cholecystokinin (CCK), is a gastrointestinal hormone that enhances gut maturation, promotes glucose-induced insulin release, is released mainly in response to fat in the diet, enhances sedation, and is thought to play a role in regulating food intake by signaling satiety (Marchini & Linden, 1992). Breastfed infants have higher plasma concentrations of CCK during the first 5 days than do formula-fed infants (Marchini et al., 1993). During the breastfeeding episode, CCK has the effect of inducing sleepiness in both the mother and the infant (Uvnas-Moberg et al., 1987). CCK levels in infants demonstrate two peaks related to breastfeeding. The first increase is seen immediately after breastfeeding, most likely due to activation of the vagal nerve; it is followed by a decline at 10 minutes and then a secondary rise at 30–60 minutes after feeding due to the stimulation effect of food on the CCK-producing cells (Uvnas-Moberg et al., 1993). The interval between these two peaks, especially at about 10 minutes after the feed on the first side, may subsequently determine the optimal timing for placing the infant on the second breast, because he or she may more easily arouse at that point in the CCK cycle. Interventions to help sleepy infants to breastfeed depend on the contributing factors and may change over time (Box 5-2).

Fussy Infant

An infant who is fussy at the breast or who fusses and is fretful after a feeding is a cause of significant anxiety in a new mother. Many mothers interpret a fussing infant or one who is not satisfied after a feeding to mean an insufficient milk supply (Hillervik-Lindquist et al., 1991; Sjolin et al., 1977, 1979; Verronen, 1982). In fact, the major cause of supplementation and premature weaning is perceived (or real) insufficient milk (Bevan et al., 1984; Bloom et al., 1982; Hill, 1991). Newborns may temporarily lack the refined skills for abundant milk transfer and indeed remain hungry after a feeding. Normal fluctuations in milk supply, growth or appetite spurts, or infant temperament can also influence an infant's behavior surrounding the feeding process. Maternal analgesia during labor has been described to have an effect on infant behavior, including increased crying (Ransjo-Arvidson et al., 2001). Maternal smoking during pregnancy has also been reported as contributing to infants who have more fussy periods and more intense reactions to events surrounding them (Kelmanson et al., 2002). Exposure to tobacco smoke and its metabolites have been linked to increased levels of plasma

BOX 5-2   Problem of the Sleepy Baby

Problem Description

- Baby does not wake or fuss on a regular enough basis to indicate hunger.
- Baby falls asleep at breast after a few sucks.
- Baby sucks sporadically at breast, falls asleep, wakes when put down, but continues to feed poorly.
- Baby falls asleep before taking second breast.

Contributing Factors

- maternal illness or certain prenatal medications
- birth complications with increased levels of endorphins
- prematurity
- neonatal illness
- congenital anomalies
- operative delivery
- birth trauma
- maternal labor medications with resulting state disorganization
- overstimulating environment
- invasive procedures
- prolonged crying
- increased levels of CCK
- hyperbilirubinemia
- phototherapy

Management	Rationale
Keep mother and baby together.	This decreases crying, which is a behavioral sign of stress. Separated infants cry 10 times more often than when kept with their mother (Michelsson et al., 1996).
Suggest skin-to-skin contact as much as possible: Baby can be carried in a sling once home so that breastfeeding cues are immediately recognized.	Mothers can respond immediately to these subtle cues. This helps to repattern the baby to suck at breast if artificial nipples have been used or if the mother was medicated during labor and delivery.

(continues)

Management

Teach alerting techniques to use when feeding cues are observed:

- talk to the baby with variable pitch
- tickle or stroke the palms or soles
- rub the baby's face
- put his hand to his mouth
- allow him to smell a nursing pad with colostrum on it
- sit the baby upright
- unwrap the baby; change the diaper
- move in any direction with uneven rhythms

Provide incentives at breast to entice the baby to wake and feed:

- Place a dropper of colostrum or D5 into the side of the baby's mouth while latching.
- Use a feeding tube device, butterfly tubing taped to breast and connected to a 10 cc syringe, gavage tubing taped to breast, or periodontal syringe (Figure 5-22) to deliver boluses at breast.

Rationale

These activities stimulate the trigeminal nerve (5th cranial nerve), which is the sensory arm for rooting and sucking. The trigeminal has input into the reticular activating system—the alarm clock of the brain.

Sucking action decreases above 80°F room temperature.

Allows baby's movements to awaken him.

Establishing flow of fluid will often initiate and help sustain sucking.

Figure 5-22   Periodontal Syringes

Management	**Rationale**
If the baby is overstimulated and is shutting out the noise and light by sleeping, modify the environment and attempts at stimulation:	Helps supply behavioral organization to a disorganized or dysmature baby.

- provide a quiet, dim room
- do some gentle walking
- pat baby's back at the rate of his heartbeat, gradually slowing the patting to 72 per minute
- feed the baby for short periods of time with timeouts
- avoid talking to the baby or rubbing his head while at breast
- avoid jiggling the baby
- tug back gently on the nipple to induce a suck as long as the nipples are not sore
- use alternate massage if baby dozes at breast between sucking bursts
- avoid caretaking behaviors that promote sleep such as tight wrapping, solitary sleeping in a bassinet, use of a pacifier, rocking the bassinet, high ambient temperature, ignoring cries or feeding cues

Management	**Rationale**
If baby refuses the second breast at a feeding, suggest that the mother offer it after 10 minutes or again after about an hour or when she sees feeding cues again.	Cholecystokinin levels usually fall at these times and baby may start to cycle into a lighter sleep state.
To help parents and clinicians keep track of feedings and diaper counts, a log can be given to parents to fill out for a week or so until the problem is resolved (Figure 5-23).	Helps parents recognize when to seek help and avoid more serious problems such as dehydration and jaundice.

(continues)

First Week Diaper Diary

1. Circle the hour closest to when your baby starts each breastfeeding.
2. Circle a **W** when your baby makes a wet diaper.
3. Circle a **P** when your baby makes a poopy diaper.
   Some babies make more diapers each day than shown. This is great!

Sample Record for Day 4

Feedings: 12 1 2 3 4 5 6 7 8 9 10 11 Noon 1 2 3 4 5 6 7 8 9 10 11
Wet Diapers: W W W W W W
Green or Yellow Poops: P P P P

In this sample, the baby had nine feedings, six wet diapers, and three poopy diapers. By Day Four, most babies breastfeed 8 to 12 times each day.

Birth Date: ___/___/___ Time: _____ AM PM
Birth Weight: _____ Discharge Weight: _____
Baby's weight at one week: _____
For breastfeeding help call:

Call your doctor, nurse, midwife, or breastfeeding helper if:
1. **Your baby is not making enough wet or poopy diapers**
2. **There is dark colored pee after Day 3**
3. **There is dark colored poop after Day 5**

Day 1
Feedings: 12 1 2 3 4 5 6 7 8 9 10 11 Noon 1 2 3 4 5 6 7 8 9 10 11
Wet Diapers: W
Black Tarry Poops: P

Day 2
Feedings: 12 1 2 3 4 5 6 7 8 9 10 11 Noon 1 2 3 4 5 6 7 8 9 10 11
Wet Diapers: W W
Black Tarry Poops: P P

Day 3
Feedings: 12 1 2 3 4 5 6 7 8 9 10 11 Noon 1 2 3 4 5 6 7 8 9 10 11
Wet Diapers: W W W
Green Poops: P P

Day 4
Feedings: 12 1 2 3 4 5 6 7 8 9 10 11 Noon 1 2 3 4 5 6 7 8 9 10 11
Wet Diapers: W W W W
Green or Yellow Poops: P P P P

Day 5
Feedings: 12 1 2 3 4 5 6 7 8 9 10 11 Noon 1 2 3 4 5 6 7 8 9 10 11
Wet Diapers: W W W W W
Yellow Poops: P P P

Day 6
Feedings: 12 1 2 3 4 5 6 7 8 9 10 11 Noon 1 2 3 4 5 6 7 8 9 10 11
Wet Diapers: W W W W W
Yellow Poops: P P

Day 7
Feedings: 12 1 2 3 4 5 6 7 8 9 10 11 Noon 1 2 3 4 5 6 7 8 9 10 11
Wet Diapers: W W W W W
Yellow Poops: P P P P

Orders: Barbara Wilson-Clay, 12710 Burson Drive, Manchaca, TX 78652
Phone: 512-292-7227   Fax: 512-292-7228   E-Mail: bwc@lactnews.com
50 sheets/pad. $15 per pad. Bulk rate in quantities of 20. $13 per pad. Plus shipping

Figure 5-23 First Week Diaper Diary *Source:* © 2002 Kay Hoover, M Ed, IBCLC, and Barbara Wilson-Clay, BS, IBCLC.

and intestinal motilin (peptide that stimulates contractions in the gastrointestinal tract) in infants whose mothers smoked during pregnancy or who are exposed to second-hand smoke. Elevated levels of motilin have been linked with an increased risk of gastrointestinal dysregulation, including colic and acid reflux (Shenassa & Brown, 2004). There is a common perception that breastfed infants cry more, which may be related to the faster emptying of the stomach when it contains breastmilk, leading to the signal of fussing or crying as a hunger cue. However, changing an infant over to formula feeding may not reduce crying but may merely redistribute it away from evening and nighttime hours, giving the impression that the breastfed infant was not fed enough (Barr et al., 1989). Failure to address the cause of an unhappy breastfed infant can quickly lead to a downward spiral of formula supplementation, true insufficient milk, and weaning (Box 5-3).

BOX 5-3   Problem of the Fussy Baby

Problem Description

- Baby may fuss during a feeding.
- Baby may fuss following a feeding or fall asleep at the breast and fuss when put down.
- Baby may fuss between feedings, startle easily, or appear irritable.
- Baby may resist being put to the breast, arch away from the breast, push back with the arms, extend the head, or turn away from the breast.
- Once latched, baby may choke, gag, or repeatedly come on and off the breast.
- Baby may stiffen when approaching the breast or flail his or her arms and legs.

Contributing Factors

- birth trauma or pain (fractured clavicle/humerus), vacuum extraction, forceps, cephalahematoma
- intracranial hemorrhage
- oral aversion (suctioning, intubation, gloved finger)
- prenatal or perinatal medications
- illicit drug use by mother or chemically dependent mother
- sensory sensitivity
- sensory overload
- faulty imprinting on an artificial nipple
- baby may be hungry due to poor feeding skills or limited milk transfer
- insufficient milk supply
- gastroesophageal reflux

(continues)

Management	Rationale
Fussing or arching during feeding may indicate air in the baby's stomach, signaling that the baby needs to burp.	Babies swallow air when they cry; burping the baby may relieve his stomach discomfort.
If baby is overhungry, mother can express a small amount of colostrum or milk and feed the baby prior to latching attempts.	This helps to calm the baby by taking the edge off of hunger.
Offer more nighttime breastfeedings.	Many babies feed better at night because they prefer the darker, quieter environment.
Babies with birth injuries may be fussy; mothers should be instructed to: • position baby to avoid further trauma or pain to injury • provide appropriate pain medication to a baby who is in pain	Pain relief contributes to better organized feeding skills.
Note: Many of the interventions for methadone-exposed babies (see Table 5-3) are effective with the fussy baby as well.	

On the other end of the spectrum, infant fussiness may be related to a cluster of symptoms variously described as hyperlactation (oversupply) and/or overactive letdown reflex, which often occur together, usually well after the mother has established an abundant milk supply. Sometimes an infant is fussy at breast and between feeds because of gastroesophageal reflux.

The sleepy infant, the reluctant nurser, and the fussy infant may all describe the same infant at different times. The fussy infant may respond to any of the interventions described for the sleepy infant or an infant who is reluctant to breastfeed. An infant who is fussy and reluctant to latch can be the infant with birth trauma who falls asleep at the breast. Too often, one intervention is attempted one time for one problem but does not work immediately, so another approach is tried, confusing the infant and the parents, leaving the problem unresolved, and allowing the situation to continue to deteriorate. Inconsistent information combined with recommendations to keep trying a variety of interventions with no systematic evaluation and follow-up is a recipe for early weaning.

A written care plan for infants and mothers experiencing problems, which is modified as needed until the problem resolves, is a more logical approach to early problematic breastfeeding situations (Box 5-4). During the time a mother and infant are in the hospital, charting systems should record breastfeeding progress and expected outcomes (Bassett, 2001) (Figure 5-24). Variances from the expected

BOX 5-4 Care Plan for the Infant Who Won't Latch On

Occasionally, there are times when an infant has difficulty latching on to the breast. Having a step-by-step plan to guide you will help you through those feeds. The goals are to stimulate milk production and make sure your infant has adequate nourishment.

Suggestions

1. Work with your infant in short increments of time.

2. Undress the infant to the diaper; take off your top and bra to maximize skin-to-skin contact. This will help keep infant awake and more alert during feeds.

3. Spend time snuggled with your infant skin-to-skin, with no attempt to latch on.

4. Make sure you are comfortable, with supporting pillows all around.

5. Watch closely for feeding cues. When your infant demonstrates interest in feeding, attempt to put him or her to breast. Wait until infant's mouth opens wide (you can gently tickle the lower lip with your nipple) and the tongue is down. Express a bit of breastmilk onto the nipple to entice infant. Quickly pull your infant to the breast, leading with the chin so that he or she gets a big mouthful of breast tissue.

6. Use your dominant hand to pull your infant to the breast quickly:
   Right handed:
   - Football (clutch) hold on the right side
   Left handed:
   - Cross-cradle (transverse) hold on the left side

7. If your infant cries, arches away, or pulls back, stop immediately; calm him or her by allowing infant to suck on your finger (nail side against the tongue). When infant's suck becomes rhythmical and infant is calm, try again. Try ventral positioning by leaning back at a 35 degree angle and placing the baby on his tummy to feed. If he or she is crying and arching away, try only three times at that feeding.

8. Work with your infant as long as he or she is calm and willing to work to go to breast. Do not push infant's tolerance level or try to get him or her to attach to the breast while screaming. You can try each breast and each position—you never know which one will work.

9. Use verbal positive reinforcement when your infant latches on.

10. If your infant does not latch on at that time, feed expressed breastmilk with a small cup or hollow-handled medicine spoon. Pump your breasts and save the milk for the next feed (breastmilk is safe at room temperature for 8–10 hours).

11. When your infant shows interest in the breast, try again. As long as you continue to pump your breasts, attempt to put your infant to breast, and feed him or her without a bottle nipple, you will maintain your milk supply.

12. Attempt to put your infant to breast at every feeding: at least ____ times in 24 hours.

13. Attempt feeding your infant before your infant is fully awake or crying to feed. A successful latch-on during the night is common.

Mother's signature   Date

Lactation consultant's signature   Date

Source: Adapted from parental care plan for infants who won't latch hand-out developed for Breastfeeding Support Consultants, 1996.

Nutrition & Elimination
Criteria for assessment of newborn infant at the breast position:
- Mother states that she is comfortable: back, feet, & arms supported (head supported in side-lying)
- Infant's head and body supported at the level of the breast (pillows usually helpful with cradle and football to support mother's arm that is holding infant's head and body)
- Infant turned completely on side with nose, chin, chest, abdomen, and knees touching mother (cradle and side lying)
- Infant's head in neutral position (hip, shoulder, and ear aligned)
- Infant kept close by support from mother's arm and hand along the infant's back and buttock
- Mother's breast supported with cupped hand; thumb and fingers will be back from areola

Latch:
- Mouth wide open (like a yawn)
- Lips visible and flanged outward
- ¾–1" of areola covered by the infant's lips (usually most or all of the areola)
- Tongue over lower gum line
- No clicking or smacking sounds
- No indrawing or dimpling of cheek
- Mother states she is comfortable (no persistent nipple pain)

Suck and Swallow:
- Chin moves in rhythmic motion
- Bursts of sucking, swallowing, and rests

⏱ First Side X Second Side		Date															
		Time															
	Breast																
RIGHT SIDE – POSITION	Reverse arm hold																
	Cradle																
	Football																
	Sidelying																
RIGHT SIDE – BABY RESPONSE	Latch achieved																
	Minimal sucking																
	Sustained sucking																
	Sucking & swallowing																
	No latch achieved																
	Too sleepy																
	Reluctant																
LEFT SIDE – POSITION	Reverse arm hold																
	Cradle																
	Football																
	Sidelying																
LEFT SIDE – BABY RESPONSE	Latch achieved																
	Minimal sucking																
	Sustained sucking																
	Sucking & swallowing																
	No latch achieved																
	Too sleepy																
	Reluctant																
ASSISTANCE	Independent																
	Minimum																
	Moderate																
	Maximum																
	Feeding observed by nurse																
	Feeding reported by patient																
	Formula																
	R.N. initials																
STOOLS	Meconium																
	Transitional																
	Curdy																
	Yellow																
	Green																
	⏱ for each stool																
URINE	Normal																
	Uric acid crystals																
	⏱ for each void																

Figure 5-24   Assessment of Newborn at Breast

Source: Adapted from original developed by the Ottawa Hospital, ON, Canada.

behaviors are recorded, and a feeding plan should be devised to address outstanding issues. Some hospitals use care plans or care maps to organize teaching within short hospital maternity stays (Zander, 1991, 1992). A pathway is a collaborative plan of care that

- Identifies critical components of intervention and care that must occur to achieve a predetermined length of stay
- Sequences major interventions to achieve the anticipated length of stay
- States the desired patient outcomes
- Ensures consistency of patient care
- Eliminates duplication or omission of information
- Provides objectives that are to be met each day to avoid information overload on the day of discharge
- Becomes a systematic plan of care so that each nurse has responsibility for a part of the total patient education plan

Accompanying a pathway would be a list of criteria for referral to a lactation consultant (Backas, 1998) for more specialized and intensive work with the mother and baby to create the in-hospital and discharge feeding plan (Tables 5-7 and 5-8).

Mothers of infants who do not respond to a standard feeding plan need individualized plans with interventions based on what the infant responds to best during feedings. Because the mother is a partner in the development of feeding plans, any plans that are formulated should be done so with her input and assurances that the plan can be carried out (Cadwell & Turner-Maffei, 2004). Critical thinking (Bandman & Bandman, 1988) is necessary to start the problem-solving process (Burns & Grove, 1993) for the creation of a feeding plan tailored to each mother–baby unit's unique needs. The problem-solving process involves the following steps:

- Gathering and evaluating data
- Defining the problem
- Determining and evaluating potential options
- Choosing an approach and taking action
- Evaluating the outcomes of the action (Nichols & Zwelling, 1997)

TABLE 5-7   Criteria for Referral to In-Hospital Lactation Consultant

---

- Low birth weight (<2,500 g)
- Infant in special care nursery
- Multiple birth
- Maternal history of breast surgery (reduction, augmentation, biopsy)
- Maternal–infant separation related to maternal illness
- Maternal breast or nipple pathology/anomaly
- Maternal insulin-dependent diabetes mellitus
- Repeated newborn blood sugar/low body temperature
- History of previous unsuccessful breastfeeding experience
- Infant less than 37 weeks gestation
- Non–English-speaking mother
- Infant who fails to latch on
- Repeated difficulty latching to breast
- No suckling
- Sore nipples

Source: Beth Allen RNC, IBCLC, Perinatal and Lactation Center Manager, Northside Hospital, Atlanta, GA, 1998.

TABLE 5-8   Situations in Which Consultation With an Expert in Lactation Management May Be Helpful

---

- Maternal request/anxiety
- Previous negative breastfeeding experience
- Mother has flat/inverted nipples
- Mother has history of breast surgery
- Multiple births (twins, triplets)
- Infant is premature (<37 weeks gestation)
- Infant has congenital anomaly, neurological impairment, or other medical condition that affects the infant's ability to breastfeed
- Maternal or infant medical condition for which breastfeeding must be temporarily postponed or for which milk expression is required
- Documentation, after the first few feedings, that there is difficulty in establishing breastfeeding (e.g., poor latch-on, sleepy infant)

Source: Clinical Protocol Number 5: Peripartum breastfeeding management for the healthy mother and infant at term. Academy of Breastfeeding Medicine, 2008. Retrieved March 21, 2009, from www.bfmed.org.

A feeding plan also includes short- and long-term goals, outcome criteria, evaluation of the plan, and revisions as needed. For example, a common occurrence during a 48-hour hospital stay for many newborns and their mothers is an infant with ineffective latch and feeding, with the resulting question of "how long should the infant go before we supplement?" There is no one right answer to this question or situation; it depends on the status of the infant and the availability of skilled intervention. A feeding plan could resemble the sample in Box 5-4 depending on the factors contributing to the problem.

Decision Trees

Many hospital maternity units and outpatient settings use clinical algorithms (Babic et al., 1999a; Babic et al., 1999b) or decision trees as guidelines, tools for decision support, and strategies to strengthen the intervention choice process. The decision trees featured in Figures 5-25, 5-26, 5-27, and 5-28 are examples of comprehensive and effective breastfeeding and postpartum checklists and flowcharts.

Problem of Hypoglycemia

Hypoglycemia is a common metabolic concern in the newborn infant and represents a continuum of blood glucose concentration, falling immediately after delivery and rising thereafter. Hypoglycemia is not a single number. Transient hypoglycemia in the first 3 hours after birth is normal with spontaneous recovery. Although breastfeeding in the first hour after birth is very important to the course of lactation, feeding a normal healthy newborn in the first hour after birth does not cause the blood glucose levels to rise (Sweet et al., 1999). Therefore an infant who misses this opportunity at breast does not require supplementation, nor does a healthy full-term breastfeeding infant require routine blood glucose monitoring (American Academy of Pediatrics, 1993). Adaptation in normal circumstances progresses in a pattern.

Physiological Adaptation After Birth

- The brain derives almost all of its energy from glucose.
- During gestation glucose is stored in the fetus as glycogen, mostly in the liver but also in cardiac and skeletal muscle.
- Delivery terminates the glucose supply obtained from the mother in utero.

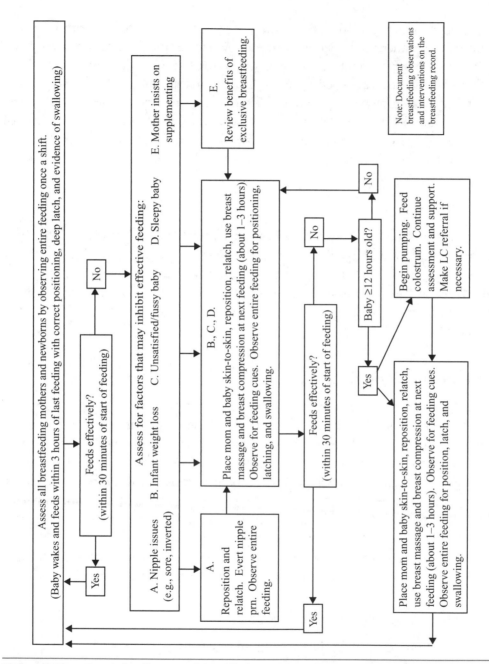

Figure 5-25   Breastfeeding Decision Tree and Checklist For use with normal newborns of more than 37 weeks gestational age. *(continues)*

Source: © Presbyterian Hospital of Dallas, 2003. Used with permission.

Checklist

Normal breastfeeding:
- ☐ Baby wakes and breastfeeds about every 1½ to 3 hours
- ☐ Baby nurses 8–12 times in 24 hours
- ☐ Baby may have frequent nursing sessions over a 4- to 5-hour period followed by a 4- to 5- hour sleep
- ☐ Baby wakes more frequently to nurse at night compared to daytime, during the early days
- ☐ Baby nurses better during quiet alert state
- ☐ Baby learns to nurse more effectively when kept skin-to-skin with mom
- ☐ When feeding cues are observed, place baby skin-to-skin with mom and offer breast
- ☐ Avoid pacifier unless requested by mom. Pacifiers are associated with masked feeding cues, fewer breastfeeding sessions per day, lower breastmilk intake, and shorter breastfeeding duration
- ☐ Rooming-in associated with shorter time to effective latch, increased milk supply, and longer breastfeeding duration

Signs of milk transfer:
- ☐ Mom has contractions
- ☐ Mom is thirsty
- ☐ Mom gets drowsy
- ☐ Baby switches from non nutritive suck to long "suck/swallows"
- ☐ Baby has one or more wet diapers and one or more stools during the first 24 hours
- ☐ Baby has two or more wet diapers and two or more stools during the second 24 hours
- ☐ Baby has three or more wet diapers and two or more stools during the third 24 hours
- ☐ Baby has four or more wet diapers and two or more stools during the fourth 24 hours

Exclusive breastfeeding in the early postpartum period is associated with:
- ☐ Shorter time to effective latch
- ☐ Greater milk supply and longer breastfeeding duration
- ☐ Decreased exposure to foreign proteins

The American Academy of Pediatrics (AAP) recommends exclusive breastfeeding for about 6 months, with the gradual introduction of iron-rich solid foods combined with breastmilk during the second half of the first year. The AAP recommends that breastfeeding continue for at least 12 months and, thereafter, for as long as mutually desired.

If there is a compelling clinical indication for supplementation, quantity should mimic the average intake of a breastfed baby:

Age in Hours	Amount/Feed	24-Hour Total*
<24	4–5 cc	1 oz
<48	15–20 cc	3–4 oz
<72	30 cc	8 oz
<96	60 cc	16 oz

*Based on 8 feedings/day

Figure 5-25   Breastfeeding Decision Tree and Checklist For use with normal newborns of more than 37 weeks gestational age. *(continued)*

Source: © Presbyterian Hospital of Dallas, 2003. Used with permission.

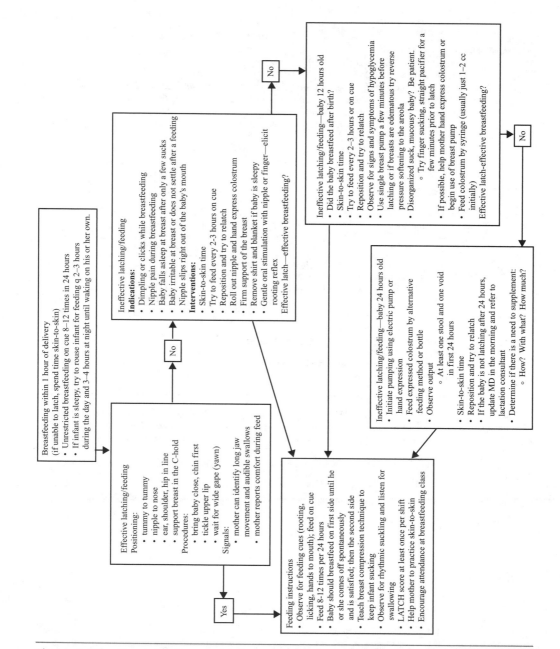

Figure 5-26 Breastfeeding Guidelines for the First 24 Hours Through Discharge for a Healthy 37+ Week Infant

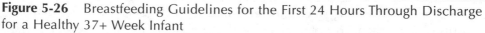

Source: Developed by Joy Hughes, RN, IBCLC; Teresa Shannon, BSN, IBCLC; and Martha McCarty, MD. Used with the permission of Winchester Hospital, Winchester, MA.

Figure 5-27   Breastfeeding Flowchart

Source: Eliott Hospital, Manchester, NH. Used with permission.

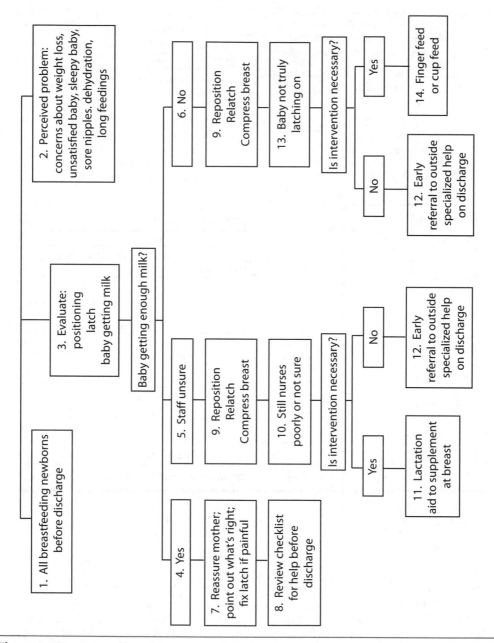

Figure 5-28   Immediate-Postpartum Decision Tree

Source: Adapted by Jeannette Crenshaw for the Lamaze International Breastfeeding Support Specialist Training Program from: Newman J. Decision tree and postpartum management for preventing dehydration in the breastfed baby. *J Hum Lact.* 1996;12:129–135. Used with permission.

- Hepatic breakdown of the stored glycogen is triggered within minutes of the umbilical cord being cut by a surge in glucoregulatory hormones:
  - Increased epinephrine
  - Increased insulin
  - Increased norepinephrine
  - Increased catecholamines
  - Increased glucagon
  - Increased corticosteroids
  - Net effect is mobilization of glycogen and fatty acids
- Liver glycogen stores are 90% depleted by 3 hours and gone by 12 hours (Hagedorn & Gardner, 1999).
- Activities that maintain glucose homeostasis are collectively called counterregulation and consist of
  - Glycogenolysis—the mobilization and release of glycogen from body stores to form glucose
  - Gluconeogenesis—the production of glucose by the liver and kidneys from noncarbohydrate substrates such as fatty acids and amino acids
    - Rate of glucose production is 4–6 mg/kg/min.
    - 3.7 mg/kg/min are needed to meet the energy requirements of the brain.
    - Approximately 70% of energy requirement is provided by glucose oxidation; the rest is provided by alternative fuels.
- Production of alternative brain fuels such as ketone bodies and lactate.
  - The lowest blood glucose values typically occur between 1 and 2 hours after birth (World Health Organization, 1997).
  - After 12 hours the infant depends on glucose made from milk components (20–50%) and gluconeogenesis to maintain blood glucose (galactose, amino acids, glycerol, lactate) as well as free fatty acids from fat stores and milk.
  - Sixteen percent of infant's body weight is fat.
  - Breastmilk is more ketogenic (promotes production of ketones as an alternate brain fuel) than formula.
  - Breastfed infants produce ketones as an adaptive mechanism. This may explain the healthy breastfed newborn with relatively low blood sugar who remains asymptomatic.

A number of conditions or situations that put an infant at risk for hypoglycemia are as follows:

Preterm (AGA)	Discordant twin	Postmaturity
Preterm (SGA)	LGA	Hyperinsulinemia
Full term (SGA)	Erythroblastosis fetalis	Endocrine disorders
Asphyxia	Polycythemia	Inborn errors of metabolism
Cold stress	Microphallus or midline defect	Diabetic mother
Congestive heart failure	Respiratory distress	Maternal toxemia
Sepsis	Maternal glucose IV	Intrapartum fever (Depuy et al., 2009)
Rh disease	Maternal epidural	

Schaefer-Graf et al. (2002) studied risk factors for hypoglycemia in large for gestational age newborns of nondiabetic mothers. The antenatal 1-hour glucose test given during pregnancy was shown to be predictive of hypoglycemia in the newborn. An incremental risk of newborn hypoglycemia was seen with increasing 1-hour oral glucose tolerance test values with hypoglycemia rates of 2.5%, 9.3%, 22.0%, and 50% that were associated with maternal 1-hour glucose values of <120, 120–179, 180–239, and ≥240 mg/dL, respectively. Infants of mothers with high values may benefit from increased vigilance and placement in an at-risk category.

Signs and symptoms of hypoglycemia are subtle, nonspecific, and variable (Table 5-9). Jitteriness is a very common and usually benign finding in otherwise healthy full-term infants (D'Harlingue & Durand, 1993). In a study of 102 infants described as jittery, sucking on the clinician's finger stopped the jitteriness in 80% of infants. Of the other infants whose jitteriness did not stop, five were hypoglycemic and the rest were hypocalcemic (Linder et al., 1989). Nicholl (2003) recommended that if an infant appears jittery, first allow the infant to suck on a finger. The infant could also be put to breast to see if sucking would reduce the jitteriness. If the jitteriness remains, blood glucose and calcium should be measured, with blood glucose concentrations less than 1.5 mmol/L (<27 mg/dL) being addressed immediately.

Problems With Glucose-Level Measurements

Whole blood glucose-level measurements are generally 10–15% lower than the corresponding plasma values. The normal blood glucose range for newborns during the first week is 27–108 mg/dL (1.5–6 mmol/L). The optimal method for measuring plasma glucose is the hexokinase method performed in a laboratory, but this method is often too slow for timely treatment. Therefore "point of care" devices are often used for measuring whole blood glucose concentration in the newborn nursery or neonatal intensive care units. Point of care glucose monitoring systems need to be accurate, precise, and versatile (Sirkin et al., 2002). Reagent strips and bedside machines will, on average, wrongly identify hypoglycemia in one of four infants who are, in fact, normoglycemic (World Health Organization, 1997). Low birth weight, low hematocrit, and parenteral feeding decrease the accuracy of point of care devices (Bellini et al., 2007). Anemia falsely raises and polycythemia falsely depresses glucometer readings. Most current point of care glucometers are sufficient only for initial screening, and their values need to be confirmed with laboratory measurements and clinical assessment of the infant (Ho et al., 2004) (Box 5-5). Future improvements on glucose monitoring include subcutaneous microdialysis for long-term monitoring in the neonatal intensive care unit (Baumeister et al., 2001) and near infrared spectroscopy (Gabriely et al., 1999) as a noninvasive method of glucose screening for all infants.

TABLE 5-9 Signs and Symptoms of Hypoglycemia

Abnormal cry	Vomiting
Apathy	Diaphoresis
Apnea	Tremors
Cardiac arrest	Tachypnea
Seizures	Exaggerated reflexes
Cyanosis	Irritability
Congestive heart failure	Irregular breathing
Abnormal eye movements	Temperature instability
Hypothermia	Vasomotor instability (pallor)
Hypotonia	Poor suck
Jitteriness	Refusal to feed
Lethargy	

BOX 5-5   Glucose Screening Techniques and Equipment

Sampling techniques and their effect on glucose values when using bedside screening tools:

- Once in the sample tube, red blood cells continue to metabolize glucose.

- Bedside tools measure whole blood glucose concentrations, which can be 15% lower than plasma concentrations (which is where blood glucose is measured in a laboratory).

- Blood samples that are allowed to sit at room temperature for long periods of time may result in a glucose concentration drop of 18 mg/dL per hour.

- To avoid sampling errors, blood samples should be transported quickly to the laboratory, put on ice, or placed in a tube containing a glycolytic inhibitor.

- The infant's heel should be warmed to prevent venous stasis in heelstick samples that can lead to falsely low glucose values.

Screening Equipment

- Bedside or "point-of-care" glucose screening devices are commonly used as a rapid screening tool for neonatal hypoglycemia.

- One class of these devices is photometers that rely on reflectance-based technology to read reagent strips.

- The Dextrostix reagent strips were commonly used for many years to screen for neonatal hypoglycemia, despite the fact that this product was never intended to be used on neonates as stated on the package insert and that the results were inaccurate below 50 mg/dL. They were removed from the market in 1997.

- Meloy et al., in a study on the Accu-Check III reflectance meter, documented that the machine could correctly identify neonatal hypoglycemia only 76% of the time.

- More accurate and reliable equipment is available that utilizes electrochemical techniques or quantitative analysis, such as glucose oxidase meters.

- Even with reliable bedside screening devices, operational threshold values should be validated by laboratory analysis.

Sources: Cornblath M, Ichord R. Hypoglycemia in the neonate. *Semin Perinatol.* 2000;24:136–149; Cowett R. Neonatal hypoglycemia: a little goes a long way [editorial]. *J Pediatr.* 1999;134:389–391; Meloy L, Miller G, Chandrasekaran M, et al. Accuracy of glucose reflectance testing for detecting hypoglycemia in term newborns. *Clin Pediatr.* 1999;38:717–724; National Association of Neonatal Nurses. Neonatal Hypoglycemia Guidelines for Practice. Neonatal Netw, Petaluma, CA; 1994; Noerr B. State of the science: neonatal hypoglycemia. *Adv Neonatal Care.* 2001;1:4–21; Thomas C, Critchley L, Davies M. Determining the best method for first-line assessment of neonatal blood glucose levels. *J Paediatr Child Health.* 2000;36:343–348.

There are a number of considerations when interpreting glucose measurements and choosing a course of action:

- Chemical reagent strips such as Dextrostix were not designed for use with a neonate but for use with adult diabetics.

- These methods usually underestimate blood glucose by ±5–15 mg/dL, especially in the lower ranges.

- Laboratory follow-up and confirmation of glucose levels are necessary before treatment.

- Hematocrit should be considered because decreased glucose readings occur with a high hematocrit.

- Use of maternal glucose intravenously (seen in older studies) contributed to the risk of hypoglycemia in the infant.

- Repeated heelsticks/venipunctures increase stress hormone response from pain and decrease blood glucose levels.

- Squeezing the heel causes hemolysis, which interferes with the assay, producing falsely low values (blood samples must be free flowing).

Diwakar and Sasidhar (2002) demonstrated that term breastfed infants have their own distinct plasma glucose levels, which tend to show little significant variation between 3 and 72 hours of age. Prelacteal feeds were unnecessary, and satisfactory glucose levels were maintained even when infants remained unfed for up to 6 hours of age. Blood glucose concentrations tend to be lower during the first 24 hours. However, Hoseth et al. (2000) reported that with frequent effective breastfeeding, normal, healthy, full-term infants with no risk factors, who showed the lowest blood sugar levels at 1 hour of age, 1.4 mmol/L (25.2 mg/dL) to 1.9 mmol/L (28.7 mg/dL), developed no clinical signs of hypoglycemia. Defining hypoglycemia as a specific number does not take into account the multiple variables affecting blood glucose levels in the newborn. If a number such as 40 mg/dL were chosen as the cutoff point for treatment, this value could produce as much as a 20% incidence of diagnosis of hypoglycemia in full-term infants (Sexon, 1984).

Rather than a specific number, the concept of operational thresholds has been suggested to refine diagnosis and better handle glycemic changes in the newborn. Operational thresholds (i.e., blood glucose levels at which clinical interventions should be considered) have been delineated by Cornblath et al. (2000). These threshold values described for surveillance and intervention are different and should be separated from the targeted therapeutic values, which should be in the range of 72–90 mg/dL (4–5 mmol/L) (Kalhan & Peter-Wohl, 2000). They delineate a range of blood glucose values based on parameters that account for the status and age of the infant (Box 5-6).

Term Infant

- Healthy full-term infants from normal pregnancy and delivery and who have no clinical signs do not require routine monitoring of glucose concentrations (Eidelman, 2001).

Breastfed Term Infant

- These infants tend to have lower concentrations of blood glucose than formula-fed infants but higher concentrations of ketone bodies.
- The breastfed infants who lose the most weight have the highest ketone bodies concentration.
- Provision of alternative fuels is a normal adaptive response to low nutrient intake during the establishment of breastfeeding.
- Breastfed infants may well tolerate lower plasma glucose levels without any significant clinical manifestation or sequelae.

Infant With Abnormal Clinical Signs

Symptomatic infant

- Plasma glucose should be measured
- If the value is less than 45 mg/dL (2.5 mmol/L), clinical intervention should be started.

At-risk infants

- At-risk infants should be screened before any symptoms manifest (Wight, 2006).
- Routine measurements should occur as soon as possible after birth, either on admission to the unit or within 30–60 minutes after birth.
- Screening should occur every 30 minutes for infants being treated for hypoglycemia and before feeding or any time there are abnormal signs.
- Plasma glucose of less than 36 mg/dL (2.0 mmol/L) requires close surveillance.

BOX 5-6 Neonatal Hypoglycemia and Operational Thresholds for Clinical Intervention

Age	Threshold Glucose Infant Parameters	Postbirth Values for Intervention
Asymptomatic		
Full or near term (34–37 weeks)	1st 24 hours	<30–35 mg/dL
Healthy	After 24 hours	<40–50 mg/dL
Full enteral feedings		
No risk factors		
Ill infant		
Low birth weight	1st 24 hours	<45–50 mg/dL
Preterm	After 24 hours	<40–50 mg/dL
Sepsis		
Asphyxia		
RDS		
Symptomatic infant		
Signs of hypoglycemia	Any age	<45 mg/dL
Any gestational age		
At-risk infant		
Infant of diabetic mother	Any age	<36 mg/dL
Sepsis		
Asphyxia		
SGA		
Hyperinsulin		
Endocrine disorders		
Metabolic disorders		
Infants with glucose levels	Any age close monitoring	IV glucose therapy and <20–25 mg/dL

Sources: Adapted from Noerr B. State of the science: neonatal hypoglycemia. *Adv Neonatal Care.* 2001;1:4–21; Cornblath M, Ichord R. Hypoglycemia in the neonate. *Semin Perinatol.* 2000;24: 136–149.

- Intervention is required if plasma glucose remains below this level, if the level does not increase after a feed, or if abnormal clinical signs develop.
- At very low glucose concentrations, less than 20–25 mg/dL (1.1–1.4 mmol/L), IV glucose infusion should aim to raise levels above 45 mg/dL (2.5 mmol/L).
- The therapeutic objective of 45 mg/dL is different from the threshold for intervention—36 mg/dL (2.0 mmol/L).

Breastfeeding Management: Reducing the Likelihood of Hypoglycemia

Breastfeeding protocols and caretaking activities during the hours after delivery should be designed to proactively reduce the likelihood of inducing hypoglycemia. Chertok et al. (2009) studied the effects of breastfeeding immediately after delivery compared with later initiation of breastfeeding on neonatal glucose levels of term infants born to mothers with gestational diabetes. The study also compared the glycemic levels of infants who breastfed with those who received formula for their first feed. The results showed that infants who were breastfed right after delivery had a significantly lower rate of borderline hypoglycemia than those not breastfed in the early minutes after birth. Infants breastfed immediately after birth had significantly higher mean blood glucose levels compared to infants who were not breastfed early. Breastfed infants additionally had a significantly higher mean blood glucose level compared to those who were fed formula for their first feed. Early breastfeeding when the infant is swallowing colostrum helps facilitate glycemic stability in infants, especially in those born to diabetic mothers. The clinician is well advised to see that effective breastfeeding takes places as soon as possible after delivery and ensure that the infant is swallowing colostrum at this time. Prevention activities also include the following:

- Breastfeed frequently, on cue, before sustained crying occurs, and avoid long intervals between feedings.
- Infants separated from their mothers have lower body temperatures, cry more, and have decreased blood glucose levels (Christensson et al., 1992; Durand et al., 1997). Christensson et al. (1992) reported that newborn infants separated from their mothers had blood sugar levels that were 10 mg/dL lower than infants kept in skin-to-skin contact at 90 minutes after birth. Environmental stress, such as hypothermia, can increase the energy demands of a newborn, which could exceed the infant's capacity to generate energy

substrate (Kaplan & Eidelman, 1985). Walters et al. (2007) demonstrated that healthy term infants placed skin-to-skin within 1 minute of birth had temperatures that rose and blood glucose levels in a satisfactory range (43–85 mg/dL), even in infants who had not fed before the study's glucose measurement at 60 minutes after birth (43–118 mg/dL).

- Keep the infant in skin-to-skin contact with the mother during the early hours after birth. Skin-to-skin care heats the infant's entire body (peripheral and trunk) rather than just the trunk which occurs under a radiant warmer (Christidis et al., 2003). This avoids the possibility of chilling during the early hours as does delaying the infant bath.
  - Keep the mother and infant together (even at night).
  - Do not allow the infant to cry.
  - Immediately respond to any cries.
- There is a normal dip in blood glucose in the first 1 to 4 hours after birth.
  - Avoid giving sugar water by mouth, because it is metabolized rapidly, often before the infant can mount effective counterregulatory activities. This may cause rebound hypoglycemia.
  - Avoid testing blood sugar during this time with reagent strips (in asymptomatic, low-risk infants).
  - Provide unlimited access to the breast and ensure colostrum/milk transfer.
- Feed expressed colostrum if the infant is unable to latch or feeds poorly. Infants with risk factors for hypoglycemia should be fed frequently.
  - The protein and fat in colostrum provide substrates for gluconeogenesis.
  - Colostrum and breastmilk enhance ketogenesis.
  - Colostrum increases gut motility and gastric emptying time, causing rapid absorption of nutrients.
  - If the infant is unable to latch or effectively transfer colostrum, have the mother hand express colostrum into a spoon and spoon-feed it to the infant (using a pump often results in little to no colostrum being retrievable to feed to the infant, because it sticks to the sides of the bottle).

Consider using an evidence-based hypoglycemia protocol to protect breastfeeding and appropriately manage hypoglycemia in the breastfed infant. The Academy of Breastfeeding Medicine developed a clinical protocol to use as a guideline for obtaining blood glucose levels in neonates who are at risk for developing hypoglycemia and to delineate appropriate interventions (Wight et al.,

2006). The Academy of Breastfeeding Medicine's clinical management is based on four basic principles:

1. Monitoring those infants at highest risk

2. Confirming that plasma glucose concentration is low and indeed responsible for the clinical manifestations present

3. Demonstrating that the symptoms have responded after glucose therapy with restoration of the blood glucose to normoglycemic levels

4. Observing and carefully documenting all of the above

Summary: The Design in Nature

Individual infants and their unique circumstances can present a challenge to breastfeeding that many mothers may not have anticipated. Birth trauma is not limited to the infant. Up to 34% of mothers have reported experiencing a traumatic delivery. The impact of this trauma can lead mothers down two very different breastfeeding paths. Some mothers are determined to persevere with breastfeeding to make up for a devastating childbirth, whereas others meet impediments to breastfeeding that cause sufficient distress for them to abandon breastfeeding attempts (Beck & Watson, 2008).

Clinicians may need to use their years of experience and tap into their knowledge base to initiate and preserve breastfeeding in difficult situations. Nature has programmed infants to be anatomically, physiologically, and metabolically competent to feed at the breast and consume mother's milk, but anatomy, perinatal events, and unforeseen circumstances may interfere with this process. Infants were born to be breastfed, but sometimes nature presents a different path that requires carefully selected interventions to reach the goal of an infant at the breast or breastmilk being provided to the infant.

References

Abadie, V., Andre, A., Zaouche, A., et al. (2001). Early feeding resistance: A possible consequence of neonatal oro-oesophageal dyskinesia. *Acta Paediatr., 90,* 738–745.

Abdel-Latif, M. E., Pinner, J., Clews, S., Cooke, F., Lui, K., & Oei, J. (2006). Effects of breast milk on the severity and outcome of neonatal abstinence syndrome among infants of drug-dependent mothers. *Pediatrics, 117,* e1163–e1169.

Als, H. (1995). *Manual for the naturalistic observation of newborn behavior, Newborn Individualized Developmental Care and Assessment Program (NIDCAP).* Boston: Harvard Medical School.

Als, H., Tronick, E., Adamson, L., & Brazelton, T. B. (1976). The behavior of the full-term but underweight newborn infant. *Dev Med Child Neurol., 18,* 590–602.

American Academy of Pediatrics, Committee on the Fetus and Newborn. (1993). Routine evaluation of blood pressure, hematocrit, and glucose in newborns. *Pediatrics, 92,* 474–476.

Anderson, G. C. (1991). Current knowledge about skin-to-skin (kangaroo) care for preterm infants. *J Perinatol., 11,* 216–226.

Anderson, M. E., Johnson, D. C., & Batal, H. A. (2005). Sudden infant death syndrome and prenatal maternal smoking: Rising attributed risk in the Back to Sleep era. *MBC Medicine, 3,* 4.

Auerbach, K. G. (1990). The effect of nipple shields on maternal milk volume. *JOGNN, 19,* 419–427.

Ayers, A. J. (1977). *Sensory integration and learning disorders.* Los Angeles: Western Psychological Services.

Babic, S. H., Kokol, P., & Stiglic, M. M. (1999). Fuzzy decision trees in the support of breastfeeding. Presented at the 12th IEEE Symposium on Computer Based Medical Systems, June 18–20, Stamford, Connecticut.

Babic, S. H., Sprogar, M., Zorman, M., et al. (1999). Evaluating breastfeeding advantages using decision trees. Presented at the 12th IEEE Symposium on Computer Based Medical Systems, June 18–20, Stamford, Connecticut.

Backas, N. (1998). *Working your way through the reimbursement maze. Medela rental roundup: The Medela messenger.* McHenry, IL: Medela.

Bandman, E. L., & Bandman, B. (1988). *Critical thinking in nursing.* Norwalk, CT: Appleton & Lange.

Barr, R. G., Kramer, M. S., Pless, I. B., et al. (1989). Feeding and temperament as determinants of early infant crying/fussing behavior. *Pediatrics, 84,* 514–521.

Bassett, V. (2001). How one Canadian hospital developed a newborn critical path and documentation tool that supports moms and babies. *AWHONN Lifelines, 5,* 48–54.

Baumeister, F. A. M., Rolinski, B., Busch, R., et al. (2001). Glucose monitoring with long-term subcutaneous microdialysis in neonates. *Pediatrics, 108,* 1187–1192.

Beck, C. T., & Watson, S. (2008). Impact of birth trauma on breastfeeding: A take of two pathways. *Nurs Res., 57,* 228–236.

Begg, E. J., Malpas, T. J., Hackett, L. P., & Ilett, K. F. (2001). Distribution of R- and S-methadone into human milk during multiple, medium to high oral dosing. *Br J Clin Pharmacol., 52,* 681–685.

Bellini, C., Serra, G., Risso, D., Mazzella, M., & Bonioli, E. (2007). Reliability assessment of glucose measurement by HemoCue analyzer in a neonatal intensive care unit. *Clin Chem Lab Med., 45,* 1549–1554.

Bevan, M., Mosley, D., Lobach, K., & Salimano, G. (1984). Factors influencing breastfeeding in an urban WIC program. *J Am Diet Assoc., 84,* 563–567.

Black, L. S. (1993). *Baby-friendly newborn care.* Workshop for Lactation Specialists, Series VIII. Chicago: La Leche League International.

Blair, A., Cadwell, K., Turner-Maffei, C., & Brimdyr, K. (2003). The relationship between positioning, the breastfeeding dynamic, the latching process and pain in breastfeeding mothers with sore nipples. *Breastfeeding Rev., 11,* 5–10.

Bloom, K., Goldbloom, R., Robinson, S., & Stevens, F. II. (1982). Factors affecting breastfeeding. *Acta Paediatr Scand., 300*(Suppl), 9–14.

Bodley, V., & Powers, D. (1996). Long-term nipple shield use—A positive perspective. *J Human Lact., 12,* 301–304.

Bosma, J. F. (1988). Functional anatomy of the upper airway during development. In O. Mathew & G. Sant'Ambrogio (Eds.), *Respiratory function of the upper airway* (pp. 44, 47–86). New York: Marcel Dekker.

Boukydis, C. F. Z., Bigsby, R., & Lester, B. M. (2004). Clinical use of the neonatal intensive care unit network neurobehavioral scale. *Pediatrics, 113,* 679–689.

Brandt, K. A., Andrews, C. M., & Kvale, J. (1998). Mother-infant interaction and breastfeeding outcome 6 weeks after birth. *JOGNN, 27,* 169–174.

Brigham, M. (1996). Mothers' reports of the outcome of nipple shield use. *J Human Lact., 12,* 291–297.

Brussel, C. (2001). Considering craniosacral therapy in difficult situations. *Leaven, 37,* 82–83.

Burns, N., & Grove, S. K. (1993). *The practice of nursing research: Conduct, critique and utilization.* Philadelphia: WB Saunders.

Butte, N. F., Jensen, C. L., Moon, J. K., et al. (1992). Sleep organization and energy expenditure of breast-fed and formula-fed infants. *Pediatr Res., 32,* 514–519.

Cadwell, K. (2007). Latching-on and suckling of the healthy term neonate: Breastfeeding assessment. *J Midwifery Women's Health, 52,* 638–642.

Cadwell, K., & Turner-Maffei, C. (2004). *Case studies in breastfeeding: Problem-solving skills and strategies.* Sudbury, MA: Jones and Bartlett.

Castrucci, B. C., Hoover, K. L., Lim, S., & Maus, K. C. (2006). A comparison of breastfeeding rates in an urban birth cohort among women delivering infants at hospitals that employ and do not employ lactation consultants. *J Public Health Management Pract., 12,* 578–585.

Chertok, I. R., Raz, I., Shoham, I., Haddad, H., & Wiznitzer, A. (2009). Effects of early breastfeeding on neonatal glucose levels of term infants born to women with gestational diabetes. *J Hum Nutr Diet, 22,* 166–169.

Chertok, I. R., Schneider, J., & Blackburn, S. (2006). A pilot study of maternal and term infant outcomes associated with ultrathin nipple shield use. *J Obstet, Gynecol Neonatal Nurs., 35,* 265–272.

Christensson, K., Siles, C., Moreno, L., et al. (1992). Temperature, metabolic adaption and crying in healthy full-term newborns cared for skin-to-skin or in a cot. *Acta Paediatr., 81,* 488–493.

Christidis, I., Zotter, H., Rosegger, H., Engele, H., Kurz, R., & Kerbel, R. (2003). Infrared thermography in newborns: The first hour after birth. *Bynakol Geburtshilfliche Rundsch, 43,* 31–35.

Chute, G. E. (1992). Promoting breastfeeding success: An overview of basic management. *NAACOG's Clinical Issues in Perinatal & Women's Health Nursing: Breastfeeding, 3,* 570–582.

Clum, D., & Primomo, J. (1996). Use of a silicone nipple shield with premature infants. *J Hum Lact., 12,* 287–290.

Cohen, S. M. (1998). Congenital hypotonia is not benign: Early recognition and intervention is the key to recovery. *MCN, 23,* 93–98.

Colson, S. D., de Pooy, L., & Hawdon, J. M. (2003). Biological nurturing increases duration of breastfeeding for a vulnerable cohort. *MIDIRS Midwifery Digest, 13,* 92–97.

Colson, S. D., Meek, J. H., & Hawdon, J. M. (2008). Optimal positions for the release of primitive neonatal reflexes stimulating breastfeeding. *Early Hum Dev., 84,* 441–449.

Cornblath, M., Hawdon, J. M., Williams, A. F., et al. (2000). Controversies regarding definition of neonatal hypoglycemia: Suggested operational thresholds. *Pediatrics, 105,* 1141–1145.

Dahlstrom, A., Ebersjo, C., & Lundell, B. (2004). Nicotine exposure in breastfed infants. *Acta Paediatr., 93,* 810–816.

Dahlstrom, A., Ebersjo, C., & Lundell, B. (2008). Nicotine in breast milk influences heart rate variability. *Acta Paediatr., 97,* 1075–1079.

Danner, S. C., & Cerutti, E. R. (1984). *Nursing your neurologically impaired baby.* Waco, TX: Childbirth Graphics.

DeNicola, M. (1986). One case of nipple shield addiction. *J Hum Lact., 2,* 28–29.

Depuy, A. M., Coassolo, K. M., Som, D. A., & Smulian, J. C. (2009). Neonatal hypoglycemia in term, non-diabetic pregnancies. *Am J Obstet Gynecol., 200,* e45–51.

Desmarais, L., & Browne, S. (1990). *Inadequate weight gain in breastfeeding infants: Assessments and resolutions.* Lactation Consultant Series Unit 8. Garden City Park, NY: Avery.

D'Harlingue, A. E., & Durand, D. J. (1993). Recognition, stabilization and transport of the high-risk newborn. In M. H. Klaus & A. A. Fanaroff (Eds.), *Care of the high risk neonate* (pp. 62–85). Philadelphia: Saunders.

DiFranza, J. R., Aligne, C. A., & Weitzman, M. (2004). Prenatal and postnatal environmental tobacco smoke exposure and children's health. *Pediatrics, 113,* 1007–1015.

DiGirolamo, A. M., Grummer-Strawn, L. M., & Fein, S. B. (2003). Do perceived attitudes of physicians and hospital staff affect breastfeeding decisions? *Birth, 30,* 94–100.

DiGirolamo, A. M., Grummer-Strawn, L. M., & Fein, S. B. (2008). Effect of maternity-care practices on breastfeeding. *Pediatrics, 122*(Suppl 2), S43–S49.

Di Scipio, W., Kaslon, J. K., & Ruben, R. J. (1978). Traumatically acquired conditioned dysphagia in children. *Ann Otol Rhinol Laryngol., 87,* 509–514.

Diwakar, K. K., & Sasidhar, M. V. (2002). Plasma glucose levels in term infants who are appropriate size for gestation and exclusively breastfed. *Arch Dis Child Fetal Neonatal Ed., 87,* F46–F48.

Doucet, S., Soussignan, R., Sagot, P., & Schaal, B. (2007). The "smellscape" of mother's breast: Effects of odor masking and selective unmasking on neonatal arousal, oral, and visual responses. *Dev Psychobiol., 49,* 129–138.

Driscoll, J. W. (1992). Breastfeeding success and failure: Implications for nurses. *NAACOG's Clinical Issues in Perinatal & Women's Health Nursing: Breastfeeding, 3,* 565–569.

Dryden, C., Young, D., Hepburn, M., & Mactier, H. (2009). Maternal methadone use in pregnancy: Factors associated with the development of neonatal abstinence syndrome and implications for healthcare resources. *BJOG, 116,* 665–671.

Durand, R., Hodges, S., LaRock, S., et al. (1997, March/April). The effect of skin-to-skin breastfeeding in the immediate recovery period on newborn thermoregulation and blood glucose values. *Neonatal Intensive Care,* 23–29.

Ebersold, S. L., Murphy, S. D., Paterno, M. T., Sauvager, M. D., & Wright, E. M. (2007). Nurses and breastfeeding: Are you being supportive? *Nurs Womens' Health, 11,* 482–487.

Eidelman, A. I. (2001). Hypoglycemia and the breastfed neonate. *Pediatr Clin North Am., 48,* 377–387.

Elder, M. S. (1970). The effects of temperature and position on the sucking pressure of newborn infants. *Child Dev., 41,* 95–102.

Escott, R. (1989, May). Positioning, attachment and milk transfer. *Breastfeeding Rev.,* 31–36.

Ferber, S. G., & Makhoul, I. R. (2004). The effect of skin-to-skin contact (kangaroo care) shortly after birth on neurobehavioral responses of the term newborn: A randomized controlled trial. *Pediatrics, 113,* 858–865.

Ferreira, E., Carceller, A. M., Agogue, C., et al. Effects of selective serotonin reuptake inhibitors and venlafaxine during pregnancy in term and preterm neonates. *Pediatrics, 119,* 52–59.

Frantz, K. B., & Kalmen, B. A. (1979, December). Breastfeeding works for cesareans too. *RN,* 39–47.

Freudigman, K., & Thoman, E. B. (1994). Ultradian and diurnal cyclicity in the sleep states of newborn infants during the first two postnatal days. *Early Hum Dev., 38,* 67–80.

Freudigman, K. A., & Thoman, E. B. (1998). Infants' earliest sleep/wake organization differs as a function of delivery mode. *Early Hum Dev., 32,* 293–303.

Gabriely, I., Wozniak, R., Mevorach, M., et al. (1999). Transcutaneous glucose measurement using near-infrared spectroscopy during hypoglycemia. *Diabetes Care, 22,* 2026–2032.

Genna, C. W. (2001). Tactile defensiveness and other sensory modulation difficulties. *Leaven, 37,* 51–53.

Genna, C. W. (2008). *Supporting sucking skills in breastfeeding infants.* Sudbury, MA: Jones and Bartlett.

Gewolb, I. H., Fishman, D., Qureshi, M. A., & Voce, F. L. (2004). Coordination of suck-swallow-respiration in infants born to mothers with drug-abuse problems. *Dev Med Child Neurol., 46,* 700–705.

Gill, S. L. (2001). The little things: Perceptions of breastfeeding support. *JOGNN, 30,* 401–409.

Goldade, K., Nichter, M., Nichter, M., Adrian, S., Tesler, L., & Muramoto, M. (2008). Breastfeeding and smoking among low-income women: Results of a longitudinal qualitative study. *Birth, 35,* 230–240.

Goldberg, H., & Nissim, R. (1994). Psychotropic drugs in pregnancy and lactation. *Intl J Psychiatry Med., 2,* 129–149.

Gomez, R. L., Bootzin, R. R., & Nadel, L. (2006). Naps promote abstraction in language-learning infants. *Psychol Sci., 17,* 670–674.

Graffy, J., & Taylor, J. (2005). What information, advice, and support do women want with breastfeeding? *Birth, 32,* 179–186.

Green, C., Martin, C. W., Bassett, K., & Kazanjian, A. (1999). *A systematic review and critical appraisal of the scientific evidence on craniosacral therapy.* British Columbia Office of Health Technology Assessment.

Hagedorn, M. I. E., & Gardner, S. L. (1999). Hypoglycemia in the newborn, part 1: Pathophysiology and nursing management. *Mother and Baby Journal, 4,* 15–21.

Hankins, G. D. V., Clark, S., & Munn, M. B. (2006). Cesarean section on request at 39 weeks: Impact on shoulder dystocia, fetal trauma, neonatal encephalopathy, and intrauterine fetal demise. *Sem Perinatol., 30,* 276–287.

Harris, H. (1994). Remedial co-bathing for breastfeeding difficulties. *Breastfeeding Rev., 2*(10), 465–468.

Healow, L. K., & Hugh, R. S. (2000). Oral aversion in the breastfed neonate. *Breastfeeding Abs., 20,* 3–4.

Hewitt, E. G. (1999). Chiropractic care for infants with dysfunctional nursing: A case series. *J Clin Chiropractic Pediatr., 4,* 241–244.

Hill, P. (1991). The enigma of insufficient milk supply. *MCN, 16,* 312–316.

Hill, P. D., & Aldag, J. C. (1996). Smoking and breastfeeding status. *Res Nurs Health, 19,* 125–132.

Hillervik-Lindquist, C., Hofvander, Y., & Sjolin, S. (1991). Studies on perceived breast milk insufficiency. III. Consequences for breast milk consumption and growth. *Acta Paediatr Scand., 80,* 297–303.

Ho, H. T., Yeung, W. K. Y., & Young, B. W. Y. (2004). Evaluation of "point of care" devices in the measurement of low blood glucose in neonatal practice. *Arch Dis Child Fetal Neonatal Ed.,* F356–F359.

Holtrop, D. P. (2000). Resolution of suckling intolerance in a 6-month-old chiropractic patient. *J Manipulative Physiol Therapy, 23,* 615–618.

Hong, T. M., Callister, L. C., & Schwartz, R. (2003). First-time mothers' views of breastfeeding support from nurses. *MCN, 28,* 10–15.

Hopkinson, J. M., Schanler, R. J., Fraley, J. K., & Garza, C. (1992). Milk production by mothers of premature infants: Influence of cigarette smoking. *Pediatrics, 90,* 934–938.

Horne, R. S. C., Parslow, P. M., Ferens, D., et al. Comparison of evoked arousability in breast and formula fed infants. *Arch Dis Child.,* 22–25.

Hoseth, E., Joergensen, A., Ebbesen, F., & Moeller, M. (2000). Blood glucose levels in a population of healthy, breastfed, term infants of appropriate size for gestational age. *Arch Dis Child Fetal Neonatal Ed., 83,* F117–F119.

Humenick, S. S., Hill, P. D., & Hart, A. M. (1998). Evaluation of a pillow designed to promote breastfeeding. *J Perinat Ed., 7,* 25–31.

Inoue, N., Sakashita, R., & Kamegai, T. (1995). Reduction of masseter muscle activity in bottle-fed infants. *Early Hum Dev., 42,* 185–193.

Jansson, L. M., Choo, R., Velez, M. L., Lowe, R., & Huestis, M. A. (2008). Methadone maintenance and long-term lactation. *Breastfeed Med., 3,* 34–37.

Jansson, L., Velez, M., & Harrow, C. (2004). Methadone maintenance and lactation: A review of the literature and current management guidelines. *J Hum Lact.,* 62–71.

Jean, A. (2001). Brain stem control of swallowing: Neuronal network and cellular mechanisms. *Physiol Rev., 81,* 929–969.

Jonas, W., Johansson, L. M., Nissen, E., Ejdeback, M., Ransjo-Arvidson, A. B., & Uvnas-Moberg, K. (2009). Effects of intrapartum oxytocin administration and epidural analgesia on the concentration of plasma oxytocin and prolactin in response to suckling during the second day postpartum. *Breastfeeding Med., 4.*

Jordan, A. E., Jackson, G. L., Deardorff, D., Shivakumar, G., McIntire, D. D., & Dashe, J. S. (2008). Serotonin reuptake inhibitor use in pregnancy and the neonatal behavioral syndrome. *J Maternal Fetal Neonat Med., 21,* 745–751.

Kalhan, S., & Peter-Wohl, S. (2000). Hypoglycemia: What is it for the neonate? *Am J Perinatol., 17,* 11–18.

Kandall, S. (1995). Treatment options for drug-exposed infants. *NIDA Res Monogr., 149,* 78–99.

Kaplan, M., & Eidelman, A. I. (1985). Improved prognosis in severely hypothermic newborns treated by rapid rewarming. *J Pediatr., 105,* 515–518.

Karl, D. J. (2004). Using principles of newborn behavioral state organization to facilitate breastfeeding. *MCN, 29,* 292–298.

Karl, D. J., Beal, J. A., O'Hare, C. M., & Rissmiller, P. N. (2006). Reconceptualizing the nurse's role in the newborn period as an "attacher." *MCN, 31,* 257–262.

Kelmanson, I. A., Erman, L. V., & Litvina, S. V. (2002). Maternal smoking during pregnancy and behavioural characteristics in 2–4 month-old infants. *Klinische Padiatrie, 214,* 359–364.

King, J. C. (1997). Substance abuse in pregnancy: A bigger problem than you think. *Postgraduate Medicine, 102,* 135–137, 140–145, 149–150.

Kutner, L. (1986). Nipple shield consent form: A teaching aid. *J Hum Lact., 2,* 25–27.

Lattimore, K. A., Donn, S. M., Kaciroti, N., et al. (2005). Selective serotonin reuptake inhibitor (SSRI) use during pregnancy and effects on the fetus and newborn: A meta-analysis. *J Perinatol., 25,* 595–604.

Law, K. L., Stroud, L. R., LaGasse, L. L., et al. Smoking during pregnancy and newborn neurobehavior. *Pediatrics, 111,* 1318–1323.

Lester, B. M., Tronick, E. Z., in collaboration with T. Berry Brazelton. (2004). The neonatal intensive care unit network neurobehavioral scale procedures. *Pediatrics, 113,* 641–667.

Lester, B. M., Tronick, E. Z., LaGasse, L. L., et al. (2002). The Maternal Lifestyle Study (MLS): Effects of substance exposure during pregnancy on neurodevelopmental outcome in 1-month old infants. *Pediatrics, 110,* 1182–1192.

Levrini, L., Merlo, P., & Paracchini, L. (2007). Different geometric patterns of pacifiers compared on the basis of finite element analysis. *J Paediatr Dent., 8,* 173–178.

Linder, N., Maser, A. M., Asli, I., et al. Suckling stimulation test for neonatal tremor. *Arch Dis Child, 64,* 44–46.

Liu, J., Rosenberg, K. D., & Sandoval, A. P. (2006). Breastfeeding duration and perinatal cigarette smoking in a population-based cohort. *Am J Public Health, 96,* 309–314.

Lothian, J. A. (1995). It takes two to breastfeed: The baby's role in successful breastfeeding. *J Nurse Midwifery, 40,* 328–334.

Macfarlane, A. (1975). Olfaction in the development of social preferences in the human neonate. In R. Porter & M. O'Connor (Eds.), *Parent-infant interaction* (pp. 103–113). Ciba Foundation Symposium 33. New York: Elsevier.

Macknin, M. L., Medendorp, S. V., & Maier, M. C. (1989). Infant sleep and bedtime cereal. *Am J Dis Child, 143,* 1066–1068.

Makin, J. W., & Porter, R. H. (1989). Attractiveness of lactating females' breast odors to neonates. *Child Dev., 60,* 803–810.

Mannel, R., & Mannel, R. S. (2006). Staffing for hospital lactation programs: Recommendations from a tertiary care teaching hospital. *J Hum Lact., 22,* 409–417.

Mantha, S., Davies, B., Moyer, A., & Crowe, K. (2008). Providing responsive nursing care to new mothers with high and low confidence. *MCN, 33,* 307–314.

Marchini, G., & Linden, A. (1992). Cholecystokinin, a satiety signal in newborn infants? *J Dev Physiol., 17,* 215–219.

Marchini, G., Simoni, M. R., Bartolini, F., & Linden, A. (1993). The relationship of plasma cholecystokinin levels to different feeding routines in newborn infants. *Early Hum Dev., 35,* 31–35.

Marmet, C., & Shell, E. (2008). Therapeutic positioning for breastfeeding. In C. W. Genna (Ed.), *Supporting sucking skills in breastfeeding infants.* Sudbury, MA: Jones and Bartlett.

Matheson, I., & Rivrud, G. N. (1989). The effect of smoking on lactation and infantile colic. *JAMA, 261,* 42–43.

Matthews, M. K. (1991). Mothers' satisfaction with their neonates' breastfeeding behaviors. *JOGNN, 20,* 49–55.

McDermott, C. M., Lahoste, G. J., Chen, C., Musto, A., Bazan, N. G., & Magee, J. C. (2003). Sleep deprivation causes behavioral, synaptic, and membrane excitability alterations in hippocampal neurons. *J Neurosci., 23,* 9687–9695.

McInnes, R. J., & Chambers, J. A. (2008). Supporting breastfeeding mothers: Qualitative synthesis. *J Adv Nurs., 62,* 407–427.

McKenna, J. J., Mosko, S., Dungy, C., & McAninch, J. (1990). Sleep and arousal patterns of co-sleeping human mother/infant pairs: A preliminary physiological study with implications for the study of sudden infant death syndrome (SIDS). *Am J Phys Anthropol., 83,* 331–347.

Medoff-Cooper, B. (1991). Changes in nutritive sucking patterns with increasing gestational age. *Nurs Res., 40,* 245–247.

Medoff-Cooper, B., Weininger, S., & Zukowsky, K. (1989). Neonatal sucking as a clinical assessment tool: Preliminary findings. *Nurs Res., 38,* 162–165.

Meier, P. P., Brown, L. P., Hurst, N. M., et al. (2000). Nipple shields for preterm infants: Effect on milk transfer and duration of breastfeeding. *J Hum Lact., 16,* 106–113.

Mennella, J. A., & Beauchamp, G. K. (1998). Smoking and the flavor of breast milk. *N Engl J Med., 339,* 1559–1560.

Mennella, J. A., Yourshaw, L. M., & Morgan, L. K. (2007). Breastfeeding and smoking: Short-term effects on infant feeding and sleep. *Pediatrics, 120,* 497–502.

Meyer, K., & Anderson, G. C. (1999). Using kangaroo care in a clinical setting with full term infants having breastfeeding difficulties. *MCN, 24,* 190–192.

Michelsson, K., Christensson, K., Rothganger, H., et al. (1996). Crying in separated and non-separated newborns: Sound spectrographic analysis. *Acta Paediatr., 85,* 471–475.

Millard, A. V. (1990). The place of the clock in pediatric advice: Rationales, cultural themes, and impediments to breastfeeding. *Soc Sci Med., 31,* 211–221.

Minchin, M. (1998). *Breastfeeding matters* (4th ed., pp. 84–89, 142–147). St. Kilda, Victoria, Canada: Alma.

Mizuno, K., Fujimaki, K., & Sawada, M. (2004). Sucking behavior at breast during the early newborn period affects later breastfeeding rate and duration of breastfeeding. *Pediatr Int., 46,* 15–20.

Mizuno, K., Nishida, Y., Mizuno, N., Taki, M., Murase, M., & Itabashi, K. (2008). The important role of deep attachment in the uniform drainage of breast milk from mammary lobe. *Acta Paediatr., 97,* 1200–1204.

Mizuno, K., & Ueda, A. (2004). Antenatal olfactory learning influences infant feeding. *Early Hum Dev., 76,* 83–90.

Mobbs, E. G. (1989, May). Human imprinting and breastfeeding—Are the textbooks deficient? *Breastfeeding Review,* 39–41.

Morton, J. A. (1992). Ineffective suckling: A possible consequence of obstructive positioning. *J Hum Lact., 8,* 83–85.

Mozingo, J. N., Davis, M. W., Droppleman, P. G., & Merideth, A. (2000). "It wasn't working": Women's experiences with short-term breastfeeding. *MCN, 25,* 120–126.

Neifert, M. R., Lawrence, R., & Seacat, J. (1995). Nipple confusion: Toward a formal definition. *J Pediatr., 126,* S125–S129.

Nicholl, R. (2003). What is the normal range of blood glucose concentrations for healthy term newborns? *Arch Dis Child, 88,* 238–239.

Nichols, F. H., & Zwelling, E. (1997). *Maternal-newborn nursing: Theory and practice.* Philadelphia: Saunders.

Nowak, A. J., Smith, W. L., & Erenberg, A. (1995). Imaging evaluation of breast-feeding and bottle-feeding systems. *J Pediatr., 126,* S130–S134.

Nyqvist, K. H. (2001). The development of preterm infants' milk intake during breastfeeding: Influence of gestational age. *J Neonat Nurs., 7,* 48–52.

Ozkan, H., Tuzan, F., Kumral, A., Yesilirmak, D., & Duman, N. (2008). Increased sleep tendency in jaundiced infants: Role of endogenous CO. *Medical Hypotheses, 71,* 879–880.

Pinilla, T., & Birch, L. L. (1993). Help me make it through the night: Behavioral entrainment of breast-fed infants' sleep patterns. *Pediatrics, 91,* 436–444.

Porter, R. H., Makin, J. W., Davis, L. B., & Christensen, K. M. (1991). An assessment of the salient olfactory environment of formula-fed infants. *Physiol Behav., 50,* 907–911.

Porter, R. H., & Winberg, J. (1999). Unique salience of maternal breast odors for newborn infants. *Neurosci Biobehav Rev., 23,* 439–449.

Powers, D., & Tapia, V. B. (2004). Women's experiences using a nipple shield. *J Hum Lact., 20,* 327–334.

Prasad, A. N., & Prasad, C. (2003). The floppy infant: Contribution of genetic and metabolic disorders. *Brain and Development, 25,* 457–476.

Ransjo-Arvidson, A. B., Matthiesen, A. S., Lilja, G., et al. Maternal analgesia during labor disturbs newborn behavior: Effects on breastfeeding, temperature, and crying. *Birth, 28,* 5–12.

Reisman, J. (2002). Sensory processing disorders. *Minnesota Medicine, 85.* Retrieved September 4, 2005, from www.mmaonline.net/publications/MNMed2002/November/Reisman.html

Righard, L., & Alade, M. O. (1990). Effect of delivery room routines on success of first breast-feed. *Lancet, 336,* 1105–1107.

Roffwarg, H. P., Muzio, J. N., & Dement, W. C. (1966). Ontogenetic development of the human sleep-dream cycle. *Science, 152,* 604–619.

Ruchala, P. L. (2000). Teaching new mothers: Priorities of nurses and postpartum women. *J Obstet Gynecol Neonat Nurs., 29,* 265–273.

Sadeh, A., Dark, I., & Vohr, B. R. (1996). Newborns' sleep-wake patterns: The role of maternal, delivery and infant factors. *Early Hum Dev., 44,* 113–126.

Schaefer-Graf, U. M., Rossi, R., Buhrer, C., et al. (2002). Rate and risk factors of hypoglycemia in large-for-gestational-age newborn infants of nondiabetic mothers. *Am J Obstet Gynecol., 187,* 913–917.

Schechtman, V. L., Harper, R. M., Wilson, A. J., & Southall, D. P. (1992). Sleep state organization in normal infants and victims of the sudden infant death syndrome. *Pediatrics, 89,* 865–870.

Sexon, W. R. (1984). Incidence of neonatal hypoglycemia: A matter of definition. *J Pediatr., 105,* 149–150.

Shenassa, E. D., & Brown M.-J. (2004). Maternal smoking and infantile gastrointestinal dysregulation. *Pediatrics, 114,* e497–e505.

Sherer, D. M., Metlay, L. A., & Woods, J. R. (1995). Lack of mandibular movement manifested by absent fetal swallowing: A possible factor in the pathogenesis of micrognathia. *Am J Perinatol., 12,* 30–33.

Shrago, L., & Bocar, D. (1990). The infant's contribution to breastfeeding. *JOGNN, 19,* 209–215.

Sirkin, A., Jalloh, T., & Lee, L. (2002). Selecting an accurate point-of-care testing system: Clinical and technical issues and implications in neonatal blood glucose monitoring. *J Spec Pediatr Nurs., 7,* 104–112.

Sjolin, S., Hofvander, Y., & Hillervik, C. (1977). Factors related to early termination of breastfeeding. A retrospective study in Sweden. *Acta Paediatr Scand., 66,* 505–511.

Sjolin, S., Hofvander, Y., & Hillervik, C. (1979). A prospective study of individual courses of breastfeeding. *Acta Paediatr Scand., 68,* 521–529.

Smith, L. (2004). Physics, forces, and mechanical effects of birth on breastfeeding. In M. Kroeger (Ed.), *Impact of birthing practices on breastfeeding: Protecting the mother and baby continuum* (pp. 119–145). Sudbury, MA: Jones and Bartlett.

Stephens, J., & Kotowski, J. (1994). The extrusion reflex—Its relevance to early breastfeeding. *Breastfeeding Review, 2,* 418–421.

Stroud, L. R., Paster, R. L., Papandonatos, G. D., et al. (2009). Maternal smoking during pregnancy and newborn behavior: Effects at 10 to 27 days. *J Pediatr., 154,* 10–16.

Sweet, D. G., Hadden, D., & Halliday, H. L. (1999). The effect of early feeding on the neonatal blood glucose level at 1 hour of age. *Early Hum Dev., 55,* 63–66.

Taveras, E. M., Li, R., Grummer-Strawn, L., et al. (2004). Opinions and practices of clinicians associated with continuation of exclusive breastfeeding. *Pediatrics, 113,* e283–e290. Retrieved September 4, 2005, from www.pediatrics.org/cgi/content/full/113/4/e283

Thompson, C. E. (2002). Benign congenital hypotonia is not a diagnosis. *Letters in Dev Med Child Neurol., 44,* 283–284.

Turney, J. (2002). Tackling birth trauma with cranio-sacral therapy. *Practicing Midwife, 5,* 17–19.

Upledger, J. E. (2003a). Applications of craniosacral therapy in newborns and infants, Part I. Massage Today.com, May. Retrieved September 4, 2005, from www.massagetoday.com/archives/2003/05/08.html

Upledger, J. E. (2003b). Applications of craniosacral therapy in newborns and infants, Part II. Massage Today.com, June. Retrieved September 4, 2005, from www.massagetoday.com/archives/2003/06/13.html

Uvnas-Moberg, K., Marchini, G., & Winberg, J. (1993). Plasma cholecystokinin concentrations after breastfeeding in healthy 4 day old infants. *Arch Dis Child., 68,* 46–48.

Uvnas-Moberg, K., Widstrom, A. M., Marchini, G., & Winberg, J. (1987). Release of GI hormones in mother and infant by sensory stimulation. *Acta Paediatr Scand., 76,* 851–860.

Vallone, S. (2004). Chiropractic evaluation and treatment of musculoskeletal dysfunction in infants demonstrating difficulty breastfeeding. *Pediatrics, 6, J Clin Chiropractic Pediatr.,* 349–361.

Varendi, H., & Porter, R. H. (2001). Breast odour as the only maternal stimulus elicits crawling towards the odour source. *Acta Paediatr., 90,* 372–375.

Varendi, H., Porter, R. H., & Winberg, J. (1994). Does the newborn baby find the nipple by smell? *Lancet, 344,* 989–990.

Verronen, P. (1982). Reasons for giving up and transient lactational crises. *Acta Paediatr Scand., 71,* 447–450.

Volmanen, P., Valanne, F., & Alahuhta, S. (2004). Breastfeeding problems after epidural analgesia for labour: A retrospective cohort study of pain, obstetrical procedures and breastfeeding practices. *Int J Obstet Anesthesia, 13,* 25–29.

Walker, M. (1997). Breastfeeding the sleepy baby. *J Hum Lact., 13,* 151–153.

Wall, V., & Glass, R. (2006). Mandibular asymmetry and breastfeeding problems: Experience from 11 cases. *J Hum Lact., 22,* 328–334.

Walters, M. W., Boggs, K. M., Ludington-Hoe, S., Price, K. M., & Morrison, B. (2007). Kangaroo care at birth for full term infants: A pilot study. *MCN, 32,* 375–381.

Weiss-Salinas, D., & Williams, N. (2001). Sensory defensiveness: A theory of its effect on breastfeeding. *J Hum Lact., 17,* 145–151.

Wescott, N. (2004). The use of cranial osteopathy in the treatment of infants with breastfeeding problems or sucking dysfunction. *Australian J Holist Nurs., 11,* 25–32.

Widstrom, A.-M., Ransjo-Arvidson, A. B., Christensson, K., et al. (1987). Gastric suction in healthy newborn infants. *Acta Paediatr Scand., 76,* 566–572.

Widstrom, A.-M., & Thringstrom-Paulsson, J. (1993). The position of the tongue during rooting reflexes elicited in newborn infants before the first suckle. *Acta Paediatr., 82,* 281–283.

Wiessinger, D. (1998). A breastfeeding teaching tool using a sandwich analogy for latch-on. *J Hum Lact.,* *14,* 51–56.

Wight, N., Marinelli, K. A., & ABM Protocol Committee. (2006). ABM clinical protocol #1: Guidelines for glucose monitoring and treatment of hypoglycemia in breastfed neonates. *Breastfeeding Med., 3,* 178–184.

Wight, N. E. (2003). Breastfeeding the borderline (near-term) preterm infant. *Pediatric Annals, 32,* 329–336.

Wight, N. E. (2006). Hypoglycemia in breastfed neonates. *Breastfeeding Med., 1,* 253–262.

Wilson-Clay, B. (1996). Clinical use of silicone nipple shields. *J Hum Lact., 12,* 279–285.

Wilson-Clay, B. (2003). Nipple shields in clinical practice: A review. *Breastfeeding Abstracts, 22,* 11–12.

Wilson-Clay, B., & Hoover, K. (2002). *The breastfeeding atlas* (2nd ed.). Austin, TX: LactNews Press.

Wolf, L. S., & Glass, R. P. (1992). *Feeding and swallowing disorders of infancy: Assessment and management.* Tucson, AZ: Therapy Skill Builders.

Woodworth, M., & Frank, E. (1996). Transitioning to the breast at six weeks: Use of a nipple shield. *J Hum Lact., 12,* 305–307.

World Health Organization. (1997). *Hypoglycemia of the newborn: Review of the literature* (pp. 30–31). Geneva: WHO.

Zander, K. (1991). Care maps: The core of cost/quality care. *New Definition, 6,* 9–11.

Zander, K. (1992). Quantifying, managing, and improving quality: How CareMaps link CQI to the patient. *New Definition, 7,* 1–3.

Zeskind, P. S., & Stephens, L. E. (2004). Maternal selective serotonin reuptake inhibitor use during pregnancy and newborn neurobehavior. *Pediatrics, 113,* 368–375.

Additional Reading/Resources

The Academy of Breastfeeding Medicine has developed protocols on common clinical issues, including the one on hypoglycemia referenced in this chapter, as guidelines for the care of breastfeeding infants and their mothers. Full text versions of all the Academy of Breastfeeding Medicine's protocols are available at http://www.bfmed.org/protocols.htm

The Baby-Friendly Hospital Initiative published new guidelines on developing hypoglycemia policies. This document offers guidance on developing or amending policies relating to the prevention and treatment of hypoglycemia in newborn infants. It includes key issues for consideration, including how to identify infants who could be considered at risk, basic principles that should underpin all guidelines related to the management of such infants, and a sample flow chart and checklist to ensure that all key aspects are included. http://www.babyfriendly.org.uk/pdfs/hypo_policy.pdf

In-Utero Drug Exposure

Neonatal Drug Withdrawal guidelines from the American Academy of Pediatrics, Sample Withdrawal Scoring Sheet—from Lucile Packard Children's Hospital, and a video clip of neonatal abstinence syndrome: http://newborns.stanford.edu/InUteroDrugs.html

◖ Appendix 5-1 ◗

Summary Interventions on Shield Use

Situations for Which Shield Use Is Commonly Advised

Latch Difficulty

- Nipple anomalies (flat, retracted, fibrous, inelastic)
- Mismatch between small infant mouth and large nipple
- Infant from heavily medicated mother
- Birth trauma (vacuum extraction, forceps)
- Oral aversion (vigorous suctioning)
- Artificial nipple preference (pacifiers, bottles)
- Infant with weak or disorganized suck (slips off nipple, preterm, neurological problems)
- Infant with high or low tone
- Delay in putting infant to breast

Oral Cavity Problems

- Cleft palate
- Channel palate (Turner syndrome, formerly intubated)
- Bubble palate
- Lack of fat pads (preterm, small for gestational age)
- Low-threshold mouth
- Poor central grooving of the tongue
- Micrognathia (recessed jaw)

Upper Airway Problems
- Tracheomalacia
- Laryngomalacia

Damaged Nipples
- When all else fails and the mother states she is going to quit breastfeeding

Instructions for Shield Use

- Choose an appropriate size shield.
- Drip expressed milk onto the outside of the teat to encourage the infant to latch.
- Warm the shield to help it stick.
- Apply the shield (may moisten the edges to help it adhere better) by turning it almost inside out.
- Hand express a little milk into the teat if necessary.
- Use a periodontal syringe to pre-fill the teat if the mother is unable to express colostrum or milk into the teat.
- Use alternate massage to help drain the breast.
- Tubing can be placed inside or outside of the shield for supplementation.
- Check the infant's latch with the shield: The mouth must not close on the shaft of the teat.
- Check that the infant is not just sucking on the tip of the teat.
- Some mothers may need more than one shield.
- Some mothers may need to pump after each feeding.
- Mothers should carefully check their breasts for plugged ducts and areas that are not draining well.
- If yeast is present on the areola, the shield should be boiled; otherwise, the shield should be washed in hot soapy water after each use and rinsed thoroughly, and air dried.
- Perform an infant weight check about every 3 days until the mother's milk supply is stable and the infant is gaining well.

Chapter 6

Beyond the Initial 48–72 Hours: Infant Challenges

Introduction

A number of breastfeeding problems and issues must be addressed immediately and throughout the initial hospital stay, whereas other issues may have their origins in the early days, becoming apparent after discharge. Some are conditions that require an ongoing need for specialized lactation support postdischarge. This chapter discusses situations that require close follow-up and intense support, including hyperbilirubinemia (jaundice), dehydration, weight gain/loss issues, and breastfeeding late preterm and preterm infants.

Neonatal Jaundice

Neonatal jaundice is a common condition in the newborn. It is estimated that 60–70% of term infants will become visibly jaundiced, that is, serum bilirubin levels exceeding 5–7 mg/dL (85–119 mmol/L), in the first week of life (MacMahon et al., 1998). Neonatal hyperbilirubinemia increases during the hours after birth and usually peaks at ages 96–120 hours after discharge from the hospital. Approximately 5% reach levels >17 mg/dL (290.7 mmol/L) (Harris et al., 2001), and around 2% of these newborns reach a total serum bilirubin level of ≥20 mg/dL (342 mmol/L) (Newman et al., 1999). Estimated rates of high-risk bilirubin levels (≥25 mg/dL [427 mmol/L]) vary from 1:700 (Newman et al., 1999) to 1:1,000 (Bhutani et al., 1999a). Jaundice is a frequent reason for readmission to the hospital during the first 2 weeks of life (Hall et al., 2000; Maisels & Kring, 1998). Most jaundice in healthy full-term newborns is a benign condition that resolves over the first week or 2. However, extremely high levels of bilirubin (>25–30 mg/dL [427.5–513 mmol/L]) can be toxic to the brain, producing a condition known as kernicterus. Kernicterus involves bilirubin toxicity to the basal ganglia and various brainstem nuclei when extreme amounts of bilirubin cross the blood–brain barrier, infiltrate, and destroy nerve cells.

Bilirubin Metabolism

Bilirubin is an orange or yellow pigment, 80–90% of which is derived from the breakdown of hemoglobin from aged or hemolyzed red blood cells. Heme is a constituent of hemoglobin that is released in association with the breakdown of aging red blood cells. Most heme in the newborn originates from fetal erythrocytes, is initially converted to biliverdin through the action of the enzyme heme oxygenase, and then is reduced further to bilirubin that is transported in the circulation tightly bound to albumin. In the liver, bilirubin is conjugated by another enzyme, uridine diphosphoglucuronosyl transferase (UDPGT); released into the bile duct; and delivered to the intestinal tract for elimination through the stool (also termed direct bilirubin). However, some unconjugated (indirect) bilirubin remains unbound to albumin and circulates as free bilirubin. Unbound, unconjugated bilirubin passes easily through lipid-containing membranes, like the blood–brain barrier, where in high amounts it is neurotoxic and can transiently or permanently affect neurons (Volpe, 2001).

The production, conjugation, and excretion of bilirubin are affected by conditions unique to the newborn that cause an imbalance in this metabolic process, predisposing the newborn to hyperbilirubinemia. As the newborn moves from the low oxygen environment of the uterus to the relatively high oxygen environment of room air, excess fetal red blood cells are no longer needed. Infants produce more bilirubin than they can eliminate, a situation exacerbated by prematurity, bruising or hematoma formation, infection, maternal glucose intolerance, and all types of hemolysis. Alterations in this process include the following:

- Production: High bilirubin production (twice that of an adult) occurs because fetal erythrocytes are overabundant, have a short life span, and their breakdown rapidly creates an excess of heme for the newborn liver to process.
- Conjugation: Conjugation undergoes delays because the activity of UDPGT is limited and hepatic uptake of bilirubin is decreased.

- Excretion: The small intestine of the newborn delays bilirubin excretion through the activity of the enzyme beta-glucuronidase, which converts conjugated bilirubin back to its unconjugated state, allowing bilirubin to be reabsorbed back into the circulation (enterohepatic circulation) (Steffensrud, 2004). The newborn sterile bowel only slowly becomes colonized with the bacteria needed to degrade bilirubin into urobilinogen that cannot be reabsorbed. The longer direct (conjugated) bilirubin remains in the intestine, the greater the likelihood of its conversion back to indirect bilirubin (unconjugated), which is sent back to the liver for reprocessing (Blackburn, 1995). At birth, the intestines can contain as much as 200 g of meconium, including up to 175 mg of bilirubin, half of which is in the indirect form, an amount that is four to seven times the daily rate of bilirubin production at term (Bartoletti et al., 1979).

- Genetic predisposition: There are racial variations in bilirubin metabolism among the normal population (Beutler et al., 1998). Mutation of the gene for the enzyme required for bilirubin conjugation accounts for the increased predisposition of some Asian infants (~20%) for severe neonatal hyperbilirubinemia (Akaba et al., 1998).

Classifications of Newborn Jaundice

Clinicians see jaundice in an infant when bilirubin pigment is deposited in subcutaneous tissue, producing the characteristic yellowing of the skin and sclera. The type of jaundice typically seen in full-term neonates is termed physiological jaundice, where bilirubin levels rise steadily during the first 3–4 days of life, peak around the fifth day, and decline thereafter. In preterm infants bilirubin levels may peak on day 6 or 7 and resolve over a more extended period of time. Total serum bilirubin levels are influenced by a number of factors such as race, gestational age, type of feeding, and drugs or medications given to the mother or infant. The newborn's age in hours is commonly used as the criteria to decide if a particular bilirubin level is acceptable or if further monitoring is necessary (Bhutani et al., 1999a). Other contributing factors to physiological jaundice include a previous sibling with jaundice, lack of effective breastfeeding, excessive weight or water loss after birth, infection, mother with diabetes, and bruising/hematoma (Dixit & Gartner, 2000).

Jaundice that is not physiological or that is not related to breastfeeding or breastmilk is classified as pathological. Infants with risk factors should be monitored closely during the first days to weeks of life (Porter & Dennis, 2002). Characteristics of pathological jaundice include the following (Dennery et al., 2001; Melton & Akinbi, 1999):

- Appearance of jaundice within the first 24 hours after birth.
- Fast rising bilirubin levels (>5 mg/dL/day [85 mmol/L]).
- Total serum bilirubin level higher than 17 mg/dL (290.7 mmol/L) in a full-term newborn.
- Bilirubin levels greater than 8 mg/dL (136 mmol/L) in the first 24 hours may be hemolytic in origin (Maisels, 2001).

Pathological causes may include

- Sepsis.
- Rubella.
- Toxoplasmosis.
- Hemolytic disease (Rh isoimmunization, ABO blood group incompatibility).
- Erythrocyte disorders (glucose-6-phosphate-dehydrogenase deficiency). Glucose-6-phosphate-dehydrogenase deficiency occurs in 11–13% of African Americans (Kaplan & Hammerman, 2000) and is more common among mothers from Mediterranean countries and Southeast Asia. Screening for this disorder is not routinely performed and is associated with an increased incidence of hyperbilirubinemia and the need for phototherapy (Kaplan et al., 2004). It has also been associated with cases of kernicterus in the United States (Johnson & Brown, 1999; Penn et al., 1994; Washington et al., 1995).
- Extravasation of blood (cephalohematoma or subgaleal hemorrhage, such as from vacuum extraction, bruising).
- Inborn errors of metabolism.
- Hypothyroidism.
- Polycythemia (such as from delayed cord clamping, twin–twin transfusion).
- Intestinal defect or obstruction.
- Macrosomic infant of a diabetic mother.

Whereas total serum bilirubin levels of 15–20 mg/dL (255–340 μmol/L) are not that unusual in some healthy full-term normal infants, extreme hyperbilirubinemia, although rare, is of concern. Strong predictors of total serum bilirubin levels of at least 25 mg/dL are gestational age, bruising, family history, and a rapid rise in total serum bilirubin levels (Kuzniewicz et al., 2008). There is a set of common clinical risk factors for severe hyperbilirubinemia. The more risk factors present, the greater the risk for severe hyperbilirubinemia (Table 6-1).

Newman et al. (1999) studied the incidence of extremes in bilirubin levels in a sample of 50,000 term and near-term infants and found the following:

- Levels greater than 20 mg/dL (340 μmol/L) in 2% of the sample (1 in 50 infants)

- Levels of 25 mg/dL (425 μmol/L) or greater in 0.15% (1 in 650 infants)

- Levels of 30 mg/dL (510 μmol/L) or greater in 0.01% (1 in 10,000 infants)

TABLE 6-1   Common Clinical Risk Factors for Severe Hyperbilirubinemia

- Jaundice in the first 24 hours of life.

- Visible jaundice before discharge (48 hours)—Dermal icterus is not visibly noticed as yellowing of the skin below total serum bilirubin levels of 4 mg/dL (68 umol/L) (Kramer, 1969). It progresses in a cephalocaudal pattern (Knudsen & Ebbesen, 1997) and is noticed in the face at 5 mg/dL, progressing to the upper chest at 10 mg/dL (171 umol/L), followed by visibility on the abdomen at 12 mg/dL, and finally on the palms and soles when bilirubin levels are greater than 15 mg/dL. Although these observations do not replace transcutaneous measurements or laboratory blood analysis, they give the clinician an idea of how closely an infant should be monitored.

- Previous jaundiced sibling.

- Gestational age of 35–38 weeks—Late preterm infants are between 2.4 and 5.7 times more likely to develop significant hyperbilirubinemia (Newman et al., 2000; Sarici et al., 2004), with serum bilirubin levels peaking later, at 5 to 7 days, necessitating a longer period of follow-up; readmission for hyperbilirubinemia is much more likely in these infants when discharged at less than 48 hours of age (Hall, Simon, & Smith, 2000).

- Exclusive breastfeeding—Clinically, this is usually an infant who is not efficiently transferring milk.

- East Asian ethnicity.

- Bruising, cephalohematoma.

- Maternal age greater than 25 years.

- Male infant.

Source: Adapted from American Academy of Pediatrics, Subcommittee on Neonatal Hyperbilirubinemia. Neonatal jaundice and kernicterus. *Pediatr.* 2001;108:763–765.

Bilirubin levels in some infants can infrequently rise high enough to cause neurological consequences if not monitored closely or if interventions are not implemented to lower bilirubin levels. The term *bilirubin encephalopathy* is often used to describe the clinical manifestations of bilirubin toxicity, and the American Academy of Pediatrics (AAP, 2004a) recommends that the term *acute bilirubin encephalopathy* be used to describe the acute manifestations of toxicity seen in the first weeks after birth and the term *kernicterus* be used as a pathological description of the yellow staining of the brainstem nuclei and basal ganglia (Cashore, 1998). The AAP (2004a) recommends that the term *kernicterus* be reserved for the chronic and permanent clinical sequelae of bilirubin toxicity.

No exact bilirubin level or duration of hyperbilirubinemia exposure has been defined to locate the exact point at which neurotoxicity could occur. Furthermore, evidence to date cannot explicitly account for why some infants with extremes of bilirubin levels develop kernicterus and others do not, or why early signs of bilirubin encephalopathy appear reversible in some infants and are permanent in others (Hanko et al., 2001). Bilirubin entry into the brain is facilitated by numerous conditions, including displacement of bilirubin from its albumin binding, reduced albumin binding capacity, and increased permeability of the blood–brain barrier. Bilirubin is oxidized in the brain by an enzyme whose activity increases with greater postnatal age (Hansen, 2000). The brain may be able to protect itself to an extent through bilirubin oxidation (Hansen et al., 1999) that may be subject to genetic variability (Hansen, 2001). This protective effect may vary among infants, possibly accounting for the differing outcomes in infants with high bilirubin levels. Bilirubin encephalopathy proceeds along a continuum (Table 6-2), where early signs and symptoms may be subtle, nonspecific, transient, and potentially reversible to an advanced and chronic stage of permanent neurological injury (Volpe, 2001).

Although extreme levels of bilirubin have the potential to be neurotoxic, it actually has a physiological role in the body as an antioxidant (McDonagh, 1990). Bilirubin "protection" may be seen in infants with illnesses associated with free radical production such as circulatory failure, neonatal asphyxia, aspiration, and sepsis, where the rate of bilirubin rise appears less in these infants, because bilirubin is consumed to cope with oxidative stress (Sedlak & Snyder, 2004). Neonatal blood plasma is better protected against oxidative stress due in part to the elevated levels of bilirubin (Wiedemann et al., 2003). Shekeeb et al. (2008) showed that bilirubin acts as a physiological antioxidant until it reaches a concentration of 20 mg/dL in full-term normal neonates. Beyond that concentration

TABLE 6-2   Continuum of Bilirubin Encephalopathy

Early (first 3 to 4 days after birth)	After First Week	Chronic (kernicterus)
Lethargy	Increasing lethargy	Athetoid cerebral palsy
Decreased alertness	Increased irritability	High-frequency hearing loss
Poor feeding	Minimal feeding	Developmental delays
Weak suck	Fever	Motor delays
Excessive sleepiness	Shrill cry	Paralysis of upward gaze
High-pitched cry	Opisthotonus*	Dental dysplasia
Hypotonia	Seizures	Mild mental retardation
	Apnea	
	Retrocollis**	
	Oculogyric crisis***	
	Hypertonia	
	Stupor, coma	
	Rigidity	

*opisthotonus = a spasm in which the heels and head are bent backward and the body is bowed forward
** retrocollis = torticollis with spasms affecting the posterior neck muscles
*** oculogyric crisis = a spasm causing upward fixation of the eyeballs lasting several minutes or hours

Sources: Adapted from: Connelly AM, Volpe JJ. Clinical features of bilirubin encephalopathy. *Clin Perinatol.* 1990;17:371–379; Dennery PA, Seidman DS, Stevenson DK. Neonatal hyperbilirubinemia. *N Eng J Med.* 2001;344:581–590; Maisels MJ, Newman TB. Kernicterus in otherwise healthy, breastfed term newborns. *Pediatr.* 1995;96(4pt1):730–733; Volpe JJ. Bilirubin and brain injury. In: Volpe JJ, ed. *Neonatal Neurology.* Philadelphia, PA: Saunders; 2001.

it is conjectured that bilirubin no longer acts as an antioxidant and cannot be considered physiological. For bilirubin to disrupt brain function, it must gain entry into the brain. Normally, the blood–brain barrier functions to block the passage of bilirubin into the brain, but this action is less mature in newborn infants. Bilirubin, once it has entered the brain, has a short half-life and is cleared from the brain by the action of an enzyme. However, this enzyme's activity is lower in the neonate and is subject to interindividual differences and genetic variability, suggesting that vulnerability to bilirubin toxicity may in part have a genetic basis (Hansen, 2002). A number of factors can disrupt the blood–brain barrier, which is normally closed to albumin and bilirubin as long as it is bound to albumin (Hansen, 1994). These include hyperosmolality, hypercarbia, hypoxia, hyperoxemia, asphyxia, acidosis, prematurity, hypoalbuminemia, and bilirubin-displacing drugs.

Breastfeeding and Jaundice

Stevenson et al. (2001) consider breastfeeding as the "normal driving influence on the transitional pattern of hyperbilirubinemia with formula feeding representing an iatrogenic perturbation of the normal influences of human milk on the entero-hepatic circulation of bilirubin." Neonatal jaundice is connected to breastfeeding in three situations seen in clinical practice:

1. The exclusively breastfed, healthy term infant during the first week after birth

2. Newborns who do not receive adequate amounts of breastmilk and have high concentrations of indirect bilirubin during the first postnatal week (referred to as nonfeeding jaundice, starvation jaundice, lack of breastfeeding jaundice)

3. Breastfed infants who experience a situation of prolonged unconjugated hyperbilirubinemia (called breastmilk jaundice)

Breastfeeding has long been associated with higher bilirubin levels and a more prolonged duration of jaundice compared with formula feeding (Dahms et al., 1973; Osborn, Reiff, & Bolus, 1984; Schneider, 1986). Breastfeeding practices at the time of these studies, however, may have contributed to this impression. Infants in the early studies may have experienced restricted milk intake from

- Hospital policies that ordered nothing by mouth for the first 24 hours
- Limited access to breastfeeding from restrictive schedules that allowed feedings only every 4 hours and usually not at night
- Short access times to the breast from advice that limited feedings to only a couple of minutes per side
- Supplementation with sterile water or sugar water that provided few to no calories

Fasting (lack of calories) can enhance the enterohepatic circulation of bilirubin as can the continued presence of a reservoir of bilirubin contained in unpassed meconium. Bertini et al. (2001) demonstrated that the development of early jaundice was not associated with breastfeeding per se but rather with increased weight loss after birth subsequent to fasting or insufficient milk intake. A subpopulation of breastfed infants in their study experienced a high bilirubin level peak that was associated with mixed feeding (supplemented infants) and a higher weight loss. They also found a strong association between significant hyperbilirubinemia and vacuum extraction. Thus what is sometimes termed early-onset breastfeeding jaundice is most likely a manifestation of inadequate breastfeeding that causes the exaggerated pattern of hyperbilirubinemia in the first 5 days of life (Gartner, 2001; Neifert, 1998). Infrequent, inefficient breastfeeding reduces caloric intake, increases weight loss, delays meconium passage, and can drive bilirubin to levels where clinical intervention becomes necessary.

Hyperbilirubinemia that peaks between 6 and 14 days has been termed late-onset or breastmilk jaundice and can develop in up to one-third of healthy breastfed infants (AAP, 1994). Total serum bilirubin levels may range from 12 to 20 mg/dL (205.2–342 mmol/L) and are considered nonpathological. It can persist for up to 3 months (Gartner, 2001). The underlying cause of breastmilk jaundice is not clearly understood and may be multifactorial. It has been suggested that substances in breastmilk such as beta-glucuronidases and nonesterified fatty acids might inhibit normal bilirubin metabolism (Brodersen & Herman, 1963; Gartner & Herschel, 2001; Melton & Akinbi, 1999; Poland, 1981). Maruo et al. (2000) suggested that a defect or mutation in the bilirubin UDPGT gene may cause an infant with such a mutation to be susceptible to jaundice that components in the mother's milk may trigger.

Managing Hyperbilirubinemia

Numerous methods are used to prevent or manage hyperbilirubinemia:

- One of the most successful methods for preventing hyperbilirubinemia has been the administration of high-titer anti-D immunoglobulin G, or RhoGAM, to reduce the incidence and severity of Rh isoimmunization disease.

- Phototherapy is the most common therapy for high bilirubin levels. Its use is designed to prevent bilirubin toxicity, but it does not treat the underlying cause of the hyperbilirubinemia. Phototherapy has a number of side effects (Blackburn & Loper, 1992), some of which can affect breastfeeding (separation, lethargy, poor feeding, increased fluid requirement, poor state control). Phototherapy has been shown to induce DNA damage in lymphocytes, with the DNA damage increasing significantly with longer durations of phototherapy (Tatli et al., 2008). A fiberoptic blanket or band may be used—in lower urgency situations—allowing parents to hold, care for, and breastfeed the infant.

- Exchange transfusion is used in more extreme situations, usually for infants with hemolytic disease.

- Pharmacological agents have been tried over the years, with most being discarded as ineffective. A number of chemoprevention and treatment therapies have included heme oxygenase inhibitors such as metal meso- and protoporphyrins. Tin-mesoporphyrin (SnMP), blocks the action of heme oxygenase in converting hemoglobin to bilirubin. Its action is designed to shut off production of bilirubin at its source rather than remove it after it has been formed. It reduces blood bilirubin levels for 7–10 days after administration (Kappas, 2004). Its safety, indications for use, efficacy, and side effects of whole scale inhibition of bilirubin production remain to be determined (Blackmon et al., 2004; Hansen, 2003). l-aspartic acid, a beta-glucuronidase inhibitor (and component in hydrolyzed infant formula), has been given experimentally to breastfed newborns. Gourley et al. (2005) reported on a small number of infants whose fecal bilirubin excretion increased and jaundice decreased when given 5-mL doses of l-aspartic acid six times a day for 7 days after birth.

Changes in the Approach to and Prevalence of Hyperbilirubinemia and Kernicterus

The root cause for the development of kernicterus has been identified as a systems failure in neonatal care, especially during the first week after birth. A convergence of a number of changes and factors began contributing to an increasing number of infants being readmitted to the hospital for hyperbilirubinemia and an increase in reports of the development of acute bilirubin encephalopathy and kernicterus (Ross, 2003):

- A more relaxed approach to jaundice because studies did not reveal adverse developmental outcomes in infants who had experienced mild to moderate jaundice (Newman & Maisels, 1992; Watchko & Oski, 1983)

- More liberal treatment guidelines that postponed phototherapy in infants older than 72 hours of age until the total serum bilirubin level reached 20 mg/dL and for infants between 49 and 72 hours old until it reached 18 mg/dL (AAP, 1994)

- The practice of discharging healthy term newborns within 48 hours of birth, before many infants appear clinically jaundiced and after which bilirubin levels are most likely to rise (Braveman et al., 1995, 1997; Britton et al., 1994; Liu et al., 1997)
  - Early hospital discharge is associated with increased hospital readmissions for jaundice (Brown et al., 1999; Grupp-Phelan et al., 1999).
  - Short hospital stays, minimal staffing, and lack of provider expertise in breastfeeding management provide limited time and often little guidance for mothers and infants to become proficient at breastfeeding.
  - Minimum criteria for discharge within 48 hours of birth includes an infant who has completed at least two successful feedings, with documentation that the infant is capable of coordinating sucking, swallowing, and breathing. The breastfeeding mother and infant should be assessed by trained staff regarding positioning, latch-on, and adequacy of swallowing (AAP, 2004a), criteria that are not routinely performed in many hospital settings.
  - The shift in locus of care surrounding hyperbilirubinemia from the hospital to the community that has created a need for early postdischarge observation (Palmer et al., 2003).
- The typical pattern of newborn follow-up care that persists and consists of a 1- to 2-week postdischarge visit, occurring long after the period of high risk and the time for effective intervention has passed (Eaton, 2001); lack of adherence to an evidence-based follow-up schedule that recommends healthcare provider examinations and observations at age 72 hours if discharged before age 24 hours, a visit at 96 hours of age if discharged between 24 and 47.9 hours of age, and a visit at 120 hours of age if discharged between 48 and 72 hours of age (AAP, 2004b)
- An increase in reports of kernicterus (Johnson & Bhutani, 2003; Johnson & Brown, 1999)
  - Severe hyperbilirubinemia and kernicterus were the subjects of a report (Carter & Dixon, 2001).
  - Kernicterus was the subject of a sentinel event alert by the Joint Commission on Accreditation of Healthcare Organizations (2001) and a second alert of revised guidelines (2004).
  - Hyperbilirubinemia and kernicterus were discussed in a commentary by the AAP's subcommittee on hyperbilirubinemia (Eaton, 2001), emphasizing that many of the infants experiencing these conditions did

not have obvious hemolytic disease and were healthy breastfeeding newborns (frequently not receiving adequate nutrition and hydration, most likely due to inefficient feeding skills), a significant portion of whom were less than 38 weeks gestational age (near-term).

- In July 2003 the National Institute of Child Health and Human Development convened a group of experts to review the existing knowledge base regarding neonatal hyperbilirubinemia and the barriers to preventing kernicterus (Palmer et al., 2004).
- A 5-year consortium funded by the Agency for Healthcare Research and Quality explored the barriers to implementing the 1994 AAP jaundice guideline in healthcare systems. Some of the major problems included discharge before breastfeeding was established, cumbersome reimbursement policies for blood tests, clinicians who would not see infants until 2 weeks postdischarge, and insurance carriers rejecting claims for the early visit (Ip et al., 2003).

More recent reports show that the diagnosis of kernicterus has decreased to an estimated incidence of approximately 1.5 per 100,000 term newborn births and 4 per 100,000 births of preterm infants (Burke et al., 2009). Preterm infants with jaundice require close monitoring and a consistent breastfeeding plan of care with access to lactation consultant services.

Clinical Approaches to Breastfeeding Support: Practice Suggestions

Because all infants have an initial rise in bilirubin levels as they transition to extrauterine life, the goal of breastfeeding management strategies revolves around optimizing the skill sets mothers and newborns need to prevent bilirubin levels from becoming serious and to preserve breastfeeding if they do. Short postpartum stays provide increasingly less time for clinicians to teach and assess and for mothers and infants to practice their newly learned skills. The following measures optimize breastfeeding from the start and reduce the likelihood of severe hyperbilirubinemia from inadequate intake:

- Facilitate contact between mother and infant and avoid separation.
  - Encourage 24-hour rooming-in and breastfeeding at night to hasten excretion of bilirubin-laden meconium.
  - Minimize visitors who may cause a mother to delay or eliminate breastfeedings during their presence (Kovach, 2002).

- Recommend and ensure a minimum of 8 and a goal of 10–12 feedings each 24 hours (AAP, 2004b) (especially important for near-term infants and infants of mothers with diabetes or who are overweight or obese).
  - This takes advantage of the laxative effect of colostrum that stimulates gut motility and prevents the reabsorption of bilirubin.
  - Frequent feedings reduce the likelihood of large weight losses and dehydration that drive up bilirubin levels. The greater the frequency of feedings in the first days, the lower the peak bilirubin level (De Carvalho et al., 1982; Varimo et al., 1986; Yamauchi & Yamanouchi, 1990).
  - Jaundice can contribute to or exacerbate early breastfeeding problems. Increased serum bilirubin levels can cause lethargy, excessive sleepiness, and poor feeding (Gartner & Herschel, 2001).
  - Sleepy infants or infants who are closed down should be placed skin-to-skin with their mother and moved to the breast when demonstrating behavioral feeding readiness cues.
- Assess for infant swallowing at breast. Frequent attempts at feedings by themselves will not ensure adequate intake unless the infant is actually swallowing colostrum/milk. Document if and when swallowing takes place, making sure that the mother can state when the infant is swallowing.
  - If the infant is latched but not swallowing, recommend alternate massage to initiate and sustain a suck-swallow feeding pattern. If the infant pauses for an excessive amount of time between sucking bursts, the mother can use a nipple tug (i.e., simulate that she is going to remove the nipple from the infant's mouth by either pushing down on the areola enough to cause the infant to pull the nipple–areola back into his or her mouth or pull the infant slightly away from the breast without breaking suction). This is similar to the technique used to stimulate the suck of a bottle-fed infant by pulling back on the bottle but not breaking suction. As long as the mother's nipples are not sore or the tug does not create pain or damage, this may be a simple method of sustaining a sucking rhythm for an infant unable to do so. A tube-feeding device can also be taped or held at the breast to deliver colostrum/milk and prevent caloric deprivation from contributing to increased bilirubin levels (Auerbach & Gartner, 1987).
  - If the infant cannot latch or is unable to transfer milk, have the mother hand express colostrum into a spoon and spoon-feed this to the infant.

- Avoid supplementation with formula, if possible, because this reduces feeding frequency, decreases milk intake, and diminishes milk production (unless the mother is concurrently expressing milk). Nondehydrated breastfed infants should not receive water or dextrose water because this practice does not reduce total serum bilirubin levels or prevent hyperbilirubinemia (AAP, 2004b; De Carvalho et al., 1981; Nicoll et al., 1982).

- Occasionally, a breastfed infant may require supplementation due to the effects of phototherapy, the inability to effect breastmilk transfer, or the unavailability of the mother. The mother's colostrum/milk or banked human milk is the first option of choice (Herschel, 2003). If human milk is not on hand, a hydrolyzed casein formula may be a logical choice for use until the mother's colostrum/milk is accessible. A casein-hydrolysate formula has been shown to better contribute to reduced bilirubin levels than standard infant formulas (Gourley et al., 1999), perhaps because it contains a beta-glucuronidase inhibitor (Gourley et al., 1997). It also reduces the risk of provoking allergies and diabetes in susceptible infants. Mothers should be instructed to pump milk to preserve lactation and provide milk for future supplementation if needed.

- A bilirubin nomogram is currently in use to predict an infant's risk of developing clinically significant hyperbilirubinemia by plotting the total serum bilirubin level against the infant's age in hours predischarge (Bhutani et al., 1999b, 2000). Hyperbilirubinemia is defined as a bilirubin level greater than the 95th percentile at any age. Infants above the 75th percentile generally require an immediate total serum bilirubin measurement, whereas infants below the 40th percentile are at very low risk for developing subsequent hyperbilirubinemia. Although used to determine the timing and strategies of early interventions for lowering bilirubin levels (Bhutani et al., 2004), the nomogram, along with clinical risk factors, should be used to identify the need for increasingly intensive breastfeeding assistance. A significant number of infants in the low and intermediate risk zones on a bilirubin nomogram remain at risk for readmission for high bilirubin levels signaling the need for early postdischarge follow-up (Slaughter et al., 2009).

- The basic minimum criteria for discharge before 48 hours is the completion of two successful breastfeedings with documented swallowing and the ability of the mother to demonstrate competency regarding positioning, latch, and recognizing swallowing (AAP, 2004a). Breastfeeding technique, maternal competency, and documentation of swallowing, with corrective strategies implemented if needed, should be initiated before weight loss and jaundice become excessive.

The third and fourth days after birth are critical times for assessment of breastfeeding adequacy and for initiating interventions to correct problems. Interestingly, hospital stays of at least 3 days (including cesarean-born infants) were associated with a reduced risk of readmission for hyperbilirubinemia (Hall et al., 2000). Presumably, the extra time spent in the hospital improves the chances of skilled lactation services being made available and timely intervention for continued breastfeeding problems. As many as 22% of infants can still be experiencing suboptimal breastfeeding (≤10 on the Infant Breastfeeding Assessment Tool) on day 3 and up to 22% of mothers may encounter delayed lactogenesis II after discharge (i.e., greater than 72 hours with no evidence of the onset of copious milk production or engorgement) (Dewey et al., 2003). With early discharge, follow-up must take place in the primary care provider's office, in a hospital outpatient setting, in a clinic, or in the home (Egerter et al., 1998). The responsibility for detecting and monitoring jaundice has shifted to the parents, with some failing to keep follow-up appointments and many lacking a basic understanding of jaundice and how to recognize it. Although telephone follow-ups may answer early questions, they may fail to capture information from parents who are unable to assess if breastfeeding is adequate. A parent describing an infant as sleepy, lethargic, irritable, or not feeding well presents a dilemma to a clinician who cannot visually assess the infant and the breastfeeding parameters. These descriptors should not be summarily dismissed as typical newborn behaviors (Stokowski, 2002a). When mothers are taught to do so, they are capable of recognizing the progression of jaundice as well as the presence of significant jaundice (Madlon-Kay, 1997, 2002), but visual assessment is still unreliable in judging the intensity of worsening jaundice. Even nurses cannot rely on visual assessment of cephalocaudal progression of jaundice to estimate bilirubin levels, especially in late preterm infants.

Jaundice extent also has poor overall accuracy for predicting the risk of development of significant hyperbilirubinemia (Keren et al., 2009). Transcutaneous bilirubin measurement is a noninvasive screening tool that eliminates a large number of unnecessary skin punctures and is more reliable than visual assessment. However, it cannot replace laboratory measurement of serum bilirubin (Carceller-Blanchard et al., 2009). Placing the infant in sunlight will not treat high bilirubin levels and may bleach the skin to the point where visual assessment of the skin is impeded. A better approach is to objectively teach parents about jaundice, providing them with a printed resource to refer to at home (Stokowski, 2002b).

Effect of Jaundice on Continued Breastfeeding and Maternal Behaviors

Earlier studies of the effect of neonatal jaundice on maternal behaviors suggested that the experience of neonatal jaundice and its treatments were associated with a set of behaviors described as the vulnerable child syndrome, in which mothers perceived their infant's current and subsequent medical conditions as more serious, resulting in a pattern of high healthcare use and diminished reliance on their own ability to remedy minor problems themselves. The blood tests, phototherapy, separation, supplementation or replacement of breastmilk with formula, and prolonged hospitalization also had an adverse effect on breastfeeding, resulting in the increased likelihood of early termination of breastfeeding (Elander & Lindberg, 1984; Kemper et al., 1989, 1990). Mothers who lack an understanding of jaundice, who have language barriers, or whose healthcare provider does not provide clear explanations to eliminate maternal misconceptions may feel guilty, believing that they caused the jaundice (Hannon et al., 2001). Interactions with healthcare professionals are a crucial factor in mediating the impact of jaundice on the mother and the breastfeeding relationship. Conflicting orders, offhand comments about the mother's milk (or lack of milk), and recommendations to supplement or stop breastfeeding engender confusion, discontent, anger, and guilt, creating the impression that the mother is responsible for making her baby sick (Willis et al., 2002). Clinicians' actions that favor continued breastfeeding demonstrate that a high value is placed on breastfeeding and result in interventions that do not provoke premature weaning.

Use of a clinical pathway may work toward preserving breastfeeding and maternal confidence when an infant is readmitted. Spatz and Goldschmidt (2006) created a clinical pathway when it was noted that many breastfeeding infants admitted for jaundice, dehydration, or weight loss were admitted when no specialized lactation services were available (nights, weekends, holidays). The pathway provides the bedside nurse with an evidence-based, current, and consistent framework for clinical decision making and achieving the goals of effective milk transfer and preservation of the maternal milk supply. Clinicians will need to determine the infant's ability to effectively feed at breast; observe for milk transfer; select technology needed to assist latch and milk transfer, such as a tube feeding device or nipple shield; and initiate maternal pumping 8–10 times each 24 hours with a goal of 500–1,000 mL/day. If the infant is being treated with phototherapy, breast-feeding should continue on a frequent basis.

Hypernatremic Dehydration

A breastfed infant with effective feeding skills receives adequate amounts of fluid when nursing frequently, transferring milk, gaining weight appropriately, and producing urine and stools within normal age-expected parameters. Young infants are especially susceptible to volume depletion because the immature kidney does not yet maximally concentrate urine or reserve water. This is commonly seen in conditions that involve acute excessive fluid loss such as gastroenteritis. However, case reports of hypernatremic dehydration in otherwise healthy breastfed infants continue to appear in the medical literature (Neifert, 2001) and usually present around 7–10 days of age, with a range of 3–21 days (Oddie et al., 2001). Dehydration may coexist with high bilirubin levels (Tarcan et al., 2005), because the common thread between the two may have an iatrogenic etiology with parents unaware of their infant's deteriorating condition. Weight loss in an infant of greater than 7% should alert the clinician to an increased risk for hypernatremia and signal the need for more intensive breastfeeding evaluation and interventions (Unal et al., 2008; Uras et al., 2007). Percentage of weight loss from birth weight can be quite high, ranging from 14% to 32% (Cooper et al., 1995). Although jaundice is usually the most frequent diagnosis in early neonatal presentations to the emergency department, dehydration in infants less than 8 days old is also not uncommon (Manganaro et al., 2001), especially because there seems to be a correlation between early discharge and an increase in emergency department visits by neonates (Liu et al., 2000; Millar et al., 2000). The incidence of rehospitalization for dehydration in the immediate neonatal period ranges from 1.2 to 3.4 per 1,000 live births, with about 5% of these dehydrated infants presenting with a cause for dehydration as something other than feeding problems; sepsis or meningitis, for example (Escobar et al., 2002). Escobar et al. (2002) noted that the following were the most important risk factors for dehydration:

- First-time mother
- Exclusive breastfeeding (no validation of effectiveness of feeding)
- A mother older than 35 years
- Infant's gestational age less than 39 weeks
- Cesarean-born infants whose initial hospital stay was less than 48 hours

They also noted that serious sequelae were avoided in their institution due to an integrated healthcare system that provided early and easy access to follow-up and that the most effective preventive measure is to ensure successful initiation and continuation of breastfeeding, particularly among first-time mothers. Other risk factors include a delay in the first feeding after birth and a lack of attention to poor latch, delayed lactogenesis II, and nipple problems (Caglar et al., 2006).

Dehydration usually has its origins in the initial hospital stay, with fewer than eight breastfeedings each 24 hours, ineffective feedings with poor latch and little to no swallowing, maternal complaints of sore nipples, use of pacifiers, separation, and an infant at discharge who has experienced reduced colostrum intake and whose mother is unable to determine when swallowing occurs. A number of maternal and infant factors serve as red flags that can provide the setting for dehydration to occur and can alert the clinician of the need for close follow-up:

- Maternal
  - Issues with the breasts (previous insufficient milk; flat or retracted nipples; asymmetrical, hypoplastic, or tubular breasts; previous breast surgery; cracked or bleeding nipples).
  - Perinatal and delivery issues (urgent cesarean section, significant postpartum hemorrhage, hypertension, infection, diabetes, overweight/obesity, cystic fibrosis, heart disease, separation from the infant). Konetzny et al. (2009) reported that infants born by cesarean section had a 3.4 times higher risk for hypernatremia than those born vaginally.
  - Delay of lactogenesis II (copious milk production not evident by day 4, unrelieved severe engorgement).
- Infant
  - Gestational age issues (preterm infants—especially the near-term, 35- to 37-week-old infant who is discharged in 48 hours or less, small for gestational age, postterm infants)
  - Oral anomalies (cleft lip, cleft of the hard or soft palate, bubble palate, micrognathia, ankyloglossia)
  - Infant state control problems (near-term, maternal labor medications, closed down)
  - Birth issues (vacuum extraction, birth injuries)
  - Neuromotor issues (hypotonic, hypertonic, dysfunctional sucking)
  - Health issues (cardiac defect, infection, respiratory instability)
  - Newborn care issues (separation, pacifier use, crying)

Additional criteria can be used after discharge to evaluate the potential for or existence of dehydration:

- Sleepy, nondemanding infant who sleeps for long periods of time and is described by the parents as quiet or who rarely cries

- An infant who is fussy or unsettled after breastfeedings or who takes an excessive amount of time at each feeding

- Diminished urine and stool outputs; persistence of meconium-like stools on day 4, urate crystals in the diaper after day 3, dark yellow or concentrated urine

- Greater than a 7% weight loss along with other indicators, such as fewer than three stools per day, dry mucous membranes, feeding difficulties, and excessive sleeping

- Birth weight not regained by 10–14 days of age; mild dehydration may coexist with a 3–5% weight loss, moderate dehydration may become apparent at 6–10% weight loss, and weight loss greater than 10% could be an indication of severe dehydration (Manganaro et al., 2001). However, some infants appear to lose a great deal of weight before discharge because they diurese excess fluid (especially if the mother has had a large amount of intravenous fluids) and/or pass a large meconium stool.

Clinical signs of dehydration can be subtle at first and may go unnoticed by parents who might only be aware of a sleepy infant who may be difficult to feed. Dehydration may not be noted until laboratory evaluation. Infants with hypernatremic dehydration have better preserved extracellular volume with less pronounced clinical signs of dehydration. Weight loss and inadequate stooling are sensitive indicators of dehydration among breastfed infants (Moritz et al., 2005). As dehydration progresses, the clinician may observe the following signs:

- Clammy skin
- Skin turgor that goes from elastic to tenting
- Skin color that may be pale, with pallor progressing to gray or mottled skin
- Delayed capillary refill
- Decreased tears in eyes, progressing to sunken looking
- Dry lips and buccal mucosa
- Sunken anterior fontanel
- Fever (Maayan-Metzger et al., 2003; Ng et al., 1999)

- Lethargy
- Increased pulse rate progressing to tachycardia
- High serum bilirubin concentrations (Liu et al., 2000)

The popular media has reported tragic consequences in a small number of infants who suffered severe hypernatremic dehydration, painting breastfeeding as the dangerous cause of this unfortunate outcome (Helliker, 1994). These situations are preventable and due to the lack of adequate breastfeeding, clinical mismanagement, a delay in seeking help, and failure of proper follow-up on the part of the healthcare system (Laing & Wong, 2002). Clinicians may mistakenly ascribe high sodium levels in breastmilk as the causative factor, reasoning that excessive intake of high sodium breastmilk resulted in hypernatremic dehydration (Rand & Kolberg, 2001). Usually, poor breastfeeding management, lack of milk transfer, and inadequate follow-up contribute to poor intake in the infant and lack of milk drainage from the breast, with the resulting milk exhibiting high sodium levels indicative of involution. It is unlikely to be the direct cause of neonatal hypernatremia (Sofer et al., 1993). Retrospective studies of dehydration usually identify problems with milk synthesis, difficulty with breastmilk removal, and low daily breastmilk intake as the overarching factors associated with the development of hypernatremia (Livingstone et al., 2000). There appears to be an association between the degree of weight loss and the degree of hypernatremia (Macdonald et al., 2003). Mild hypernatremia (146–150 mmol/L) is commonly seen and has been documented in almost one-third of breastfed infants with all degrees of recorded weight loss (Marchini & Stock, 1997). Yaseen et al. (2004) described decreased diaper output in the clinical presentation of exclusively breastfed infants admitted for dehydration. These infants were significantly more likely to have less than six voids and less than three stools in the 24 hours before admission. Failure to screen for the problems prenatally and immediately postdelivery and a lack of adequate follow-up combine to set the stage for poor outcomes (Moritz et al., 2005; Yildizdas et al., 2005). Weighing infants at 72–96 hours along with appropriate and timely lactation support facilitates early recognition of problems and helps decrease the incidence of hypernatremia as well as the severity while preserving breastfeeding (Iyer et al., 2008).

Treatment

Because hypernatremia in breastfed infants typically develops over a longer period of time as compared with acute dehydration from gastroenteritis, it is usually corrected over a longer period of time. If the dehydration is severe, the infant may be admitted into the hospital and receive intravenous fluids to improve cardiovascular function, making sure that the brain and kidneys are perfused while avoiding a too rapid infusion that could lead to seizures or cerebral edema (Molteni, 1994). An infant who is only mildly dehydrated may not be hospitalized. Both types of situations still require that the infant be fed, preferably pumped breastmilk from the mother. If human milk is not available and the mother is not producing sufficient amounts, formula supplementation is needed until her milk production can meet the needs of the infant.

Clinical Approaches to Breastfeeding Support: Practice Suggestions

Lactation usually can and should be preserved, even if the underlying cause precludes full milk production.

- To improve milk production, the mother should be instructed to pump both breasts simultaneously with a high-quality electric breast pump at least 8–10 times per day (in the absence of an infant at breast or after breastfeedings). This pumped milk (or other supplement) should be offered to the infant during or after each breastfeeding. If the infant is hospitalized, the mother should be able to room-in with the infant and offer the breast frequently.

- If the infant is able to latch, supplemental milk can be provided to the infant through a tube-feeding device placed on the breast to improve sucking and increase milk production during the breastfeeding. The amount of supplement needed can initially be calculated by weighing the infant before and after a breastfeeding and offering the amount of supplement after each breastfeed that would provide a daily intake of 150–200 mL/kg/day. As the infant's sucking improves and the milk supply builds, more milk will be left in the supplementer or less supplement will be taken by other means. Although use of a bottle to deliver supplements is not precluded, sucking on an artificial nipple weakens the suck or may further weaken a poor suck. A tube-feeding device can be placed on the breast in such a way as to make the delivery of milk easy enough to avoid stress in the mother and infant while not causing a too rapid delivery of milk that overwhelms the infant. Supplementing at breast and pumping also demonstrate the value clinicians place on breastfeeding, human milk, and the mother's efforts to preserve lactation and the breastfeeding experience.

- Weight gain of 56 g per day (double the normal daily weight increment) or more is not unusual during the period of catch-up growth and indicates sufficient intake. Infant formula can be replaced with breastmilk as the mother's supply improves. Pumping should continue until the infant no longer needs supplements and is gaining weight adequately on exclusive breastfeeding.

- Pacifiers should be avoided, because sucking efforts need to be channeled toward improving milk transfer from the breasts.

Slow Weight Gain

The definition of normative weight loss in the healthy, full-term, breastfeeding infant has generated conflicting opinions regarding what is normal and when interventions are required such as supplemental feedings. Methodological inconsistencies among numerous studies make it difficult to determine between physiological weight loss and a red flag. MacDonald et al. (2003) demonstrated that a weight loss of up to 12% is experienced by about 95% of neonates. Noel-Weiss et al. (2008) conducted a systematic review of the literature and within the 11 studies meeting the inclusion criteria, mean weight loss ranged from 5.7% to 6.6% with a standard deviation of about 2%. Most infants in these studies regained their birth weight within the first 2 weeks postpartum, with the second and third days after birth being the days of maximum weight loss. Martens and Romphf (2007) showed that the mean in-hospital weight loss of 812 healthy full-term newborns was 5.09% ± 2.89%, varying by feeding category. Exclusively breastfed infants' in-hospital weight loss was 5.49% ± 2.6%, partially breastfed infants' 5.52% ± 3.02%, and formula-fed infants' 2.43% ± 2.12%. Factors that significantly increased the percentage of weight loss included higher birth weight, female gender, epidural use, and longer hospital stay. Maternal obesity has also been associated with excess infant weight loss when compared with infants whose mothers are not obese (Mok et al., 2008).

Other factors can contribute to early newborn weight loss in the breastfed infant that are not indicators of insufficient feeding (normal diuresis, loss of meconium, hospital and birthing practices, large amounts of maternal intravenous fluid). Although weight loss per se is important to monitor, bowel output has been suggested as another indicator of sufficient breastmilk intake. Shrago et al. (2006) found that more bowel movements per day during the first 5 days after birth were significantly associated with less initial weight loss, earlier transition to yellow bowel movements, earlier return to birth weight, and heavier weight at 14 days of age. Optimal bowel output in this study was a mean of four to five bowel movements per day with transition to yellow bowel movements at a mean of 6.8 days.

However, relying on stool output alone may yield many false positives. Nommsen-Rivers et al. (2008) demonstrated that diaper outputs when measured in the home setting showed too much overlap between infants with adequate versus inadequate breastmilk intake. This made it problematic to rely on diaper output as the only indicator of sufficient milk intake. These authors recommended that the parameters of fewer than four bowel movements on day 4 or delay of lactogenesis II beyond 72 hours after birth is suggestive of breastfeeding insufficiency. Monitoring of diaper output may provide an advance warning of pending weight loss or dehydration even though newborn diaper counts show wide variation.

After the initial weight loss during the first few days after birth, most breastfed infants regain their birth weight by 2 weeks. Up to 12% of infants may experience excess weight loss during this period (greater than 10%), which has been closely linked with delayed lactogenesis II and suboptimal infant breastfeeding skills (Dewey et al., 2003). For the mother of an infant who does not demonstrate appropriate weight gain or who continues to lose weight, the expectation of a thriving infant and a successful breastfeeding experience is abruptly challenged. Between 2 and 6 weeks of age, the average breastfed female infant is expected to gain approximately 34 g/day and the male breastfed infant should gain about 40 g/day, with the minimum expected gain for both boys and girls being about 20 g/day (Nelson et al., 1989). After this, the weight, length, and head circumference of infants are followed on growth charts.

In the United States between 1977 and 2000 the 1977 National Center for Health Statistics growth charts were used. These charts had a number of limitations, including the very few breastfed infants who were included in the reference data upon which the charts were constructed. Discrepancies were revealed when data became available on the normal growth of exclusively breastfed infants. In comparison with these charts, breastfed infants have a relatively rapid weight gain in the first 2–3 months followed by a drop in percentile ranking thereafter (Dewey et al., 1992, 1995), leading some healthcare providers to recommend supplementation for perceived growth faltering. The Centers for Disease Control and Prevention (CDC) produced new growth charts in 2000 to address some of the major concerns with the National Center for Health Statistics charts (Ogden et al., 2002). These charts, however, still fail to address the normal growth of the reference infant—one fed exclusively on breastmilk until about age 6 months and thereafter breastfed while receiving appropriate complementary foods (Dewey, 2001). With this in mind the World Health Organization (WHO) released new standards in April 2006 for assessing the growth and development of children from birth to age 5 years (de Onis et al., 2006a; WHO, 2006). These new standards are designed to describe how all children should grow rather than providing a more limited snapshot of how children grew at a specified time and place (Garza & de Onis, 2004).

There are differences between the WHO and CDC charts, with the main differences occurring in infancy. The mean weight of infants included in the WHO standards is above the CDC median during the first 6 months of infancy, crosses it at approximately 6 months, and remains below the CDC median until about 32 months (de Onis et al., 2007). These weight-for-age differences are especially important during infancy. The CDC charts cannot account for the rapidly changing weights of early infancy because the study design lacked empirical weight data between birth and 2 months of age. The infancy section of the WHO standard is based on a greater sample size and shorter measurement intervals, allowing it to account for the rapidly changing growth in early infancy and the physiological weight loss during the first few days. The WHO standards are based on exclusively breastfed infants, whereas the CDC charts included relatively few infants who were breastfed for more than a couple of months. Underweight will be higher when based on the WHO standard compared with the CDC reference during the first 6 months of infancy (de Onis et al., 2006b). When using the CDC charts, breastfed infants will show an apparent decline in weight for age after 6 months (van Dijk & Innis, 2009).

Danner et al. (2009) developed weight gain velocity charts to help align the differences between the CDC and WHO charting systems. In general, children on the WHO growth charts gain at a faster rate during the first 6 months of life, after which time the children on the CDC growth charts gain weight faster. The charts from the Danner study provide a reference for grams/day and grams/month weight gain in five different percentiles. These weight velocity charts are helpful in assessing adequacy of weight gain in short time intervals. Clinicians may find these growth velocity charts a helpful tool for assessing weight gain adequacy, especially if it appears that a breastfed infant is faltering anywhere on either of the charting systems. The WHO system may result in false positives for underweight in some breastfed infants during the first 6 months with the potential of unnecessary supplementation or early use of complementary foods (Binns et al., 2008; Cattaneo & Guoth-Gumberger, 2008). Adequate growth and the need for supplementing breastfeeding should be based on more than a single measurement from either of the growth charting systems. Clinical, developmental, and behavioral assessments are also paramount in assessing growth adequacy. Changes in growth velocity as determined by three measurements over a suitable period of time may be a more reliable indicator of growth faltering (Cattaneo & Guoth-Gumberger, 2008).

A number of authors have conceptualized the problem from various starting points, with some offering schema or flow charts to provide a more encompassing framework.

- Desmarais and Browne (1990) coined the term "impending failure to thrive" to differentiate between infants who are normal but slow growing, those who are failing to thrive, and those who are at risk for inadequate weight gain without appropriate intervention. Overlapping maternal and infant conditions may result in a complex cause-and-effect scenario that clinicians must unravel to identify the root cause or causes of the problem.

- Lawrence and Lawrence (2005) use a schema to classify causes associated with infant behavior from those related to maternal problems. Infant causes were broadly classified as poor intake, low net intake, and high energy requirements. Maternal classifications included poor milk production and poor release of milk.

- Ramsay, Gisel, and Boutry (1993) related weight-gain problems to a history of alterations in normal feeding skills and behaviors. Infants in their study with growth faltering had a history of abnormally long durations of feeding times, poor appetite (did not provide clear hunger signals), delayed texture tolerance (in older infants), and difficult feedings (infants had difficulty latching to the breast, pushed out the nipple, and had frequent feedings that lasted an hour or more). They discussed the possibility that growth faltering correlated to a subgroup of infants with what was termed a "feeding skills disorder" and that mothers of these infants did not display faulty interactions with their infants. The term "nonorganic failure to thrive" is still sometimes used to refer to infants whose lack of expected weight gain is unrelated to underlying pathology. Failure to thrive has traditionally conjured a negative connotation of poor maternal–infant interaction, but these authors found that maternal–infant interaction was not related to poor intake.

Common in many studies of postnatal factors associated with slow infant weight gain are several elements: a history of feeding problems, a description of being a slow feeder, reports of weak sucking, poor appetite, and taking in only small quantities of milk at a time (McDougall et al., 2008). Emond et al. (2007b) found that weak sucking was equally important in breastfed and bottle-fed infants. One in six infants in a cohort of 11,900 infants was reported by their parents to have weak sucking. Growth faltering was almost twice as likely in this group. These authors caution that early onset and persistence of slow or difficult feeding may be a signal of inadequate intake, leading to possible growth faltering. Growth faltering may be transient or temporary. Subtle oromotor dysfunction has also been mentioned to be associated with some weight faltering as parents have described retrospectively that their infants with weight faltering were more likely to have had sucking difficulty and problems chewing and swallowing (Wright et al., 2006). Some early feeding difficulties may possibly be a marker of subtle neurological impairments and serve as a precursor to eventual poor weight gain. There is also some evidence that slow weight gain over the first 2 months is associated with developmental delay (Drewett et al., 2005; Emond et al., 2007a). Emond et al. (2007a) showed a three-point IQ deficit in the slowest gaining 5% of term infants in the first 8 weeks, demonstrating that IQ deficit is associated with early rather than later growth faltering. With weak sucking associated with growth faltering, early weight gain issues in some infants may be a feeding skills problem of neurophysiological origin. On the other hand, if the early weeks of life are a critical period for nutritional adequacy, then insufficient nutrition could impact brain growth and later cognitive functioning. Although this effect does not appear to be large, it is comparable in size with the effects of other variables that impinge on IQ such as bottle-feeding, prenatal cocaine use, and low birth weight (Corbett & Drewett, 2004; Anderson et al., 1999). Clearly, early growth faltering is an issue that requires close monitoring.

Failure to thrive not only has a negative undertone (neglect or abuse) but also has differing definitions:

- A fall of two standard deviations on the weight chart in the first 8 weeks or a fall below the third percentile for weight (Kien, 1985)

- The rate of weight gain is less than –2 standard deviation value during an interval of 2 months or longer for infants less than 6 months of age or for 3 months for an infant over 6 months and the weight for length is less than the 5th percentile (Foman & Nelson, 1993)

- The infant continues to lose weight after 10 days of life, does not regain birth weight by 3 weeks of age, or gains at a rate below the 10th percentile for weight gain beyond 1 month of age (Lawrence & Lawrence, 1999)

Because slow weight gain or growth faltering in a breastfed infant may be interpreted differently depending on which growth charts and parameters are used

(Olsen, 2006), Powers (2001) suggested using a set of criteria to differentiate when a breastfed infant is gaining appropriately and when a feeding problem requires intervention:

1. Newborn infant less than 2 weeks of age who is more than 10% below birth weight
2. An infant whose weight is less than birth weight at 2 weeks of age
3. After an initial void, an infant who has no urine output in any given 24-hour period
4. An infant who does not have yellow milk stools by the end of the first week
5. An infant who has clinical signs of dehydration
6. Infants 2 weeks to 3 months of age whose weight gain is less than 20 g/day
7. Unexplained weight loss at any age
8. Completely flat growth curves at any age

Sometimes infants older than 3 or 4 months of age will be identified as suddenly experiencing growth faltering. It is important to differentiate whether this is the normal downward crossing of percentile rankings (i.e., the change in growth velocity and weight gain patterns typical for a healthy, well-nourished, breastfed infant when using standard growth charts) or a true problem. Lukefahr (1990) reported that when infants over 1 month of age presented with growth faltering, organic causes were actually present in about 50% of the cases. Growth faltering in length velocity or length-for-age may also indicate an organic cause or a nutrient deficiency such as a low vitamin B6 status (Heiskanen et al., 1995). Sucking becomes voluntary rather than reflexive around 3 or 4 months of age, and older infants can be highly distractible at breast. The clinician should check a number of issues, including organic or disease-based causes, as well as more common issues (Frantz, 1992) such as follows:

- Displacing sucking to fingers or other objects
- Changes in feeding patterns such as
    - Limitations on the length and frequency of feedings if an infant is teething
    - Parents are using an infant training program or a sleep-through-the-night regimen that limits or reduces the number of feeds per 24 hours
    - Infant becomes so distractible that he or she shortens the feedings to the point of inadequate intake

- · Busy maternal schedule or return to employment that reduces milk intake
- · Early introduction of less calorie-dense solid foods that displace breastmilk from the diet
- · Mother experiences illness or severe dieting
- · Mother begins taking oral contraceptives

Sometimes when an older infant who has been thriving at the breast slows or stops gaining weight, the etiology emerges as a combination of a mother with an abundant milk supply and rapid milk ejection reflex that allows an infant who is either a poor feeder, or who develops into a poor feeder, to easily obtain milk with minimal effort. When the milk production diminishes and the infant must execute correct and strong suckling, this oral motor skill emerges as less than optimal, reducing milk transfer and contributing to a flattening growth curve (Newman, 2004). Use of alternate massage may prove helpful. Breast compression can improve the pressure gradient between the breast and the infant's mouth, assisting in milk transfer.

In the presence of a slow-gaining breastfed infant, both infant (Table 6-3) and maternal (Table 6-4) assessments must be conducted to formulate a differential diagnosis, construct a problem-oriented management strategy, preserve the lactation and breastfeeding experience, and support the mother through an anxiety-provoking period of time (Powers, 1999). Slow weight gain per se is usually not "the problem" but is most often the result or manifestation of a problem. Simple faulty management should be assessed and corrected first, such as poor positioning, incorrect latch, insufficient number of feedings per 24 hours, or use of a pacifier to stretch out feeding times. Late recognition of problems results in high rates of mothers abandoning breastfeeding (Harding et al., 2001; Oddie et al., 2001).

Once a history, physical exam, and breastfeeding assessment have been completed, the clinician may have formed an opinion of what factors may be contributing to the problem. A number of interacting maternal and infant factors may need to be accounted for or corrected as the feeding plan is developed. Mothers may have a sufficient milk supply but the infant is unable to transfer this milk effectively. Mothers may have low milk production with or without an infant who demonstrates effective feeding skills. The clinician will also need to determine if supplementation is necessary and how this would be accomplished while preserving lactation and breastfeeding. Powers (2005) suggested that supplementation may be considered or indicated by the clinical condition of the infant, by the amount of weight loss (greater than 10% in a newborn or young infant),

TABLE 6-3 Infant Factors That May Contribute to Slow Weight Gain

Factor	Effect
Gestational age and growth	Preterm, near-term, postterm, SGA, IUGR, and LGA infants may lack mature feeding skills. Provision of breast-milk is especially important for SGA infants because it promotes better catch-up growth in head circumference (brain growth) than supplementing with a standard formula (Lucas et al., 1997).
Alterations in oral anatomy	Alterations such as ankyloglossia, cleft lip, cleft of hard or soft palate, bubble palate, facial growth anomalies such as micrognathia, or congenital syndromes that affect the oral structure may contribute to poor milk intake.
Alterations in oral functioning	Hypotonia, hypertonia, neurologic pathology, or physiology may interfere with the performance, strength, or stamina of the structures involved in the suck, swallow, breathe cycling.
High energy requirements	Cardiac disease, respiratory involvement (bronchopulmonary dysplasia—BPD), metabolic disorders that create a need for increased caloric intake or volume restriction that place limits on intake.
Known illness	Infection, trisomy 21, cystic fibrosis, or cardiac defects often put the infant at risk for poor growth because of the combination of a low endurance for feeding and high metabolic demands. Growth faltering may be apparent in the early months due to atopic dermatitis (Agostoni et al., 2000).
Maternal medications	Certain prenatal prescription medications or recreational drugs may interfere with normal sucking physiology.
Intrapartum factors	Cesarean delivery, hypoxia, anoxia, labor medications, state control difficulties, epidural analgesia, forceps, and vacuum extraction that affect brain function, anatomical structures, and nerves, contributing to ineffective milk transfer.
Iatrogenic factors	Hospital routines that separate mothers and infants, provide inappropriate supplementation, offer pacifiers, or provide conflicting or poor breastfeeding instruction leave both mothers and infants lacking needed feeding skills.
Gastrointestinal or metabolic/malabsorption problems	Gastroesophageal reflux or other conditions that limit nutrient intake or metabolism.

TABLE 6-4   Maternal Factors That May Contribute to Slow Infant Weight Gain

Factors	Effect
Breast abnormalities	Previous breast surgery, insufficient glandular development, augmentation, reduction, and trauma may influence the ultimate volume of milk that the breasts will produce but do not preclude breastfeeding.
Nipple anomalies	Flat, retracted, inverted, oddly shaped, or dimpled nipples may make latching more difficult and reduce milk intake. Improper suckling on nipples may also damage them, further reducing infant milk intake.
Ineffective or insufficient milk removal	Improperly positioned/latched infant, ineffective suckling, unresolved engorgement leave residual milk and reduce supply, making less milk available to the infant.
Delayed lactogenesis II	Mother who is overweight, obese, or diabetic may experience an initial delay in lactogenesis II. With copious milk production delayed, frequency of feedings must increase to offset volume deficit.
Poor breastfeeding management	Delayed or disrupted early feeding opportunities, separation, too few feedings, and illness reduce feeding opportunities at breast. Failure to pump milk in the absence of an infant suckling at breast may interfere with proliferation and sensitivity of prolactin receptors.
Medications/drugs	Prescription or recreational drugs, labor medications, and IV fluids may delay lactogenesis II or interfere with infant suckling. Oral contraceptives can reduce lactose content and overall milk volume (Hale, 2004). Smoking may also decrease volume (Vio, Salazar, & Infante, 1991) and fat content of milk (Hopkinson et al., 1992).
Hormonal alterations	Hypothyroid, retained placenta, superimposed pregnancy, pituitary disorders, polycystic ovarian syndrome, theta lutein cysts (Hoover, Barbalinardo, & Platia, 2002), oral contraceptives, diabetes insipidus, assisted reproduction/difficulty conceiving, or other endocrine-related problems may interfere with the normal progression of milk production.
Milk ejection problems	Drugs, alcohol, smoking, stress, pain, or other factors that inhibit the let-down reflex reduce the amount of milk available to the infant.
Miscellaneous factors	Lack of vitamin B12 in a vegetarian diet, parenting programs that limit feedings, ineffective breast pump or pumping schedule, inadequate weight gain during pregnancy, postpartum hemorrhage, anemia, cesarean delivery (Evans et al., 2003).

failure to return to birth weight later than 2–3 weeks of age, average daily weight gain of less than 20 g, any amount of unexplained weight loss, weight and length curves that are completely flat at any age, and deceleration of head circumference that consecutively crosses percentiles.

In complicated situations, if an infant is being monitored for intake and output or if amounts of supplements are being calculated, intake at a feeding can be determined, if necessary, by taking a pre- and postfeed weight of the infant on an electronic scale sensitive to within 2 g (Meier et al., 1994). This can be useful in determining the intake at that particular feeding. Sometimes a mother can pump her breasts after a feeding and take a postfeed weight to determine the approximate total amount of milk that was available at that particular feeding and determine if a supplement is required at that time (Meier et al., 1990). These procedures are not indicative of 24-hour intakes and milk production but may help the clinician to gather data regarding whether the milk production is appropriate and the infant is unable to effect milk transfer or to help estimate recommended amounts of supplements based on approximate intake at a feeding. Because infants demonstrate a large feed-to-feed intake variability, a closer picture of intake and milk production would involve the mother performing a prefeed weight, breastfeeding her infant, performing a postfeed weight, pumping both breasts, and totaling the amounts over a 24-hour period of time. In a more urgent situation this may not be practical, and the clinician would work to correct mismanagement or feeding techniques while supplementing the infant during or after each breastfeeding with as much pumped milk or formula as the infant will take. In a less urgent situation, Powers (2005) recommended starting amounts of supplement that represent approximately 25% of normal intake and adjust up or down as weight gain improves. For example, a 6 lb, 9 oz (3.0 kg) infant would require 15–20 oz (450–600 mL) as a total daily intake. Supplementing with 4 oz divided into six to eight feedings over a 24-hour period represents a conservative starting point.

Determining what and how to supplement can be considered on a basis of the most to least physiological. Supplements in order of preference are the mother's own expressed milk, mother's hindmilk if the supply permits, pasteurized donor milk (if indicated for an ill, preterm, or severely immune compromised infant), and infant formula (type based on the family history of the presence of allergies or diabetes). Hindmilk, which is obtained farther into a breastfeeding, is also the fat-rich cream layer seen in stored breastmilk. This cream layer can be especially calorie-dense with up to 28–30 calories or more per ounce (Lucas et al., 1978). Although milk volume is most often the major factor affecting weight gain of exclusively breastfed infants (Aksit et al., 2002), the use of the hindmilk cream layer can boost caloric intake significantly while delivering a physiological volume of milk (Valentine et al., 1994). Infants over 6 months of age can be supplemented with calorie-dense semisolid foods. The method of supplementation would preferably be directly at the breast using a tube-feeding device or tubing run through a nipple shield if the infant was unable to latch to the breast. If short-term or occasional supplements were indicated, other devices could be selected such as a cup, syringe, dropper, spoon, or bottle. During the creation of the feeding plan the clinician has a number of techniques and equipment (see Appendix 6-1) from which to choose and, in conjunction with the mother, determine which combinations best suit the situation.

Clinical Approaches to Breastfeeding Support: Practice Suggestions

The creation of the feeding plan and choice of interventions reflect the etiology of the problem (Box 6-1). The overarching goals of the management guidelines are to protect the milk supply and provide adequate nourishment to the infant to restore and support normal growth. Written feeding guidelines with short- and long-term goals for the parents are important to reinforce teaching and provide a mechanism for parents to remember the multiple tasks that must be accomplished. Feeding plans can be as simple as increasing the number of feedings and adding alternate massage on each breast at each feeding until weight gain improves. Other situations may be more complex as described in the following sections.

Breastfeeding Preterm Infants

In 2007, the premature birth rate (before 37 weeks gestation) in the United States was 12.7% of live births (Hamilton et al., 2009). Non-Hispanic black infants are more than three times as likely to be born extremely preterm (<28 weeks gestation; 1.9%) compared with non-Hispanic white and Hispanic infants (0.6%) (Martin et al., 2007). Rates of preterm birth vary by state, with a low of 9.2% in Vermont to a high of 18.3% in Mississippi. The preferred feeding modality for the more than 530,000 preterm infants born each year is human milk and breast-feeding (AAP, 2005). Whereas breastfeeding rates for term infants remain low, breastfeeding rates for preterm or low-birth-weight infants are even lower. In a survey of 124 neonatal intensive care units (NICUs), 50.3% of the 42,891 premature infants were not receiving any breastmilk when they were discharged from the hospital (Powers et al., 2001).

BOX 6-1   Case Study of Baby Briana

Date	Age (wk)	Weight	Comments
6/5	Birth	9 lb	41 1/7 weeks
6/7	Discharge 2 days	8 lb 3.8 oz	8% weight loss
6/22	2	8 lb 10 oz	2-week checkup
7/7	4+	9 lb	1-month checkup
8/10	9	8 lb 10 oz	2-month checkup
8/12	9+		Lactation consultant visit

Briana had begun sleeping through the night at 4 weeks of age, fed about six times each 24 hours, took 1 hour to feed at breast, and took an hour to consume 2 oz of formula from a bottle. She had been seen by her family practice physician with no reports of organic or pathological conditions. Briana had been seen by a feeding team at a children's hospital who recommended that she be switched to high-calorie formula and fed by a fast-flow bottle nipple. She was also noted to have a tongue thrust. She produced four to five wet diapers per day and a bowel movement every few days.

A breastfeeding was observed showing good positioning and latch, but Briana took between 17 and 34 sucks per swallow. She would swallow only after a letdown. Briana's mother stated that she wished to continue breastfeeding and providing as much of her milk as possible for Briana but that she could pump little to no milk at that point. A phone call to the infant's physician revealed that if the weight loss could not be rectified, Briana would be admitted into the hospital for further testing. If formula supplementation was indicated, a standard formula could be used.

The initial goal was to reverse the weight loss immediately and avoid admission into the hospital. The longer-term goal was to maximize milk production and help Briana improve her suckling to the point that she could consume most of her feedings at the breast within a reasonable length of time.

Techniques chosen: nipple tug, alternate massage

Equipment chosen: Supplemental Nutrition System (SNS) tube-feeding device, electric breast pump with double collection kit, feeding and weight log, infant formula if no breastmilk was available for supplementation

Plan

1. Briana was to be fed 8–10 times each 24 hours with a 2:00 am night feeding to be added temporarily. This would add more opportunities for increasing intake.

2. The SNS (with the medium-size tubing) was to be used during each feeding, with 3–4 oz of formula as the supplement until pumped milk was available. Supplements were reduced to 1–2 ounces as Briana consumed more milk from the breast and left more supplement in the SNS. Nipple tug and alternate massage were chosen as initial techniques to strengthen the suck, maximize fat intake, and increase breastmilk volume. Supplementing at the breast would serve to stimulate milk production and reduce the amount of time for each feeding. The choice of these techniques and equipment was also designed to improve sucking efficiency so that a more efficient suck-to-swallow ratio was demonstrated. Because flow regulates suck, the SNS was chosen to initiate and maintain flow.

3. Briana's mother was to pump her breasts after as many feedings as possible during the day to maximize milk production. She pumped between two to six times per day with total 24-hour volume pumped between 2 and 8 ounces.

Date	Age (wk)	Weight	Comments
8/13	9		Began using the SNS during every feeding, eight to nine feedings were recorded each 24 hours with a 2:00 am feeding, and pumping five to six times per day
8/14	10	9 lb 2 oz	
8/21	11	9 lb 12 oz	
8/28	12	10 lb 6 oz	
9/1			Began using the SNS at the end of each feeding, after Briana had breastfed with the tubing pinched off
9/3	13	10 lb 9 oz	
9/10	14	11 lb 8 oz	
9/11			Began using the SNS at the end of every other feeding; discontinued 2:00 am feeding
9/16	15	11 lb 11 oz	
9/17			Discontinued SNS
9/23	16	11 lb 8 oz	
9/24			Resumed SNS after every two feedings
9/29	17	12 lb 1 oz	
10/7	18	12 lb 14 oz	4-month checkup
10/8			Began using the SNS following every third feeding and was lost to follow-up

Parents benefit from receiving factual information regarding the therapeutic effects that human milk and breastfeeding will have on their infant so that their feeding decision is evidence based (Meier, 2001; Meier & Brown, 1997). The healthcare professional has an ethical responsibility to avoid withholding information because of the unfounded concern that to inform mothers of research-based options may make them feel guilty if they choose not to breastfeed (Hurst & Meier, 2005). A study of preterm mothers whose initial intent was to formula feed but subsequently initiated lactation after the encouragement of NICU care providers found the mothers denied feeling forced or pressured into breastfeeding by staff who presented an unequivocal message regarding the importance of breastfeeding (Miracle et al., 2004a). Women who are subsequently made aware of the nutritional and immunological properties of human milk in relation to improved infant health outcomes often express anger and frustration with the healthcare professionals who failed to share this knowledge with them (Miracle et al., 2004b). Scrutiny of a number of other non–evidence-based assumptions has shown that clinicians need not fear encouraging the mother of a preterm infant to breastfeed (Rodriguez et al., 2005).

Why use human milk for preterm infants? Feeding human milk to preterm infants has a number of important short- and long-term health outcomes that are vital to share with the mother (Table 6-5). Knowing the importance of breast-milk to their infant may help mothers to not only provide their milk for their infants but also act as a motivator to continue pumping milk during discouraging times of long hospitalizations. Necrotizing enterocolitis is a devastating and potentially lethal disease that is seen predominantly in preterm infants. The preterm fetal gut has not completed its maturation process; human milk contains

---

TABLE 6-5   Health Outcomes of Preterm Infants When Not Fed Their Own Mother's Milk

- Achievement of full enteral feedings later (Sisk et al., 2008)
- Experience a significant increase in nosocomial infections (Schanler, 2007)
- More likely to develop necrotizing enterocolitis (Meinzen-Derr et al., 2009)
- Lower scores on tests of visual acuity (Morales & Schanler, 2007)
- Decreased neurocognitive performance (Horwood et al., 2001)
- Altered immune system function (Tarcan et al., 2004)
- Increased intestinal permeability and slower intestinal maturation (Taylor et al., 2009)

components that enhance this maturation, whereas infant formula does not. The gastrointestinal system plays a major role in serving as a barrier to pathogens and allergens and as a vehicle for nutrient absorption. Artificially fed infants lack human milk components that promote the closure of the tight junctions between cells, increasing the risk that certain volumes of infant formula act as a toxic dose for the premature intestine (Taylor et al., 2009). Because preterm infants cannot fully digest carbohydrates and proteins, human milk provides components that aid this process. When fed infant formula undigested casein can reach the gut, attract neutrophils that provoke inflammation and the opening of the tight junctions between cells, allow intact proteins to engage in systemic invasion, and further damage a fragile gut, leading to necrotizing enterocolitis (Claud & Walker, 2001). Vohr et al. (2006) found that every 10 mL/kg/day increase in breastmilk intake contributed 0.53 points to the Bayley Mental Development Index, conferring a 5.3 IQ point advantage for infants consuming 110 mL/kg/day. This long-term advantage may optimize cognitive potential and decrease the need for costly early intervention and special education services in childhood.

Maternal Stresses

Some believe there is little value in investing the time and energy for mothers to provide their milk for a preterm infant; however, the large body of published evidence on the effects of human milk feeding in preterm infants shows that mother's milk is the milk of choice for the premature infant (Schanler & Atkinson, 1999). Scientific and medical advances have created a population of extremely low-birth-weight infants who are often critically ill. The use of human milk for these infants fills the gaps in their undeveloped host defenses and metabolic and gastrointestinal immaturity and produces long-term advantages in vision and neurodevelopment. Human milk provides protection from the conditions that preterm infants are most prone to develop, such as infection and necrotizing enterocolitis (Schanler, 2001).

If the assumption is that providing breastmilk is too stressful to the mother, evidence shows that the provision of breastmilk provides a mechanism for the mother to regain an element of control over an overwhelming situation. Fear, grief, remorse, anger, and guilt can be refocused into activities that allow the mother to exercise her unique role in the intimate care of her newborn. Rather than being considered as a visitor, the mother is part of the team who cares for her infant. Her milk provides both medication and nutrition, a contribution that is uniquely hers

(Kavanaugh et al., 1997; Lang, 2002; Spanier-Mingolelli et al., 1998; Whiteley, 1996). Breastfeeding (or pumping breastmilk) is an oxytocin-releasing condition that further contributes to decreased stress and improved maternal–infant attachment (Feldman et al., 1999). Expressing breastmilk for her tiny infant acts as a connection between mother and baby, conferring maternal identity in a time of stress. A hospitalized preterm infant provides limited opportunities to engage in the mothering role, whereas expressing milk helps fill a void in the maternal experience (Sweet, 2008). Although milk expression is time consuming and does not give the pleasurable feedback of an infant suckling at the breast, mothers find hope through this act. Mothers may also feel pressured to produce sufficient quantities of milk and may feel guilt if unable to do so. Therefore it is important that breastfeeding and the provision of breastmilk be treated as a priority by hospital staff in the early days after a preterm birth. Failure to acknowledge the importance of milk expression and monitor it increases the risk of low milk production and interpretation by the mother that her milk is not valued.

Mothers and Medication

Occasionally, there is the assumption that the mother's medical condition and/or requirement for medications is incompatible with breastfeeding or pumping milk. However, there are few contraindications to breastfeeding (Lawrence, 1997; Lawrence & Lawrence, 2001) and few medications that are not compatible with breastfeeding (AAP, 2001b). Medications that are not compatible may frequently be changed to those that are (Anderson et al., 2003). Maternal medications that preclude breastfeeding include antimetabolite or cytotoxic medications—anticancer drugs, I^{131}, and drugs of abuse such as heroin, cocaine, amphetamines, and phencyclidine (AAP, 2001b; Hale 2003).

Maternal illnesses that preclude breastfeeding include HIV/AIDS (although pasteurization of the expressed milk inactivates the virus), human T-cell lymphotropic virus types I and II, and active tuberculosis before treatment (AAP, 2003). Cytomegalovirus (CMV) is ubiquitous and the most common cause of intrauterine and perinatal infections in the world (Numazaki, 1997). CMV infections transmitted through breastmilk are usually asymptomatic in term infants but may pose a potential problem for immunocompromised or extremely preterm infants. CMV DNA can be detected in the breastmilk of seropositive mothers and can be transmitted to an infant through breastmilk, with most preterm infants not manifesting clinical symptoms (Yasuda, Kimura, Hayakawa, et al., 2003). However, if a number of conditions are simultaneously present, symptomatic CMV infections are possible (i.e., a high viral load in the milk, high CMV IgG in the mother, extreme prematurity with few transplacentally acquired maternal antibodies, and whether the breastmilk of a seropositive mother had been heat treated or frozen and for how long) (Jim et al., 2004). Lactoferrin in breastmilk is often protective against CMV in the early weeks when levels are high in colostrum and milk, but once these levels fall and/or viral loads increase beyond a certain threshold, transmission may occur. Local inflammation in the breast may also decrease lactoferrin levels when large amounts of virus are present in breastmilk.

Concomitant viral replication in the breast itself may lead to a local inflammation and passage of the virus into the milk (Lonnerdal & Iyer, 1995; van der Strate et al., 2001). Most breastmilk of seropositive mothers becomes positive for CMV DNA 2 weeks after delivery (Yasuda et al., 2003). DNA copy numbers increase to a peak at 3–6 weeks postpartum (Vochem et al., 1998; Yasuda et al., 2003), with CMV excretion into breastmilk declining to undetectable levels by 8–12 weeks postpartum (Hamprecht et al., 2008; Yasuda et al., 2003). Freezing breastmilk at –20°C (4°F) for 3–7 days usually decreases viral titers below the transmission threshold (AAP, 2003); however, freezing does not totally eliminate the risk of CMV transfer into the milk. The viral titer at the time of freezing, not the length of time frozen, correlates with the risk of transmission. Heat treatment or pasteurization eliminates CMV but alters some of the anti-infective properties of the milk (Lawrence, 2006).

Very low gestational age and infants with preexisting chronic diseases are conditions associated with symptomatic infection (Capretti et al., 2009). There is an apparent absence of long-term adverse outcomes in the small number of preterm infants who acquire CMV from breastmilk (Neuberger et al., 2006). CMV infection acquired through breastmilk seems to be transient, mild, and self-limiting. Given that the peak time of CMV transmission into milk is 3–4 weeks postpartum, colostrum (the first week of milk) may be used fresh or frozen. If the mother is CMV seropositive, all maternal breastmilk should be frozen for at least 24 hours before feeding until the infant is greater than 32 weeks corrected age or feeding directly at the breast (California Perinatal Quality Care Collaborative, 2008).

Sufficient and Appropriate Milk

Some assume that the mother will be unable to produce a sufficient amount of milk that is appropriate to the needs of a preterm infant. True, the conditions surrounding a preterm birth may contribute to a less-than-optimal initiation of lactation, especially if this is to be accomplished in the absence of an infant suckling at the breast. Lactogenesis II may be delayed in some preterm mothers, causing low milk production in the early days (Cregan et al., 2002). The volume of milk was further reduced when antenatal corticosteroids were administered between 28 and 34 weeks gestation and delivery occurred 3–9 days later (Henderson et al., 2008). However, pumping protocols that consider the physiology of milk production can compensate for this by initiating early and frequent pumping (Hill et al., 2001). Written pumping instructions should be provided for the mother (Walker, 1992).

Preterm mother's milk is generally adequate for growth in infants weighing 1,500–1,800 g (about 3.5–4 lb), with increased concentrations of nutrients associated with the degree of prematurity (Atkinson, 2000). If growth of infants weighing less than 1,500 g is deemed inadequate on human milk alone, powdered or liquid fortifiers are added to the mother's milk (Guerrini, 1994; Schanler, 1998; Schanler et al., 1997) and have been shown to improve growth and decrease hospital stays (Bhat & Gupta, 2003). Some controversy exists regarding the use of fortifiers due to the neutralization of preterm milk's bacteriocidal activities when fortifiers high in iron are combined with human milk (Chan, 2003). Fortification has been reported to cause azotemia, hypercalcinuria, increased infections, and increased necrotizing enterocolitis (Lucas et al., 1996).

The addition of preterm cow milk–based formula to human milk decreased lysozyme activity by 41–74% (Quan et al., 1994). Mixing excessive amounts of powdered fortifier into human milk (beyond one packet per 25 mL of milk) can result in hypercalcemia or further complications of cardiac arrhythmia. Adding human milk fortifier to breastmilk increases the osmolality after mixing, which creates a greater risk for necrotizing enterocolitis (Janjindamai & Chotsampancharoen, 2006). Protein is often the limiting factor in preterm nutrition and is important for developing healthy lean body mass. Although fortifiers may result in short-term growth advantages, powdered formula products, powdered fortifiers, and powdered specialty infant formulas are not sterile. Intrinsic contamination of powdered infant formula with *Enterobacter sakazakii* and the subsequent morbidity and mortality in some preterm infants consuming these products have been reported (CDC, 2002). Fortification of human milk has been shown to result in increased bacterial colony counts, especially when held at room temperature during continuous feeding (Jocson et al., 1997). Commercial fortifiers are concentrated forms of protein and essential minerals such as calcium and phosphorus, not a source of additional calories. Prolonged storage of fortified human milk decreases the availability of epidermal growth factor and other beneficial molecules to the infant. Fortified milk should be used immediately after its preparation (Askin & Diehl-Jones, 2005).

Fortified human milk, however, is more beneficial than preterm infant formula. Infants may gain more slowly on fortified human milk but remain healthier (Schanler et al., 1999a). Many nurseries fractionate human milk to use the high-fat hindmilk as a concentrated source of lipids and additional calories, while staying within any volume tolerance limitations of an individual infant. The lipid content in human milk correlates with the caloric density of the milk, making it relatively simple to determine the lipid and caloric content of a mother's milk by using a measure called the creamatocrit (Lucas et al., 1978). Small point-of-care machines rather than cumbersome laboratory procedures can accurately determine lipid and calorie content of milk (Meier et al., 2006), allowing more individualized nutrition for these tiny infants.

Infant Stresses

Preterm infants are at a great feeding disadvantage due to their neurological immaturity, muscle hypotony, short awake times, and nascent feeding skills. Many healthcare providers have traditionally thought that feeding at breast was harder work than feeding from a fast-flow artificial nipple. Prerequisites for feeding at breast were (and still are in some nurseries) based on attaining a certain weight or gestational age or demonstrating the ability to consume an entire bottle-feeding before being permitted to feed at breast. These clinical practices should be reexamined (Callen et al., 2005) as closer scrutiny showed that preterm infants demonstrate better oxygenation during feedings at breast as compared with feeding from a bottle. These infants exhibit fewer episodes of desaturation, bradycardia, temperature instability, and apnea and are physiologically ready to breastfeed before they are ready to bottle-feed (Blaymore-Bier, 1997; Meier, 1988; Meier & Anderson, 1987; Meier & Pugh, 1985). This is primarily related to their ability to pace their own feeding by controlling the milk flow rate to allow time for breathing between sucking bursts.

Cardiorespiratory patterns of preterm infants during bottle-feeding can show decreases in minute ventilation, decreased breathing frequency, prolonged airway closure, decreased $tcpO_2$, increased apnea, increased bradycardia, and decreased sucking pressures (Koenig et al., 1990; Matthew, 1988, 1991; Shivpuri et al., 1983).

The risk of bottle-feeding to the preterm infant's physiological regulation and stability extends right up to the days immediately before discharge from the NICU. Preterm infants continue to have desaturation events during bottle-feeding, spending as much as 20% of their feeding time with oxygen levels less than 90% (Thoyre & Carlson, 2003). Under optimal conditions, many preterm infants have the capacity for intake of adequate volumes of breastmilk that are sufficient for appropriate growth at the time, irrespective of attaining fully mature sucking patterns (Nyqvist, 2008).

Hospital Lactation Care and Services

Care of the preterm infant can be quite complex. Many NICUs use care paths or clinical pathways (California Perinatal Quality Care Collaborative, 2008; Dougherty & Luther, 2008; Forsyth et al., 1998); specific breastfeeding protocols; records that support intentional, planned, and prevention-focused interventions (Baker & Rasmussen, 1997); or a combination of approaches to address the challenges of providing mother's milk for these infants while transitioning them to breast. Early transfer of care to the infant's parents eases the transition from NICU to home (Nyqvist & Kylberg, 2008). Multiple activities occur simultaneously that include provisions for maternal milk expression, feeding of mother's milk to the infant, transitioning the infant to feedings at the breast, and provision of discharge guidelines to extend the duration of breastfeeding or the use of mother's milk.

Coordinated and comprehensive services have been established by some nurseries to prevent fragmented attempts at breastfeeding an infant shortly before discharge and to avoid the common problem of insufficient milk production (Hurst, 2007). Concerted efforts by NICUs to improve breastfeeding outcomes often result in more infants fed increased amounts of human milk, including banked human milk, and more infants discharged home breastfeeding (Montgomery et al., 2008). Structured and successful hospital models base their interventions on evidence so that all NICU staff comply with policies that are directed or coordinated by a nurse or physician (Hurst et al., 1998; Meier et al., 1993). Carstrucci et al. (2007) reported that delivering at a hospital where an International Board Certified Lactation Consultant (IBCLC) was present increased the odds of breastfeeding among mothers of infants admitted to the NICU by 34%. Introduction of an IBCLC service in an NICU increased the proportion of infants given their own mother's milk from 31% to 47% (Gonzalez et al., 2003). Mannel and Mannel

(2006) recommend 1 full-time equivalent IBCLC per 235 infant admissions to the NICU to provide the following level of services:

- Direct consult times that include direct patient interaction, documentation, and staff interaction
- First visit after delivery: 60 minutes (promote milk expression, review milk expression, facilitate acquisition of breast pump)
- Follow-up visit at 4–5 days postpartum: 60 minutes (assess milk production, pumping efficacy, infant status, kangaroo care)
- Follow-up visit at 10–14 days: 30 minutes (assess milk production, infant status, kangaroo care)
- Follow-up visit to initiate direct breastfeeding: 90 minutes
- Follow-up visit before discharge: 90 minutes (assess breastfeeding, discharge teaching)

NICUs with optimal breastfeeding support engage in a set of practices that are known to result in improved levels of mothers initiating breastfeeding and successfully expressing milk volumes adequate for infant needs both in-hospital and after discharge (Table 6-6) (Nyqvist & Kylberg, 2008; Spatz, 2004). Some units have instituted a care-by-parent program before discharge to improve readiness for independent parenting (Costello & Chapman, 1998). A large component of discharge readiness on the part of both parent and infant centers around feeding issues. Most mothers express some anxiety regarding caring for the infant and breastfeeding at home without the constant presence of a trained NICU staff. Follow-up phone calls are especially important during the first 24–72 hours postdischarge (Elliott & Reimer, 1998) because mothers of preterm infants are more likely to abandon breastfeeding efforts earlier than mothers of term infants (Furman et al., 1998; Lefebvre & Ducharme, 1989). Two impediments to breastfeeding durations beyond a few weeks are compromised milk production and failure to transition the infant to the breast, both of which have their origins in hospital practices and policies (Bier et al., 1993; Hill et al., 1994, 1997; Kavanaugh et al., 1995). Mothers' reports of dwindling volumes of pumped milk, the infant's resistance or refusal to latch, uncertainty regarding whether the infant received enough milk at each feeding, and a weak suck that fails to transfer sufficient amounts of milk, with the further reduction of breast stimulation, provide continuing challenges postdischarge. Mothers' concerns over an inadequate milk

---

TABLE 6-6   Hospital Practices Supportive of NICU Breastfeeding Care

---

- Provide evidence-based information about breastfeeding, breastmilk, and infant formula for informed decision making
- Communicate staff's value of breastfeeding
- Have a written breastfeeding policy communicated to and followed by all staff (nurses and physicians)
- Provide current and consistent breastfeeding/pumping guidelines
- Involve the mother in all feeding plans
- Encourage mothers to assume responsibility for feeding tasks such as performing pre- and postfeed weights and fractionating their milk
- Teach, assess, and monitor milk expression, storage, and transport
- Initiate skin-to-skin care (kangaroo care)
- Introduce the breast early with frequent learning opportunities
- Use a demand or semidemand breastfeeding strategy
- Teach positioning, assess latch, sucking, and swallowing
- Use assistive devices as needed
- Measure milk transfer
- Supplement without bottles if possible
- Support the father's presence and provide guidelines for his help with breastfeeding
- Create a feeding plan for the postdischarge period
- Refer parents to community sources for breastfeeding support

Sources: Nyqvist KH, Kylberg E. Application of the baby friendly hospital initiative to neonatal care: suggestions by Swedish mothers of very preterm infants. *J Hum Lact.* 2008;24:252-262; Spatz DL. Ten steps for promoting and protecting breastfeeding for vulnerable infants. *J Perinat Neonat Nurs.* 2004;18:385-396; Rodriguez NA, Miracle DJ, Meier PP. Sharing the science on human milk feedings with mothers of very-low-birth-weight infants. *JOGNN.* 2005;34:109-119; Meier PP, Engstrom JL, Mingolelli SS, Miracle DJ, Kiesling S. The Rush Mothers' Milk Club: breastfeeding interventions for mothers with very-low-birth-weight infants. *J Obstet Gynecol Neonatal Nurs.* 2004;33:164-174.

---

supply and whether the infants consumed an adequate volume of milk at a feeding are different problems requiring different approaches to resolve.

Barriers to continued breastfeeding change across time. Callen et al. (2005) reported that nipple and breast problems were most prevalent at NICU discharge, as was low milk volume, whereas poor breastfeeding technique of the infant was

most prevalent at 1 month. From discharge to 3 months many infants had difficulty breastfeeding because they were difficult to arouse, slept through feedings,
or fell asleep at the breast before completing a feeding. Some infants would fight
at the breast and have difficulty latching. Many of these problems are interrelated.
A focus on assisting mothers and infants to fully establish breastfeeding before
discharge would help reduce the problems of faulty breastfeeding technique.

   A prospective, nonrandomized trial in 71 infants ranging in age from 26 to 36
weeks gestation assessed the development of breastfeeding skills as a mechanism
to develop feeding recommendations. Efficient rooting and latching were
observed as early as 28 weeks and nutritive sucking at 30.6 weeks, with 80% of
these infants establishing full breastfeeding at a mean of 36 weeks and as early as
33.4 weeks. Although maturation is important for preterm infants to establish
mature patterns of sucking, swallowing, and breathing, experience or practice
feeding at the breast also seems important for these infants to acquire early breastfeeding skills (Hedberg Nyqvist, 2001).

Clinical Approaches to Breastfeeding Support: Practice Suggestions

Breastfeeding for the preterm infant and mother is different from a healthy term
infant. Length of the infant's stay in the hospital is significantly correlated to the
probability of being breastfed at discharge. The shorter the stay, the higher the
probability of being breastfed at the time of final discharge (Kirchner et al., 2009).
A number of barriers and complex medical situations can present themselves on
the route from birth to breastfeeding. This journey may take time, commitment,
and adjustment to a very different reality from what was imagined. Strategies for
the clinician are as follows:

1. Initiate and sustain milk production. In the absence of an infant at the breast,
   mothers of preterm infants may need to pump milk (Auerbach & Walker, 1994)
   for weeks or months until their infant is fully established at breast or to
   provide as much breastmilk as possible under very trying circumstances.
   Mothers will need to do the following:
   - Secure an efficient breast pump. The most efficient pumps have been
     shown to be fully automated, multiuser (hospital-grade) pumps that cycle
     about 48–50 times per minute, with vacuums that do not exceed 240 mm
     Hg and that use a double collection kit to pump both breasts
     simultaneously (Hill et al., 1999; Mitoulas et al., 2002). Mothers should
     be instructed in how to use the pump and receive specific guidelines for

cleaning the collection kit. Although these pumps can be rented, many low-income women cannot afford the expense and their health insurance (if they have it) may reject such a claim. Local WIC agencies may have electric pumps to loan. Some institutions may have a grant-funded program to ensure such pumps are available to all women who need them (Philipp et al., 2000).

- Use a double collection kit. Mothers tend to pump a greater quantity of milk with simultaneous pumping in a shorter period of time. Simultaneous breast pumping with added breast massage while pumping yields more milk per expression session than sequential pumping with no breast massage (Jones et al., 2001).

- Select a properly fitted flange or breastshield. When the vacuum is exerted on the maternal nipple, it is drawn into the tunnel of the breastshield and must be able to move freely. The tunnel can vary in size from 21.0 to 40.0 mm depending on the manufacturer and the number of breastshield options available with each pump (Walker, 2005). Nipple sizes can range from less than 12 mm at the base to more than 23 mm (Stark, 1994; Wilson-Clay & Hoover, 2002; Ziemer & Pidgeon, 1993). Nipples swell during pumping (Wilson-Clay & Hoover, 2002). If blanching at the nipple–areolar junction is observed or pain is experienced by the mother, reduced milk flow could occur. A standard size breastshield is 24–25 mm, but many women actually require a larger shield of 27–30 mm for pain-free and effective pumping, especially during the early weeks of frequent milk expression (Meier et al., 2004). The clinician should observe a milk expression session to determine if the breastshield is properly fitted, especially in the presence of pain or reduced milk removal.

- Begin milk expression within 6 hours of delivery. Early initiation of pumping (Meier & Brown, 1996; Neifert & Seacat, 1988) is associated with lactation continuing after the infant reaches 40 weeks corrected age (Furman et al., 2002).

2. Pump milk frequently. Frequent pumping during the first week after birth is important to optimize the eventual amount of milk that will be available to the infant. Good milk production has been associated with five or more expressions and at least 100 minutes of pumping per day (Hopkinson et al., 1988). Fewer pumping sessions per 24 hours may produce sufficient amounts of milk for mothers intending to provide milk for preterm infants of higher

gestational ages, for mothers intending to provide milk for short periods of time, or for mothers who plan to combine breastfeeding with formula use. However, clinical experience has shown that mothers who intend to produce a full milk supply, exclusively breastfeed at discharge, breastfeed multiples, or have a sufficient volume to fractionate and use hindmilk need to pump about 8–12 times per 24 hours during the first 10–14 days after birth (Hurst & Meier, 2005). Hill and colleagues (1999) showed that optimal milk output has been associated with the following:

- An output of greater than 3,500 mL/wk (500 mL/day [17–18 oz/day]) that is achieved with more than 44 pumping sessions per week.

- Adequate milk production in weeks 4 and 5 if milk volumes of 3,500 mL/wk have been achieved by week 2.

- High milk production by 10–14 days of 800–1,000 mL to provide a 50% oversupply. This can help compensate for the typical milk volume decrease seen during the second month of milk expression (Hill et al., 1995; Hurst et al., 1998). The maternal prolactin response to a breast pump, although evident, may not be the same as how prolactin release responds to a vigorously nursing infant, necessitating more frequent pumping during the early phase of lactation where the breasts calibrate how much milk they will eventually be able to produce. Many mothers will not be able to produce the high volume of milk known to optimize the chances for full lactation during the entire course of the infant's hospitalization as well as for the many months postdischarge (Bishara et al., 2009). Additional interventions may be necessary. Morton et al. (2007a) reported that pump-dependent mothers of preterm infants who hand expressed greater than five times per day as well as used an electric pump approximately five times per day during the first 3 days postpartum produced significantly larger volumes of milk than mothers who only used an electric pump. Breast massage while pumping has been shown to significantly increase the amount of milk pumped at each session, suggesting that milk volumes appear to be associated with the completeness of breast emptying rather than with increased frequency or duration of pumping (Morton et al., 2007b).

If a mother is producing 1,700 mL of milk per week by week 2, her likelihood of reaching the minimum volume of 3,500 mL/wk is only 50%. If she is producing less than 1,700 mL/week at week 2, the mother may need intensive help in salvaging the milk supply (Ehrenkranz & Ackerman, 1986).

- Monitor pumping frequency and milk volumes. A pumping log should be maintained that accounts for the number of times a mother pumps, what time of day, and the volume pumped from each breast. This allows for quick intervention if milk production falters.

3. Address low milk volume immediately. Some suggestions follow:

  - Add another pumping session at night when prolactin levels are highest. Preterm mothers tend to have lower basal prolactin levels than full-term mothers (Hill et al., 2009). Additional pumping sessions expose the breasts to higher than basal levels of prolactin multiple times during the day, perhaps compensating for the uncompleted preparation of the breasts provoked by an early delivery. Frequent pumping is extremely important for its effect on prolactin exposure. Pumping no more than five times per day may not provide sufficient prolactin exposure for many mothers.

  - Massage each breast methodically while pumping to maximize the volume and fat content per expression. Thorough breast draining is important because the degree of emptiness influences the amount of milk that is replaced (Daly et al., 1996). Milk remaining in the breast can lead to both a down-regulation in milk volume and an increased risk for milk stasis, engorgement, and mastitis. Mothers can continue pumping for 2 minutes after what appears to be the final drops of milk to ensure as complete drainage as possible. Most mothers have one breast that produces more milk than the other, and this breast dominance continues over time. Pumping instructions should specify to continue pumping for 2 minutes after both breasts have stopped flowing to ensure the nondominant breast is adequately drained (Hill et al., 2007).

  - Pump at the infant's bedside or while holding the infant skin-to-skin.

  - Facilitate kangaroo care, which has been shown to contribute to higher milk volumes (Hurst et al., 1997).

  - Check that the breastshield/flange of the pump is not constricting or strangulating the nipple. If necessary, change to a larger breastshield, especially if the mother states that her nipples are sore.

  - Check that the mother is using a fully automated hospital-grade electric breast pump and that it is working correctly and efficiently.

  - Mothers should be instructed to use their own maximum comfortable vacuum setting as soon as the first letdown is detected because most of the milk is removed during the first two milk ejections (Kent et al., 2008).

- Assess for breaks in the pumping schedule or a worsening of the infant's condition.
- Ask if the mother is using oral or injected contraceptives because these have the capacity to diminish milk production.
- If there is an impaired letdown response, milk removal may become inefficient. An infant at breast takes about 56 ± 4 seconds to elicit the letdown response. A breast pump can take up to 147 ± 13 seconds (Kent et al., 2003). Stress and fatigue may further delay milk letdown. Relaxation rituals (Fehrer et al., 1989) or breast massage before pumping may contribute to milk release. Oxytocin nasal spray before pumping can provide a temporary boost to milk ejection. Compounding pharmacies can mix oxytocin into a nasal spray form (Gross, 1995).
- Other medications and interventions (Gabay, 2002) include the use of metoclopramide (Reglan) (Ehrenkranz & Ackerman, 1986; Toppare et al., 1994), acupuncture (Clavey, 1996), domperidone (Motilium) where available (da Silva et al., 2001), and human growth hormone (Gunn et al., 1996). Metoclopramide stimulates prolactin release from the pituitary and is dose related. Metoclopramide is a dopamine antagonist and increases serum prolactin by blocking the inhibitory effect of dopamine on prolactin secretion. Doses of 30–45 mg/day are most effective, with many studies showing 66–100% increases in milk production. Other studies report conflicting results and varying methodologies (Anderson & Valdes, 2007), with some showing no improvement in milk production when mothers take sufficient doses of metoclopramide (Hansen et al., 2005). Mothers who do not respond to metoclopramide therapy may already have elevated levels of prolactin, may be overweight or obese with a blunted prolactin response to suckling, or have other factors that affect the response to prolactin enhancing therapy. Parity may also influence the effect of metoclopramide on prolactin response (Brown et al., 2000). Hale (2008) suggested ascertaining serum prolactin levels before commencing metoclopramide therapy to determine the advisability of instituting such an intervention. Maternal gastric cramping and diarrhea are infrequent side effects, and therapy for longer than 4 weeks may be accompanied by depression in some mothers. Domperidone is a peripheral dopamine antagonist, but unlike metoclopramide it does not enter the brain compartment and it has few central nervous system side effects such as

depression. It is effective in raising serum prolactin levels and increasing milk production in many but not all women (da Silva et al., 2001; Wan et al., 2008).

- Many herbal remedies such as fenugreek and milk thistle have been proposed as popular remedies for low milk production but lack the rigor of studies showing safety, proper dosing, and both intended and unintended effects in mothers of preterm infants. However, Di Pierro et al. (2008) reported that standardized *Silybum marianum* (milk thistle) extract (micronized silymarin, 420 mg/day) improved the milk production in term mothers who were producing marginally adequate amounts of milk.

- The use of mothers' colostrum/milk from days 4 to 14 for early trophic feedings (to stimulate intestinal maturity) yielded an unexpected association with improved breastmilk production (Schanler et al., 1999b). This serves to point out the powerful influence of psychological effects on maternal milk production. Just knowing that her milk is being used for her own baby shows that there may be a two-part effect in beginning early feedings with breastmilk instead of formula (Morton, 2002). Trophic feeds with breastmilk not only improve infant feeding tolerance (Schanler et al., 1999) but also enhance the maternal milk supply.

- Primiparous mothers or mothers with no prior lactation experience may produce lower volumes of milk. Hill et al. (2005) reported that preterm mothers with no prior nursing experience produced 25% less milk than did mothers with previous nursing experience during days 6 and 7 and that lower gestational ages resulted in lower milk output. Therefore mothers with no prior lactations and whose infants are of lower gestational ages constitute a subgroup that requires more vigilant monitoring of their milk production.

- A technique called "power pumping" can be recommended for improving milk output or to rescue a faltering milk supply. The mother pumps for 10–12 minutes, rests for 10–12 minutes, and repeats this process for 1 hour once a day. Some mothers do this twice a day. Power pumping takes advantage of the fact that almost half of the available milk is presented during the first letdown. Pumping five or six times within an hour with breaks in between "tricks" the breast into making this large amount of milk available at each of these minipumping sessions.

Facilitating Early and Frequent Skin-to-Skin Contact Between Mother and Infant

"The relationship between skin-to-skin contact and breastfeeding is fundamental," say Kirsten and colleagues (2001). In industrialized countries structured interventions that focus on kangaroo care and support in the establishment of an abundant milk supply improve the rates of breastfeeding at discharge (Bell et al., 1995). Evidence of the effects of skin-to-skin contact or kangaroo care on breastfeeding shows that

- Breastfeeding duration is extended (Charpak et al., 2001; Ludington-Hoe et al., 1994; Whitelaw et al., 1988).

- Breastmilk production is enhanced (Blaymore-Bier et al., 1996; Hurst et al., 1997; Thompson, 1996).

- The number of breastfeeds per day is increased (Syfrett et al., 1993).

- The breastfeeding competence of the infant is greatly improved (Hedberg Nyqvist, 2001; Koepke & Bigelow, 1997; Widstrom et al., 1988).

- More preterm infants are discharged on exclusive breastfeeding (Cattaneo et al., 1998b; Hann et al., 1999; Hurst et al., 1997).

- With a mean contact of 4.47 hours per day, exclusive breastfeeding is increased at discharge, as well as at 1.5, 3, and 6 months (Hake-Brooks & Anderson, 2008).

- The stability of the cardiorespiratory system is enhanced, hypoglycemia is decreased, and hypothermia is reduced (Bergman et al., 2004).

Implementing Suckling at the Drained Breast

To avoid delays in a preterm infant going to breast, many NICUs have abandoned the requirement of a certain age or weight attainment and simply place the infant at a recently pumped breast when the infant is stable and extubated (Meier, 2001; Narayanan et al., 1991). Guidelines from the international network on kangaroo mother care recommend that direct breastfeeding be started as soon as the infant shows a sucking ability (Cattaneo et al., 1998a). Infants engage in non-nutritive suckling, mouthing, and licking the nipple tip with no expectation of measurable intake but enjoy an introduction to the breast and a taste of their mother's milk. The infant also experiences the positive benefits of non-nutritive suckling (as with a pacifier) but without the side effects of an artificial nipple (Pinelli & Symington,

2000). Infants can next engage in non-nutritive suckling at the breast during gavage feedings. These experiences help shape the desired behavior and make progress toward sucking on a partially full breast with the expectation of a small intake. Even infants weighing less than 1,000 g who are on nasal continuous positive airway pressure can be placed in skin-to-skin contact at the breast and be encouraged to engage in non-nutritive suckling before and during gavage feedings (Hurst & Meier, 2005).

The capacity for increasing intake at the breast develops over time (Hedberg Nyqvist, 2001). It is a function of a number of combined parameters that include gestational age, age in days since birth, the presence or absence of medical complications, maturation of sucking behavior, and especially unlimited access to the breast for repeated learning opportunities. Using the Preterm Infant Breastfeeding Behavior Scale to describe the maturational steps to full breastfeeding, Hedberg Nyqvist et al. (1999) found that healthy preterm infants demonstrated rooting and sucking on the first contact with the breast. Effective rooting, areolar grasp, and latching were observed as early as 28 weeks, and repeated bursts of 10 or more sucks and maximum bursts of 30 or more sucks were seen as early as 32 weeks. Infants pace their feeds by controlling the length of sucking bursts and pauses between bursts to avoid oxygen desaturation and bradycardia from the repeated swallowing seen with artificial nipples. These researchers discussed this type of functional behavior in relation to the repeated opportunities for oral contact with the maternal nipple, exposure to the taste and smell of breastmilk, and the natural extension and modification of activities already performed in utero. The responses elicited by this type of stimulation can alter the trajectory for breastfeeding behaviors that is in line with the assumption that appropriate contingent stimuli and contextual support may reveal an infant's motor behavior that would not otherwise be apparent at a particular time.

Transitioning to Full Feedings at the Breast

Breastfeeding outcomes are optimal if infants transition to the breast before or shortly after discharge. Mothers should be advised of why feedings at the breast are more advantageous than continuing to provide pumped milk by bottle or to supplement with formula (Buckley & Charles, 2006). The sheer amount of time involved in slow feeding sessions at the breast, pumping milk, and monitoring adequate intake may overwhelm a mother as she attempts to transition her infant to exclusive feedings at the breast.

Proper positioning and support at the breast helps to compensate for a number of feeding skill deficits experienced by preterm infants.

1. Place the infant in a clutch (football) or cross-cradle position. These positions afford the best visualization for the mother; support the infant's head, neck, and trunk; allow the mother to adjust the angle of the infant's head to keep the airway from collapsing; and promote maximum chest expansion so the infant is not curled forward, restricting breathing movements.

2. The breast should be supported and "held" in the infant's mouth, because preterm infants generate low levels of vacuum, frequently losing grasp on the nipple–areola. The dancer hand position provides jaw and breast support, and the mother can slightly compress the infant's cheeks if necessary to keep the mouth in contact with the nipple.

3. Weak sucking pressures are not unusual and can result in difficulties staying attached to the nipple as well as initiating and sustaining milk flow and transfer. To compensate for low generation of vacuum, a small ultra-thin silicone nipple shield has been shown to reduce the frequent losing of the nipple and increase the amount of milk transferred per feeding (Clum & Primomo, 1996; Meier et al., 2000). Once the nipple has been drawn into the shield, a vacuum in the semirigid teat keeps the nipple elongated, reducing the workload on the infant of having to repeatedly draw the nipple–areola back into the mouth. A pool of milk remains available at the tip of the shield, rewarding the infant for any compression or vacuum exerted (Wilson-Clay & Hoover, 2002). Many NICUs use non-nutritive sucking opportunities and oral stimulation programs that have been shown to improve breastfeeding rates at discharge and through the first 6 months (Pimenta et al., 2008).

Ensuring Adequate Intake

•   If the infant needs additional milk or a mother has a low milk supply, expressed milk or formula can be provided with a tube-feeding device run under a nipple shield or placed next to the breast.

•   Supplementary or complementary feedings may be necessary until the infant is taking in all the requirements at breast. Test weighing (pre- and postfeed weights) has been used in some nurseries and research settings where accurate measurements of intake are necessary to determine how much supplement to provide (Meier et al., 1994, 1996; Scanlon et al., 2002). Pre- and postfeed weighing is an accurate mechanism to ascertain the amount of breastmilk ingested at the breast, making the calculation for supplementation more precise (Haase et al., 2009).

- To avoid using a bottle to supplement, especially in the absence of the mother, some nurseries follow protocols for providing additional milk through a nasogastric tube (Kliethermes et al., 1999; Stine, 1990) or by cup feeding (Lang et al., 1994). When compared with bottle-feeding, cup feeding is less physiologically stressful (Howard et al., 1999; Marinelli et al., 2001), but spillage or drooling of milk can be a problem (Dowling et al., 2002) if not accounted for. Abouelfettoh et al. (2008) demonstrated that infants cup fed in the hospital showed significantly more mature breastfeeding behaviors for 6 weeks after discharge compared with those who were supplemented with bottles. Cup-fed preterm infants had higher Preterm Infant Breastfeeding Behavior Scale scores than infants supplemented with bottles and had a significantly higher number of breastfeedings 1 week after discharge.

- Nutrition after discharge is designed to avoid growth failure. Some recommendations include fortifying pumped mother's milk with powdered preterm discharge formula, which may be an off-label use of the product. Little data exist as to the safety and efficacy of this practice (Griffin & Cooke, 2007).

Creating a Feeding Plan for Postdischarge Management

In preparation for discharge, infants are usually transitioned to cue-based feedings when they can consume about 50% or more of their feedings, either at the breast or through a combination of breastfeeding and supplementation (Meier, 2003). Cue-based oral feedings often result in an earlier transition to full oral feedings (Kirk et al., 2007). As the time for discharge approaches, feeding plans can be modified to arrange for the mother to stay for a longer visit of perhaps 8 hours during which time the infant is fed on cue, intake per feed is measured by pre- and post-feed weights, and any needed supplementation is provided as an extra feeding or divided over the following feedings in the absence of the mother (Spatz, 2004). Any equipment needed for discharge is secured at this point, including a rented scale. Some mothers find that the use of a tube feeding device at the breast helps their infant to consume the required amount of milk while improving sucking skills, eliminating the need for bottles. Many mothers are given a 24-hour minimum intake that their infant should consume and use the scale to calculate when and if the infant should be supplemented. Once the infant demonstrates the ability to take all feedings from the breast, the scale may be used twice weekly until the infant consistently shows an average daily weight gain of 15–30 g. If the mother has rented a breast pump, she should be instructed to keep it until the infant is fully established at breast. This may actually be 2–4 weeks after discharge when the infant reaches approximately term-corrected age (Hill et al., 1994, 1997).

Although a major concern of mothers of term infants is whether they are producing sufficient amounts of milk, preterm mothers' anxiety centers around whether their infant is consuming adequate amounts of milk (Kavanaugh et al., 1995). Even though the infant may be home, immature feeding skills may still persist—slipping off the nipple, falling asleep at breast at the beginning of a feeding, undependable feeding cue signals, and fussing after a feeding—that indicate to the mother her infant may not be getting enough. Mothers may find that they can use alternate massage at this point to increase the volume and fat content per feeding and use the nipple tug to strengthen the infant's suck. Mothers may also find that hand expressing or pumping just until the milk lets down facilitates improved milk intake by the infant. The infant's low sucking pressure could be inadequate for some mothers to trigger the letdown reflex, resulting in little to no milk transfer (Hurst, 2005).

Breastfeeding Late Preterm Infants

The fastest growing segment of preterm births is that of infants born between 34 0/7 and 36 6/7 weeks. This group represented 72% of the preterm births in 2005 (Hamilton et al., 2007). These infants are not just smaller versions of a full-term infant. Research and clinical experience are finding that preterm birth, by even just 1 week, raises the risk for neonatal morbidity and mortality (Kramer et al., 2000; Raju et al., 2006; Wang et al., 2004). In July 2005 a National Institutes of Health panel recommended that this group of infants be referred to as late preterm rather than near term to better convey their greater vulnerabilities and need for closer monitoring and follow-up. The designation "near term" was thought to mislead parents and clinicians into thinking that these infants are almost term and could thus be treated similar to term infants (Raju et al., 2006). Defining this population of infants helps clarify expectations of parents and clinicians as to how these infants behave and how better to anticipate care based on their unique vulnerabilities. Late preterm infants are at an increased risk for airway instability, apnea, bradycardia, excessive sleepiness, large weight loss, dehydration, feeding difficulties, weak sucking, jaundice, hypoglycemia, hypothermia, immature self-regulation, respiratory distress, sepsis, prolonged artificial milk supplementation, hospital readmission, and breast-feeding failure during the neonatal period (Adamkin, 2006; Engle et al., 2007). Even though some late preterm infants may look like full-term infants, late preterm infants are physiologically, metabolically, and neurologically immature and have limited compensatory mechanisms to adjust to the extrauterine environment.

The last 6 weeks of gestation are a unique period of growth and development for the fetus. At birth, the brain mass of 34- to 35-week late preterm infants is approximately 60% that of term infants, myelinization is markedly underdeveloped, and neuronal connections and synaptic junctions are not fully developed. At the end of 36 weeks of gestation, the brain weight of a premature infant is about 80% that of a term infant's brain weight (Kinney, 2006), affecting such functions as arousal, sleep-wake behavior, and the coordination of feeding with breathing. The immature brainstem adversely impacts upper airway and lung volume control, laryngeal reflexes, and the chemical control of breathing and sleep mechanisms. Ten percent of these infants experience significant apnea of prematurity (Darnall et al., 2006). With their diminished muscle tone, late preterm infants are more prone to positional apnea due to airway obstruction. Their immature autonomic system may demonstrate exaggerated responses to stressful stimuli with rapid or lower heart rates, abnormal breathing, skin mottling, frequent startling, regurgitation, or simply shutting down. Their ability to self-regulate may be limited. They may appear to be irritable, difficult to console, and/or not very responsive to their parents' overtures.

Mothers of late preterm infants may be at increased risk for delayed lactogenesis II. Preterm birth itself often compromises the initiation of lactation, delaying the onset of copious milk production (Cregan et al., 2002) and presenting a prolonged colostral phase to an infant with immature feeding skills. Late preterm infants with limited breastfeeding skills and reduced breastfeeding efficiency and whose mothers present colostrum for an extended period of time are at risk for slow or no weight gain, dehydration, and hyperbilirubinemia. Their mothers are at risk for insufficient milk production.

Late preterm infants are at a disadvantage in terms of feeding skills. They are born with low energy stores (both subcutaneous and brown fat). They have high energy demands, poor feeding abilities, and are sleepy, with fewer and shorter awake periods. They tire easily when feeding, have a weak suck and low tone, demonstrate an inability to sustain sucking, and may have a small mouth, with uncoordinated oral-motor movements. They are easily overstimulated and may shut down before consuming adequate amounts of colostrum or milk. They may take only small volumes of milk during the early days in the hospital, which are often sufficient for that period of time, but exhibit feeding difficulties and slow weight gain when higher volumes of milk intake become necessary for normal growth. Although some infants may demonstrate adequate muscle tone initially, this tone may be rapidly depleted during a feeding, indicating decreased endurance. Postural stability may be immature, creating a less efficient feeding pattern. Late preterm infants experience reduced tone in the muscles involved with feeding, which coupled with neurological immaturity of the suck-swallow-breathe cycle can result in uncoordinated and ineffective milk intake at the breast. If treated like a normal term newborn, they are at an increased risk for inadequate nourishment. They may go through the motions of feeding but may transfer little if any milk for their efforts.

The creation of a breastfeeding plan of care for late preterm infants is directed by their vulnerabilities (Walker, 2008). Breastfeeding management options for this population are often extrapolated from those used with either full-term infants or with infants less than 34 weeks of gestation, neither of which may be completely appropriate for the unique needs of the late preterm population. An in-hospital feeding plan appears in Table 6-7. Breastfeeding interventions are designed to accomplish three goals: prevent adverse outcomes, establish the mother's milk supply, and ensure adequate infant intake.

Careful positioning for breastfeeding is necessary to avoid apnea, bradycardia, or desaturation, especially for younger infants with decreased muscle tone. They are more prone to positional apnea due to airway obstruction and should not be fed in positions that cause excessive flexion of the neck or trunk. The traditional cradle hold is one of the positions to avoid early on, because infants can become so flexed that full rib cage expansion is impeded and the risk of airway collapse is increased. Some infants may prefer slight extension in their neck to keep their airway open. Clutch holds are a better choice for the late preterm infant (Meier et al., 2007). If infants have poor muscle tone, mothers may find that using the dancer hand position helps stabilize the jaw so the infant does not keep slipping off the nipple or does not bite or clench the jaws to keep from sliding off the breast (Danner & Cerutti, 1984). Some infants may need assistance in opening their mouth wide enough to draw in the entire nipple plus part of the areola because they do not exhibit spontaneous mouth opening or do not open their mouth wide enough. Eliciting the rooting reflex may help, as mouth opening is a central component of this reflex. For some infants, mothers can be instructed to gently exert downward pressure on the chin to open the mouth and turn out the lower lip (Wolf & Glass, 1992).

Colson et al. (2003) described a strategy called biological nurturing that involved holding late preterm newborn infants so that their chest, abdomen, and legs were closely flexed around a maternal body contour and unrestricted access to the breast

TABLE 6-7   Sample In-Hospital Breastfeeding Plan for Mothers

Plan	Details
Feed your infant frequently. This helps keep infant's blood sugar from falling and bilirubin from becoming too high.	Within 1 hour after birth Once every hour for the next 3–4 hours Every 2–3 hours until 12 hours of age At least 8 times each 24 hours during the hospital stay
Place infant skin-to-skin on your chest.	This keeps infant warm and the blood sugar from falling. It lets you breastfeed at the first sign of feeding cues.
Watch for rapid eye movements under the eyelids.	This is a sign that infant may be ready to feed.
Move infant to breast when infant shows feeding cues. This helps increase the amount of milk infant takes at a feeding.	Sucking movements of the mouth and tongue Rapid eye movements under the eyelids Hand-to-mouth movements Body movements Small sounds
Make sure you know how to tell when infant is swallowing.	Infant's jaw drops and holds for a second. You hear a "ca" sound. You feel a drawing action on the areola and see it move toward infant's mouth. You hear infant swallow. You feel the swallow when you place a finger on infant's throat. Your nurse hears the swallow when a stethoscope is placed on infant's throat.
Use alternate massage if infant doesn't swallow after every 1–3 sucks.	Massage and squeeze the breast each time infant stops between sucks. Do this on each breast at each feeding. This helps get more colostrum into the infant, avoids fatigue, and keeps him or her sucking longer.
If your infant does not swallow when at the breast, hand express colostrum into a teaspoon and spoon feed 2 teaspoons to your infant using the above guidelines.	Using a breast pump sometimes makes it hard to collect the small amounts of expressed colostrum. Spoon feeding your infant makes sure that he or she is well nourished until able to efficiently feed at your breast.

Source: Adapted from: Walker M. *Breastfeeding the Late Preterm Infant: Improving Care and Outcomes.* Amarillo, TX: Hale Publishing; 2009.

was offered, with abundant skin-to-skin contact. Mothers were encouraged to hold the infant in a biological nurturing position between feedings. The authors suggested that during the 40 weeks of a full-term pregnancy, mothers cannot put their infants down, so physiologically the infant could continue to be incubated or gestated in the mothers' arms during the early days after a late preterm birth. When mothers picked up on feeding cues, infants who appeared to be asleep were observed to be actively sucking at the breast. After the infant was seen to complete a suck-swallow cycle, another cycle was more easily triggered, suggesting that flow regulates suck and that the more swallows achieved, the more sucking that followed. This study suggested that mothers assume an approximately 30-degree semireclining position with the entire frontal aspect of the infant's body draped prone around a natural contour of the mother's body. Breastfeeding in a ventral or abdominal position elicited a system of primitive neonatal reflexes that avoided arching away from the breast and aided latch and sucking as gravity pulled the chin and tongue forward (Colson et al., 2008). Ventral positioning elicited more primitive neonatal feeding reflexes than traditional dorsal positions and triggered antigravity reflexes that inhibited erratic movements of arms and legs or flailing at the breast. Ventral positioning may be tried if the infant arches from the breast, flails, shows erratic movements of the arms and legs, cannot latch to the breast, or if it appears that gravity is overcoming the infant's ability to attach to the breast.

If the infant cannot obtain adequate colostrum or milk directly from the breast with the use of frequent cue-based feeds, with the addition of alternate massage, with help from milk incentives at the breast, or with a nipple shield in place, supplementation may be required. The best supplement is expressed colostrum/milk or banked human milk if available. Feeding volumes of 5–10 mL every 2–3 hours on the first day, 10–20 mL on day 2, and 20–30 mL on day 3 are suggested (Stellwagen et al., 2007). Mothers can hand express colostrum into a spoon and spoon feed this to the infant (Hoover, 1998). One teaspoon equals 5 mL. If a pump is used to express colostrum, small amounts may cling to the sides of the collection container, leaving little for actual use. Pumping into a small container, such as an Ameda diaphragm or the Medela colostrum collection container that has been placed between the valve and the collection bottle of either an Ameda or Medela breast pump, may yield a greater quantity of usable colostrum.

Clinicians and mothers find it beneficial to mutually create an individualized breastfeeding plan for use after discharge. A sample plan appears in Table 6-8. It can and should be modified to best provide mothers with the tools they need to successfully breastfeed their infants.

TABLE 6-8 Sample Discharge Breastfeeding Plan for Your Late Preterm Infant

---

Your milk and feeding at the breast are very important to your late preterm infant. Even though your infant may look full-term, he or she is not fully developed and may need some extra help and time learning to breastfeed. Your milk contains ingredients that provide protection from disease and help promote your infant's brain development that was interrupted by an early birth. Your infant may tire easily before a feeding is finished and may seem to sleep a lot. These guidelines will help get breastfeeding off to a good start.

Feed your infant on cue 8–12 times each 24 hours. Early infants are not always reliable in telling you when they need to feed. Sleeping is not an indication that infant is getting enough. Use these signs as a cue to feed if your infant is very sleepy:

- Sucking movements of the mouth and tongue
- Rapid eye movements under the eyelids
- Hand-to-mouth movements
- Body movements
- Small sounds

Place your infant in a clutch or cross-cradle position. If your infant has difficulty attaching to the breast, flails at the breast, or arches away from the breast, use a semireclining position. Recline to a 30-degree angle, place your infant on his or her tummy with mouth directly over the nipple. This allows gravity to bring his or her chin and tongue forward and help the infant latch.

As your infant latches on, make sure his or her mouth is wide open.

You should hear or feel your infant swallowing every 1–3 sucks during most of the feeding.

Use alternate massage on each breast at each feeding to keep infant sucking and increase the amount of milk he or she receives at each feeding. Thoroughly massage and compress each part of the breast so that milk does not back up and set the stage for plugged ducts or an infection.

If you are not sure how much milk your infant is getting at each feeding, you can weigh infant before and after a feeding. This will help you know if you need to offer a supplement.

Record each feeding, whether a supplement is used, the amount of pumped milk, the number of wet diapers, and the number of bowel movements on your feeding log until infant is reliably feeding and gaining weight.

(continues)

TABLE 6-8   Sample Discharge Breastfeeding Plan for Your Late Preterm Infant *(continued)*

If your infant does not latch to the breast, try the following:

- Gently roll your nipple between your fingers to make it easier for the infant to grasp.
- As you bring your infant to breast, have a helper place a tube feeding device or dropper in the corner of the infant's mouth and deliver a small amount of milk as the infant attempts to latch. If the infant swallows and attempts to latch again, another small amount of milk can be given. Repeat until infant no longer attempts to latch. These practice sessions should not last longer than 10 minutes to avoid tiring both you and your infant.
- Finish the feeding by finger or cup feeding.
- If the attempts at latching do not work, you may find that a silicone nipple shield allows the infant to latch and sustain sucking at the breast. Moisten the shield with warm water, turn almost inside-out as you apply it to the breast, apply a little breastmilk to the outside of the shield, hand express milk into the shield tunnel, and bring the infant to breast. If the infant latches, continue using alternate massage throughout the feeding.

Infant should have at least 6 wet diapers and 3 or more bowel movements each day by the fifth day. Bowel movements should start turning yellow by day 4. Meconium diapers on day 5 may indicate that infant is not getting enough milk. Uric acid crystals (red stains) on day 4 in wet diapers may also indicate that infant is not transferring enough milk at the breast.

Take your infant to the physician's office 2 days after coming home from the hospital for a weight check and to make sure he or she is not jaundiced. A weight check every 3 days or so ensures that your infant continues to gain about ½ to 1 ounce per day.

If infant cannot feed long enough at each feeding or is not gaining well, supplements of expressed breastmilk can be given by tube feeding at the breast, finger feeding, cup feeding, or bottle-feeding. If you do not have enough milk to use as a supplement, a hydrolyzed formula can be used until your milk production has increased.

Continue to pump your milk 2–3 times each day to use as a supplement and to improve your milk supply. Try "power pumping" for an hour once or twice each day. Pump for 5–10 minutes until the milk stops spraying from the first letdown. Wait 10 minutes or so and pump again until the milk stops spraying. Almost half of the milk that is available in the breast is pumped with the first letdown. Power pumping takes advantage of these "first" letdowns to mimic frequent feedings and helps increase your milk production. Depending on how your infant is doing at the breast, pumping should continue until he or she is 40–42 weeks corrected age, weaning off the pump over the first month home.

Source: Adapted from: Walker M. *Breastfeeding the Late Preterm Infant: Improving Care and Outcomes.* Amarillo, TX: Hale Publishing; 2009.

Summary: The Design in Nature

Whereas many breastfeeding problems remain iatrogenic, others are created by circumstances surrounding the birth of the infant. Mothers and clinicians require patience and persistence, because there is frequently no quick fix for some of these issues. Most of these problems and situations do not require avoiding or abandoning breastfeeding, just better breastfeeding management.

References

Abouelfettoh, A. M., Dowling, D. A., Dabash, S. A., Elguindy, S. R., & Seoud, I. A. (2008). Cup versus bottle feeding for hospitalized late preterm infants in Egypt: A quasi-experimental study. *Int Breastfeeding J. 3*, 27.

Adamkin, D. H. (2006). Feeding problems in the late preterm infant. *Clin Perinatol., 33*, 831–837.

Agostoni, C., Grandi, F., Scaglioni, S., et al. (2000). Growth pattern of breastfed and nonbreastfed infants with atopic dermatitis in the first year of life. *Pediatrics, 106*, e73.

Akaba, K., Kimura, T., Sasaki, A., et al. (1998). Neonatal hyperbilirubinemia and mutation of the bilirubin uridine diphosphate-glucuronosyltransferase gene: A common missense mutation among Japanese, Koreans and Chinese. *Biochem Mol Biol Int., 46*, 21–26.

Aksit, S., Ozkayin, N., & Caglayan, S. (2002). Effect of sucking characteristics on breast milk creamatocrit. *Paediatr Perinat Epidemiol., 16*, 355–360.

American Academy of Pediatrics [AAP]. (1994). Practice parameter: Management of hyperbilirubinemia in the healthy term newborn. *Pediatrics, 94*(4 pt 1), 558–562.

American Academy of Pediatrics [AAP]. (2001a). Neonatal jaundice and kernicterus. *Pediatrics, 108*, 763–765.

American Academy of Pediatrics [AAP], Committee on Drugs. (2001b). The transfer of drugs and chemicals into human milk. *Pediatrics, 108*, 776–789.

American Academy of Pediatrics [AAP]. (2003). *Red book. Report of the committee on infectious diseases* (26th ed.). Elk Grove Village, IL: Author.

American Academy of Pediatrics [AAP]. (2004a). Policy statement: Hospital stay for healthy term newborns. *Pediatrics, 113*, 1434–1436.

American Academy of Pediatrics [AAP], Subcommittee on Hyperbilirubinemia. (2004b). Clinical practice guideline: Management of hyperbilirubinemia in the newborn infant 35 or more weeks of gestation. *Pediatrics, 114*, 297–316.

American Academy of Pediatrics [AAP], Section on Breastfeeding. (2005). Breastfeeding and the use of human milk. *Pediatrics, 115*, 496–506.

Anderson, J. W., Johnstone, B. M., & Remley, D. T. (1999). Breastfeeding and cognitive development: A meta-analysis. *Am J Clin Nutr., 70*, 525–535.

Anderson, P. O., Pochop, S. L., & Manoguerra, A. S. (2003). Adverse drug reactions in breastfed infants: Less than imagined. *Clin Pediatr., 42*, 325–340.

Anderson, P. O., & Valdes, V. (2007). A critical review of pharmaceutical galactagogues. *Breastfeeding Med., 2*, 229–242.

Askin, D. B., & Diehl-Jones, W. L. (2005). Improving on perfection: Breast milk and breast-milk additives for preterm neonates. *Newborn Infant Nurs Rev., 5*, 10–18.

Atkinson, S. A. (2000). Human milk feeding of the micropremie. *Clin Perinatol., 27*, 235–247.

Auerbach, K. G., & Gartner, L. M. (1987). Breastfeeding and human milk: Their association with jaundice in the neonate. *Clin Perinatol., 14,* 89–107.

Auerbach, K. G., & Walker, M. (1994). When the mother of a premature infant uses a breast pump: What every NICU nurse needs to know. *Neonatal Network, 13,* 23–29.

Baker, B. J., & Rasmussen, T. W. (1997). Organizing and documenting lactation support of NICU families. *JOGNN, 26,* 515–521.

Bartoletti, A. L., et al. (1979). Pulmonary excretion of carbon monoxide in the human infant as an index of bilirubin production. Part I: Effects of gestational age and postnatal age and some common neonatal abnormalities. *J Pediatr., 94,* 952–955.

Bell, E. H., Geyer, J., & Jones, L. (1995). A structured intervention improves breastfeeding success for ill or preterm infants. *MCN, 20,* 309–314.

Bergman, N. J., Linley, L. L., & Fawcus, S. R. (2004). Randomized controlled trial of skin-to-skin contact from birth versus conventional incubator for physiological stabilization in 1200 g to 2199 g neonates. *Acta Paediatr., 93,* 779–785.

Bertini, G., Dani, C., Tronchin, M., & Rubaltelli, F. F. (2001). Is breastfeeding really favoring early neonatal jaundice? *Pediatrics, 107,* e41. Retrieved September 14, 2005, from www.pediatrics.org/cgi/content/full/107/3/e41

Beutler, E., Gelbart, T., & Demina, A. (1998). Racial variability in the UDP-glucuronosyltransferase 1 (UGT1A1) promoter: A balanced polymorphism for regulation of bilirubin metabolism? *Proc Natl Acad Sci USA, 95,* 8170–8174.

Bhat, B. A., & Gupta, B. (2003). Effects of human milk fortification on morbidity factors in very low birth weight infants. *Annals of Saudi Medicine, 23,* 28–31.

Bhutani, V. K., Gourley, G. R., Adler, S., et al. (2000). Noninvasive measurement of total serum bilirubin in a multiracial predischarge newborn population to assess the risk of severe hyperbilirubinemia. *Pediatrics, 106,* e17. Retrieved September 14, 2005, from www.pediatrics.org/cgi/content/full/106/2/e17

Bhutani, V. K., Johnson, L. H., & Keren, R. (2004). Diagnosis and management of hyperbilirubinemia in the term neonate: For a safer first week. *Pediatr Clin North Am., 51,* 843–861.

Bhutani, V. K., Johnson, L. H., & Sivieri, E. M. (1999a). Risk assessment of hyperbilirubinemia in near-term newborns. *Pediatrics, 104*(Suppl 3), 741.

Bhutani, V. K., Johnson, L., & Sivieri, E. M. (1999b). Predictive ability of a predischarge hour-specific serum bilirubin for subsequent significant hyperbilirubinemia in healthy term and near-term newborns. *Pediatrics, 103,* 6–14.

Bier, J. B., Ferguson, A., Anderson, L., et al. (1993). Breastfeeding of very low birth-weight infants. *J Pediatr., 23,* 773–778.

Binns, C., James, J., & Lee, M. K. (2008). Why the new WHO growth charts are dangerous to breastfeeding. *Breastfeeding Rev., 16,* 5–7.

Bishara, R., Dunn, M. S., Merko, S. E., & Darling, P. (2009). Volume of foremilk, hindmilk, and total milk produced by mothers of very preterm infants born at less than 28 weeks of gestation. *J Hum Lact., 25,* 272–279.

Blackburn, S. (1995). Hyperbilirubinemia and neonatal jaundice. *Neonatal Network, 14,* 15–25.

Blackburn, S. T., & Loper, D. L. (1992). *Maternal, fetal, and neonatal physiology: A clinical perspective.* Philadelphia: W.B. Saunders.

Blackmon, L. R., Fanaroff, A. A., & Raju, T. N. K. (2004). Research on prevention of bilirubin-induced brain injury and kernicterus: National Institute of Child Health and Human Development conference executive summary. *Pediatrics, 114,* 229–233.

Blaymore-Bier, J. A. (1997). Breastfeeding infants who were extremely low birth weight. *Pediatrics, 100,* e3.

Blaymore-Bier, J. A., Ferguson, A. E., Morales, Y., et al. (1996). Comparison of skin-to-skin contact with standard contact in low-birth-weight infants who are breastfed. *Arch Pediatr Adolesc Med., 150,* 1265.

Braveman, P., Egerter, S., Pearl, M., et al. (1995). Early discharge of newborns and mothers: A critical review of the literature. *Pediatrics, 96*, 716–726.

Braveman, P., Kessel, W., Egerter, S., & Richmond, J. (1997). Early discharge and evidence-based practice: Good science and good judgment. *JAMA, 278*, 334–336.

Britton, J. R., Britton, H. L., & Beebe, S. A. (1994). Early discharge of the term newborn: A continued dilemma. *Pediatrics, 94*, 291–295.

Brodersen, R., & Herman, L. S. (1963). Intestinal reabsorption of unconjugated bilirubin. *Lancet, 1*, 1242.

Brown, A. K., Damus, K., Kim, M. H., et al. (1999). Factors relating to readmission of term and near-term neonates the first two weeks of life. Early discharge survey group of the health professional advisory board of the greater New York chapter of the March of Dimes. *J Perinat Med., 27*, 263–275.

Brown, T. E., Fernandes, P. A., Grant, L. J., Hutsul, J. A., & McCoshen, J. A. (2000). Effect of parity on pituitary prolactin response to metoclopramide and domperidone: Implications for the enhancement of lactation. *J Soc Gynecol Investig., 7*, 65–69.

Buckley, K. M., & Charles, G. E. (2006). Benefits and challenges of transitioning preterm infants to at-breast feedings. *Int Breastfeeding J., 1*, 13.

Burke, B. L., Robbins, J. M., MacBird, T., Hobbs, C. A., Nesmith, C., & Tilford, J. M. (2009). Trends in hospitalizations for neonatal jaundice and kernicterus in the United States, 1988–2005. *Pediatrics, 123*, 524–532.

Caglar, M. K., Ozer, I., & Altugan, F. S. (2006). Risk factors for excess weight loss and hypernatremia in exclusively breastfed infants. *Brazilian Journal of Medical and Biological Research, 39*, 539–544.

California Perinatal Quality Care Collaborative. (2008). Nutritional support of the very low birth weight infant. Retrieved April 11, 2009, from www.cpqcc.org/quality_improvement/qi_toolkits/nutritional_support_of_the_vlbw_infant_rev_december_2008

Callen, J., Pinelli, J., Atkinson, S., & Saigal, S. (2005). Qualitative analysis of barriers to breastfeeding in very-low-birthweight infants in the hospital and postdischarge. *Adv Neonat Care, 5*, 93–103.

Capretti, M. G., Lanari, M., Lazzarotto, T., et al. (2009). Very low birth weight infants born to cytomegalovirus-seropositive mothers fed with their mother's milk: A prospective study. *J Pediatr., 154*:842–848.

Carceller-Blanchard, A., Cousineau, J., & Delvin, E. E. (2009). Point of care testing: Transcutaneous bilirubinometry in neonates. *Clin Biochem., 42*, 143–149.

Carter, K., & Dixon, K. (2001). Morbidity and Mortality Weekly Report. Kernicterus in full-term infants—United States, 1994–1998. *MMWR, 50*, 491–494.

Cashore, W. J. (1998). Bilirubin metabolism and toxicity in the newborn. In P. A. Polin & W. W. Fox (Eds.), *Fetal and neonatal physiology*. Philadelphia: W.B. Saunders.

Castrucci, B. C., Hoover, K. L., Lim, S., & Maus, K. C. (2007). Availability of lactation counseling services influences breastfeeding among infants admitted to neonatal intensive care units. *Am J Health Promotion, 21*, 410–415.

Cattaneo, A., Davanzo, R., Uxa, F., & Tamburlini, G., for the International Network on Kangaroo Mother Care. (1998a). II. Recommendations for the implementation of the kangaroo mother care for low birthweight infants. *Acta Paediatr., 87*, 440–445.

Cattaneo, A., Davanzo, R., Worku, B., et al. (1998b). Kangaroo mother care for low birthweight infants: A randomized controlled trial in different settings. *Acta Paediatr., 87*, 976–985.

Cattaneo, A., & Guoth-Gumberger, M. (2008). The new WHO child growth standards: Possible effects on exclusive breastfeeding in the first six months. *Breastfeeding Rev., 16*, 9–12.

Centers for Disease Control and Prevention [CDC]. (2002). *Enterobacter sakazakii* infections associated with the use of powdered infant formula—Tennessee, 2001. *MMWR, 51*, 298–300.

Chan, G. (2003). Effects of powdered human milk fortifiers on the antimicrobial actions of human milk. *J Perinatol., 23*, 620–623.

Charpak, N., Ruiz-Pelaez, J. G., de Figueroa, C. Z., & Charpak, Y. (2001). A randomized, controlled trial of kangaroo mother care: Results of follow-up at 1 year of corrected age. *Pediatrics, 108,* 1072–1079.

Claud, E. C., & Walker, A. (2001). Hypothesis: Inappropriate colonization of the premature intestine can cause neonatal necrotizing enterocolitis. *FASEB Journal, 15,* 1398–1403.

Clavey, S. (1996). The use of acupuncture for the treatment of insufficient lactation. (Que Ru). *Am J Acupuncture, 24,* 35–46.

Clum, D., & Primomo, J. (1996). Use of a silicone nipple shield with premature infants. *J Hum Lact., 12,* 287–290.

Colson, S. D., de Rooy, L., & Hawdon, J. M. (2003). Biological nurturing increases duration of breast-feeding for a vulnerable cohort. *MIDIRS Midwifery Digest, 13,* 92–97.

Colson, S. D., Meek, J. H., & Hawdon, J. M. (2008). Optimal positions for the release of primitive neonatal reflexes stimulating breastfeeding. *Early Hum Dev., 84,* 441–449.

Cooper, W. O., Atherton, H. D., Kahana, M., & Kotagal, U. R. (1995). Increased incidence of severe breast-feeding malnutrition and hypernatremia in a metropolitan area. *Pediatrics, 96*(5 pt 1), 957–960.

Corbett, S. S., & Drewett, R. F. (2004). To what extent is failure to thrive in infancy associated with poorer cognitive development? A review and meta-analysis. *J Child Psychol Psychiat, 45,* 641–654.

Costello, A., & Chapman, J. (1998). Mothers' perceptions of the care-by-parent program prior to hospital discharge of their preterm infants. *Neonatal Network, 17,* 37–42.

Cregan, M. D., De Mello, T. R., Kershaw, D., et al. (2002). Initiation of lactation in women after preterm delivery. *Acta Obstetricia et Gynecologica Scandinavica, 81,* 870–877.

Dahms, B. B., Krauss, A. N., Gartner, L. M., et al. (1973). Breastfeeding and serum bilirubin values during the first 4 days of life. *J Pediatr., 83,* 1049–1054.

Daly, S. E., Kent, J. C., Owens, R. A., & Hartmann, P. E. (1996). Frequency and degree of milk removal and the short-term control of human milk synthesis. *Exp Physiol., 81,* 861–875.

Danner, S. C., & Cerutti, E. R. (1984). *Nursing your neurologically impaired baby.* Rochester, NY: Childbirth Graphics.

Danner, E., Joeckel, R., Michalak, S., Phillips, S., & Goday, P. S. (2009). Weight velocity in infants and children. *Nutr Clin Pract., 24,* 76–79.

Darnall, R. A., Ariagno, R. L., & Kinney, H. C. (2006). The late preterm infant and the control of breathing, sleep, and brainstem development: A review. *Clin Perinatol., 33,* 883–914.

Da Silva, O. P., et al. (2001). Effect of domperidone on milk production in mothers of premature newborns: A randomized double blind, placebo-controlled trial. *CMAJ, 164,* 17–21.

De Carvalho, M., Hall, M., & Harvey, D. (1981). Effects of water supplementation on physiological jaundice in breastfed infants. *Arch Dis Child, 56,* 568–569.

De Carvalho, M., Klaus, M. H., & Merkatz, R. B. (1982). Frequency of breastfeeding and serum bilirubin concentration. *Am J Dis Child, 136,* 737–738.

De Onis, M., Garza, C., Onyango, A. W., & Borghi, E. (2007). Comparison of the WHO Child Growth Standards and the CDC 2000 growth charts. *J Nutr., 137,* 144–148.

De Onis, M., Garza, C., Onyango, A. W., & Martorell, R. (Eds.). (2006a). WHO Child Growth Standards. *Acta Paediatr Suppl., 450,* 1–101.

De Onis, M., Onyango, A. W., Borghi, E., Garza, C., & Yang, H. (2006b). Comparison of the World Health Organization (WHO) Child Growth Standards and the National Center for Health Statistics/WHO International Growth Reference: Implications for child health programmes. *Public Health and Nutrition, 9,* 942–947.

Dennery, P. A., Seidman, D. S., & Stevenson, D. K. (2001). Neonatal hyperbilirubinemia. *N Engl J Med., 344,* 581–590.

Desmarais, L., & Browne, S. (1990). Inadequate weight gain in breastfeeding infants: Assessments and resolutions. In K. G. Auerbach (Ed.), *Lactation consultant series*. Garden City Park, NY: Avery Publishing Group.

Dewey, K. G. (2001). Nutrition, growth and complementary feeding of the breastfed infant. *Pediatr Clin North Am., 48*, 87–104.

Dewey, K. G., Heinig, M. J., Nommsen, L. A., et al. (1992). Growth of breastfed and formula-fed infants from 0 to 18 months: The DARLING study. *Pediatrics, 89*, 1035–1041.

Dewey, K. G., Nommsen-Rivers, L. A., Heinig, M. J., & Cohen, R. J. (2003). Risk factors for suboptimal infant breastfeeding behavior, delayed onset of lactation, and excess neonatal weight loss. *Pediatrics, 112*, 607–619.

Dewey, K. G., Peerson, J. M., Brown, K. H., et al. (1995). WHO working group on infant growth: Growth of breastfed infants deviates from current reference data: A pooled analysis of US, Canadian, and European data sets. *Pediatrics, 96*, 495–503.

Di Pierro, F., Callegari, A., Carotenuto, D., & Tapia, M. M. (2008). Clinical efficacy, safety and tolerability of BIO-C (micronized Silymarin) as a galactagogue. *Acta Biomedica, 79*, 205–210.

Dixit, R., & Gartner, L. (2000). The jaundiced newborn: Minimizing the risks. *Patient Care, 34*, 45–69.

Dougherty, D., & Luther, M. (2008). Birth to breast—a feeding care map for the NICU: Helping the extremely low birth weight infant navigate the course. *Neonatal Network, 27*, 371–377.

Dowling, D. A., et al. (2002). Cup feeding for preterm infants: Mechanics and safety. *J Hum Lact., 18*, 13–20.

Drewett, R. F., Emond, A., Blair, P., & Emmett, P. (2005). The importance of slow weight gain in the first 2 months in identifying children who fail to thrive. *J Reprod Infant Psychol., 23*, 309–317.

Eaton, A. P. (2001). Early postpartum discharge: Recommendations from a preliminary report to Congress [commentary]. *Pediatrics, 107*, 400–404.

Egerter, S. A., Braverman, P. A., & Marchi, K. S. (1998). Follow-up of newborns and their mothers after early hospital discharge. *Clin Perinatol., 25*, 471–481.

Ehrenkranz, R., & Ackerman, B. (1986). Metoclopramide effect on faltering milk production by mothers of premature infants. *Pediatrics, 78*, 614–619.

Elander, G., & Lindberg, T. (1984). Hospital routines in infants with hyperbilirubinemia influence the duration of breastfeeding. *Acta Paediatr Scand., 73*, 708–712.

Elliott, S., & Reimer, C. (1998). Postdischarge telephone follow-up program for breastfeeding preterm infants discharged from a special care nursery. *Neonatal Network, 17*, 41–45.

Emond, A. M., Blair, P. S., Emmett, P. M., & Drewett, R. F. (2007a). Weight faltering in infancy and IQ levels at 8 years in the Avon Longitudinal Study of Parents and Children. *Pediatrics, 120*, e1051–e1058.

Emond, A., Drewett, R., Blair, P., & Emmett, P. (2007b). Postnatal factors associated with failure to thrive in term infants in the Avon Longitudinal Study of Parents and Children. *Arch Dis Child, 92*, 115–119.

Engle, W. A., Tomashek, K. M., Wallman, C., & Committee on Fetus and Newborn, American Academy of Pediatrics. (2007). "Late-preterm" infants: A population at risk. *Pediatrics, 120*, 1390–1401.

Escobar, G. J., Gonzales, V. M., Armstrong, M. A., et al. (2002). Rehospitalization for neonatal dehydration. *Arch Pediatr Adolesc Med., 156*, 155–161.

Evans, K. C., Evans, R. G., Royal, R., et al. (2003). Effect of caesarean section on breast milk transfer to the normal term newborn over the first week of life. *Arch Dis Child. Fetal and Neonatal Edition, 88*, F380–F382.

Fehrer, S., Berger, L., Johnson, J., & Wilde, J. (1989). Increasing breastmilk production for premature infants with a relaxation/imagery audiotape. *Pediatrics, 83*, 57–60.

Feldman, R., Weller, A., Leckman, J. F., et al. (1999). The nature of the mother's tie to her infant: Maternal bonding under conditions of proximity, separation, and potential loss. *J Child Psychol Psychiatr., 40*, 929–939.

Foman, S. J., Nelson, S. E. (1993). Size and growth. In S. J. Foman (Ed.), *Nutrition of normal infants*. St. Louis, MO: Mosby.

Forsyth, T. J., Maney, L. A., Ramirez, A., et al. (1998). Nursing case management in the NICU: Enhanced coordination for discharge planning. *Neonatal Network, 17*, 23–34.

Frantz, K. B. (1992). The slow-gaining breastfeeding infant. *NAACOG's Clinical Issues in Perinatal and Women's Health Nursing: Breastfeeding, 3*, 647–655.

Furman, L., Minich, N. M., & Hack, M. (1998). Breastfeeding of very low birth weight infants. *J Hum Lact., 14*, 29–34.

Furman, L., Minich, N., & Hack, M. (2002). Correlates of lactation in mothers of very low birth weight infants. *Pediatrics, 109*, 695–696.

Gabay, M. P. (2002). Galactagogues: Medications that induce lactation. *J Hum Lact., 18*, 274–279.

Gartner, L. M. (2001). Breastfeeding and jaundice. *J Perinatol., 21*, S25–S29.

Gartner, L. M., & Herschel, M. (2001). Jaundice and breastfeeding. *Pediatr Clin North Am., 48*, 389–399.

Garza, C., & de Onis, M. (2004). WHO Multicentre Growth Reference Study Group. Rationale for developing a new international growth reference. *Food and Nutrition Bulletin, 24*(Suppl 1), S5–S14.

Gonzalez, K. A., Meinzen-Derr, J., Burke, B. L., et al. (2003). Evaluation of a lactation support service in a children's hospital neonatal intensive care unit. *J Hum Lact., 19*, 286–292.

Gourley, G. R., Kreamer, B. L., & Cohnen, M. (1997). Inhibition of beta-glucuronidase by casein hydrolysate formula. *J Pediatr Gastroenterol., 25*, 267–272.

Gourley, G. R., Kreamer, B., Cohnen, M., & Kosorok, M. R. (1999). Neonatal jaundice and diet. *Arch Pediatr Adolesc Med., 153*, 184–188.

Gourley, G. R., Zhanhai, L., Kreamer, B. L., & Kosorok, M. R. (2005). A controlled, randomized, double-blind trial of prophylaxis against jaundice among breastfed newborns. *Pediatrics, 116*, 385–391.

Griffin, I. J., & Cooke, R. J. (2007). Nutrition of preterm infants after hospital discharge. *J Pediatr Gastroenterol Nutr., 45*(Suppl 3), S195–S203.

Gross, M. S. (1995). Letter. *ILCA Globe, 3*, 5.

Grupp-Phelan, J., Taylor, J. A., Liu, L. L., & Davis, R. L. (1999). Early newborn hospital discharge and readmission for mild and severe jaundice. *Arch Pediatr Adolesc Med., 153*, 1283–1288.

Guerrini, P. (1994). Human milk fortifiers. *Acta Paediatr., 402*(Suppl), 37–39.

Gunn, A. J., et al. (1996). Growth hormone increases breast milk volumes in mothers of preterm infants. *Pediatrics, 98*, 279–282.

Haase, B., Barreira, J., Murphy, P. K., Mueller, M., & Rhodes, J. (2009). The development of an accurate test weighing technique for preterm and high-risk hospitalized infants. *Breastfeeding and Medicine*, 4: 151–156.

Hake-Brooks, S. J., & Anderson, G. C. (2008). Kangaroo care and breastfeeding of mother-preterm infant dyads 0–18 months: A randomized, controlled trial. *Neonatal Network, 27*, 151–159.

Hale, T. W. (2003). Medications in breastfeeding mothers of preterm infants. *Pediatric Annals, 32*, 337–347.

Hale, T. W. (2008). *Medications and mothers' milk* (13th ed.). Amarillo, TX: Hale Publishing.

Hall, R. T., Simon, S., & Smith, M. T. (2000). Readmission of breastfed infants in the first 2 weeks of life. *J Perinatol., 20*, 432–437.

Hamilton, B. E., Martin, J. A., & Ventura, S. J. (2007). *Births: Preliminary data for 2006*. National Vital Statistics Reports, vol. 56, no. 7. Hyattsville, MD: National Center for Health Statistics.

Hamilton, B. E., Martin, J. A., & Ventura, S. J. (2009). *Births: Preliminary data for 2007*. National Vital Statistics Reports, vol. 57, no. 12. Hyattsville, MD: National Center for Health Statistics. Retrieved April 10, 2009, from www.cdc.gov/nchs/data/nvsr/nvsr57/nvsr57_12.pdf

Hamprecht, K., Maschmann, J., Jahn, G., Poets, C. F., & Goelz, R. (2008). Cytomegalovirus transmission to preterm infants during lactation. *J Clin Virol., 41*, 198–205.

Hanko, E., Lindemann, R., & Hansen, T. W. R. (2001). Spectrum of outcome in infants with extreme neonatal jaundice. *Acta Paediatr., 90,* 782–785.

Hann, M., Malan, A., Kronson, M., et al. (1999). Kangaroo mother care. *South African Medical Journal, 89,* 37.

Hannon, P. R., Willis, S. K., & Scrimshaw, S. C. (2001). Persistence of maternal concerns surrounding neonatal jaundice: An exploratory study. *Arch Pediatr Adolesc Med., 155,* 1357–1363.

Hansen, T. W. (2000). Bilirubin oxidation in the brain. *Molecular and Genetic Metabolism, 71,* 411–417.

Hansen, T. W. (2001). Bilirubin brain toxicity. *J Perinatol., 21,* S48–S51.

Hansen, T. W. (2003). Recent advances in the pharmacotherapy for hyperbilirubinemia in the neonate. *Expert Opinion in Pharmacotherapy, 4,* 1939–1948.

Hansen, T. W., Allen, J. W., & Tommarello, S. (1999). Oxidation of bilirubin in the brain—Further characterization of a potentially protective mechanism. *Molecular and Genetic Metabolism, 68,* 404–409.

Hansen, T. W. R. (1994). Bilirubin in the brain. *Clin Pediatr., 33,* 452–459.

Hansen, T. W. R. (2002). Mechanisms of bilirubin toxicity: Clinical implications. *Clin Perinatol., 29,* 765–778.

Hansen, W. F., McAndrew, S., Harris, K., & Zimmerman, M. B. (2005). Metoclopramide effect on breastfeeding the preterm infant: A randomized trial. *Obstet Gynecol., 105,* 383–389.

Harding, D., Cairns, P., Gupta, S., et al. (2001). Hypernatremia: Why bother weighing breastfed babies? *Arch Dis Child. Fetal and Neonatal Edition, 85,* F145.

Harris, M. C., Bernbaum, J. C., Polin, J. R., et al. (2001). Developmental follow-up of breastfed term and near-term infants with marked hyperbilirubinemia. *Pediatrics, 107,* 1075–1080.

Hedberg Nyqvist, K. (2001). The development of preterm infants' milk intake during breastfeeding. *J Neonat Nurs., 7,* 48–52.

Hedberg Nyqvist, K., Sjoden, P.-O., & Ewald, U. (1999). The development of preterm infants' breastfeeding behavior. *Early Hum Dev., 55,* 247–264.

Heiskanen, K., Siimes, M. A., & Salmenpera Perheentupa, J. (1995). Low vitamin B_6 status associated with slow growth in healthy breastfed infants. *Pediatr Res., 38,* 740–746.

Helliker, K. (1994). Dying for milk. Some mothers try in vain to breastfeed, starve their infants. *Wall Street Journal,* July 22, pp. 1, 4.

Henderson, J. J., Hartmann, P. E., Newnham, J. P., & Simmer, K. (2008). Effect of preterm birth and antenatal corticosteroid treatment on lactogenesis II in women. *Pediatrics, 121,* e92–e100.

Herschel, M. (2003). *Jaundice and Breastfeeding.* Independent study module #12. Schaumburg, IL: La Leche League International.

Hill, P. D., Aldag, J. C., & Chatterton, R. T. (1999). Effects of pumping style on milk production in mothers of non-nursing preterm infants. *J Hum Lact., 15,* 209–216.

Hill, P. D., Aldag, J. C., & Chatterton, R. T. (2001). Initiation and frequency of pumping and milk production in mothers of non-nursing preterm infants. *J Hum Lact., 17,* 9–13.

Hill, P. D., Aldag, J. C., Chatterton, R. T., & Zinaman, M. (2005). Primary and secondary mediators' influence on milk output in lactating mothers of preterm and term infants. *J Hum Lact., 21,* 138–150.

Hill, P. D., Aldag, J. C., Demirtas, H., et al. (2009). Association of serum prolactin and oxytocin with milk production in mothers of preterm and term infants. *Biolog Res Nurs., 10,* 340–349.

Hill, P. D., Aldag, J. C., Zinaman, M. D., & Chatterton, R. T. (2007). Comparison of milk output between breasts in pump-dependent mothers. *J Hum Lact., 23,* 333–337.

Hill, P. D., Brown, L. P., & Harker, T. L. (1995). Initiation and frequency of breast expression in breastfeeding mothers of LBW and VLBW infants. *Nurs Res., 44,* 352–355.

Hill, P. D., Hanson, K. S., & Mefford, A. L. (1994). Mothers of low birthweight infants: Breastfeeding patterns and problems. *J Hum Lact., 10,* 169–176.

Hill, P. D., Ledbetter, R. J., & Kavanaugh, K. (1997). Breastfeeding patterns in low-birth-weight infants after hospital discharge. *JOGNN, 26,* 190–197.

Hoover, K. (1998). Supplementation of the newborn by spoon in the first 24 hours. *J Hum Lact., 14,* 245.

Hoover, K. L., Barbalinardo, L. H., & Platia, M. P. (2002). Delayed lactogenesis II secondary to gestational ovarian theca lutein cysts in two normal singleton pregnancies. *J Hum Lact., 18,* 264–268.

Hopkinson, J. M., Schanler, R. J., Fraley, J. K., & Garza, C. (1992). Milk production by mothers of premature infants: Influence of cigarette smoking. *Pediatrics, 90,* 934–938.

Hopkinson, J. M., Schanler, R. J., & Garza, C. (1988). Milk production by mothers of premature infants. *Pediatrics, 81,* 815–820.

Horwood, L. J., Darlow, B. A., & Mogridge, N. (2001). Breast milk feeding and cognitive ability at 7–8 years. *Arch Dis Child. Fetal and Neonatal Edition, 84,* F23–F27.

Howard, C. R., de Blieck, E. A., ten Hoopen, C. B., et al. (1999). Physiologic stability of newborns during cup- and bottle-feeding. *Pediatrics, 104,* 1204–1207.

Hurst, N. (2005). Assessing and facilitating milk transfer during breastfeeding for the premature infant. *Newborn Infant Nurs Rev., 5,* 19–26.

Hurst, N. M. (2007). The 3 M's of breastfeeding the preterm infant. *J Perinat Neonat Nurs., 21,* 234–239.

Hurst, N. M., & Meier, P. P. (2005). Breastfeeding the preterm infant. In J. Riordan (Ed.), *Breastfeeding and human lactation* (3rd ed.). Sudbury, MA: Jones and Bartlett.

Hurst, N. M., Myatt, A., & Schanler, R. J. (1998). Growth and development of a hospital-based lactation program and mother's own milk bank. *JOGNN, 27,* 503–510.

Hurst, N. M., Valentine, C. J., Renfro, L., et al. (1997). Skin-to-skin holding in the neonatal intensive care unit influences maternal milk volume. *J Perinatol., 17,* 213–217.

Ip, S., Glicken, S., Kulig, J., et al. (2003, January). Management of neonatal hyperbilirubinemia. Evidence Report/Technology Assessment No. 65 (prepared by Tufts-New England Medical Center Evidence-Based Practice Center under contract No. 290-97-0019). AHRQ Publication No. 03-E011. Rockville, MD: U.S. Department of Health and Human Services, Agency for Healthcare Research and Quality.

Iyer, N. P., Srinivasan, R., Evans, K., Ward, L., Cheung, W. Y., & Matthes, J. W. (2008). Impact of an early weighing policy on neonatal dehydration and breastfeeding. *Arch Dis Child, 93,* 297–299.

Janjindamai, W., & Chotsampancharoen, T. (2006). Effect of fortification on the osmolality of human milk. *Journal of the Medical Association of Thailand, 89,* 1400–1403.

Jim, W.-T., Shu, C.-H., Chiu, N.-C., et al. (2004). Transmission of cytomegalovirus from mothers to preterm infants by breast milk. *Pediatric Infectious Disease Journal, 23,* 9.

Jocson, M. A. L., Mason, E. O., & Schanler, R. J. (1997). The effects of nutrient fortification and varying storage conditions on host defense properties of human milk. *Pediatrics, 100,* 240–242.

Johnson, L., & Bhutani, V. K. (2003). Reply to the editor. *J Pediatr., 142,* 214–215.

Johnson, L., Bhutani, V. K., Karp, K., Sivieri, E. M., Shapiro, S. M. (2009). Clinical report from the pilot USA Kernicterus Registry (1992 to 2004). *J Perinatol., 29,* S25–S45.

Johnson, L., & Brown, A. K. (1999). A pilot registry for acute and chronic kernicterus in term and near-term infants. *Pediatrics, 104,* 736.

Joint Commission on Accreditation of Healthcare Organizations. (2001). Kernicterus threatens healthy newborns. Sentinel Event Alert, 18(April).

Joint Commission on Accreditation of Healthcare Organizations. (2001). Revised guidance to help prevent kernicterus. Sentinel Event Alert, 31(April).

Jones, E., Dimmock, P. W., & Spencer, S. A. (2001). A randomized controlled trial to compare methods of milk expression after preterm delivery. *Arch Dis Child. Fetal and Neonatal Edition, 85,* F91–F95.

Kaplan, M., & Hammerman, C. (2000). Glucose-6-phosphate dehydrogenase-deficient neonates. A potential cause for concern in North America. *Pediatrics, 106,* 1478–1480.

Kaplan, M., Herschel, M., Hammerman, C., et al. (2004). Hyperbilirubinemia among African American, glucose-6-phosphate dehydrogenase-deficient neonates. *Pediatrics, 114,* e213–e219.

Kappas, A. (2004). A method for interdicting the development of severe jaundice in newborns by inhibiting the production of bilirubin. *Pediatrics, 113,* 119–123.

Kassing, D. (2002). Bottle-feeding as a tool to reinforce breastfeeding. *J Hum Lact., 18,* 56–60.

Kavanaugh, K., Mead, L., Meier, P., & Mangurten, H. H. (195). Getting enough: Mother's concerns about breastfeeding a preterm infant after discharge. *JOGNN, 24,* 23–32.

Kavanaugh, K., Meier, P., Zimmermann, B., & Mead, L. (1997). The rewards outweigh the efforts: Breastfeeding outcomes for mothers of preterm infants. *J Hum Lact., 13,* 15–21.

Kemper, K., Forsyth, B., & McCarthy, P. (1989). Jaundice, terminating breastfeeding, and the vulnerable child. *Pediatrics, 84,* 773–778.

Kemper, K. J., Forsyth, B. W., & McCarthy, P. L. (1990). Persistent perceptions of vulnerability following neonatal jaundice. *Am J Dis Child, 144,* 238–241.

Kent, J. C., Mitoulas, L. R., Cregan, M. D., et al. (2008). Importance of vacuum for breastmilk expression. *Breastfeeding Med., 3,* 11–19.

Kent, J. C., Ramsay, D. T., Doherty, D., et al. (2003). Response of breasts to different stimulation patterns of an electric breast pump. *J Hum Lact., 19,* 179–186.

Keren, R., Luan, X., Tremont, K., & Cnaan, A. (2009). Visual assessment of jaundice in term and late preterm infants. *Arch Dis Child. Fetal and Neonatal Edition, 94,* F317–F322.

Kien, C. L. (1985). Failure to thrive. In W. A. Walher & J. B. Watkins (Eds.), *Nutrition in pediatrics.* Boston: Little, Brown.

Kinney, H. C. (2006). The near-term (late preterm) human brain and risk for periventricular leuko-malacia: A review. *Seminars in Perinatology, 30,* 81–88.

Kirchner, L., Jeitler, V., Waldhor, T., Pollak, A., & Wald, M. (2009). Long hospitalization is the most important risk factor for early weaning from breast milk in premature babies. *Acta Paediatr., 98,* 981–984.

Kirk, A. T., Alder, S. C., & King, J. D. (2007). Cue-based oral feeding clinical pathway results in earlier attainment of full oral feeding in premature infants. *J Perinatol., 27,* 572–578.

Kirsten, G. F., Bergman, N. J., & Hann, F. M. (2001). Kangaroo mother care in the nursery. *Pediatr Clin North Am., 48,* 443–452.

Kliethermes, P. A., Cross, M. L., Lanese, M. G., et al. (1999). Transitioning preterm infants with nasogas-tric tube supplementation: Increased likelihood of breastfeeding. *JOGNN, 28,* 264–273.

Knudsen, A., & Ebbesen, F. (1997). Cephalocaudal progression of jaundice in newborns admitted to neonatal intensive care units. *Biology of the Neonate, 71,* 357–361.

Koenig, J. S., et al. (1990). Coordination of breathing, sucking, and swallowing during bottle-feedings in human infants. *J Appl Physiol., 69,* 1623–1629.

Koepke, J. E., & Bigelow, A. E. (1997). Observations of newborn suckling behavior. *Infant Behavior and Development, 20,* 93.

Konetzny, G., Bucher, H. U., & Arlettaz, R. (2009). Prevention of hypernatraemic dehydration in breastfed newborn infants by daily weighing. *Eur J Pediatr., 168,* 815–818.

Kovach, A. C. (2002). A 5-year follow-up study of hospital breastfeeding policies in the Philadelphia area: A comparison with the ten steps. *J Hum Lact., 18,* 144–154.

Kramer, L. I. (1969). Advancement of dermal icterus in the jaundiced newborn. *Am J Dis Child., 118,* 454–458.

Kramer, M. S., Demissie, K., Yang, H., Platt, R.W., Sauvé, R., & Liston, R. (2000). The contribution of mild and moderate preterm birth to infant mortality. Fetal and Infant Health Study Group of the Canadian Perinatal Surveillance System. *JAMA, 284,* 843–849.

Kuzniewicz, M. W., Escobar, G. J., Wi, S., Liljestrand, P., McCulloch, C., & Newman, T. B. (2008). Risk factors for severe hyperbilirubinemia among infants with borderline bilirubin levels: A nested case-control study. *J Pediatr., 153,* 234–240.

Laing, I. A., & Wong, C. M. (2002). Hypernatraemia in the first few days: Is the incidence rising? *Arch Dis Child. Fetal and Neonatal Edition, 87,* F158–F162.

Lang, S. (2002). *Breastfeeding special care babies* (2nd ed.). Edinburgh, Scotland: Bailliere Tindall.

Lang, S., Lawrence, C. J., & Orme, R. L. (1994). Cup feeding: An alternative method of infant feeding. *Arch Dis Child, 71,* 365–369.

Lawrence, R. A. (1997). *A review of the medical benefits and contraindications to breastfeeding in the United States.* Maternal and Child Health Technical Information Bulletin. Arlington, VA: National Center for Education in Maternal and Child Health.

Lawrence, R. A., & Lawrence, R. M. (2005). *Breastfeeding: A guide for the medical profession* (6th ed.). St. Louis, MO: Mosby.

Lawrence, R. M. (2006). Cytomegalovirus in human breast milk: Risk to the premature infant. *Breastfeeding and Medicine, 1,* 99–107.

Lawrence, R. M., & Lawrence, R. A. (2001). Given the benefits of breastfeeding, what contraindications exist? *Pediatr Clin North Am., 48,* 235–251.

Lefebvre, F., & Ducharme, M. (1989). Incidence and duration of lactation and lactational performance among mothers of low-birth-weight and term infants. *CMAJ, 140,* 1159–1164.

Liu, L. L., Clemens, C. J., Shay, D. K., et al. (1997). The safety of newborn early discharge: The Washington State experience. *JAMA, 278,* 293–298.

Liu, S., Wen, S. W., McMillan, D., et al. (2000). Increased neonatal admission rate associated with decreased length of hospital stay at birth in Canada. *Can J Public Health, 91,* 46–50.

Livingstone, V. H., Willis, C. E., Abdel-Wareth, L. O., et al. (2000). Neonatal hypernatremic dehydration associated with breastfeeding malnutrition: A retrospective survey. *CMAJ, 162,* 647–652.

Lonnerdal, B., & Iyer, S. (1995). Lactoferrin: Molecular structure and biological function. *Ann Rev Nutr., 15,* 93–110.

Lucas, A., Fewtrell, M. S., Davies, P. S. W., et al. (1997). Breastfeeding and catch-up growth in infants born small for gestational age. *Acta Paediatr., 86,* 564–569.

Lucas, A., Fewtrell, M. S., Morley, R., et al. (1996). Randomized outcome trial of human milk fortification and developmental outcome in preterm infants. *Am J Clin Nutr., 64,* 142–151.

Lucas, A., Gibbs, J. A., Lyster, R. L., et al. (1978). Creamatocrit: Simple clinical technique for estimating fat concentration and energy value of human milk. *BMJ, 1,* 1018–1020.

Ludington-Hoe, S. M., Thompson, C., Swinth, J., et al. (1994). Kangaroo care: Research results, and protocol implications and guidelines. *Neonatal Network, 13,* 19–27.

Lukefahr, J. L. (1990). Underlying illness associated with failure to thrive in breastfed infants. *Clin Pediatr., 29,* 468–470.

Maayan-Metzger, A., Mazkereth, R., & Kuint, J. (2003). Fever in healthy asymptomatic newborns during the first days of life. *Arch Dis Child. Fetal and Neonatal Edition, 88,* F312–F314.

Macdonald, P. D., Ross, S. R. M., Grant, L., & Young, D. (2003). Neonatal weight loss in breast and formula fed infants. *Arch Dis Child. Fetal and Neonatal Edition, 88,* F472–F476.

MacMahon, J. R., Stevenson, D. K., & Oski, F. A. (1998). Physiologic jaundice. In H. W. Taeusch & R. A. Ballard (Eds.), *Avery's diseases of the newborn* (7th ed.). Philadelphia: W.B. Saunders.

Madlon-Kay, D. J. (1997). Recognition of the presence and severity of newborn jaundice by parents, nurses, physicians, and icterometer. *Pediatrics, 100,* e3.

Madlon-Kay, D. J. (2002). Maternal assessment of neonatal jaundice after discharge. *J Fam Pract., 51,* 445–448.

Maisels, M. J. (2001). Neonatal hyperbilirubinemia. In M. H. Klaus & A. A. Fanaroff (Eds.), *Care of the high-risk neonate*. Philadelphia: W.B. Saunders.

Maisels, M. J., & Kring, E. (1998). Length of stay, jaundice, and hospital readmission. *Pediatrics, 101,* 995–998.

Malhotra, N., Vishwambaran, L., Sundaram, K. R., & Narayanan, I. (1999). A controlled trial of alternative methods of oral feeding in neonates. *Early Hum Dev., 54,* 29–38.

Manganaro, R., Mami, C., Marrone, T., et al. (2001). Incidence of dehydration and hypernatremia in exclusively breastfed infants. *J Pediatr., 139,* 673–675.

Mannel, R., & Mannel, R. S. (2006). Staffing for hospital lactation programs: Recommendations from a tertiary care teaching hospital. *J Hum Lact., 22,* 409–417.

Marchini, G., & Stock, S. (1997). Thirst and vasopressin secretion counteract dehydration in newborn infants. *J Pediatr., 130,* 736–739.

Marinelli, K. A., Burke, G. S., & Dodd, V. L. (2001). A comparison of the safety of cupfeedings and bottle-feedings in premature infants whose mothers intend to breastfeed. *J Perinatol., 21,* 350–355.

Marquis, G. S., Penny, M. E., Diaz, J. M., & Marin, R. M. (2002). Postpartum consequences of an overlap of breastfeeding and pregnancy: Reduced breast milk intake and growth during early infancy. *Pediatrics, 109,* e56.

Martens, P. J., & Romphf, L. (2007). Factors associated with newborn in-hospital weight loss: Comparisons by feeding method, demographics, and birthing procedures. *J Hum Lact., 23,* 233–241.

Martin, J. A., Hamilton, B. E., Sutton, P. D., Ventura, S. J., Menacker, F., Kirmeyer, S., & Munson, M. L. (2007). *Births: Final data for 2005*. National Vital Statistics Reports, vol. 56, no. 6. Hyattsville, MD: National Center for Health Statistics.

Maruo, Y., Nishizawa, K., Sato, H., et al. (2000). Prolonged unconjugated hyperbilirubinemia associated with breast milk and mutations of the bilirubin uridine diphosphate-glucuronosyltransferase gene. *Pediatrics, 106,* e59.

Matthew, O. (1988). Respiratory control during nipple feeding in preterm infants. *Pediatric Pulmonology, 5,* 220–224.

Matthew, O. (1991). Breathing patterns of preterm infants during bottle-feeding: Role of milk flow. *J Pediatr., 119,* 960–965.

McDonagh, A. F. (1990). Is bilirubin good for you? *Clin Perinatol., 17,* 359–369.

McDougall, P., Drewett, R. F., Hungin, P., & Wright, C. M. (2008). The detection of early weight faltering at the 6–8 week check and its association with family factors, feeding and behavioral development. *Arch Dis Child., 94,* 549–552.

Meier, P. P. (1988). Bottle- and breastfeeding: Effects on transcutaneous oxygen pressure and temperature in preterm infants. *Nurs Res., 37,* 36–41.

Meier, P. P. (2001). Breastfeeding in the special care nursery. Prematures and infants with medical problems. *Pediatr Clin North Am., 48,* 425–442.

Meier, P. P. (2003). Supporting lactation in mothers with very low birth weight infants. *Pediatr Ann., 32,* 317–325.

Meier, P. P., & Anderson, G. C. (1987). Responses of small preterm infants to bottle- and breastfeeding. *MCN, 12,* 97–105.

Meier, P. P., & Brown, L. P. (1996). State of the science: Breastfeeding for mothers and low birth weight infants. *Nurs Clin North Am., 31,* 351–365.

Meier, P. P., & Brown, L. P. (1997). Defining terminology for improved breastfeeding research. *J Nurse Midwifery, 42,* 65–66.

Meier, P. P., Brown, L., Hurst N., et al. (2000). Nipple shields for preterm infants: Effect on milk transfer and duration of breastfeeding. *J Hum Lact., 16,* 106–114.

Meier, P. P., Engstrom, J. L., Crichton, C. L., et al. (1994). A new scale for in-home test-weighing for mothers of preterm and high risk infants. *J Hum Lact., 10,* 163–168.

Meier, P. P., Engstrom, J. L., Fleming, B., et al. (1996). Estimating milk intake of hospitalized preterm infants who breastfeed. *J Hum Lact., 12,* 21–26.

Meier, P. P., Engstrom, J. L., Mangurten, H. H., et al. (1993). Breastfeeding support services in the neonatal intensive care unit. *JOGNN, 22,* 338–347.

Meier, P. P., Engstrom, J. L., Mingolelli, S. S., Miracle, D. J., & Kiesling, S. (2004). The Rush Mothers' Milk Club: Breastfeeding interventions for mothers with very-low-birth-weight infants. *J Obstet Gynecol Neonatal Nurs., 33,* 164–174.

Meier, P. P., Engstrom, J. L., Zuleger, J. L., et al. (2006). Accuracy of a user-friendly centrifuge for measuring creamatocrits on mothers' milk in the clinical setting. *Breastfeeding Med., 1,* 79–87.

Meier, P. P., Firman, L. M., & Degenhardt, M. (2007). Increased lactation risk for late preterm infants and mothers: Evidence and management strategies to protect breastfeeding. *J Midwifery Women's Health, 52,* 579–587.

Meier, P. P., Lysakowski, Y., Engstrom, J. L., et al. (1990). The accuracy of test weighing for preterm infants. *J Pediatr Gastroenterol Nutr., 10,* 62–65.

Meier, P. P., Motykowski, J. E., & Zuleger, J. L. (2004). Choosing a correctly-fitted breastshield for milk expression. *Medela Messenger, 21,* 1, 8–9.

Meier, P. P., & Pugh, E. J. (1985). Breastfeeding behavior of small preterm infants. *MCN, 10,* 396–401.

Meinzen-Derr, J., Poindexter, B., Wrage, L., Morrow, A. L., Stoll, B., & Donovan, E. F. (2009). Role of human milk in extremely low birth weight infants' risk of necrotizing enterocolitis or death. *J Perinatol., 29,* 57–62.

Melton, K., & Akinbi, H. T. (1999). Neonatal jaundice: Strategies to reduce bilirubin-induced complications. *Postgraduate Medicine, 106,* 167–168, 171–174, 177–178.

Millar, K. R., Gloor, J. E., Wellington, N., & Joubert, G. I. E. (2000). Early neonatal presentations to the pediatric emergency department. *Pediatric Emergency Care, 16,* 145–150.

Miracle, D. J., Meier, P. P., & Bennett, P. A. (2004a). Making my baby healthy: Changing the decision from formula to human milk feedings for very-low-birth-weight infants. *Adv Experimental Med Biol., 554,* 317–319.

Miracle, D. J., Meier, P. P., & Bennett, P. A. (2004b). Mothers' decisions to change from formula to mother's milk for very-low-birth-weight infants. *JOGNN, 33,* 692–703.

Mitoulas, L. R., Lai, C. T., Gurrin, L. C., et al. (2002). Efficacy of breast milk expression using an electric breast pump. *J Hum Lact., 18,* 344–352.

Mok, E., Multon, C., Piguel, L., et al. (2008). Decreased full breastfeeding, altered practices, perceptions, and infant weight change of prepregnant obese women: A need for extra support. *Pediatrics, 121,* e1319–e1324.

Molteni, K. H. (1994). Initial management of hypernatremic dehydration in the breastfed infant. *Clin Pediatr., 33,* 731–740.

Montgomery, D., Schmutz, N., Baer, V. L., et al. (2008). Effects of instituting the "BEST Program" (Breast Milk Early Saves Trouble) in a level III NICU. *J Hum Lact., 24,* 248–251.

Morales, Y., & Schanler, R. J. (2007). Human milk and clinical outcomes in VLBW infants: How compelling is the evidence of benefit? *Semin Perinatol., 31,* 83–88.

Morbidity and Mortality Weekly Report. (2001). Kernicterus in full-term infants—United States, 1994–1998. *MMWR, 50,* 491–494.

Moritz, M. L., Manole, M. D., Bogen, D. L., & Ayus, J. C. (2005). Breastfeeding-associated hypernatremia: Are we missing the diagnosis? *Pediatrics, 16,* e343–e347. Retrieved September 15, 2005, from www.pediatrics.org/cgi/doi/10.1542/peds.2004-264

Morton, J. A. (2002). Strategies to support extended breastfeeding of the premature infant. *Adv Neonat Care, 2,* 267–282.

Morton, J., Hall, J. Y., Thairu, L., et al. (2007a). Early hand expression affects breastmilk production in pump-dependent mothers of preterm infants. Retrieved April 25, 2009, from www.abstracts2view.com/pasall/view.php?nu=PAS07L1_37

Morton, J., Hall, J. Y., Thairu, L., et al. (2007b). Breast massage maximizes milk volumes of pump-dependent mothers. Retrieved April 25, 2009, from www.abstracts2view.com/pasall/view.php?nu=PAS07L1_32

Narayanan, I., et al. (1991). Sucking on the "emptied" breast: Non-nutritive sucking with a difference. *Arch Dis Child, 66,* 241–244.

Neifert, M. (1998). The optimization of breastfeeding in the perinatal period. *Clin Perinatol., 25,* 303–326.

Neifert, M. A., & Seacat, J. (1988). Practical aspects of breastfeeding the premature infant. *Perinatol Neonatol., 12,* 24–30.

Neifert, M. R. (2001). Prevention of breastfeeding tragedies. *Pediatr Clin North Am., 48,* 273–297.

Nelson, S. E., Rogers, R. R., Ziegler, E. E., et al. (1989). Gain in weight and length during early infancy. *Early Hum Dev., 19,* 223–239.

Neuberger, P., Hamprecht, K., Vochem, M., et al. (2006). Case-control study of symptoms and neonatal outcome of human milk-transmitted cytomegalovirus infection in premature infants. *J Pediatr., 148,* 326–331.

Newman, J. (2004). Case study: Slow weight gain after initial rapid gain. *ABM News and Views, 10,* 23–24.

Newman, T. B., Escobar, G. J., Gonzalez, V. M., et al. (1999). Frequency of neonatal bilirubin testing and hyperbilirubinemia in a large health maintenance organization. *Pediatrics, 104,* 1198–1203.

Newman, T. B., & Maisels, M. J. (1992). Evaluation and treatment of jaundice in the term newborn: A kinder, gentler approach. *Pediatrics, 89,* 809–818.

Newman, T. B., Xiong, B., Gonzales, V. M., & Escobar, G. J. (2000). Prediction and prevention of extreme neonatal hyperbilirubinemia in a mature health maintenance organization. *Arch Pediatr Adolesc Med., 154,* 1140–1147.

Ng, P. C., Chan, H. B., Fok, T. F., et al. (1999). Early onset hypernatraemic dehydration and fever in exclusively breastfed infants. *J Pediatr Child Health, 35,* 585–587.

Nicholl, A., Ginsburg, R., & Tripp, J. H. (1982). Supplementary feeding and jaundice in newborns. *Acta Paediatr Scand., 71,* 759–761.

Noel-Weiss, J., Courant, G., & Woodend, A. K. (2008). Physiological weight loss in the breastfed neonate: A systematic review. *Open Medicine, 2,* e11–e22.

Nommsen-Rivers, L. A., Heinig, M. J., Cohen, R. J., & Dewey, K. G. (2008). Newborn wet and soiled diaper counts and timing of onset of lactation as indicators of breastfeeding inadequacy. *J Hum Lact., 24,* 27–33.

Numazaki, K. (1997). Human cytomegalovirus infection of breast milk. *FEMS Immunology and Medical Microbiology, 18,* 91–98.

Nyqvist, K. H. (2008). Early attainment of breastfeeding competence in very preterm infants. *Acta Paediatr., 97,* 776–781.

Nyqvist, K. H., & Kylberg, E. (2008). Application of the Baby Friendly Hospital Initiative to neonatal care: Suggestions by Swedish mothers of very preterm infants. *J Hum Lact., 24,* 252–262.

Oddie, S., Richmond, S., & Coultard, M. (2001). Hypernatremic dehydration and breastfeeding: A population study. *Arch Dis Child, 85,* 318–320.

Ogden, C. L., Kuczmarski, R. J., Flegal, K. M., et al. (2002). Centers for Disease Control and Prevention 2000 growth charts for the United States: Improvements to the 1977 National Center for Health Statistics version. *Pediatrics, 109,* 45–60.

Olsen, E. M. (2006). Failure to thrive: Still a problem of definition. *Clin Pediatr., 45*, 1–6.

Osborn, L. M., Reiff, M. I., & Bolus, R. (1984). Jaundice in the full term neonate. *Pediatrics, 73*, 520–525.

Palmer, R. H., Clanton, M., Ezhuthachan, S., et al. (2003). Applying the "10 simple rules" of the Institute of Medicine to management of hyperbilirubinemia in newborns. *Pediatrics, 112*, 1388–1393.

Palmer, R. H., Keren, R., Maisels, M. J., & Yeargin-Allsopp, M. (2004). National Institute of Child Health and Human Development (NICHD) conference on kernicterus: A population perspective on prevention of kernicterus. *J Perinatol., 24*, 723–725.

Penn, A. A., Enzmann, D. R., Hahn, J. S., & Stevenson, D. K. (1994). Kernicterus in a full term infant. *Pediatrics, 93*, 1003–1006.

Philipp, B. L., Brown, E., & Merewood, A. (2000). Pumps for peanuts: Leveling the playing field in the NICU. *J Perinatol., 4*, 249–250.

Pimenta, H. P., Moreira, M. E., Rocha, A. D., Gomes, S. C. Jr., Pinto, L. W., & Lucena, S. L. (2008). Effects of non-nutritive sucking and oral stimulation on breastfeeding rates for preterm, low birth weight infants: A randomized clinical trial. *J Pediatr., 84*, 423–427.

Pinelli, J., & Symington, A. (2000). Non-nutritive sucking for promoting physiologic stability and nutrition in preterm infants. *Cochrane Database System Review, 2*.

Poland, R. L. (1981). Breast-milk jaundice. *J Pediatr., 99*, 86–88.

Porter, M. L., & Dennis, B. L. (2002). Hyperbilirubinemia in the term newborn. *Am Fam Phys., 65*, 599–606, 613–614.

Powers, N., Clark, R. H., Bloom, B. T., et al. (2001). Site variation in rates of breastmilk feedings in neonates discharged from intensive care units [abstract]. *Academy of Breastfeeding Medical News and Views, 7*, 37.

Powers, N. G. (1999). Slow weight gain and low milk supply in the breastfeeding dyad. *Clin Perinatol., 26*, 399–430.

Powers, N. G. (2001). How to assess slow growth in the breastfed infant: Birth to 3 months. *Pediatr Clin North Am., 48*, 345–363.

Powers, N. G. (2005). Low intake in the breastfed infant: Maternal and infant considerations. In J. Riordan (Ed.), *Breastfeeding and human lactation* (3rd ed.). Sudbury, MA: Jones and Bartlett.

Quan, R., et al. (1994, June). The effect of nutritional additives on anti-infective factors in human milk. *Clin Pediatr.*, 325–328.

Raju, T. N., Higgins, R. D., Stark, A. R., & Leveno, K. J. (2006). Optimizing care and outcome for late-preterm (near-term) infants: A summary of the workshop sponsored by the National Institute of Child Health and Human Development. *Pediatrics, 118*, 1207–1214.

Ramsay, M., Gisel, E. G., & Boutry, M. (1993). Non-organic failure to thrive: Growth failure secondary to feeding-skills disorder. *Dev Med Child Neurol., 35*, 285–297.

Rand, S. E., & Kolberg, A. (2001). Neonatal hypernatremic dehydration secondary to lactation failure. *J Am Board Fam Pract., 14*, 155–158.

Rodriguez, N. A., Miracle, D. J., & Meier, P. P. (2005). Sharing the science on human milk feedings with mothers of very-low-birth-weight infants. *JOGNN, 34*, 109–119.

Ross, G. (2003). Hyperbilirubinemia in the 2000s: What should we do next? *Am J Perinatol., 20*, 415–424.

Sarici, S. U., Serdar, M. A., Korkmaz, A., et al. (2004). Incidence, course, and prediction of hyperbilirubinemia in near-term and term newborns. *Pediatrics, 113*, 775–780.

Scanlon, K. S., et al. (2002). Assessment of infant feeding: The validity of measuring milk intake. *Nutrition Review, 60*, 235–251.

Schanler, R. J. (1998). Fortified human milk: Nature's way to feed premature infants. *J Hum Lact., 14*, 5–11.

Schanler, R. J. (2001). The use of human milk for premature infants. *Pediatr Clin North Am., 48*, 207–219.

Schanler, R. J. (2007). Mother's own milk, donor human milk, and preterm formulas in the feeding of extremely premature infants. *J Pediatr Gastroenterol Nutr., 45*(Suppl 3), S175–S177.

Schanler, R. J., & Atkinson, S. A. (1999). Effects of nutrients in human milk on the recipient premature infant. *Journal of Mammary Gland Biology and Neoplasia, 4,* 297–307.

Schanler, R. J., Shulman, R. J., & Lau, C. (1997). Growth of premature infants fed fortified human milk. *Pediatr Res., 41,* 240A.

Schanler, R. J., Shulman, R. J., & Lau, C., et al. (1999a). Feeding strategies for premature infants: Beneficial outcomes of feeding fortified human milk versus preterm formula. *Pediatrics, 103,* 1150–1157.

Schanler, R. J., Shulman, R. J., Lau, C., et al. (1999b). Feeding strategies for premature infants: Randomized trial of gastrointestinal priming and tube-feeding methods. *Pediatrics, 103,* 434–439.

Schneider, A. P. II. (1986). Breast milk jaundice in the newborn. A reality. *JAMA, 255,* 3270–3274.

Sedlak, T. W., & Snyder, S. H. (2004). Bilirubin benefits: Cellular protection by a biliverdin reductase antioxidant cycle. *Pediatrics, 113,* 1776–1782.

Shekeeb, S. M., Kumar, P., Sharma, N., Narang, A., & Prasad, R. (2008). Evaluation of oxidant and antioxidant status in term neonates: A plausible protective role of bilirubin. *Molecular and Cellular Biochemistry, 317,* 51–59.

Shivpuri, C. R., et al. (1983). Decreased ventilation in preterm infants during oral feeding. *J Pediatr., 103,* 285–289.

Shrago, L. C., Reifsnider, E., & Insel, K. (2006). The neonatal bowel output study: Indicators of adequate breast milk intake in neonates. *Pediatr Nurs., 32,* 195–201.

Sisk, P. M., Lovelady, C. A., Gruber, K. J., Dillard, R. G., & O'Shea, T. M. (2008). Human milk consumption and full enteral feeding among infants who weigh < 1250 grams. *Pediatrics, 121,* e1528–e1533.

Slaughter, J., Annibale, D., & Suresh, G. (2009). False-negative results of pre-discharge neonatal bilirubin screening to predict severe hyperbilirubinemia: A need for caution. *Eur J Pediatr.,* 10.1007/500431-009-0950-2

Sofer, S., Ben-Ezer, D., & Dagan, R. (1993). Early severe dehydration in young breastfed newborn infants. *Israeli Journal of Medical Science, 29,* 85–89.

Spanier-Mingolelli, S. R., Meier, P. P., & Bradford, L. (1998). "Making the difference for my baby." A powerful breastfeeding motivator for mothers of preterm and high risk infants [abstract]. *Pediatr Res., 43,* 269.

Spatz, D. L. (2004). Ten steps for promoting and protecting breastfeeding for vulnerable infants. *J Perinat Neonat Nurs., 18,* 385–396.

Spatz, D. L., & Goldschmidt, K. A. (2006). Preserving breastfeeding for the rehospitalized infant: A clinical pathway. *MCN, 31,* 45–51.

Stark, Y. (1994). Human nipples: Function and anatomical variations in relationship to breastfeeding. Master's thesis. Pasadena, CA: Pacific Oaks College.

Steffensrud, S. (2004). Hyperbilirubinemia in term and near-term infants: Kernicterus on the rise? *Newborn and Infant Nursing Review, 4,* 191–200.

Stellwagen, L. M., Hubbard, E. T., & Wolf, A. (2007). The late preterm infant: A little baby with big needs. *Contemporary Pediatrics.* Retrieved September 18, 2009, from http://contemporarypediatrics.modernmedicine.com/contpeds/Features/The-late-preterm-infant-A-little-baby-with-big-nee/Article Standard/Article/detail/483620

Stevenson, D. K., Dennery, P. A., & Hintz, S. R. (2001). Understanding newborn jaundice. *J Perinatol., 21,* S21–S24.

Stokowski, L. A. (2002a). Early recognition of neonatal jaundice and kernicterus. *Adv Neonat Care, 2,* 101–114.

Stokowski, L. A. (2002b). Family teaching toolbox. Newborn jaundice. *Adv Neonat Care, 2,* 115–116.

Syfrett, E. B., Anderson, G. C., Behnke, M., et al. (1993). Early and virtually continuous kangaroo care for lower risk preterm infants: Effect on temperature, breastfeeding, supplementation, and weight. Presented at the Proceedings of the Biennial Conference of the Council of Nurse Researchers, American Nurses Association, November, Washington, DC.

Stine, M. J. (1990). Breastfeeding the premature newborn: A protocol without bottles. *J Hum Lact., 6,* 167–170.

Sweet, L. (2008). Expressed breast milk as "connection" and its influence on the construction of "motherhood" for mothers of preterm infants: A qualitative study. *International Breastfeeding Journal, 3,* 30.

Tarcan, A., Gurakan, B., Tiker, F., & Ozbek, N. (2004). Influence of feeding formula and breast milk fortifier on lymphocyte subsets in very low birth weight premature newborns. *Biology of the Neonate, 86,* 22–28.

Tarcan, A., Tiker, F., Vatandas, N. S., Haberal, A., & Gurakan, B. (2005). Weight loss and hypernatremia in breastfed babies: Frequency in neonates with non-hemolytic jaundice. *J Pediatr Child Health, 41,* 484–487.

Tatli, M. M., Minnet, C., Kocyigit, A., & Karadag, A. (2008). Phototherapy increases DNA damage in lymphocytes of hyperbilirubinemic neonates. *Mutation Research, 654,* 93–95.

Taylor, S. N., Basile, L. A., Ebeling, M., & Wagner, C. L. (2009). Intestinal permeability in preterm infants by feeding type: Mother's milk versus formula. *Breastfeeding Med., 4,* 11–15.

Thompson, N. M. (1996). Relactation in a newborn intensive care setting. *J Hum Lact., 12,* 233–235.

Thoyre, S. M., & Carlson, J. (2003). Occurrence of oxygen desaturation events during preterm infant bottle feeding near discharge. *Early Hum Dev., 72,* 25–36.

Toppare, M. F., et al. (1994). Metoclopramide for breast milk production. *Nutr Res., 14,* 1019–1029.

Unal, S., Arhan, E., Kara, N., Uncu, N., & Aliefendioglu, D. (2008). Breastfeeding-associated hypernatremia: Retrospective analysis of 169 term newborns. *Pediatrics International, 50,* 29–34.

Uras, N., Karadag, A., Dogan G, Tonbul, A., & Tatli, M. M. (2007). Moderate hypernatremic dehydration in newborn infants: Retrospective evaluation of 64 cases. *J Matern Fetal Neonatal Med., 20,* 449–452.

Valentine, C. J., Hurst, N. M., & Schanler, R. J. (1994). Hindmilk improves weight gain in low birth weight infants fed human milk. *J Pediatr Gastroenterol Nutr., 18,* 474–477.

Van der Strate, B. W. A., Harmsen, M. C., Schafer, P., et al. (2001). Viral load in breast milk correlates with transmission of human cytomegalovirus to preterm neonates, but lactoferrin concentrations do not. *Clinical and Diagnostic Laboratory Immunology, 8,* 818–821.

Van Dijk, C. E., & Innis, S. M. (2009). Growth-curve standards and the assessment of early excess weight gain in infancy. *Pediatrics, 123,* 102–108.

Varimo, P., Simila, S., Wendt, L., & Kolvisto, M. (1986). Frequency of breastfeeding and hyperbilirubinemia [letter]. *Clin Pediatr., 25,* 112.

Vio, F., Salazar, G., & Infante, C. (1991). Smoking during pregnancy and lactation and its effects on breast milk volume. *Am J Clin Nutr., 54,* 1011–1016.

Vochem, M., Hamprecht, K., Jahn, G., & Speer, C. P. (1998). Transmission of cytomegalovirus to preterm infants through breast milk. *Pediatr Infect Dis J., 17,* 53–58.

Vohr, B. R., Poindexter, B. B., Dusick, A. M., et al. (2006). Beneficial effects of breast milk in the neonatal intensive care unit on the developmental outcome of extremely low birth weight infants at 18 months of age. *Pediatrics, 118,* e115–e123.

Volpe, J. J. (2001). Bilirubin and brain injury. In J. J. Volpe (Ed.), *Neonatal neurology.* Philadelphia: W.B. Saunders.

Walker, M. (1992). Breastfeeding the premature infant. *NAACOG's Clinical Issues in Perinatal and Women's Health Nursing, 3,* 620–633.

Walker, M. (2005). Breast pumps and other technologies. In J. Riordan (Ed.), *Breastfeeding and human lactation.* Sudbury, MA: Jones and Bartlett.

Walker, M. (2008). Breastfeeding the late preterm infant. *JOGNN, 37,* 692–701.

Wan, E. W., Davey, K., Page-Sharp, M., Hartmann, P. E., Simmer, K., & Ilett, K. F. (2008). Dose-effect study of domperidone as a galactagogue in preterm mothers with insufficient milk supply, and its transfer into milk. *British Journal of Clinical Pharmacology, 66,* 283–289.

Wang, M. L., Dorer, D. J., Fleming, M. P., & Catlin, E. (2004). Clinical outcomes of near-term infants. *Pediatrics, 114,* 372–376.

Washington, E. C., Ector, W., & Abboud, M. (1995). Hemolytic jaundice due to G6PD deficiency causing kernicterus in a female newborn. *Southern Medical Journal, 88,* 776–779.

Watchko, J. F., & Oski, F. A. (1983). Bilirubin 20 mg/dL: Vingintiphobia. *Pediatrics, 71,* 660–663.

Whitelaw, A., Histerkamp, G., Sleath, K., et al. (1988). Skin to skin contact for very low birthweight infants and their mothers. *Arch Dis Child., 63,* 1377.

Whiteley, W. (1996). A parent's experience of a special care baby unit. Emotional dimensions of prematurity. *Prof Care Mother Child, 6,* 141–142.

WHO Multicentre Growth Reference Study Group. (2006). *WHO Child Growth Standards: Length/height-for-age, weight-for-age, weight-for-length, weight-for-height and body mass index-for-age: Methods and development.* Geneva: World Health Organization.

Widstrom, A. M., Marchini, G., Matthiesen, A. S., et al. (1988). Nonnutritive sucking in tube-fed preterm infants: Effects on gastric motility and gastric contents of somatostatin. *J Pediatr Gastroenterol Nutr., 7,* 517.

Wiedemann, M., Kontush, A., Finckh, B., et al. (2003). Neonatal blood plasma is less susceptible to oxidation than adult plasma owing to its higher content of bilirubin and lower content of oxidizable fatty acids. *Pediatr Res., 53,* 843–849.

Willis, S. K., Hannon, P. R., & Scrimshaw, S. C. (2002). The impact of the maternal experience with a jaundiced newborn on the breastfeeding relationship. *J Fam Pract., 51,* 465.

Wilson-Clay, B., & Hoover, K. (2002). *The breastfeeding atlas.* Austin, TX: LactNews Press.

Wolf, L. S., & Glass, R. P. (1992). *Feeding and swallowing disorders in infancy.* Tucson, AZ: Therapy Skill Builders.

Wright, C. M., Parkinson, K. N., & Drewett, R. F. (2006). How does maternal and child feeding behavior relate to weight gain and failure to thrive? Data from a prospective birth cohort. *Pediatrics, 117,* 1262–1269.

Yamauchi, Y., & Yamanouchi, I. (1990). Breastfeeding frequency during the first 24 hours after birth in full-term neonates. *Pediatrics, 86,* 171–175.

Yaseen, H., Salem, M., & Darwich, L. (2004). Clinical presentation of hypernatremic dehydration in exclusively breastfed neonates. *Indian J Pediatr., 71,* 1059–1062.

Yasuda, A., Kimura, H., Hayakawa, M., et al. (2003). Evaluation of cytomegalovirus infections transmitted via breast milk in preterm infants with a real-time polymerase chain reaction assay. *Pediatrics, 111,* 1333–1336.

Yildizdas, H. Y., Satar, M., Tutak, E., et al. (2005). May the best friend be an enemy is not recognized early: Hypernatremic dehydration due to breastfeeding. *Pediatric Emergency Care, 21,* 445–448.

Ziemer, M., & Pidgeon, J. (1993). Skin changes and pain in the nipple during the first week of lactation. *JOGNN, 22,* 247–256.

Additional Reading/Resources

Breastfeeding Preterm Infants

California Perinatal Quality Care Collaborative. Nutritional support of the VLBW infant: Part II. Retrieved from www.cpqcc.org.

Callen J, Pinelli J. A review of the literature examining the benefits and challenges, incidence and duration, and barriers to breastfeeding in preterm infants. *Adv Neonatal Care.* 2005;5:72–88.

Callen J, Pinelli J, Atkinson S, Saigal S. Qualitative analysis of barriers to breastfeeding in very-low-birthweight infants in the hospital and postdischarge. *Adv Neonatal Care.* 2005;5:93–103.

Hoover K, Wilson-Clay B. Pumping milk for your premature baby and pumping record. Patient teaching sheets available from www.lactnews.com.

Hurst N. Assessing and facilitating milk transfer during breastfeeding for the premature infant. *Newborn Infant Nurs Rev.* 2005;5:19–26.

Meier PP, Engstrom JL, Mingolelli SS, et al. The Rush Mothers' Milk Club: breastfeeding interventions for mothers of very low birth weight infants. *JOGNN.* 2004;33:164–174.

Nyqvist KH. Breastfeeding support in neonatal care: an example of the integration of international evidence and experience. *Newborn Infant Nurs Rev.* 2005;5:34–48.

Wight NE, Morton JA, Kim JH. *Best medicine: human milk in the NICU.* Amarillo, TX: Hale Publishing; 2008.

Resources on Jaundice

For Health Providers

California Perinatal Quality Control Collaborative
http://www.cpqcc.org/quality_improvement/qi_toolkits/
severe_hyperbilirubinemia_prevention

CDC jaundice materials for clinicians to distribute to patients
http://www.cdc.gov/ncbddd/dd/kernicterus/materials.htm

BiliTool for jaundice risk assessment
http://bilitool.org/

American Academy of Pediatrics
Predischarge Assessment of the Risk for Severe Hyperbilirubinemia
in Newborns 35 or More Weeks of Gestation
http://practice.aap.org/public/Hyperbilirubinemia_SAMPLE.pdf

A Clinician's Guide: Suggested Questions to Assess Breastfeeding in Primary
Care Practice
http://practice.aap.org/public/Breastfeeding_SAMPLE.pdf

For Parents

Jaundice and Your Newborn
http://www.aap.org/family/Jaundicefaq.htm

Newborns and Jaundice
http://www.aap.org/family/healthychildren/07school/HC-07School-Jaundice.pdf

Question and Answers: Jaundice and Your Newborn
http://www.aap.org/family/jaundicefaq.htm

Resources on Premature Infants

For Parents

PreemieCare
http://www.preemiecare.org/

The Premature Baby Book: Everything You Need to Know About Your Premature Baby from Birth to Age One. Sears et al., Little, Brown & Co.

Webpage for parents of premature infants from the American Academy of Pediatrics
http://www.aap.org/sections/perinatal/families.html

For Providers

DVDs
Breastmilk Solutions, Dr. Jane Morton
http://www.breastmilksolutions.com/index.html

Stanford School of Medicine
Getting Started with Breastfeeding
http://newborns.stanford.edu/Breastfeeding/

Human Milk Banking Association of North America
For ordering banked human milk
http://www.hmbana.org/

Resources on Late Preterm Infants

For Parents

Parent Guide: Going home with your late preterm infant
Contemporary Pediatrics, retrieved August 29, 2008, from
www.modernmedicine.com/modernmedicine/Parent+Guides/Parent-Guide-
Going-home-with-your-late-preterm-inf/ArticleStandard/Article/detail/
473739?contextCategoryId=6465

Late Preterm (Near-Term) Infant: What Parents Need to Know
AWHONN, retrieved August 29, 2008, from www.awhonn.org/awhonn/
content.do?name=02_PracticeResources/2C3_Focus_NearTermInfant.htm

ILCA's Inside Track: Breastfeeding Your Baby Who Arrived Slightly Early
Journal of Human Lactation 2007;23:269–270, retrieved from
www.ilca.org/membership/JHL/nov07/07NovemberITBW.pdf

The Diaper Diary (for keeping track of output) and Pumping Milk for Your
Premature Baby. Retrieved April 28, 2009, from www.lactnews.com/ddiary.html

Guoth-Gumberger M. *Breastfeeding with the supplementary nursing system.*
Rosenheim, Germany; 2006. Retrieved from www.breastfeeding-support.de

Name and contact information of a lactation consultant with the IBCLC credential
Retrieved April 28, 2009, from www.ilca.org/falc.html

Massachusetts Breastfeeding Coalition Zip Milk: to locate lactation consultants
and other sources of breastfeeding support in Massachusetts
Retrieved April 28, 2009, from www.massbfc.org

For Providers

Care and Management of the Late Preterm Infant Toolkit
Retrieved April 28, 2009, from www.cpqcc.org/quality_improvement/
qi_toolkits/care_and_management_of_the_late_preterm_infant_toolkit

Walker, M. Breastfeeding the late preterm infant.

Summary Interventions on Slow Infant Weight Gain: Breastfeeding Techniques Useful in Slow Weight Gain Situations

Technique	Rationale
Cross-cradle or clutch position	Provides good visualization for the mother and may be easier for her to manipulate and support the infant's head and body.
Specialty positions	Prone oblique is a position used for infants with upper airway or breathing problems such as laryngomalacia or tracheomalacia.
Dancer hand position	Offers additional jaw support for hypotonia and excessive jaw movement, slightly decreases intraoral space. A variation is just a finger placed under the chin.
Sublingual pressure	The index finger is placed gently under the chin where the tongue attaches to the floor of the mouth to keep the tongue from losing contact with the nipple. It can be used when clicking or smacking sounds are heard, indicating that the tongue is losing contact with the nipple.
Nipple tug	The mother pulls back slightly on her areola when the infant pauses (or pulls infant slightly away from her) without breaking the suction and only if the nipples are not sore. This causes the infant to pull the nipple–areola back into the mouth, strengthening the suck and sustaining the suckling.

(continues)

Technique	Rationale
Alternate massage	The mother massages and compresses the breast during the pause between sucking bursts to increase the volume and fat content of the feeding, to encourage the infant to begin another sucking burst, and to sustain and increase the number of sucks and swallows per burst.
Finger feeding	A length of tubing attached to a bottle, syringe, or feeding tube device is placed on the index finger. The infant draws the finger into the mouth and receives milk after each suck.

Equipment for Use in Slow Gaining Situations

Device	Rationale
Tube-feeding device	Commercial devices such as the Medela Supplemental Nutrition System (SNS), the starter SNS, the Lact-Aid Nursing Training System from Lact-Aid International, or ones constructed from butterfly tubing (with the needle removed) attached to a syringe; a length of number 5 French tubing run from a bottle of expressed milk; or a gavage feeding setup. Any of these can be attached to the breast to deliver supplement as the infant breastfeeds. This encourages proper suckling, improves the maternal milk supply, and avoids artificial nipples. The flow of milk into the infant's mouth stimulates further sucking (flow regulates suck). If an infant is unable to latch to the breast, the tubing can be run underneath and through an opening in a nipple shield.
Nipple shield	A thin silicone nipple shield may help an infant latch to the breast, especially one with a weak suck. Sometimes milk transfer is enhanced when combined with alternate massage.
Periodontal syringe, dropper	These are usually used to provide an incentive at breast for encouraging the infant to latch on or to sustain sucking. They are a slow mechanism to provide meaningful amounts of supplementary milk, and if used as such, generally prolong feedings and exhaust the infant and the parents.

Device	*Rationale*
Cup	A small 28 cc medicine cup, a paladai (Malhotra et al., 1999), or other small cup with a smooth, rounded edge can be a quick and safe way to increase milk intake after practice sessions at the breast (Howard et al., 1999). The milk is not poured into the infant's mouth, but the infant is supported in an upright position and allowed to sip milk at his or her own pace.
Spoon or spoon-like device	The Medela Soft Feeder or a medicine-dispensing device with a spoon-like shape can be used for small amounts of supplement.
Standard bottle/nipple	Standard bottle nipples may deliver a fast flow of milk and contribute to weakening the suck of an infant who may already be demonstrating sucking variations. A slow- to medium-flow round nipple made of soft silicone may be a reasonable choice (Kassing, 2002).
Specialty bottle/nipple	A device such as the Haberman feeder from Medela has a nipple with a valve that releases milk only with sucking effort and reduces the amount of negative pressure required to withdraw milk. Adjustments are graduated from an easy to a more difficult flow to strengthen the suck and avoid flooding the infant's mouth with milk.
Breast pump (or hand expression)	A hospital-grade electric breast pump with a double collection kit can be used to increase milk production, especially helpful for use in longer term situations. Some mothers can use a personal use category of breast pump for pumping on a shorter term basis.
Electronic scale	An electronic scale that is accurate to within 2 g can be used for monitoring intake (for example, Olympic Smart Scale, Medela Baby Weigh Scale). These scales are often used during the initial assessment of the slow weight gain and can be rented by the mother to monitor intake at feedings and help determine the need for supplements after each feeding and over a 24-hour period.

(continues)

Device	*Rationale*
Feeding logs	Depending on the complexity of the situation, mothers may need to keep track of a number of parameters such as the number of feeds per 24 hours, the amount of milk transferred from the breast to the infant by pre- and postfeed weights, the amount of milk pumped, the amount of supplement consumed, daily weights, and diaper counts of urine and stool output.

Chapter 7

Physical, Medical, and Environmental Problems and Issues

Introduction

Although it is the dream of all parents and the hope of all clinicians that infants are able to sail through breastfeeding with fair winds and few obstacles, this is not always the case. A number of conditions and situations do not preclude breast-feeding but may complicate the process. Even if direct feeding at the breast is not possible for some infants, almost all infants benefit from receiving human milk.

Twins and Higher Order Multiples

It is both possible and desirable to breastfeed twins and higher order multiples. In 2006 there were 137,085 births of twins. The number of births of triplets or higher declined 2% from the previous year to the lowest reported in a decade (6,540 in 2006) and included 6,118 triplets, 355 quadruplets, and 67 quintuplets (Martin et al., 2009). Multiple births are more common with increasing maternal age and with the use of infertility therapy. There is a high risk of adverse outcomes in mul-tiple births. One of every eight twins and one of every three triplets are born very preterm (less than 32 weeks of gestation), compared with fewer than 2 of every 100 singletons. Accordingly, death during infancy is much more common among twins (29.8 per 1,000) and triplets (59.6 per 1,000) than among singletons (6.0 per 1,000). In response to the unparalleled rise in higher order multiple births during the 1980s and 1990s and their attendant risk of poor outcome, the American Society of Reproductive Medicine published guidelines intended to reduce the incidence of triplets/+ resulting from assisted reproductive therapy by limiting the number of embryos transferred (The Practice Committee of the American Society for Reproductive Technology, the American Society for Reproductive Medicine, 2006). Studies have since documented substantial declines in such transfers (Stern et al., 2007).

In an analysis of over 1,000 higher order multiples births, 74% of the members of the Mothers of Supertwins organization reported that they initiated breast-feeding, with a mean duration of 3.1 months (ranging from a few days to 28 months) (Boyle & Collopy, 2000). Increased breastfeeding rates for mothers of multiples may be achieved with highly motivated mothers who have access to lactation help and support groups (Damato et al., 2005a; Gromada & Spangler, 1998). Mothers wish to breastfeed their infants due to the improved health outcomes from the use of breastmilk but may need extensive education on the importance of providing their milk to multiple infants (Friedman et al., 2004). Although mothers of multiples elect to breastfeed at similar rates to mothers with singleton pregnancies (Bowers & Gromada, 2003), they and their infants are at an increased risk for a number of complications. The higher the plurality, the greater the likelihood of poor perinatal outcomes. These infants tend to be born both preterm and small for gestational age (Table 7-1).

Geraghty et al. (2004b) evaluated the feeding practices of four groups of mothers: mothers of term singletons, mothers of preterm singletons, mothers of term multiples, and mothers of preterm multiples. By 3 days postpartum, mothers of preterm multiples provided breastmilk less often than all other groups. This trend continued for the first 6 months of life, showing that the duration of any

TABLE 7-1   Comparison of Gestational Age and Birth Weight in Multiple Births

Plurality	Mean Gestational Age (wk)	Mean Birth Weight (g)
Singleton	38.8 (± 2.5)	3,332 (± 573) [~7 lb 4 oz]
Twins	35.3 (± 3.7)	2,347 (± 645) [~5 lb 3 oz]
Triplets	32.2 (± 3.8)	1,687 (± 561) [~ 3 lb 12 oz]
Quadruplets	29.4 (± 4.0)	1,309 (± 522) [~ 2 lb 14 oz]
Quintuplets +	28.5 (± 4.7)	1,105 (± 777) [~ 2lb 7 oz]

Values in parentheses are standard deviations

Source: Martin JA, Hamilton BE, Sutton PD, et al. *Births: Final Data for 2002.* National Vital Statistics Reports, Vol. 52. Hyattsville, MD: National Center for Health Statistics; 2003.

breastmilk feeding was significantly shorter for preterm multiples than for all other groups (12 weeks for preterm multiples, 24 weeks for term singletons, 19 weeks for preterm singletons, and 24 weeks for term multiples). The combination of multiple gestation and preterm delivery resulted in lower breastmilk feeding rates and a shorter duration of breastfeeding by mothers of preterm multiples. This suggests the need for more intensive breastfeeding support and follow-up for this especially vulnerable population.

The inability to synthesize sufficient amounts of milk for multiples does not appear to account for the less-optimal breastfeeding outcomes in preterm multiples. Milk yields in mothers of twins measured between 2 and 6 months ranged from 1,680 to 3,000 mL/day. Mothers of multiples are capable of producing sufficient amounts of milk for two or more infants over long periods of time (Biancuzzo, 1994; Liang et al., 1997). The milk yield of one mother of triplets was 3,080 mL/day at 2.5 months (Saint et al., 1986). Mean daily weight gains of quadruplets during the first month after discharge varied from 30 to 54 g, indicative of adequate milk supply as a result of optimal breastfeeding management (Mead et al., 1992). Berlin (2007) reported that a mother of quadruplets expressed 108 oz per 24 hours during the time the infants were in the neonatal intensive care unit (NICU), validating the capacity of the breasts to respond to the increased needs of multiple infants. In a case study of a mother of quintuplets, banked donor human milk was also used when the infants required more milk than the mother could provide. This allowed the infants to be fed human milk exclusively, which contributed to the relative lack of medical complications in these infants (Szucs et al., 2009).

Prenatal Preparation for Breastfeeding Multiples

Although most mothers are aware early in their pregnancy that they are carrying more than one infant, they may question their ability to breastfeed multiple infants. Clinicians should reassure parents that the provision of breastmilk and breastfeeding remains both possible and optimal (Sollid et al., 1989). Breastmilk provides the same protective factors to multiples as to singletons (Flidel-Rimon & Shinwell, 2002) and can promote the development of a close maternal attachment to each infant (Gromada, 1981). Other prenatal considerations are as follows:

- Maternal nutritional management. Because preterm birth and growth-restricted infants are two common outcomes of a multiple pregnancy, maternal nutrition and weight gain are especially important factors in optimizing the duration of the pregnancy and reducing the incidence of low or very low birth weight infants (Leonard, 1982). Mothers carrying multiple infants usually benefit from nutritional counseling to ensure adequate intake of energy and nutrients to achieve weight gain targets of 35–44 lb for a twin pregnancy (Roem, 2003) and a 50-lb weight gain for a triplet pregnancy (Brown & Carlson, 2000). Optimal rates of fetal growth and birth weights in a twin pregnancy are achieved at rates of maternal weight gain that vary by gestational period and by maternal pregravid body mass index (Luke et al., 2003) (Table 7-2).

• An identified source of breastfeeding support. A mother will need access to a lactation consultant and/or other resources for breastfeeding support who possess specific expertise in managing the breastfeeding of multiples (Leonard, 2000; Storr, 1989). She will also require information regarding prenatal classes specific to multiple births (Moxley & Haddon, 1999) and information on the extent of lactation care and services she can expect where she delivers her infants. Efforts should be made to designate a case manager or other healthcare provider that coordinates both breastfeeding management and the other support services needed by a multiple-birth family. This helps reduce confusion, miscommunication, and fragmented care that contribute to poor breastfeeding outcomes (Leonard, 2003).

TABLE 7-2 Weight Gain in Twin Pregnancies by Pregravid Weight and Gestational Period

Pregravid Weight Status	Gestational Period	Weight Gain
Underweight	0–20 wk	1.25–1.75 lb/wk
	20–28 wk	1.5–1.75 lb/wk
	28 wk to delivery	1.25 lb/wk
Normal weight	0–20 wk	1.0–1.5 lb/wk
	20–28 wk	1.25–1.75 lb/wk
	28 wk to delivery	1.0 lb/wk
Overweight	0–20 wk	1.0–1.25 lb/wk
	20–28 wk	1.0–1.5 lb/wk
	28 wk to delivery	1.0 lb/wk
Obese	0–20 wk	0.75–1.0 lb/wk
	20–28 wk	0.75–1.25 lb/wk
	28 wk to delivery	0.75 lb/wk

- Written and video resources. A mother should have a working knowledge of breastfeeding with specific written materials relevant to how multiple births affect breastfeeding (Gromada, 1999) and have viewed a video with her spouse and family so that family members understand their role. She should also be provided with community and online support sources specific to parenting multiples.

- Equipment resources. Mothers need written information on where to secure an electric breast pump, digital scale, "V" or horseshoe-shaped pillow for simultaneous feeding of two infants, equipment for transporting twins or higher order multiples, and so forth. She should also check if her health insurance covers the cost of a pump rental and lactation care and services.

- Exploring and setting breastfeeding goals. Discuss the mother's plans for how much breastfeeding she would like to accomplish (Auer & Gromada, 1998). There are many different ways to breastfeed multiples:

  - Some mothers of twins and triplets are able to provide breastmilk for and/or breastfeed exclusively all of the infants (Leonard, 2000; Liang et al., 1997).

  - Mothers may combine feeding at the breast, bottle-feeding expressed breastmilk, and/or bottle-feeding (or other alternative feeding technique) infant formula depending on the number of infants, their health status, in-hospital experience, and the mother's milk production (Biancuzzo, 1994; Hattori & Hattori, 1999). This may change over time as the infants become more proficient at the breast, the milk supply increases, or one or more infants do not tolerate infant formula or experience other health problems.

  - Even small amounts of breastmilk are important to multiple infants, especially if born preterm or with other health concerns. Some mothers use a rotation plan of feeding two triplets at the breast simultaneously (one on each breast), followed by the third infant who is given both breasts. This rotation may help the smaller infant who feeds from both breasts, which may contain the higher-fat-content milk.

- Securing at-home help. Expectant parents of multiples need to secure regular and reliable sources of ongoing help at home. This is especially important for parents of higher order multiples and if the mother has experienced a cesarean delivery, extended bedrest, or other complications of a multiple pregnancy. These sources may be family, friends, postpartum doulas, postpartum support agencies, volunteers from church organizations, or grandparent organizations. Some parents may not be able to afford at-home help and need to explore other community services for which they may be eligible, such as homemaker and home health aid services. This type of help is often necessary for many months, especially with higher order multiples.

Managing the In-Hospital Experience

Once the infants are born, a breastfeeding plan should be created, taking into account the number of infants, the status of the infants, the mother's health and comfort needs, the mother's desires, and the agreed on short- and long-term goals. Overarching goals include the initiation and maintenance of optimal milk production and establishing feeding at the breast or breastmilk feeding (if one or more infants are unable to feed directly from the breast) of all infants.

Healthy Full-Term Multiples

Flexible rooming-in should be encouraged, with the timing and amount of rooming-in individualized to each family (Leonard, 2002). Healthy twins and triplets can be kept skin-to-skin and breastfed on cue, with feeding sessions assisted and documented by a nurse, lactation consultant, or other caregiver skilled in preterm multiple breastfeeding. Cue-based feeding takes into account the differing needs and feeding skills of each infant (Gromada, 1992). Mothers benefit from the presence of the father and other helpers such as student nurses, peer counselors, or even family members who can assist with holding and positioning the infants. Each infant should have his or her own color-coded documentation forms to track intake and output and to record breastfeeding assessments. Breastfeeding should be initiated at the earliest opportunity, with one infant at a time. This allows each infant to be properly positioned and latched and to ensure that the infant is swallowing milk. It also helps in maternal attachment to each infant. Simultaneous breastfeeding is better postponed until the infants demonstrate effective breastfeeding skills that can be validated with an assessment tool. The mother thus becomes acquainted with each infant's breastfeeding style and needs, helping her acquire competence and confidence in her ability to breastfeed each baby. Simultaneous breastfeeding at this point could mask problems, especially the ability of each infant to sustain nutritive sucking and swallowing. If the infants are not in the mother's room, they should be brought to her on cue for all feedings. In the absence of maternal complications, healthy multiples should have early access to the breast and breastfeed between 8 and 12 times each 24 hours (Gromada & Spangler, 1998). Supplements, pacifiers, and bottles should be avoided except for medical reasons. Infants should not alternate between feeding at the breast and being bottle-fed. This practice has the potential to delay the acquisition of effective feeding skills at the breast and to interfere with the initiation and maintenance of an abundant milk supply.

In some situations the infants may be full term and healthy, but the mother's postpartum recovery may be affected by complications of the pregnancy or delivery. It is not unusual to encounter a mother of multiples who has pregnancy-induced hypertension or preeclampsia, is receiving magnesium sulfate ($MgSO_4$) to treat this, has experienced a cesarean delivery, is on a PCA (patient-controlled analgesia) pump for pain medication, and is experiencing weakness from extended bedrest or heavy blood loss. A mother on $MgSO_4$ (and pain medications) may be temporarily unable to orient herself and organize her time to attend to all the tasks she is expected to accomplish. She may be weak and need physical help in positioning and actually holding the infants at the breast. She may need someone else to watch for infant feeding readiness cues and initiate each breastfeeding session. If the mother is pumping for preterm or ill infants in the NICU, she may also need to be reminded about each pumping session and require someone to physically hold the breastshields to her breast and operate the pump. Many of these mothers are unable to absorb verbal teaching, keep records, or remember details about each infant's condition until the effects of the medications have worn off.

Clinicians and parents should anticipate that lactogenesis II and copious milk production may be delayed by factors common to multiple births and known to affect the timing of these events such as an urgent cesarean section (Dewey et al., 2003), extreme stress (Chen et al., 1998; Dewey, 2001), presence of diabetes, severe postpartum hemorrhage (Willis & Livingstone, 1995), anemia (Henly et al., 1995), ineffective or infrequent breast drainage, and unrelieved severe engorgement. Use of $MgSO_4$ has been suggested as a contributor to poor milk production and a later onset of lactation (Haldeman, 1993; Hale & Ilett, 2002). Although the amount of magnesium transferred to breastmilk is almost clinically irrelevant, sedation, hypotonia, and poor sucking have been reported in infants whose mothers received $MgSO_4$ prenatally or during the intrapartum period (Finnegan, 1982; Fuentes & Goldkrand, 1987; Hale, 2004; Riaz et al., 1998), adding yet another dimension to ineffective breast drainage and a delay in lactogenesis II.

Preterm Multiples

If the infants have been born preterm, they may be separated from their mother in a special care nursery or NICU, may or may not be capable of feeding at the breast, or may be too preterm or ill to be brought out to the mother. They may be placed in separate beds, separate nurseries, or transported to different hospitals depending on their acuity and availability of beds where they were born. If the infants are unable to transfer milk effectively at breast or cannot be fed at the breast, the mother should begin pumping her milk within about 6 hours of delivery. Mothers who hand express or pump within an hour or 2 of giving birth may yield enough colostrum for each infant's first feeding. After that, mothers should pump milk with an electric pump, a double collection kit, and a breast-shield large enough to accommodate the nipple comfortably within the nipple tunnel. Breastmilk production can be maximized by early pumping, expressing 8–12 times each 24 hours, and massaging and compressing the breast while pumping (Hill et al., 2001; Jones et al., 2001).

Parents can be encouraged to practice kangaroo care of their newborns, either one or two at a time and shared between the mother and father, helping to facilitate milk production, earlier feedings at the breast, and parental self-confidence (Dombrowski et al., 2000). Cobedding twins or pairs of multiples involves keeping two infants snuggled together in the same bassinet. This practice enhances stabilization, reduces stress levels, often results in better breastfeeding, and tends to keep them awake at the same time (Nyqvist & Lutes, 1998). Breastfeeding is also improved as mothers synchronize breastfeeding with the twins' behavioral states (Nyqvist, 2002). If the mother is unable to walk to the special care nursery or NICU, she should be transported in her bed or wheelchair when ready to see and touch her infants. Parents will need to discuss how the expressed colostrum should be distributed among the infants if early volumes are limited. Options include small amounts evenly distributed among all infants, all colostrum given to the sickest infant, or rotating complete colostrum feedings among each infant.

As the infants move toward direct feeding at the breast, a breastfeeding plan for each infant is necessary and adapted as needed to account for variations in their conditions, specific feeding problems, pumping schedule, equipment needs, the parents' needs, and the needs and care of older children. Within the plan would be strategies to address ineffective suckling, need for complemental or supplemental feedings, limited milk transfer, and the effect of any congenital anomalies on breastfeeding (LaFleur & Niesen, 1996). Milk transfer in healthy multiples should be carefully assessed before giving additional formula directly after or in between breastfeedings. Unnecessary formula feeding can depress the infant's appetite, prolong intervals between breastfeeds, reduce sucking efficiency, prolong feeding sessions, and extend the time it takes to establish exclusive breastfeeding (Biancuzzo, 1994).

Hospital Discharge

Before discharging the mother or any of the infants, mothers need a clear plan of how to feed and care for themselves and their infants. All household helpers and nursing equipment should be in place and/or in the home before discharge, including an electric breast pump, collection containers if milk will be transported to the infants remaining in the hospital, digital scale for pre- and postfeed intake assessments and periodic weight checks, nipple shields if needed for infants with a weak suck, alternative feeding equipment if needed, special pillow for simultaneous infant feeding, and a designated location for feedings.

Ideally, all infants would be discharged at the same time, but this is not always possible. Each infant may come home at a different time with some infants admitted into different hospitals, making visiting, breastfeeding, and milk transport a logistical nightmare. When one or more infants come home and one or more remain in the hospital the mother can use the following plans:

- Bring the at-home infants along with a caregiver to the hospital while visiting those infants who remain hospitalized; this might be very likely when the mother lives a great distance from the hospital.
- For briefer visits, the infants at home can be left with a caregiver while the mother visits the hospital.
- In the event that the mother is unwell or unable to visit the hospital, her pumped milk can be brought to the infants by the father or other helper; in some instances, hospital employees who live near the mother have transported milk to the hospitalized infants.
- A mother can breastfeed the infant at home on one side while pumping the other breast, maintaining a connection to the infant(s) still hospitalized, as mother and infant work as a team to provide milk for the absent infant.
- Mothers may feel torn between the infants at home and those in the hospital. Some units have "video conferencing" capabilities where a camera can transmit images of the infants to the mother at home.

Feeding Rotations

Mothers usually adopt a breast rotation pattern that best fits everyone's needs. Mothers can alternate breasts for each feeding, rotate infants and breasts every 24 hours, or "assign" breasts to each infant.

It is important to ensure that each breast is producing its maximum capacity of milk by avoiding the assignment of one breast to a poorly feeding infant. Most mothers offer one breast per feeding (or the third triplet can be offered both sides after two have been fed). Mothers of odd-numbered sets of multiples may need to alternate breasts and infants more frequently than each 24 hours because infants' bilateral development is enhanced when fed in different positions. Pacifiers may be a temptation to use when all infants are crying at once or to calm an infant until it is his or her turn at breast. However, pacifiers have the potential to alter an infant's mouth conformation and introduce poor breastfeeding technique into the breastfeeding plan. Mothers of multiples do not need the increased chance of problems that pacifiers could produce.

Separate and Simultaneous Feedings

Whereas some mothers with healthy full-term infants are ready for simultaneous feedings early in the postpartum period, many mothers prefer to feed one infant at a time, allowing them to become acquainted with each one individually. It may be difficult for some mothers to sort out the different feeding sensations of each infant when they are being fed simultaneously, especially if one infant is not feeding efficiently. An infant with feeding difficulties, chronic health problems, or special needs may require being fed separately until feeding skills have been mastered. Infants who cannot meet their full nutritional needs at the breast may need to be fed individually if the mother must use a nipple shield or tube-feeding device or must weigh the baby pre- and postfeed to determine supplementation quantities.

Simultaneous feeding saves time and works well when all infants are skilled at feeding, the mother enjoys it, and each infant copes well with his or her sibling at the other breast. Some mothers, however, feel awkward or do not enjoy the sensation of two infants who may be suckling with different rhythms and reserve simultaneous feedings for times when both are crying or when time constraints exist. Birth anomalies such as torticollis or plagiocephaly may also play a part in determining how some of the infants are best positioned for feedings. Plural births experience a higher incidence and risk of plagiocephaly. Breastfeeding may help prevent occipital plagiocephaly as breastfed infants are repositioned more frequently and sleep for shorter periods of time (Losee et al., 2007). When feeding simultaneously, some mothers begin with the infant with greater latching difficulties while both hands are free, followed by a more skilled infant. Occasionally, a skilled infant can be put to breast to elongate and shape the nipple–areola, elicit milk ejection, and be removed from that breast and placed on the other breast, while the less-skilled infant takes advantage of a nipple that has been elongated for him or her with milk readily available. Mothers of higher order multiples may breastfeed two infants at a time while bottle-feeding the third.

Mothers typically use a combination of single and simultaneous feedings and move from feeding on cue to more scheduled feedings, especially with three or more infants. Some mothers use a modified demand schedule where one infant is fed on cue and the other(s) simultaneously or sequentially immediately afterward. Some mothers wake the other infant or infants when the first one rouses, coordinating simultaneous feeds, or she may prefer sequential feeding of one infant right after the other.

Simultaneous feeding positions may be easier initially when using special pillows that are shaped to accommodate two infants. These are firmer than bed pillows and angled such that the infants are not flat but slightly elevated and semilying on their side. Narrow rocking chairs or recliners may not have enough room to use such pillows. There are three basic simultaneous feeding positions and many variations that mothers devise to best suit their needs:

1. Double cradle (crisscross): Each infant is held in the cradle position with their bodies crisscrossed, either one over the other or parallel to the mother's thighs.

2. Double clutch or football: Often an easier position to learn initially, each infant lies tucked under an arm or lies on a pillow perpendicular to the mother's body.

3. Combination (one infant in the cradle position, one in the clutch position): This positioning may be a little more discrete but care should be taken that the infant's head in the clutch position does not overly compress the other infant's abdomen.

Partial Breastfeeding and Breastmilk Feeding Options

Mothers of multiples are more likely to supplement or complement with bottles, infant formula, or expressed breastmilk given by bottle or alternative feeding method. This is especially common with higher order multiples and if early effective breastfeeding or breastmilk expression was adversely impacted by maternal and/or infant complications. Complements and supplements are least likely to diminish milk production if each multiple is breastfeeding 7–10 times per day. Certain feeding patterns are more likely to result in diminished milk production and early weaning unless the feeding plan includes pumping breast-milk for the complements and supplements:

- Alternating breast and bottle such that all infants feed at breast for one feeding and all are bottle-fed the next feeding
- All infants receive a complement after each breastfeeding
- Breastfeeding one or more multiples and supplement the others at each feeding
- One infant exclusively breastfeeds and the other exclusively bottle-feeds

Some infants with chronic health problems may never accomplish direct feeding at the breast but can still receive pumped human milk. Over time, most mothers are able to decrease the number of complements and supplements and may offer alternative feeds on a daily or weekly basis to sleep for a few uninterrupted hours or if milk production cannot keep pace with the increasing needs of the infants. Checklists that include feeding and pumping logs should be kept to ensure adequate intake and growth of all of the infants. Many parents will paint a fingernail or toenail a different color on each infant to easily and rapidly tell them apart if needed and to color code their individual records.

Each infant is an individual and may present a range of feeding behaviors that change over time. The infants may experience growth spurts at different times, may gain weight differently, may come to prefer one breast over the other, may start solids at different times, and may wean at different times.

Prolonging Breastfeeding and the Provision of Breastmilk

New breastfeeding issues continue to arise over the course of the breastfeeding experience. Mothers of twins list numerous explanations for the cessation of breastfeeding or expressing (Damato et al., 2005b): return to work, inadequate milk supply, breast or nipple problems, time burdens of either nursing or pumping or both, presence of older siblings, maternal illness, fatigue, poor infant feeding behaviors, infant sleepiness, and/or desire to have more time for other things. Infants from multiple births do not meet the national breastfeeding goals outlined in the Healthy People 2010 recommendations of 75% initiation rate and 50% continuation rate at 6 months. Geraghty et al. (2004a) reported a continuous decline in the amount of breastmilk received by multiples with 64% of twins receiving at least some breastmilk at 3 days of life and 25% of twin infants receiving some breastmilk at 6 months. Fifty-five percent of triplets received some breastmilk within the first month of life, with only 15% receiving any breastmilk at 6 months.

Some mothers find increasing time burdens if it becomes difficult to nurse infants simultaneously as they grow larger and must nurse one infant at a time. A major factor in continued breastfeeding is the length of time required to feed each infant (Flidel-Rimon & Shinwell, 2006). Some infants remain very slow feeders, and interventions to accelerate feedings may prove helpful (alternate massage, supplementing at breast, scheduled feedings). Mothers who have been on extended bedrest during the pregnancy may have difficulty meeting the physical demand of caring for infants, pumping, and breastfeeding due to the deconditioning that happens during prolonged periods of inactivity. Mothers may find that the large amounts of help they enjoyed during the early weeks have dwindled, making it more difficult to attend to multiple infants and other responsibilities.

Breast pumps should be checked periodically to make sure they are functioning properly. A vacuum gauge should be used to occasionally ensure that a pump is generating maximum amounts of vacuum because some pumps may lose vacuum-generating capacity, especially if a mother is not using a large hospital-grade breast pump.

Damato et al. (2005a) found that the percentage of breastmilk feedings at 1 month after expected delivery date was predictive of continued breastfeeding at 6 months after expected delivery date. Intensive breastfeeding interventions and support are frequently necessary to ensure breastfeeding continues. Often, the first 5–9 weeks of breastfeeding are the most difficult and require the most time investment. At 5 weeks the effort put into breastfeeding equals the same effort as bottle-feeding, but between 8 and 9 weeks the effort to breastfeed becomes less than that to bottle-feed. If mothers can sustain breastfeeding for 1–2 months, breastfeeding becomes less time consuming than bottle-feeding, not only with bottle preparation but also in better health and decreased trips to the pediatrician or hospital (Chay et al., 2007). Knowing this may help mothers set a goal and provide hope that things will improve. Mothers who feed solely at the breast, especially during the first 2 months postpartum, are more likely to continue feeding human milk at later time points and to feed human milk for longer durations (Geraghty et al., 2005).

Anomalies, Diseases, and Disorders That Can Affect Breastfeeding

Ankyloglossia

Ankyloglossia, or tongue-tie, is a congenital oral anomaly, whose prevalence or incidence is between 1.7% and 10.7%, or about 1 to 4 infants per 100 in consecutive births and as high as 25% in infants identified as having breastfeeding difficulties (Ballard et al., 2002; Hogan et al., 2005; Masaitis & Kaempf, 1996; Messner et al., 2000). The wide range in prevalence can be attributed to different diagnostic criteria used in the studies. There is no standard test or criteria for the definition or recognition of ankyloglossia, and it may be described in terms of physical characteristics of the infant's oral anatomy or include signs of functional impairment. It is generally described as a condition in which the normal range of motion of the tongue is restricted due to an abnormal attachment of the lingual frenulum (or frenum) toward the tip of the tongue. The lingual frenulum may be too short, thick, and taut after birth or may not have receded, remaining attached too far along the base of the tongue. The frenula are strong cords of tissue at the front and center of the mouth that guide the development of mouth structures during gestation. Development of the tongue begins in the floor of the primitive oral cavity when the embryo is 4 weeks old and the external face is developing. Important during fetal development, the frenula continue after birth to help guide and position the baby teeth as they come in. Children with tongue-tie may be unable to protrude the tongue, touch the roof of the mouth, or move the tongue from side to side. If the lingual frenum extends to the tip of the tongue, a V-shaped notch or heart shape can be seen at the tip.

Ankyloglossia is often familial, not preventable, and usually seen as an isolated condition in an otherwise normal, healthy infant. However, some malformations of the tongue that happen during embryogenesis are seen in combination with a high arched palate, recessed chin, and/or other congenital defects and syndromes (Emmanouil-Nikoloussi & Kerameos-Foroglou, 1992a, 1992b). Because tongue-tie is a midline defect and can be associated with a number of genetic syndromes, failure to see improved breastfeeding after correction of ankyloglossia may signal the need to evaluate the infant further for other causes of poor neurological or mechanical control of the tongue.

Problems Associated With Tongue-Tie

A number of pathologies may be associated with tongue-tie:

- Breastfeeding difficulties: With the rising breastfeeding initiation rates and improved assessment techniques, case studies, small uncontrolled case series, and clinician concerns regarding breastfeeding difficulties associated with tongue-tie have proliferated (Berg, 1990a; Fleiss et al., 1990; Huggins, 1990; Marmet et al., 1990; Notestine, 1990; Ward, 1990; Wilton, 1990). Ankyloglossia is associated with a 25–60% incidence of difficulties with breastfeeding. Among lactation experts, ankyloglossia has become a recognized cause of breastfeeding difficulties that include poor latching, inadequate milk transfer by the infant, slow weight gain, and distress while feeding and in the mother, sore/macerated nipples (Palmer, 2003), diminished milk production, displeasure with continuous feedings, and premature weaning (Berg, 1990b; Griffiths, 2004; Jain, 1995; Walker, 1989). For every day of maternal pain during the first 3 weeks of breastfeeding, there is a 10–26% risk of cessation of breastfeeding (Schwartz et al., 2002), making it a priority to immediately address conditions that cause maternal nipple pain such as ankyloglossia. The prevalence of persistent nipple pain in mothers whose infants have ankyloglossia is between 36% and 80%. Only 3% of mothers of normal infants have intractable pain or difficulty in achieving latch at 6 weeks, but 25% of mothers of infants with ankyloglossia have these problems (Messner et al., 2000). Some infants may also present with a high arched palate because the tongue's contact with the palate typically gives the palate its characteristic shape. A tongue that cannot assume its normal position may contribute to an alteration in the oral cavity's shape, acting as a further contributor to sore nipples in the mother and possible diminished milk transfer in the infant. Mothers themselves describe obvious differences between breastfeeding older children who are unaffected and breastfeeding a subsequent infant with tongue-tie. After tongue-tie release, most mothers note an improvement in breastfeeding and a reduction in nipple trauma (Lalakea & Messner, 2003a). Researchers reported that tongue-tie can also be associated with displacement of the epiglottis and larynx, resulting in decreased oxygen saturation during feeding (Mukai et al., 1991). Young infants with ankyloglossia are often observed to come off of the breast frequently, pause for long periods of time between sucking bursts, choke, cry, or fall asleep at the breast. Some of the improvement seen after frenotomy may also be due to the resolution of respiratory and circulatory compromise that could have been contributing to the altered breastfeeding patterns.

- Speech problems: Many of the shapes that the tongue engages in during speaking are also seen in feeding. It has been suggested that the matrix of tongue movements during human speech is derived from the wide range and variety of tongue movements found in suckling and feeding (Hiimae & Palmer, 2003). Controversy exists (even among speech therapists) regarding whether or not the anomaly interferes with speech (Messner & Lalakea, 2000). Some children with ankyloglossia develop normal speech as they learn to compensate for limited tongue mobility, even without speech therapy (Wright, 1995). Up to 50% of children with ankyloglossia referred for otolaryngology evaluation have articulation difficulties, with the rate and range of articulation errors causing their speech to be difficult to understand (Fletcher & Meldrum, 1968; Lalakea & Messner, 2003b; Messner & Lalakea, 2002). Tongue-tie impacts tongue tip mobility, affecting the sounds made by l, r, t, s, d, n, th, sh, and z. Although problematic to predict which infants with tongue-tie are likely to experience articulation problems later, the following characteristics are common in children with speech problems:

- V-shaped notch at the tip of the tongue
- Inability to protrude the tongue past the upper gums
- Inability to touch the roof of the mouth
- Difficulty moving the tongue from side to side

• Dental and orthodontic problems: Pressure from a tight lingual frenulum can cause a diastasis or gap between the two lower central incisors, just as a taut labial frenulum (under the upper lip) can result in a large gap between the two upper central incisors. Restriction of normal tongue movements may result in a tongue thrust, forcing the tongue forward during a swallow instead of moving it up and back against the roof of the mouth. This can establish a pattern of abnormal swallowing (Palmer, 2001), affecting not only breastfeeding but also the ultimate positioning of the teeth.

Controversies in Diagnosis and Management

Disagreement exists among a number of healthcare disciplines regarding both the definition and management of ankyloglossia. In a survey of medical experts, significant differences of opinion existed regarding ankyloglossia's association with breastfeeding difficulties, altered speech patterns, dental problems, and whether or not correction was needed or helpful (Messner & Lalakea, 2000). The tightness of the frenulum can vary significantly, and the degree of tightness can influence consequences and outcomes. A number of schemata have been advanced to confirm the presence of ankyloglossia and grade its severity as a mechanism to validate intervention:

• The Assessment Tool for Lingual Frenulum Function (Hazelbaker, 1993) evaluates the infant's tongue with scores of 0 to 2 on five appearance items and seven function items, with frenotomy recommended when the score totals 8 or less on appearance and 11 or less on function. However, not all items on this tool have good interrater reliability (Madlon-Kay et al., 2008). Amir et al. (2006) found that the first three items on the function score that assess the mobility of the tongue (forward extension, lateral movement, and tongue elevation) were reliable indicators for frenotomy when the score was less than or equal to 4.

- The Frenotomy Decision Rule for Breastfeeding Infants (Srinivasan et al., 2006) evaluates the need for frenotomy based on
  - Mother with nipple pain/trauma, AND/OR inability to maintain latch, AND/OR poor infant weight gain, AND a visible frenulum restricting tongue movement leading to
    - Tongue unable to touch roof of mouth, OR
    - Tongue unable to cup examining finger, OR
    - Tongue cannot protrude beyond gum line

  This approach found no relationship between actual length of the frenulum and breastfeeding problems, but the extent of breastfeeding difficulties determined if surgical correction was necessary. Frenotomy based on the above criteria improved the LATCH score, reduced nipple pain almost immediately, and extended breastfeeding.

- Ankyloglossia was described and graded in relation to abnormalities of the lingual frenulum and to variations in the origin of the free portion of the tongue (Mukai et al., 1991).

- Ankyloglossia has been categorized by the length of the free tongue (length of tongue from insertion of the lingual frenulum into the base of the tongue to the tip of the tongue). The normal range of the free tongue was defined as greater than 16 mm (Kotlow, 1999):
  - Class I: mild ankyloglossia, 12–16 mm
  - Class II: moderate, 8–11 mm
  - Class III: severe, 3–7 mm
  - Class IV: complete, less than 3 mm

Structural guidelines were also advanced that described criteria for the normal range of motion and behavior of the tongue:

- The tip of the tongue should be capable of protruding outside the mouth without clefting.
- The tip of the tongue should be able to sweep the upper and lower lips without straining.

- When the tongue is moved backward, it should not blanch the tissue behind the teeth.
- The tongue should not place excessive forces on the lower central incisors.
- The lingual frenulum should allow a normal swallowing pattern.
- The lingual frenulum should not create a gap between the lower central incisors.
- The underside of the infant's tongue should not exhibit abrasion or erosion.
- The frenulum should not prohibit the infant from achieving a proper latch to the nipple–areola.
- Speech difficulties should not be created from limited tongue movements.

- Tongue-ties were divided into four types according to how close to the tip of the tongue the leading edge of the frenulum was attached (Coryllos et al., 2004):

  1. Type 1—the frenulum is attached to the tip of the tongue, in front of the alveolar ridge.

  2. Type 2—the frenulum is attached 2–4 mm behind the tongue tip and attaches on or just behind the alveolar ridge.

  3. Type 3—the frenulum attaches to the mid-tongue and the middle floor of the mouth. This is a tighter and less elastic frenulum.

  4. Type 4—the frenulum is very thick, shiny, and highly inelastic because it is essentially attached against the base of the tongue. This situation can result in difficulties with bolus formation and swallowing because the tongue is unable to assume a cupped shape and form a central groove to channel milk to the back of the throat for the swallow. This tongue would have difficulty engaging in an anterior to posterior peristaltic wave with a resulting presentation of limited milk intake and sore or macerated maternal nipples. Although less common in occurrence, this type of tongue-tie is not immediately visible when the infant opens his or her mouth and can go unnoticed until breastfeeding problems become symptomatic.

Some practitioners may resist intervention and instead recommend waiting for the infant to outgrow the condition and/or place the infant on a bottle if breastfeeding difficulties cannot be resolved. Delays in surgical correction, even with intensive lactation counseling and education, usually do not improve breastfeeding (Hogan et al., 2005; Marmet & Shell, 1990). An infant with ankyloglossia can obtain milk from a bottle by a chewing motion that would be problematic at breast; however, placing such an infant on a bottle will not resolve the possible tongue thrust, faulty swallowing, open bite, and articulation errors that may still manifest themselves if the condition remains uncorrected. This infant might also experience problems swallowing semisolid foods when they are introduced. Visual and digital assessment of the infant's tongue reveals the extent of the problem with the mother often presenting with sore or macerated nipples (Ricke et al., 2005), poor drainage of the breasts with possible resulting milk stasis, and descriptions of feeding sessions that are frustrating and lengthy. The infant may pop on and off the breast, make a clicking or smacking sound while nursing as the tongue loses contact with the nipple–areolar complex, dribble milk from the corners of the mouth because the tongue cannot form a central groove to channel milk to the back of the throat, and fatigue quickly during feedings (Fernando, 1998).

Geddes et al. (2008) performed ultrasound scans on the oral cavities of 24 infants with ankyloglossia before and after frenotomy. Total milk production of these mothers increased significantly after frenotomy, which serves to alert the clinician to ensure milk production remains adequate before and after surgery but especially in mothers when frenotomy is not performed. Milk intake, milk transfer, and the LATCH assessment scores increased significantly and the mothers' pain decreased significantly after surgery. Ultrasound scans identified two types of tongue movements, with infants compressing either the base or the tip of the nipple. These movements resolved following frenotomy as did maternal nipple pain.

Surgical Intervention

Clipping the frenulum, or frenotomy (without repair), is a simple procedure typically used for infants under 4 months of age with a feeding improvement rate of up to 95% (Hogan et al., 2005). It is an office procedure performed by a doctor, without anesthesia or at the most perhaps topical benzocaine applied to each side of the frenulum. The procedure is usually brief and bloodless, with hemostasis (if needed) achieved by simple pressure or breastfeeding, which lengthens the tongue and acts as an analgesic and antiseptic. Frenuloplasty is a procedure often performed on older children (or in cases of severe ankyloglossia in infants) involving a more complete release of the frenulum with a plastic closure (z-plasty flap closure or a horizontal to vertical plasty). Complex cases can be referred to an oral surgeon or an ear, nose, and throat specialist. Some frenotomies can also be done by laser in a dentist's office or with an electrocautery needle (Naimer et al., 2003).

Complications of frenotomy and frenuloplasty were historically reported to include concerns about pain, infection, excessive bleeding, scarring at the surgical site and restricted mobility of the tongue, too much tongue mobility, or damage to the orifices of the submandibular and lingual salivary glands. Current practitioners, however, report few if any complications and less pain than a vaccine injection (Ballard et al., 2002; Coryllos et al., 2004; Griffiths, 2004; Lalakea & Messner, 2003a). Frenotomy is a safe and effective early intervention for problems attributed to ankyloglossia (Segal et al., 2007), especially given the association between nipple pain and the cessation of breastfeeding. Instructions for the frenotomy procedure can be found in a number of sources, including from the Academy of Breastfeeding Medicine (2004; Coryllos et al., 2004; Lalakea & Messner, 2002; Marmet et al., 1990). A video with a demonstration of the complete procedure along with follow-up breastfeeding management is also available (Jain, 1996).

Breastfeeding Management

Ankyloglossia can be initially identified in the hospital before discharge with a typical presentation of a difficult or poor latch and persistent maternal nipple pain (Ballard et al., 2002). Infants may also present with sucking blisters on the upper and/or lower lip. This combination of breastfeeding difficulties is an indication to check the infant's lingual frenulum. Parents should be advised of the condition, its possible ramifications if left uncorrected (Karabulut et al., 2008), and options for and possible side effects of correction. Clipping the frenulum at this point improves latch, strength and rhythmicity of suckling, and milk transfer and eliminates the clicking sounds and popping on and off the breast. Maternal nipple pain is significantly diminished (Dollberg et al., 2006), removing a major roadblock to maternal breastfeeding plans. Once discharged, undiagnosed or uncorrected ankyloglossia may result in significantly more and severe complications. Ricke et al. (2005) reported that breastfeeding infants who were tongue-tied were three times more likely to be exclusively bottle-fed at 1 week than matched control infants with no tongue-tie. If surgical intervention is delayed or not an option (for religious, cultural, or personal reasons) or if parents are unable to locate a healthcare professional willing to perform the procedure, a breastfeeding plan would include the following:

- Positioning of the infant that would encourage gravity assistance for the tongue to move down and forward (semiprone, completely vertical, or an upright clutch hold)
- Latch modifications that might include stroking the infant's tongue down and forward, chin or jaw support, techniques to evert flat nipples before latch
- Using a nipple shield for relief from the pain and adequate milk transfer to the infant

- Pumping milk to follow each feeding to ensure an adequate supply and to provide as a supplement if the infant is unable to transfer sufficient amounts of milk or if the maternal nipples are too sore or damaged

- Checking the weight frequently to ensure adequate infant growth; paying close attention to articulation achievements as the infant begins to vocalize

If surgical intervention is an option, the mother should be informed of the following:

- Frenotomy usually provides immediate relief from nipple pain and markedly improved infant latch and milk transfer.

- Infants engage in compensatory tongue movements, resulting in varied patterns of tongue, mouth, head, neck, and body movements while breastfeeding.

- If ankyloglossia has remained uncorrected for a period of time (usually more than 5 days), the infant may need time to retrain the tongue and develop suckling strength. To help infants learn the use of a newly mobilized tongue, they may benefit from having the tongue stroked down and forward before each feeding. To encourage extension of the tongue, tongue "exercises" can be used such as dipping a cotton swab in breastmilk or a flavoring and touching the tip and sides of the tongue to encourage forward and lateral movement. To improve suckling strength, a nipple tug can be used several times during each feeding if the maternal nipples are not sore (the mother pulls back slightly on the nipple or pulls the infant slightly away from the breast while latched, not enough to break suction but enough to cause the infant to draw the nipple–areola deeper into the mouth). If the nipples are sore, the tugging can be done with a clean finger in the infant's mouth, pulling back slightly without breaking suction to encourage the infant to exert more vacuum.

Follow-up on all maternal and infant breastfeeding complications of ankyloglossia should take place immediately after the surgical procedure until resolved and should be ongoing if no interventions are used to correct the defect. Maternal complications include the following:

- Damage or infection to the nipples may require topical medication and hand expression rather than mechanical expression, unless pumping remains comfortable. A mother with flat nipples may wish to evert the nipple before placing the infant at breast to avoid further pain or damage.

- Milk stasis or mastitis may respond well to use of alternate massage during breastfeedings and/or pumping with breast massage between feeds.

Inflammatory conditions may also respond well to systemic nonsteroidal anti-inflammatory medications.

- Diminished milk production is addressed by frequent feedings at breast with alternate massage and pumping milk until adequate production is established. The pump flange should be large enough to avoid causing pain to the nipples.

Infant issues may include the following:

- The infant should be assessed during a feeding to ensure milk transfer and adequate intake, with pre- and postfeed weights taken if needed. Weight checks should take place every 3 to 4 days until an acceptable weight gain pattern is established. Infants having difficulty with milk transfer may need to be temporarily supplemented with pumped breastmilk.

- After a frenotomy, a white patch under the tongue at the surgical site is normal for about 48 hours. Pain medication and antibiotics are rarely, if ever, required.

Cleft Lips and Palates

As the fourth most common congenital disability, oral clefting represents a significant feeding challenge to the infant, to his or her parents, and to the interdisciplinary healthcare team involved in caring for such an infant over an extended period of time (Edmondson & Reinhartsen, 1998). It may occur in isolation or as part of 150–300 syndromes (Cohen & Bankier, 1991). Up to 13% of infants with clefting have other birth defects. Some genetic influence may be present (Merritt, 2005a) as once one child is affected parents have a 40% chance of having another affected child. In the United States the prevalence for cleft lip with or without cleft palate is 2.2–11.7 per 10,000 births. Cleft palate alone results in a prevalence rate of 5.5–6.6 per 10,000 births (Forrester & Merz, 2004). It is most prevalent among Native Americans (3.6/1,000 births) and less commonly seen in Asians (1.7–2.1/1,000 births), whites (1/1,000 births), and African Americans (0.3/1,000 births) (Lewanda & Jabs, 1994).

Although cleft lip and palate are frequently associated with each other, they develop separately at differing gestational ages, allowing a child to present with one or any combination of clefting. Approximately 50% have a combined cleft lip and palate, whereas 30% have an isolated cleft palate and 20% have an isolated cleft lip. Cleft lip results when the two sides of the lip fail to fuse during the fifth to eighth week of gestation. This may also include a split in the upper gum (alveolar ridge) and upper jaw. Cleft palate occurs when the palatine processes do not join during the 6th to 12th week of gestation.

The etiology of clefting is not well understood and most likely results from a combination of genetic and environmental factors. Gene variants have been identified that may contribute to oral clefts and triple the risk of recurrence in affected families (Zucchero et al., 2004). A few of the numerous recognized teratogens have been identified as being associated with cleft defects, including alcohol consumption during the embryonic period and ingestion of drugs, such as phenytoin and retinoids, and recreational drugs, such as cocaine. Ultrasound can detect clefts as early as 17 weeks of gestation. Some data have shown that mothers who take multivitamins containing folic acid or consume vitamin-enriched cereals from 2 months before conception through the first trimester can reduce the risk of clefting by 25–50% (Shaw et al., 1995; Tolarova & Harris, 1995).

A breakdown of cleft lip and/or palate shows three groups: sporadic occurrence (75–80%), familial (10–15%), and clefting associated with syndromes (1–5%). Additional anomalies present in 44–64% of all infants with oral clefting (Sprintzen et al., 1985). Routine screening for associated malformations in infants with clefting may find cardiac, skeletal, and central nervous system anomalies along with possible effects seen in the eyes, ears, digestive system, and urogenital system (Rawashdeh & Jawdat Abu-Hawas, 2008).

Clefting is usually apparent at birth and requires sensitive and supportive care from the healthcare team. Parents need immediate help with feeding techniques and plans before discharge. Mothers need to be shown how to feed the infant, how to determine sufficient intake, what problems to anticipate, and how to handle them as provision of breastmilk for these infants tends to be of a shorter duration (Smedegaard et al., 2008). Feeding challenges are usually the first priority for parents. Many mothers discharged from the hospital lack adequate information, are in need of specific feeding instructions, and experience dissatisfaction with the type and amount of information and follow-up they received (Byrnes et al., 2003; Oliver & Jones, 1997; Trenouth & Campbell, 1996; Young et al., 2001). Mothers of infants with clefting are eager for information and quite responsive to the needs of their infant (Coy et al., 2002).

Feeding directly from the breast may be an option for infants with an isolated cleft of the lip, a narrow or small posterior clefting of the palate, or a small submucous cleft (Curtin, 1990). Reid et al. (2007) found that infants with cleft lip generate the greatest amount of suction followed by those with cleft palate and cleft lip and palate, whereas infants with cleft lip and palate generate reduced amounts of compression. However, with greater involvement of the palate, generation of intraoral suction is significantly compromised, and with a bilateral cleft palate, it may be difficult or impossible to compress the nipple between the tongue and any part of the roof of the mouth.

Poor feeding skills are common, especially if the cleft palate is associated with a syndrome or Pierre Robin sequence (Reid et al., 2006). Sucking parameters are altered in cleft-involved infants. Masarei et al. (2007) showed that sucking was less efficient in cleft-involved infants, with shorter sucks, a faster rate of sucking, more sucks per swallow, and a greater proportion of intraoral positive pressure generation than infants without clefting. This may necessitate assisted milk delivery and a modification of feeding management, including short- or long-term breastmilk expression (Stockdale, 2000).

Human milk is very important to infants with clefting. Children with cleft lip and palate are at an increased risk for otitis media and hearing, speech, language, social, dental, and academic difficulties. The greater the degree of hearing loss at 12 months, the lower the language scores for expressive skills and comprehension (Jocelyn et al., 1996). Children with clefts who are breastfed or receive breastmilk for less than a month have been shown to require special education services in significantly higher numbers, demonstrating that a short duration of breastmilk intake is associated with poorer school performance (Erkkila et al., 2005). The provision of breastmilk, even if the infant cannot feed directly from the breast, has been shown to reduce middle ear infections and improve the amount of time infants are free from effusion, contributing to the reduction of conductive hearing loss. Protection against otitis media extends well beyond the period of breastmilk feeding (Paradise et al., 1994). Aniansson et al. (2002) demonstrated a significant correlation during the first 18 months of life between a longer duration of feeding with breastmilk and a lower incidence of acute and secretory otitis media, concluding that premature cessation of human milk feeding can contribute to an increased incidence of both acute and secretory otitis media.

Feeding methods and feeding management guidelines can be selected based on the variety of sizes and positions of the clefts, the anatomical shape and size of the maternal nipple–areola, the breastmilk supply and rate of milk flow, the choice of specialized equipment and techniques, and when surgical interventions are planned. Breastfeeding is important to infants with clefts to aid in the development of muscles for feeding as well as those for speech (Merritt, 2005b).

A number of specialized feeding devices and common equipment can be selected and combined to best match the infant's needs and contribute to a tailored approach for each individual situation:

- Palatal obturator: An obturator is a silastic or acrylic device that acts as an artificial palate that when custom molded fills or occludes the palatal cleft. They are fabricated by a pediatric dentist or prosthodontist for a hard palate cleft and are not used for submucous clefts or clefts of the soft palate (Osuji, 1995). Some infants are fitted for the obturator within the first few days after birth to act as the initial orthopedic treatment in facilitating or directing the desired development of the oral cavity. The device supports the palatal shelves as they grow and keeps the tongue out of the cleft, helping to normalize tongue activity and positioning. It simultaneously acts as a feeding appliance to create a seal over the palatal cleft, providing a mechanism for generating negative intraoral pressure and a surface against which the tongue can compress the nipple (Crossman, 1998). Use of an obturator has been shown to reduce feeding times, enhance the volume of milk consumed (Turner et al., 2001), develop some weak intraoral negative pressure (Kogo et al., 1997), and allow an infant to feed directly at breast for at least some of his or her required intake. Turner and Moore (1995) and Humenczuk (1998) described highly motivated breastfeeding mothers whose infants could obtain 25–50% of their milk at the breast with early insertion of a palatal obturator, with the rest of the infants' nutritional requirements provided through the Special Needs Feeder (formerly called the Haberman bottle feeder). Checking the appliance for rough edges should be done if the mother complains of sore nipples while breastfeeding when the obturator is in place.

- The Special Needs Feeder (Haberman feeder): The Special Needs Feeder nipple has a slit rather than cross-cut opening and is attached to a milk reservoir with a one-way valve, allowing milk but not air to enter the reservoir chamber. The chamber is pliable so that milk can be gently squeezed into the infant's mouth as needed. Around the base of the nipple are markings to indicate how to position the nipple to achieve variations in flow rate. The nipple shank is available in a standard length and a shorter preemie length. Milk can be extracted from this device by compression only so that an infant who cannot generate vacuum can obtain milk through the compressive force generated by the jaw and gums (Haberman, 1988).

- Mead Johnson cleft palate nurser: This feeder has a long, soft, thin-walled nipple with a cross-cut designed to direct the milk flow past the cleft. If the nipple is too long for the infant, a standard nipple with a single hole or an orthodontic nipple can be substituted. The bottle is soft and is easily squeezed in rhythm to the infant's sucking and swallowing movements. The bottle is gently pulsed, not continually squeezed, to overcome the lack of vacuum and to ensure that milk is not aspirated from a rapid or forceful injection of milk into the back of the throat. A flexible or squeezable bottle may be easier for parents to use and results in an increased volume of milk intake and good weight outcomes when assisted feeding is needed (Shaw et al., 1999).

- Pigeon cleft palate nurser: The nipple on the pigeon feeder is Y-cut, somewhat larger and more bulbous than other types of nipples. It is firm on top and soft on the bottom for more efficient tongue compression. An air valve prevents the nipple from collapsing, and tightening or loosening the collar on the bottle controls the speed of the milk flow. A back-flow valve prevents milk from flowing back into the bottle from the nipple, reducing the amount of air the infant swallows. The bottle is not soft and pliable.

- Abbott Nutrition (Ross Laboratories) cleft palate assembly: This nipple tapers to a small narrow tube and frequently is used after surgical repair of the palate or to hasten feedings when they routinely take longer than 40 minutes. It provides a continuous flow of milk and must be used carefully to avoid milk flow that the infant is unable to handle. A catheter-tipped plunger syringe, Brecht feeder, or Asepto syringe with a length of soft tubing is also sometimes used after surgery.

- Angled bottles: These usually make it easier to feed infants in an upright position.

- Supplemental nursing system (SNS) or the Lact-Aid nursing trainer system: Both tube feeding devices deliver supplemental milk at the breast, can be squeezed to facilitate milk flow, and can be suspended around the mother's neck at varying heights for gravity-assisted flow. Some infants with a small cleft may have enough intact palate toward which the breast and tubing can be directed.

- Nipple shields: These have also been used in some situations because they provide a firm teat. Once milk is drawn into or expressed into the teat, weak suckling or compression will withdraw the milk.

- Spoons, cups, and syringes: These are sometimes used by parents for delivering extra milk.

- Hospital-grade electric breast pump with a double collection kit: Most mothers of infants with clefting, especially when the infant has a cleft palate, will need to express milk, sometimes for an extended period of time (Stockdale, 2000).

- Digital scale: A rented digital scale can be used for pre- and postfeed weights to monitor intake of the recommended amount of milk each 24 hours until feeding and weight gain are well established.

Pre- and Postoperative Considerations

Primary surgical closure of the cleft lip may take place as early as 2–3 days of age and usually within the first 3 months of life. Early lip closure has the potential to alter the palatal dimensions, which is why early lip closure may be accompanied by the use of a palatal obturator to prevent palatal collapse immediately after lip surgery (Kramer et al., 1994). Repair of the palate usually takes place in the second half of the first year. Some surgeons currently repair the palate before 6 months of age, with feeding from the breast a direct possibility as a result. A study of 21 infants undergoing palate repair within the first month of life and returning to breastfeeding or bottle-feeding after recovery from anesthesia showed no short-term adverse outcomes, although long-term effects on facial development and speech were not evaluated (Denk, 1998).

Although opinions vary (Redford-Badwal et al., 2003), most infants can feed directly from the breast immediately after cleft lip repair surgery without disrupting the integrity of the suture line (Weatherly-White et al., 1987). Returning to direct breastfeeding rather than using spoon, dropper, bottle, or tube and syringe feedings postsurgery after both cleft lip and cleft palate repair has been shown to be advantageous to infants in that they require less sedation, less intravenous fluids, fewer hospital days, and are capable of gaining weight while avoiding disruption of the surgical repair (Cohen et al., 1992; Darzi et al., 1996).

With the possibility of direct breastfeeding after cleft repair, mothers need to ensure that they have an abundant milk supply that can be sustained over a protracted period of time. It is to the infant's advantage to be put to breast before surgical repairs, even if he or she is unable to secure all the milk needed for growth. At a minimum, this facilitates familiarity with the breast and a soft soothing breast for comfort sucking, with most milk provided through assisted delivery devices as necessary. Although infants with cleft palates may not be able to support normal growth through exclusive feeding at the breast, imprinting on the breast is desirable. This keeps open the options for some feedings at the breast after lip and/or palate repair.

Feeding and Breastfeeding Management

There is a paucity of information describing breastfeeding and breastfeeding outcomes in the cleft population (Reid, 2004). Evidence-based guidelines for breastfeeding infants with clefting help increase the likelihood that these infants will receive breastmilk and enjoy feeding at the breast (Reilly et al., 2007). A combination of feeding methods is generally used to provide an optimal feeding environment for infants with clefting. Clarren and coworkers (1987) described an approach that considered the parameters of the feeding deficit in terms of the anatomical defect and then matched the deficits to the specific feeding devices or techniques. They based their recommendations on assessment of how the deficit affects the normal feeding parameters of generation of negative pressure and the ability to engage in mechanical movements. Infants with a cleft lip, cleft palate, or a combination of both who do not have concomitant health problems or other syndromes that would affect feeding generally swallow normally but suck abnormally. Reflux of milk through the nose without sequelae is not diagnostic of a swallowing problem. Infants with cleft palate can ingest excessive amounts of air because there is no separation between the nasal and oral cavities. This leads to bloating, choking, gagging, fatigue with feeding, prolonged feeding times, and spitting up (Cooper-Brown et al., 2008). Generation of negative pressure is generally precluded when there is a cleft in the lip and alveolus, the bony palate, or a combination, unless the deficit can be plugged. Problems with the actual muscular movements used by the infant in the mechanics of feeding occur in three cleft-related defects:

1. Bilateral cleft lip when there is significant anterior projection of the premaxilla. This makes it difficult for the infant to stabilize the nipple.

2. Wide or extensive palatal clefts that involve so much of the palate that there is little to no surface against which the tongue can press the nipple.

3. Retroplaced tongues may be actively inserted into the palatal cleft. They may not cup and move down and forward, contributing to an inability to perform coordinated movements.

Cleft Lip Only

Clefts of the lip can range from a small unilateral notch to bilateral clefts that extend into the nares with projection of the premaxilla. Presurgical orthopedic appliances or treatments may be placed to help mold the nose. In the absence of any coexisting problems, infants with an isolated cleft lip demonstrate appropriate mechanical movements of the tongue and jaw to compress the nipple, form a bolus, and swallow normally, but negative pressure or vacuum could be compromised by the lack of an intact upper lip to form a seal. Evidence has shown that infants with cleft lip can generate suction and breastfeed successfully (Choi et al., 1992; Garcez & Giugliani, 2005). The most frequently seen problems are the presence of weak suction, difficulty in latching to the breast, and breastmilk escaping through the nostrils.

Techniques. Positioning at the breast is most important for these infants. Typically, for a unilateral defect the breast should enter the mouth from the side on which the defect is located so that the nipple–areola approximates the section of the palate that is most intact. A cleft in the lip may be sealed by breast tissue or by the mother's thumb pushing the tissue over the gap. An infant with a bilateral defect often feeds best when directly facing the breast in a straddle position with the breast tipped down or angled slightly to one side of the mouth (Danner, 1992a). Some infants feed more efficiently when their throat is level with or slightly higher than the breast such that the nape of the neck is level with or slightly higher than the areola. Other infants can obtain more milk by having the mother lean over them, allowing gravity to assist in keeping the breast in the infant's mouth (Danner, 1997).

Because the infant with a cleft palate is usually unable to generate sufficient intraoral negative pressure to hold the breast in his or her mouth, the mother needs to support the breast and the infant's head to keep the infant from falling off the breast. Substantial chin support is needed such as with the dancer hand position.

Positioning for feeding by bottle is also a concern. Proper position of the head and neck is important, with the head usually at an angle between 40 and 60 degrees to minimize nasal regurgitation of milk. The infant's chin may need to be supported, especially with a small jaw. Infants tend to swallow a lot of air and may need to be burped frequently. The bottle is squeezed rhythmically when the infant sucks or every 3–5 sucks if the infant experiences breathing difficulties while feeding. It is important that the artificial nipple is placed on top of the tongue as it is inserted, because there is a tendency for the tongue to be pushed or drawn backward into the mouth, obstructing the airway and preventing proper sucking movements.

The use of the dancer hand position helps to stabilize the infant's mouth. If the mother presses her thumb and forefinger gently against the infant's cheeks, this causes the buccal surfaces of the cheek to maintain contact with the nipple, improving oral suction.

Some mothers with an abundant milk supply can hand express milk into the infant's mouth. This may partially meet the needs of the infant, but many infants require supplemental milk after feeding at the breast.

Listening plays a key role in breastfeeding the challenged infant. Swallowing at breast is a reassuring sign that milk intake has occurred. A nonreassuring sign is the soft hissing or "kissing" sound of air going through the cleft (Biancuzzo, 1998; Glass & Wolf, 1999).

Infants can be positioned in a clutch or very upright cradle or cross-cradle position. Some infants prefer to straddle the mother's thigh, facing the breast with the neck slightly extended and lower jaw pressing close into the breast. The mother's breast tissue may occlude the cleft with no further adjustment, or the mother may need to either cover the cleft with her thumb or press breast tissue over the cleft to prevent an air leak. If the lip curls under, the mother can lift and reposition it. The infant's head and the mother's breast need to be securely held during the entire feeding, allowing the breast tissue to conform to the defect and prevent the infant from losing his or her grip on the nipple–areola. Because the infant may be unable to generate the initial suction necessary to draw the nipple–areola far into the mouth and elongate these tissues to form a teat, some mothers report that they manually form or shape the nipple and place it into the infant's mouth as an assisted form of latching (Grady, 1977; Styer & Freeh, 1981). The mother can use alternate massage to initiate and sustain sucking and improve both volume and fat content of each feeding. If the infant tires easily, the mother can hand express milk directly into the infant's mouth.

Equipment. If feedings take longer than 30–45 minutes and/or the infant is not gaining weight adequately, a Lact-Aid nursing trainer or SNS device may be used to deliver more milk in a shorter period of time while still feeding at the breast. If weight gain is an ongoing issue, consider using pumped hindmilk in the supplementing device at breast or secured to a finger for finger feeding. Extra milk can also be delivered by periodontal syringe while sucking on the breast or on a finger, by cup, or by bottle using an artificial nipple with a large soft base that occludes the cleft and offers variable flow options.

Cleft of the Soft Palate, Submucous Cleft, or Bifid Uvula

Many infants with soft palate clefting may breastfeed normally. Others may breastfeed well until the head grows larger and the unseen gap in the underlying musculature widens. Some infants may regurgitate milk through their nose when the soft palate does not seal against the tongue. Paradise et al. (1994) rated the severity or degree of nasal regurgitation as an indicator of the degree of impairment of palatal function (none, mild, moderate, and severe) but provided no data on whether this aspect was predictive of breastfeeding outcomes. Miller (1998) anecdotally found that breastfeeding success before surgical repair of the palate seemed inversely proportional to the size of the cleft in the soft palate, not the total size of the entire cleft. When there is difficulty with palatal movement, oral suction may be interrupted prematurely, a click may be heard when the seal is broken, intermittent airway obstruction is possible with noisy breathing, the volume of fluid per suck may be reduced, and feeding can become inefficient (Wolf & Glass, 1992). Weight gain should be monitored closely, as with all types of cleft defects.

Techniques. Any feeding at the breast should be done in an upright position to reduce nasal regurgitation. Breastfeeding in a side-lying position may exacerbate this problem. Alternate massage may be helpful to improve volume and fat intake per suck and per feeding. The infant's head position may need to be adjusted and modified to reduce the possibility of airway obstruction or swallowing difficulties.

Equipment. Palatal obturators are not used for soft palate clefts. Weight gain may be monitored by pre- and postfeed weights on a digital scale. Hindmilk supplements may be needed for weight gain and can be delivered through tube-feeding devices; milk may need to be pumped if the infant is unable to obtain adequate amounts from direct feedings at the breast. If the mother chooses to use an artificial nipple, she may find that a standard nipple with a longer nipple shaft is efficient and effective. An angled bottle also allows the infant to be more easily fed in an upright position.

Isolated Cleft of the Bony (Hard) Palate

The generation of both vacuum and compression is affected depending on the location and size of the cleft. Effective vacuum and compression of the nipple–areola is not possible with a large midline cleft. With a narrow or posterior cleft, enough intact palate may exist for the generation of sufficient vacuum to position and stabilize the nipple in the anterior portion of the mouth or to the opposite side of the mouth, where the tongue would find an opposing surface against which to elongate and compress the breast. However, this may increase the likelihood of sore or damaged nipples. Feedings at breast may be sufficient enough for at least a partial intake of milk but may need to be supplemented.

Techniques. Upright positioning is recommended. The mother may need to manually shape and insert her nipple–areola into the infant's mouth if sufficient vacuum cannot be generated to draw in and hold the nipple–areola in place. Hand expression of milk directly into the infant's mouth improves intake at each feeding. If the cleft is unilateral (not midline), the infant may do better with the breast entering the mouth from the side on which the defect is located, thus directing the nipple to the area of the palate that is intact (Danner, 1992a). The breast must be held in the infant's mouth with chin support, and the infant must be held to the breast for the entire feeding.

Equipment. With a large cleft, extra milk can be provided at breast through a Lact-Aid, SNS, or tubing attached to a syringe. These devices normally require an infant to generate suction to cause the milk to flow. The SNS and Lact-Aid may need to be suspended in a higher position with the tubing straighter and of a larger size, and on the SNS, both tubes may need to be open for optimal milk flow. Pressure usually needs to be applied to the milk container suspended between the mother's breasts in rhythm with the infant's sucking. Pressure should be applied just after the gums compress the areola to sequence the milk bolus to enter the infant's mouth at the same time any milk flows from the breast (Danner, 1997). The tubing may need to be taped to the breast on the same axis that the breast enters the infant's mouth such that the tubing is placed to the side of the nipple where the intact palate is or where the nipple and tubing can be compressed along the alveolar ridge. The tubing can also be taped to the underside of the mother's areola, whichever gives the best results. A nipple shield may be used and tubing can be attached either under or on top of the shield for the delivery of additional milk. If the infant needs to be further supplemented, a Special Needs Feeder (Haberman feeder) or other flexible bottle arrangement can be used to ensure adequate intake per feeding in a reasonable amount of time.

Cleft Lip and Palate

When a cleft lip and palate are present, the cleft is usually quite large with little to no intact palate for compression, making the generation of vacuum impossible (Wolf & Glass, 1992). Some milk intake may be possible in a few infants, but the majority of milk needs to be delivered with assistive devices. Palatal obturators may be used, which occlude the cleft and allow compression and some suction. Nipple shields may also be tried. Infants may fatigue quickly when being fed or become fussy with hunger and small milk intakes. Weight checks should be frequent because weight gain can be rapidly compromised by the infant's limited ability to consume milk is a reasonable amount of time.

Techniques. The infant with a bilateral cleft can be positioned to directly face the breast by straddling the mother's lap. The breast, nipple, and areola need to be shaped and guided to the side with the most intact tissue and pointed slightly downward. The mother can elicit the milk ejection reflex and hand express milk into the infant's mouth, at least for the beginning of the feeding. She then follows with pumped milk through either a tube-feeding device at the breast or her choice of an assistive feeding device. The amount of milk needed by the infant each day should be calculated and a plan designed to ensure adequate intake. Infants have an easier time accomplishing any feeding at breast if they are at least put to the breast intermittently, even if they receive the bulk of their milk from a feeding device. Many mothers reserve the breastfeeding time as cuddle time without the pressure and expectation of large milk intakes.

Equipment. Mothers may use a digital scale for determining the amount of milk taken from the breast to calculate how much to offer as a supplement. Daily weights are taken to ensure appropriate weight gain. Mothers need an electric pump with a double collection kit, and pumping times should be built into the daily feeding plan. If the mother uses a bottle for assisted milk delivery, she should choose one with a nipple that does not deliver milk so fast that it compromises swallowing and breathing and one that works to stimulate sucking patterns as close to those of breastfeeding as possible (Noble & Bovey, 1997). The flow rate of an artificial nipple should be similar to that from the breast, 0.1–0.5 cc per suck (Wolf & Glass, 1992). Usually, a squeezable bottle with a standard-size nipple hole is sufficient. Cutting larger holes or cross-cuts into the nipple may create a rapid and irregular flow of milk. Infants showing signs of being overwhelmed by a fast flow of milk may need to rest each three to five sucks by removing the bottle from the infant's mouth or using a nipple with a smaller hole (Richard, 1991). A Special Needs Feeder (Haberman feeder) is also a good choice because it delivers milk with compression and allows the feeder to gently squeeze the milk reservoir if needed. Milk does not flow back into the bottle and ingested air is minimized.

Syndromes and Congenital Anomalies

Pierre Robin Sequence

Pierre Robin sequence (PRS) is characterized by the presence of three congenital anomalies: micrognathia or retrognathia (a small or posteriorly positioned mandible located about 10–12 mm behind the superior arch), glossoptosis (a normal-sized tongue that is displaced into the pharynx, causing obstruction of the airway), and a wide U-shaped cleft palate. It occurs in approximately 1 in 8,850 live births (Sheffield et al., 1987) and is termed a sequence rather than a syndrome.[1] In approximately 80% of newborns with PRS, the triad of anomalies occurs as part of an underlying genetic condition. About 40% of infants with PRS have Stickler syndrome (a tissue disorder that includes not only clefting but also cataracts or retinal detachment, a flat face, a small jaw, and skeletal abnormalities, hearing loss, and cardiac problems) with another 15% experiencing velocardiofacial syndrome (an autosomal dominant condition that includes not only clefting but abnormalities of the heart, learning disabilities, hearing loss, speech problems, leg pain, and behavior extremes). Hyoid bone abnormalities have been observed in some infants with PRS and are associated with swallowing dysfunction (El Amm & Denny, 2008). Infants with PRS should always be evaluated for other underlying or associated conditions (Prows & Bender, 1999).

The single defect that initiates the cascade of anomalies is micrognathia. The abnormally small mandible during fetal development displaces the tongue to such a posterior position that it prevents the palatal shelves from fusing, creating the cleft in the palate. The small mandible can be caused by mechanical factors in utero such as fibroids or a transverse position; by teratogens such as alcohol, Accutane, or tobacco; and/or by genetic factors such as chromosome abnormalities or gene mutations. The primary problem upon birth is airway obstruction, with prone positioning used to bring the tongue forward to create a patent airway. If this simple positioning is not effective, other interventions may be used as needed such as a nasopharyngeal airway, continuous positive airway pressure, surgery, or tracheostomy (Marques et al., 2001).

The chronic airway resistance caused by PRS requires infants to exert increased breathing and cardiac efforts that consume additional calories. The method of

---

[1]A syndrome is generally defined as a specific pattern of anomalies that have a common cause, such as Down syndrome, which originates from the presence of an extra copy of chromosome 21. A sequence is a pattern of anomalies resulting from a single defect during fetal development, but the etiology of the primary defect varies from person to person.

feeding is determined by the degree and type of medical interventions needed and on the general management of airway obstruction. With or without the presence of a cleft palate, airway obstruction remains a prime cause of oral feeding problems (Marcellus, 2001). Some infants may require ongoing nasogastric feedings until oral feedings are fully established. Although most airway obstruction is obvious within several hours of birth, some infants with PRS may present with late airway obstruction as evidenced by failure to thrive and oxygen desaturation, necessitating close follow-up for weight gain upon hospital discharge (Wilson et al., 2000). Mothers may wish to provide supplementation at the breast to strengthen feeding and speech muscles and to familiarize the infant with the breast, making it easier to feed at the breast in the future.

Techniques. If the micrognathia is mild and there is no cleft, some direct feeding at the breast may be possible with alternate massage, concurrent with or followed by supplement delivered through a tube-feeding device. Feedings should be limited to 15–20 minutes to avoid excessive fatigue. Lingual massage may be helpful to relax and bring the tongue forward. Positioning of the infant with micrognathia and airway instability is usually prone but is complicated when a nasopharyngeal airway is in place.

Equipment. Cleft palate feeders may be used to deliver all or part of the required milk. Some mothers use a nipple shield, which does not require suction to draw it into the infant's mouth. The mother expresses milk into the shield reservoir for the infant to remove by compression and follows with any supplement by bottle that is needed. Some infants require nasogastric feeding to accomplish adequate weight gain.

Choanal Atresia

Choanal atresia is a congenital anomaly of the anterior skull base characterized by narrowing or blockage of the nasal airway by membranous or bony tissue. It occurs in approximately 1 in 7,000 to 8,000 live births, with about 60% demonstrating unilateral blockage. Unilateral choanal atresia may be asymptomatic until a respiratory infection occurs or the mother notices that the infant exhibits periodic mouth breathing, chest retraction when breathing through the nose, difficulty coordinating breathing while suckling at the breast (sputtering, choking, coughing), or circumoral cyanosis (bluish lips). The infant may "pace" the feedings by using shorter sucking bursts and pausing longer between bursts to breathe. Mothers should be instructed to watch for circumoral cyanosis and remove the infant from the breast to allow breathing between sucking bursts if the infant does not do so. Bilateral choanal atresia is more serious because both sides of the nose are blocked and, if completely occluded, cause acute breathing problems and cyanosis. Infants may breathe through their mouths; however, the work of mouth breathing is costly to the infant and could only shortly delay, not remove, the need for surgery.

Bilateral choanal atresia is identified in the hospital shortly after birth and usually requires immediate placement of an airway. Surgery is generally performed early in the newborn period with stents placed to maintain the integrity of the surgically created airway. The length of the stents may need to be adjusted to accommodate feedings at the breast and the mother may need to experiment with positions until she and her infant find one that is comfortable and effective. Feeding at the breast with bilateral choanal atresia is usually not possible until a patent airway has been established. Until then, feedings are delivered through an oral-gastric tube. Mothers whose infants present with choanal atresia (especially bilateral) should begin pumping breastmilk as soon as possible and continue to do so until the infant is completely established at the breast.

Bilateral choanal atresia is also commonly associated as a component of other congenital anomalies, such as the CHARGE syndrome. This is a nonrandom association of anomalies that includes

C   Coloboma, a cleft of the iris plus a number of other eye malformations

H   Heart malformations

A   Atresia choanae and possibly cleft lip and palate

R   Retarded growth, although birth weights and lengths are usually normal

G   Genitourinary problems

E   Ear anomalies, along with dysfunction of cranial nerves that can result in facial palsy, swallowing problems, and reflux

Cranial nerve dysfunction is a primary clinical feature of CHARGE syndrome, which is seen as weak sucking, swallowing difficulty, gastroesophageal reflux, and aspiration (Dobbelsteyn et al., 2008; White et al., 2005). Affected infants may also demonstrate oral aversion or defensiveness either as a primary sensory disorder or as secondary to delayed or negative oral sensory and unpleasant feeding experiences (Dobbelsteyn et al., 2005). Depending on the number and severity of the problems, some infants may be able to partially breastfeed but may only be able to receive expressed milk through gastrostomy feeding tubes.

There are many other more rare craniofacial anomalies, most of which occur as components of syndromes that have greater or lesser effects on feeding management in the involved infants. Feeding problems are frequent with infants who require interventions for airway management, especially in infants with mandibular hypoplasia (Perkins et al., 1997).

Upper Airway Problems

Laryngomalacia

This generally benign congenital abnormality of the laryngeal cartilage is the most common cause of noninfective stridor in infancy (Solomons & Prescot, 1987; Wood, 1984). It accounts for 65–75% of cases of stridor in children under 1 year of age and is eight times more common than tracheomalacia. It may be accompanied by tracheomalacia, although the two have different etiology and pathophysiology (Mair & Parsons, 1992; Solomons & Prescot, 1987). The malacia, or softening, is thought to be a delay in the maturation of the structures that support the larynx, causing the epiglottis to prolapse over the larynx during inspiration. This partial obstruction typically causes stridor upon inspiration that is usually more apparent when the infant is in the supine position, crying, feeding, excited, or has an upper respiratory infection. The flexible supraglottic soft tissue structures that are drawn in during inspiration blow out passively during expiration so that there is no resistance to air escaping and no expiratory stridor.

Stridor typically is heard starting between 4 and 6 weeks of age, because until then the flow of air upon inspiration may not be strong enough to generate the typical sound of stridor. Stridor generally increases over the first 6 months with a gradual disappearance by about 2 years of age. The intensity of stridor may fluctuate during the day with periods of quiet respiration (Gibson, 2004). Infants with laryngomalacia generally breathe and sleep better prone. When sitting, they should be at least at a 30-degree angle with their head positioned to relieve or reduce the obstruction. They should be held in an upright position for 30 minutes after feedings and not fed lying down.

Infants with laryngomalacia are at an increased risk of developing gastroesophageal reflux (GER) (Belmont & Grundfast, 1984; Bibi et al., 2001), thought to occur as a result of the more negative intrathoracic pressures necessary to overcome the inspiratory obstruction. This may cause wide swings in intrathoracic and abdominal pressures that overcome the antireflux barrier. Depending on the severity of GER, failure to gain weight or weight loss can occur, heightening the anxiety of parents already concerned about their infant's noisy breathing (Milczuk & Johnson, 2000). Crying exacerbates the obstruction and increases the work of breathing. Occasionally, an infant will experience a more clinically severe lesion where there is sufficient interference with ventilation that feeding and growth are impaired. Crowing respirations may be heard, and chest retractions that are severe enough to cause chest wall deformities represent the extremes. Rarely, clinical hypoxemia may be seen with oxygen saturation below 90% and supplemental oxygen prescribed, or in severe cases nasotracheal intubation or even tracheostomy may be needed.

Breastfeeding Management

Laryngomalacia has the potential to disrupt the normal sequence of suck, swallow, and breathe as the infant attempts to coordinate breathing with sucking and swallowing. Noisy respiration may be identified before hospital discharge but may be ascribed to residual fluid in the airways that typically clears on its own. Once lactogenesis II occurs, both the increased amount of milk and the pressure from the milk ejection reflex may result in an infant who chokes, coughs, sputters, and frequently comes off the breast during a feeding. Latching and feeding in certain positions may exacerbate the problem. Infants may have difficulty gaining weight, feedings may be prolonged and difficult, infants may engage in breath holding with brief periods of circumoral cyanosis, and stridor may become more apparent over the first 3–4 weeks. The increased work of breathing may cause an infant to become fatigued at breast before accomplishing sufficient milk intake. An infant may have more prominent airway obstruction on one side if the laryngomalacia is more pronounced on that side.

Glass and Wolf (1994) suggested feeding position modifications and pacing techniques to improve feeding efficiency and to reduce the stress and work of feeding. Pacing is done by removing the breast every four to five suck-swallows to allow regular times for breathing. Pacing may only be necessary during high-flow-rate periods of the feeding (i.e., with the initial milk ejection reflex and several of the following ones) until there is less pressure and a decreased flow rate further into the feeding as the breast drains. Positioning for feeding should avoid supine positions because this allows the epiglottic soft tissues to fall backward into the laryngeal outlet. Infants may feed better when the head is allowed to extend slightly to open the airway. Mothers may wish to recline and place the infant in a prone or ventral position for feeding. Sucking bursts may be short and rest periods longer as the infant compensates.

Tracheomalacia

Tracheomalacia is a congenital developmental defect in the tracheal wall cartilage where the softened tracheal rings cannot prevent the airway from collapsing during expiration. Called type 1, it becomes apparent shortly after birth. Tracheomalacia can be acquired from events outside the trachea, such as an abnormality of the blood vessels surrounding the trachea (vascular ring) or a tumor in the neck or throat causing pressure on the airway and changes in the cartilage (type 2). Type 3 tracheomalacia is an actual breakdown of the tracheal cartilage from prolonged intubation or chronic or recurrent tracheal infections. Infants with tracheomalacia demonstrate stridor on expiration and coughing, and they have worsening breathing when crying and feeding and when an upper respiratory infection is present. They frequently have GER and begin wheezing around 4 weeks of age. Wheezing can be mistaken for asthma, cystic fibrosis, or bronchiolitis, but infants with tracheomalacia are generally healthy, happy wheezers.

Tracheomalacia, laryngomalacia, and bronchomalacia can occur in isolation or in combination with each other. Malacia lesions may occur in association with other disorders such as congenital heart disorders, tracheoesophageal fistula, and various syndromes (Masters et al., 2002). Most children outgrow type 1 tracheomalacia between the ages of 1 and 3 years but may need to be monitored more closely if they have respiratory infections—an important reason to ensure adequate breastmilk intake to reduce this risk.

Breastfeeding Management

Many of these infants breathe and sleep better when prone. Some breastfeed better in a prone or semiprone position, which both eases breathing and allows gravity to slow the flow of milk during milk ejection and when the breast is very full. Some infants also feed better with the use of a nipple shield. The shield helps control the fast flow of milk, allowing the infant to better pace swallowing with pauses for breathing. Infants should remain upright after feedings because they have a tendency to swallow air and experience GER. Most of the same feeding recommendations suggested for laryngomalacia also apply to tracheomalacia. Weight gain must be followed closely, because the work of breathing burns calories and places these infants at an increased risk for slow weight gain or weight loss.

Mothers who have infants with breathing difficulties must ensure that their breasts are adequately drained at each feeding to prevent milk stasis, engorgement, or mastitis. Whereas alternate massage is often used to assist in weight gain and to increase feeding efficiency, this technique may not be appropriate while an infant with tracheomalacia or laryngomalacia is attached to the breast. It may be more helpful to massage and compress the breast during pacing pauses as well as toward the end of a feeding when the breast has been partially drained. Mothers should check for areas of the breast that are not draining well and manually massage those areas to improve milk drainage. Some mothers may also need to express milk if the infant remains a poor feeder or needs supplements.

Tracheostomy

Tracheostomy involves a surgical procedure to place a tube into the trachea with an opening in the throat called a stoma. In severe cases of respiratory compromise or obstructed airway, this procedure may be performed so that the infant may breathe through the stoma. The stoma is kept clear and the air entering it is kept moist so that secretions do not dry and block the opening. As long as the infant is capable of breastfeeding, nursing at the breast is both possible and desirable. If the infant is unable to breastfeed directly at the breast, expressed milk should be provided. Mothers may need to express their milk during the time surrounding the surgery and recovery period until the infant can be reestablished at the breast. Care must be taken when positioning the infant at the breast such that the stoma is not obstructed by clothing, head positioning, or the mother's hand. The mother should be able to see the throat throughout the feeding, with some mothers preferring the cradle or cross-cradle hold to better visualize the stoma area (Merewood & Philipp, 2001). Some infants may prefer a more flexed head position. Many mothers will use a covering with a filter or a specially designed humidifier during feedings as insurance that dribbled milk or milk that is spit up does not inadvertently enter the stoma.

Gastrointestinal Disorders, Anomalies, and Conditions

Tracheoesophageal Fistula (TEF) and Esophageal Atresia (EA)

These are congenital anomalies of the gastrointestinal tract that occur early in fetal development. Their incidence is reported to be between 1 in 1,500 and 1 in 4,500 live births (Clark, 1999), with approximately 30–40% of these infants having other coexisting congenital defects. TEF/EA may be part of a complex known as the VATER or VACTERL association, where vertebral, anal, cardiac, radial, renal, and/or limb anomalies are also present. An infant with TEF/EA should be examined for such additional anomalies (Spoon, 2003). There is a strong association between maternal diabetes and multisystem anomalies, with the incidence of VACTERL association in infants of diabetic mothers five times greater than that of infants from nondiabetic mothers (Loffredo et al., 2001). In normal development the trachea and esophagus completely separate from each other. When they do not, a fistula (abnormal opening or connection) may be present between the esophagus and trachea or an atresia may be present, which usually involves the esophagus ending in a blind pouch with no connection to the stomach. There are five common classifications based on the esophageal configuration and the presence or absence of a fistula:

1. Type A: esophageal atresia—the proximal and distal ends of the esophagus end in blind pouches, neither connected to each other nor with a fistula present.

2. Type B: tracheoesophageal fistula—the proximal or upper segment of the esophagus is connected to the trachea.

3. Type C: esophageal atresia—a fistula in the distal section of the esophagus and the upper portion of the esophagus ending in a blind pouch. This is the most common form occurring in about 85% of all TEF cases (Ryckman & Balistreri, 2002).

4. Type D: the upper and lower portions of the esophagus are connected to the trachea but not to each other.

5. Type E: This anomaly resembles the letter H in which there is a small fistula connecting the esophagus to the trachea at about the midpoint of the esophagus. The fistula varies in size, with some no more than pinpoint size. This is the only configuration that may not be apparent at birth if the fistula is small. The esophagus and trachea are essentially intact, feeding is possible, but the infant may demonstrate frequent coughing and respiratory infections.

Infants with TEF/EA may also have tracheomalacia, abnormal esophageal peristalsis, and GER. This defect may be picked up on prenatal ultrasound and can be suspected if the mother has polyhydramnios. If polyhydramnios is present or the infant is symptomatic, a feeding tube is usually passed to ensure patency of the esophagus before the infant breastfeeds. At birth, infants may have frothy saliva and mucus in the mouth and nose and exhibit choking and coughing with noticeable drooling, respiratory distress, cyanosis, and, if fed, choking and gagging with milk regurgitated through the mouth and nose. Surgical repair is generally performed in the first few days after birth, with parenteral nutrition provided before and immediately after surgery and enteral feedings, including breastfeeding, started about 5–7 days postoperatively. Long delays before normal feeding can result in oral aversion and lack of feeding skills. The infant may be given sham feedings by mouth in conjunction with gastrostomy feeding to accustom the infant to associate oral feeding with satiety and decrease later feeding difficulties. Gastrostomy is usually placed for nutrition in more complex situations where repair can be delayed for many months, with the possibility of sham breast-feeding. Milk drains out of the stoma, but the infant experiences the process of feeding and the comfort and enjoyment of "feeding" at the breast. The mother will need to pump breastmilk for the gastrostomy feeds (Wolf & Glass, 1992).

Colic

Infantile colic is a set of behaviors typically described in healthy infants as episodes of irritability and hard, unexplained, and inconsolable crying, often with clenched fists, a red face, and drawn-up legs (Lucassen et al., 1998). It begins in the early weeks of life, peaks between 5 and 8 weeks of age, and usually resolves spontaneously between 4 and 6 months of age. The prevalence of colic is esti-mated to be between 5% and 28% (Lucassen et al., 2001). Some clinicians use the "rule of threes" as the criterion for defining colic, which states that the behaviors persist for 3 or more hours each day, for 3 or more days each week, for 3 or more weeks (Wessel et al., 1954). Colic has been attributed to various independent causes such as infant temperament (Canifet et al., 2002), type of feeding, cow milk allergies, lactose intolerance, maternal smoking (Sondergaard et al., 2001), and maternal anxiety or depression (Barr, 1996). The physiological relationship between maternal smoking (or tobacco exposure) and colic shows that smoking is linked to increased plasma and intestinal motilin (gastrointestinal hormone that stimulates gastric and intestinal motility) levels and higher than average motilin levels are linked to elevated risks of colic (Shenassa & Brown, 2004). Daily maternal smoking during pregnancy increases the risk of infant colic, with exclu-sive breastfeeding being somewhat protective (Canivet et al., 2008). The preva-lence of colic has been shown to be twofold higher in infants of smoking mothers but less among those infants who were breastfed (Reijneveld et al., 2000).

Allergy to cow milk protein in breastfed infants has been implicated in colic and GER. Bovine whey proteins are present in human milk (Axelsson et al., 1986; Cant et al., 1985; Stuart et al., 1984), and ingestion by susceptible infants could provoke symptoms of colic (Jakobsson & Lindberg, 1983; Kilshaw & Cant, 1984;

Lothe & Lindberg, 1989; Lothe et al., 1982). Eliminating cow milk protein from the maternal diet may reduce or resolve the colic (Hill et al., 1995; Jakobsson et al., 1983; Jakobsson & Lindberg, 1978). A low allergen diet with maternal elimination of common allergenic foods (cow milk, eggs, peanuts, tree nuts, wheat, soy, and fish) showed a reduction in infant distressed behavior among breastfed infants presenting with colic in the first 6 weeks (Hill et al., 2005). However, even with the reduction in crying, the infants still met the criteria for the definition of colic. Switching a fussy breastfed infant to infant formula is not recommended nor does this practice improve colic symptoms (American Academy of Pediatrics [AAP], 1997). The use of soy protein–based infant formula is also not recommended for the prevention of colic or allergy (AAP, 1998).

Although primary lactose intolerance is rare, occasionally excessive crying, gassiness, and green frothy stools may have their origin in a transient lactose intolerance as a result of disruption in lactase production. Lactase is a brush border, small intestinal enzyme that breaks down lactose. Its production could be disrupted from illness, antibiotic use, or encounters with cow milk protein. A functional lactase deficiency could result from low-fat feedings that cause rapid gastric emptying (Anon, 1986) with large quantities of lactose being presented to the small intestinal brush border for digestion. The ability of lactase to handle the high load of lactose may simply be overwhelmed (Lawlor-Smith & Lawlor-Smith, 1998). A high lactose load in breastmilk feedings has been described as occurring due to limited or timed feedings on the first breast, leading to a reduced fat and increased lactose intake (Woolridge & Fisher, 1988). If some colic symptoms are an artifact of breastfeeding routines, then management should consist of ensuring that the infant finishes the first side before being offered the second breast, the use of alternate massage should be encouraged to optimize fat intake, and perhaps offering the drained breast again to further increase fat content of the feed. Rather than substitute a lactose-free formula into the infant's diet, it is possible to add a commercial preparation of lactase to expressed breastmilk that converts lactose to simple sugars before the feeding (Buckley, 2000).

Savino et al. (2005a) found a difference in the colonization patterns of lactobacilli in the intestines of breastfed colicky and noncolicky infants. *L. brevis* and *L. lactis lactis* were found only in colicky infants, whereas *L. acidophilus* was found only in noncolicky infants. Colicky infants are also more frequently colonized by anaerobic gram-negative bacteria, but it is not known whether gut microflora differences are the cause of colic or its consequence (Savino et al., 2004). Oral administration of the probiotic *L. reuteri* improved colicky symptoms in breastfed infants within 1 week of treatment compared with simethicone, which had little effect (Savino et al., 2007). Crying time reduction was seen in breastfed colicky infants who received an extract based on *Matricariae recutita* (German chamomile), *Foeniculum vulgare* (fennel), and *Melissa officinalis* (lemon balm) (Savino et al., 2005b).

Although excessive crying usually resolves over the first 3 months of life, a subgroup of infants with persistent colic symptoms has been identified (Clifford et al., 2002). In some infants, feeding problems have been shown to occur simultaneously with crying problems (Asnes & Mones, 1982; Berkowitz et al., 1997; Dellert et al., 1993; Feranchak et al., 1994; Nelson et al., 1997). There are limited data on the association between functional measures of feeding, such as the organization of oral motor skills, as they relate to the modulation of crying during feeding interactions (Ferguson et al., 1996). Miller-Loncar et al. (2004) provided evidence of feeding-related problems in four areas for a clinic-referred sample of infants with colic. Compared with infants without colic, these infants demonstrated

1. More evidence of reflux

2. More sucking and feeding problems on the Neonatal Oral-Motor Assessment Scale (NOMAS) and Clinical Feeding Evaluation as evidenced by arrhythmic jaw movements and difficulty coordinating sucking, swallowing, and breathing

3. Less responsiveness during feeding interactions

4. More episodes of feeding discomfort

It is not known whether feeding problems contribute to colic, if colic contributes to feeding problems, or if the two often coexist. Only about 5–10% of colic is due to organic disturbances such as gastrointestinal disorders (Barr & Rappaport, 1999). Popular remedies containing simethicone are ineffective in alleviating crying associated with colic (Garrison & Christakis, 2000; Lucassen et al., 1998; Metcalf et al., 1994).

A study of children who had been referred for clinical treatment of colic during infancy demonstrated difficulties with sensory processing, emotional reactivity, and inattention at 3–8 years of age (DeSantis et al., 2004). These data, as well as other investigations, suggest an underlying dysregulation in children who present with clinical levels of colic:

- The preprandial and postprandial plasma levels of cholecystokinin are lower in colicky infants, resulting in the possible predisposition to excessive crying in the absence of the calming effect of cholecystokinin (Huhtala et al., 2003).

- A vagal tone imbalance has been suggested as a theory underlying colic symptoms.
- Cortisol (White et al., 2000) and melatonin (Weissbluth, 1994) have both been studied as contributors in the larger hormonal and neural balance that may contribute to excessive crying through the biochemical effects of inherent or induced imbalances in these substances.

Excessive crying may also indicate underlying pathology with a history and physical examination in order when an infant presents with a chief complaint of crying, irritability, fussiness, or screaming. Urinary tract infections should be ruled out (Freedman et al., 2009). Physical abuse/shaken infant syndrome is a serious medical consequence of early unremitted infant crying.

It is important to address colic as Howard et al. (2006) found that mothers of infants with a physician diagnosis of colic experienced a shorter breastfeeding duration as did mothers whose breastfeeding did not provide an effective means of comforting. Thus excessive infant crying as defined by a physician diagnosis of colic independently shortened the duration of breastfeeding possibly because infants with colic are less likely to be comforted by breastfeeding compared with crying infants without such a diagnosis. Mothers who rated breastfeeding as a highly effective means of comforting their crying infant breastfed for longer durations.

There are myriad strategies for coping with colic that include rocking, holding, use of a sling, breastfeeding, craniosacral osteopathic manipulation, infant massage, crib vibrator, sucrose, gripe water, prone positioning across an adult arm, car rides, and car ride simulators. Numerous pharmaceutical interventions have been suggested such as simethicone, dicyclomine, and methylscopolamine, which may be ineffective and/or hazardous (Joanna Briggs Institute, 2008). There is evidence that a sucrose solution can effectively treat colic in breastfed infants. In two trials, colicky infants responded positively to sucrose. The first trial found that positive effects were seen in 89% of infants receiving sucrose compared with 32% of infants receiving the placebo. In the second trial a controlled environment measured the effects of sucrose on colicky and noncolicky infants. This trial found that both groups responded positively to sucrose. However, sucrose appears to be effective for only a short time as the infants' response only lasted, on average, between 3 and 30 minutes (Garrison & Christakis, 2000). Minimal acupuncture has been shown to be an effective intervention in reducing crying and pain-related behavior in colicky infants by reducing intestinal peristaltic movements (Reinthal et al., 2008).

GER and GER Disease

GER, the involuntary passage or backwash of gastric contents into the esophagus, occurs in approximately one-half of infants 1–3 months of age, peaks around 4 months, and diminishes between 8 and 10 months of age (Nelson et al., 1997). It is common in infants with persistent crying and frequent regurgitation (Heine et al., 2006). GER manifestations vary between infants fed breastmilk and infants fed formula (Campanozzi et al., 2009). Breastfed infants demonstrate GER episodes of significantly shorter duration than formula-fed infants, possibly due to the lower pH value in breastfed infants, which stimulates peristalsis and limits the duration of reflux (Heacock et al., 1992). Transient lower esophageal sphincter relaxation is the predominant mechanism of GER in healthy infants. However, symptomatic infants with GER and complications of the condition are said to have gastroesophageal reflux disease (GERD).

GERD is much less common than GER, affecting 1 in 300 infants (Jung, 2001). Infants with GERD typically have more episodes of transient lower esophageal sphincter relaxation with acid reflux (Omari et al., 2002), which can contribute to persistent symptoms. Clinical manifestations of GERD include vomiting, poor weight gain, dysphagia, abdominal or substernal pain, esophagitis, and respiratory disorders. GERD is common in children with neurological impairments, in preterm infants, and in infants with anomalies of the gastrointestinal tract and the lower and upper airways. GER/GERD is associated with and can be induced by cow milk allergy (Salvatore & Vandenplas, 2002). It may occur secondary to a number of genetic syndromes, chromosomal anomalies, and birth defects. GERD can result from certain external factors such as supine positioning as well as medical interventions and procedures:

- Exposure to tobacco smoke (Alaswad et al., 1996)
- Administration of medications such as caffeine and theophylline (Vandenplas et al., 1986)
- Use of antenatal steroids such as betamethasone and dexamethasone (Chin et al., 2003)
- Use of nasogastric tubes for feeding premature infants (Peter et al., 2002)

GERD can contribute to ongoing feeding problems during and beyond infancy. In a study of 700 children referred to a tertiary care institution for severe feeding problems, 33% were diagnosed with GERD (Rommel et al., 2003). Infants with GERD ranging in age from 5–7 months showed significantly more feeding problems affecting swallowing, behavior, food intake, and mother–child interactions compared with control infants (Mathisen et al., 1999). Coughing, stridor, and an inflamed throat may be present, even in the absence of spitting up or vomiting. GERD is capable of contributing to severe events such as pneumonia, asthma, apnea, and bradycardia (Jadcherla, 2002). Infants with GERD may have alterations in their sleeping patterns with less daytime sleep and increased night awakenings (Ghaem et al., 1998). Swallowing dysfunction may be present with laryngeal edema or laryngomalacia from the acid reflux (Mercado-Deane et al., 2001). Pathological regurgitation, as opposed to frequent spitting up, is characterized by actual vomiting, frequent wet burps, problems with weight gain or weight loss, abdominal pain, and gagging or choking at the end of a feeding (Mason, 2000; Rudolph et al., 2001).

At the extreme end of the GERD spectrum are a number of more severe complications such as esophagitis, hematemesis, Sandifer syndrome (torticollis of the head and arching of the body) (De Ybarrondo & Mazur, 2000), Barrett esophagus (changes in the epithelial lining of the esophagus leading to malignancy), and adenocarcinoma (American Society for Gastrointestinal Endoscopy, 1999; Ault & Schmidt, 1998). Even though symptoms may improve over time for many infants, histology from esophageal biopsy may remain abnormal, raising the possibility of ongoing esophageal insult and predisposing the individual to GERD-related complications (Gold, 2006; Orenstein et al., 2006).

Breastfeeding Management

A progression of management therapies ranges from positioning and feeding modifications to pharmacological and/or surgical intervention (Henry, 2004).

Positioning Modifications

This is the first and most fundamental intervention for GER and GERD. Traditionally, the prone and elevated prone positions were used for infants with GERD. This has been modified due to the supine sleeping recommendations of the AAP (2000b) to recommending prone positioning only in special circumstances (Rudolph et al., 2001). Some parents use prone positioning during the daytime when the infant can be continuously observed. Placing preterm infants in the prone or left lateral position after eating has been shown to limit GER and esophageal acid exposure (Corvaglia et al., 2007). Infants can be seated in an upright position supported in an infant seat with about 90 degrees of hip flexion. They should not be slouched where the abdomen can be compressed such as in an infant seat, car seat, sling, or umbrella stroller. Infants can be carried in a front pack carrier, keeping them fully upright. A left lateral sleeping position is also used by some parents because it decreases reflux (Ewer et al., 1999; Tobin et al., 1997). Positioning for breastfeeding should be between a 45-degree and a 60-degree angle with no abdominal compression (Wolf & Glass, 1992). Positioning changes may be needed if the infant cries during feedings, arches from the breast, or pulls off the breasts before completing the feeding. If other feeding positions do not provide relief, the mother can try feeding the infant while standing upright. The infant should be kept in an upright position after feedings.

Thickened Feedings

Thickening the liquid feeding with rice cereal has long been used and thought to keep the stomach contents heavy enough to resist rising into the esophagus. This practice is controversial with mixed results. Although it may reduce the frequency and volume of regurgitation, acid reflux remains unaffected, with as much or more exposure of the esophagus to acidic backwash (Bailey et al., 1987). Some parents feed their infant 1–2 tablespoons of rice cereal by spoon first and then breastfeed if they see decreased episodes of spitting up by doing so. However, there is little evidence that feed thickening affects the actual acid backwash or the course of the condition (Carroll et al., 2002; Huang et al., 2003).

Small Frequent Feedings

Smaller and more frequent feedings have been associated with decreased reflux episodes (Orenstein, 1999).

Drug Therapy

Gastric acidity inhibitors and proton pump inhibitors are used for GERD treatment. However, gastric acid is a disease protective factor because it limits the survival of microorganisms ingested by the infant. Canani et al. (2006) demonstrated that the use of gastric acidity inhibitors was associated with an increased risk of acute gastroenteritis and community-acquired pneumonia.

Chiropractic Therapy

Alcantara and Anderson (2008) described improvement in GERD symptoms in a 3-month-old infant using chiropractic manipulation and craniosacral therapy.

Colitis/Proctocolitis

Inflammation of the colon (colitis) and/or rectum (proctocolitis) with mild rectal bleeding is occasionally seen in a breastfed infant, even one fed exclusively on breastmilk. The dietary-induced inflammatory reaction is usually caused by allergy to cow milk protein transferred to the infant from the maternal milk (Anvenden-Hertzberg et al., 1996; Lake et al., 1982; Odze et al., 1993; Patenaude et al., 2000). Infants usually present with mild to moderate diarrhea or grossly blood-streaked stool with mucus. Onset is between 1 week and 5 months of age, with the infant in apparently very good health other than the bleeding. Specific diagnostic criteria are lacking, but Hwang et al. (2007) suggested that certain endoscopic and histopathological findings are effective in a differential diagnosis. Smehilova et al. (2008) reported that infants with allergic colitis had significantly lower counts of bifidobacteria in their intestines compared with infants without colitis. It is not known whether this contributes to the onset of colitis or is the result of the condition.

Generally, eliminating cow milk protein from the maternal diet alleviates the bleeding, often within 72–96 hours (Pumberger et al., 2001). Most infants experience a benign course of the condition, with many showing gradual resolution even when there are no changes in the maternal diet, suggesting that this may be a self-limiting situation (Machida et al., 1994). Sometimes, eliminating all forms of cow milk products from the maternal diet fails to completely resolve the bleeding and mothers may be asked to eliminate soy protein, eggs, corn, nuts, fish, shellfish, wheat, and chocolate from their diet, because these foods may cause a similar reaction either as the sole allergen or in combination with the cow milk (Choi et al., 2005; Machida et al., 1994).

If infants do not respond to the elimination of cow milk protein, it might be due to cross-reactivity between human milk proteins and cow milk proteins. Some similarities between cow milk and human milk amino acid structures may provoke allergic symptoms in cow milk–allergic infants when they ingest human milk (Bernard et al., 2000; Restani et al., 1999). Mothers may also need to eliminate beef from their diet. Casein hydrolysate formulas (Nutramigen, Pregestimil, or elemental amino acid formulas) are sometimes given temporarily to the infant if the bleeding remains or intensifies during the time of the maternal elimination diet, with breastfeeding resuming after the bleeding ceases. If this more extreme measure is taken, the mother should pump her milk and freeze it. That milk can be given to the infant when he or she is a little older and has outgrown the problem. Although this intervention may resolve rectal bleeding, it deprives infants and mothers of the advantages of breastfeeding.

Finding blood in the stool of their infant is quite alarming to parents. Many ask why and how this could happen in an exclusively breastfed infant and in a family with no history of such occurrences. The clinician should ask if the infant received a bottle of cow milk–based formula in the hospital before discharge. Supplementation of breastfed infants is common and many times done without the knowledge or permission of the mother. In a susceptible infant, one bottle can sensitize the infant, with subsequent exposure to cow milk through the maternal diet resulting in allergic symptoms. Only small amounts of bovine beta-lactalbumin (i.e., 1 ng [a billionth of a gram]) are necessary to create the sensitizing event. Although human milk contains 0.5–32 ng/L of bovine beta-lactalbumin, a 40-mL feeding of cow milk–based formula contains the equivalent amount of beta-lactalbumin that a breastfed infant would receive from 21 years of breastfeeding (Businco et al., 1999)!

A treatment regimen has been developed that may reduce the colic symptoms, eliminate or decrease the bloody stools, facilitate breastfeeding, and avoid the use of hypoallergenic formulas. It is based on the maternal use of pancrease, a digestive enzyme that breaks down fats, proteins, and carbohydrates in the mother's diet before they circulate and enter her milk (Repucci, 1999). The three-part regimen (Schach & Haight, 2002) allows mothers to continue breastfeeding and includes the maternal elimination of dairy products, soy, nuts, strawberries, and chocolate and further eliminating wheat, eggs, and corn if this does not resolve the infant's symptoms. The mother also takes two pancrease MT-4–strength tablets with each meal and one with each snack.

Clinicians report an amazing variety of foods that have been traced back as sources for colitis. Some recommend that the mother eat foods that she has never before had in her diet as a mechanism to completely eliminate the offending food or family of foods from her system. Breastfeeding should not be abandoned, because the infant most often simply outgrows the problem.

Pyloric Stenosis

Hypertrophic pyloric stenosis is the narrowing of the pyloric orifice that connects the stomach to the duodenum due to excessive thickening of the pyloric sphincter or hypertrophy (excessive growth) of the mucosa or submucosa of the pylorus.

The enlarged pyloric musculature obstructs the gastric outlet, resulting in the classic symptom of projectile vomiting following feedings. Pyloric stenosis

- Affects 0.5–3.0 infants per 1,000 live births (Applegate & Druschel, 1995; Persson et al., 2001).

- Is the most common condition requiring surgery in the early months of life (Ohshiro & Puri, 1998).

- May have a familial or genetic component in its etiology (Everett et al., 2008; Mitchell & Risch, 1991).

- Is more common among first-born children (Dodge, 1975; Jedd et al., 1986; Webb et al., 1983) and less common in African-American infants (Wang et al., 2008).

- Occurs in a preponderance of male infants (Habbick et al., 1989; Lammer & Edmonds, 1987; Webb et al., 1983), affecting males four times more frequently than females (Everett et al., 2008).

- Is generally not congenital, because infants who eventually develop pyloric stenosis have structurally normal pylori at birth.

- Usually develops between the second and sixth week of life with intermittent vomiting at first, progressing to include vomiting that is often forceful or projectile after each feeding. The infant remains hungry, continues to feed eagerly, but weight loss and dehydration, decreased urine and stool output, irritability, and weakness may eventually result in an electrolyte imbalance and the need for corrective surgery.

The etiology of pyloric stenosis shows a strong postnatal influence on its development. A number of causal factors have been linked to or associated with the occurrence of pyloric stenosis:

- Maternal smoking: Maternal smoking has been shown to be a risk factor for pyloric stenosis, with infants of smokers being twice as likely to develop the condition. It is not known whether the association is caused by maternal prenatal smoking, exposure to second-hand smoke after birth, or exposure through breastmilk (Sorensen et al., 2002).

- *Helicobacter pylori*: This bacterium is commonly found in the human stomach, and its epidemiological and clinical features are very similar to pyloric stenosis, suggesting that some pyloric stenosis may have an infectious etiology (Paulozzi, 2000).

- Abnormalities in pyloric innervation: Some abnormalities in the intramuscular innervation of the pyloric muscle have been reported, suggesting that the reduced production of neurotrophins (nerve growth factors) may be responsible for the delay in the functional and structural maturation of pyloric innervation, leading to the abnormalities in growth (Guarino et al., 2001).

- Early postnatal exposure to erythromycin: Young infants who received erythromycin antibiotics have shown a significantly increased incidence of pyloric stenosis (Hauben & Amsden, 2002), especially when the drug was prescribed systemically (not ophthalmically) for the infant during the first 2 weeks of life (Mahon et al., 2001). Exposure to erythromycin through breastmilk also significantly increases the risk and occurrence of pyloric stenosis in breastfed infants between 0 and 90 days of age, depending on the period of postnatal exposure (Sorensen et al., 2003; Stang, 1986).

- Lack of breastfeeding: Infants with pyloric stenosis are less likely to have been breastfed during the first week of life (Pisacane et al., 1996). Although other studies are not consistent with feeding-type effects on pyloric stenosis, Pisacane et al. (1996) showed that 35% of the cases of pyloric stenosis in their study of 102 infants with surgically confirmed pyloric stenosis could be associated with the lack of exclusive breastfeeding during the early neonatal period. They speculated on the possible protective effects that breastmilk may have on the development of this condition, including the presence of high levels of hormones such as vasoactive intestinal peptide, which favors pyloric relaxation, or the increased plasma gastrin levels seen in formula-fed infants or supplemented breastfed infants (Marchini et al., 1994), which could be associated with spasm of the pylorus, pyloric hypertrophy, and the consequent damage to peptide-containing nerve fibers.

Surgical intervention (pyloromyotomy) may be performed with correction of dehydration and electrolyte imbalance. Either an open or a laparoscopic procedure may be performed, with earlier full feedings and decreased length of hospitalization seen with laparoscopic pyloromyotomy (Fugimoto et al., 1999). After an uncomplicated procedure, infants can usually begin ad lib breastfeeding once they have recovered from the anesthesia, decreasing the time spent in the hospital and reducing the stress of surgery on the family (Carpenter et al., 1999; Garza et al., 2002; Puapong et al., 2002). Mothers may need to pump their milk during the surgical period.

Breastfeeding Management

Breastfeeding management during the early course of this condition (often before it is diagnosed) usually consists of frequent feedings, often with refeeding right after the infant has spit up. As the spitting up becomes more frequent and forceful, mothers need to keep track of diaper counts, and more frequent weight checks may be in order. If weight stasis or loss becomes evident, hindmilk refeeds can be tried, but surgery may be necessary if weight loss and electrolyte imbalance become problematic. Clinicians may wish to refrain from prescribing erythromycin to lactating mothers and young infants and to explain that smoking increases the risk for this condition.

Metabolic Disorders

Abnormalities in the newborn's body chemistry that affect how food is built up or broken down are typically referred to as inborn errors of metabolism. These may take the form of amino acid disorders, fatty acid oxidation disorders, organic acid disorders, and urea cycle disorders. Most metabolic disorders are inherited as autosomal recessive traits (two copies of the defective gene are needed for the disorder to be expressed, one from each parent). All U.S. states screen newborns for two disorders: phenylketonuria (PKU) and congenital hypothyroidism. Most states also screen newborns for some other disorders, such as galactosemia, hemoglobin abnormalities, maple syrup urine disease, homocystinuria, biotinidase deficiency, congenital adrenal hyperplasia, and medium-chain Acyl-CoA dehydrogenase deficiency. Although the AAP (2000a) has recommended that all states screen for 30 specific disorders, screening varies from state to state and is inconsistent for what is screened. In 2005 the AAP (2008) endorsed a report from the American College of Medical Genetics (2006), which recommended that all states screen newborn infants for a core panel of 29 treatable congenital conditions and an additional 25 conditions that may be detected by screening. Clinicians should check with their own state for screening information.

Breastfeeding is quite possible with many inherited metabolic disorders, including not only PKU but also organic acidemias (Huner et al., 2005; MacDonald et al., 2006). Gokcay et al. (2006) reported that breastfed infants with organic acidemias experienced a decreased frequency of infections, acute metabolic episodes, and hospital admissions compared with infants with organic acidemias who were not breastfed. However, close monitoring of clinical parameters such as growth, development, and biochemistry is imperative. Mothers should be closely supported to ensure an abundant milk supply, especially if breastfeeding gets off to a slow start or there are interruptions in the infant feeding directly at the breast.

Phenylketonuria

PKU is an inherited autosomal recessive trait affecting 1 in 13,500–19,000 live births (NIH Consensus Statement, 2000). It is caused by a deficiency in the hepatic enzyme phenylalanine hydroxylase, which is required for the metabolism of the essential amino acid phenylalanine (PHE) into tyrosine. When this enzyme deficiency goes untreated, PHE accumulates in the tissues and brain where it can interfere with brain development, eventually causing mental retardation as well as a host of bizarre behaviors and failure to thrive. PKU is treated by dietary management, providing enough PHE for normal growth and development while preventing excessive amounts from accumulating.

Breastmilk is extremely important for infants with PKU, especially during the time before diagnosis and institution of dietary interventions. Riva et al. (1996) found that infants breastfed for 20–40 days during the prediagnostic stage showed improved neurodevelopment, with a 12.9-point IQ advantage over infants fed formula during the same period. Breastfeeding can successfully continue (Motzfeldt et al., 1999) once a diagnosis has been made and is done in combination with a PHE-free formula. Blood levels of PHE are monitored, with dietary adjustments as needed to keep PHE serum concentrations between 120 and 360 μmol/L (Medical Research Council Working Party on Phenylketonuria, 1993).

Because human milk is lower in PHE than commercial formulas, 40 mg/dL versus 70–85 mg/dL (McCabe et al., 1992), infants with PKU can continue to receive significant amounts of human milk in their diet. Infants fed 362 mL (first month) to 464 mL (fourth month) of breastmilk daily in addition to PHE-free formula showed a lower PHE intake than infants fed exclusively with a low-PHE formula during the first 6 months of life. These infants demonstrated normal weight, length, head circumference, and hematological indices (McCabe et al., 1989).

Breastfeeding Management

A number of feeding protocols have been used to incorporate breastfeeding into the dietary management of this condition using breastmilk as the PHE source (Kanufre et al., 2007). For instance, during the first few days after diagnosis, especially with high serum PHE levels, the infant is given limited amounts of breastmilk or only

PHE-free formula to normalize serum PHE levels quickly while the mother pumps her milk during this time to maintain her supply. When serum PHE levels normalize, breastfeeding is begun, with each feeding consisting of a measured amount of PHE-free formula first (10–30 mL) (Clark, 1992) followed by breastfeeding. Breastfeeding times are adjusted depending on the results of weekly blood tests (Purnell, 2001). PHE-free formula can be given by bottle, alternative feeding method, or by supplementer at the breast but should not be offered after a breast-feeding. Over half of the infant's diet can be breastmilk.

Breastfeeding can alternate with PHE-free formula feeds. At each feeding, the infant feeds until satiety on either the PHE-free formula or at the breast. The number of feedings at the breast is adapted to the plasma PHE concentrations. Compared with a regimen where both bottle and breast are offered at each feeding, this approach may be more convenient for parents, and the infant can fully drain the breasts to receive the full complement of fat-rich milk available as the breasts drain (van Rijn et al., 2003).

Published estimates of volume and energy of daily human milk consumption are used to calculate how much PHE-free formula to include in a 24-hour period of time. Starting with the weight of the infant, the total volume of milk needed in a 24-hour period is calculated along with the maximal amount of PHE allowed (25–45 mg/kg/day), the maximum allowable amount of human milk (based on 0.41 mg/mL of PHE in human milk), and the amount of PHE-free formula for the infant to consume such that he or she does not exceed the maximum amount of breastmilk allowed in the diet. The PHE-free formula is divided into equal amounts to be given either before each breastfeeding or during each breastfeeding with a supplementer device (Greve et al., 1994). Mothers can weigh the infant before and after feeding from the breast to determine the amount of breastmilk consumed, and the next feeding can consist of an appropriately measured amount of PHE-free formula (Yannicelli et al., 1988). This is a cumbersome but fairly accurate method of determining breastmilk intake.

The infant's intake at the breast also can be correlated with a time measurement. The infant is weighed before and after each breastfeeding over a 48-hour time period, along with recording the number of minutes the infant nurses at each feeding. These numbers are used to calculate an average of minutes per ounce consumed. The PHE recommendations are converted to the number of minutes of feeding from the breast that is allowed in a 24-hour period. Infants feed from the breast until the total time specified has been met for the day and PHE-free formula is given for the rest of the feedings. This method usually requires more frequent monitoring of serum levels of PHE because it is a less accurate method for determining the true PHE intake (Duncan & Elder, 1997).

The treatment plan for an infant is individualized and managed by a physician and dietitian specializing in metabolic disorders. Each state has one or more medical centers capable of providing consultation and treatment for metabolic defects. The clinician should be aware of each facility that has this capability and be prepared to work as part of a team to optimize the dietary management of infants with PKU. Clinicians should remind parents to avoid giving their infant any product containing aspartame. Aspartame is an artificial sweetener made from PHE and is found in foods, drinks, and medicines, in addition to products designed as sugar substitutes. Because infants with PKU are more susceptible to thrush, mothers should be vigilant for signs of *Candida* overgrowth in the infant as well as on their nipples and areolae (Lawrence & Lawrence, 2005).

Cystic Fibrosis

Cystic fibrosis (CF) is a genetic disease occurring in approximately 1 in every 3,900 live births. The gene defect causes abnormalities in the cells that line the airways, biliary tree, pancreatic ducts, vas deferens, sweat ducts, and intestines, accounting for the multiple systems and organs involved in the condition. Secretions from all these sites become thickened to the point of obstructing the hepatic ducts, blocking the flow of pancreatic digestive enzymes, and interfering with the movement of cilia in the lungs. Thick secretions from the lungs place the child at high risk for pulmonary complications due to persistent respiratory infections. Symptoms vary from person to person due in part to the more than 1,000 mutations of the CF gene. Newborns may present with meconium ileus, which is a surgical emergency, or may already have pancreatic insufficiency. Parents may remark that the infant's skin and sweat taste salty, which is a classic symptom. Weight gain can be a problem because fat and nutrient absorption is usually impaired, even though the infant may feed frequently and vigorously. The median age of survival for a person with CF is about 33 years, with many female infants with CF growing up and having infants of their own.

Breastfeeding is highly beneficial to infants with CF due to the protective factors in human milk that lower the risk of respiratory infections. Breastfeeding exclusively for 6 months is associated with a decreased need for intravenous antibiotic use, confirming a decreased incidence and severity of infections in infants with CF (Parker et al., 2004). Breastfeeding helps protect children against decline in pulmonary function and decreases the number of infections in the first 3 years (Colombo et al., 2007). Not all infants with CF are diagnosed at birth, but most infants are identified by the time they reach 12 months. Failure to gain an appropriate amount of weight may persist, respiratory problems may increase, and when solid foods are introduced, the stool may turn bulky, foul smelling, and greasy.

Breastfeeding Management

Breastfeeding should proceed as usual, because children with CF who were exclusively breastfed were found to be heavier and taller than those exclusively bottle-fed (Holliday et al., 1991). Most CF centers recommend exclusive breastfeeding, the use of pancreatic enzymes, and/or hydrolyzed formula if needed (Luder et al., 1990). Breastmilk contains lipase, an enzyme that helps digest fats, which is beneficial in working to improve fat absorption from the diet. Because about half of even asymptomatic infants show pancreatic insufficiency and nutritional deficits at diagnosis, breastmilk may be augmented with extra calories, a pancreatic replacement enzyme, and fat-soluble vitamins (Koletzko & Reinhardt, 2001). Replacement enzymes along with exclusive breastfeeding improve nutrient tolerance and weight gain, reducing or eliminating the need to use or wean to infant formula (Cannella et al., 1993). Mothers can optimize caloric intake at the breast by the use of alternate massage, good drainage of the breasts at each feeding, and frequent feedings. Fat-rich hindmilk can also be used for calorie supplementation.

Galactosemia

Galactosemia is a hereditary autosomal recessive disorder of carbohydrate metabolism, occurring in about 1 in every 60,000 live births. Figure 7-1 demonstrates that an infant who inherits two normal genes would neither be affected nor would he or she be a carrier. A carrier of classic galactosemia inherits one normal gene and one galactosemia gene, resulting in enzyme activity that is less than normal but neither requiring dietary management nor showing apparent medical complications. If an infant inherited both galactosemia genes, he or she would have classic galactosemia.

Galactosemia is an autosomal recessive disorder and a general term referring to a category of metabolic defects in which an enzyme deficiency disrupts the normal metabolism of the sugar galactose. Normally, galactose is metabolized by the body into glucose in a step-wise fashion by three specific enzyme reactions. Galactose comprises half of lactose, the sugar found in milk, whereas glucose

Figure 7-1 Genotypes Involving Classic Galactosemia

Source: Available at: www.galactosemia.org. Accessed September 19, 2005.

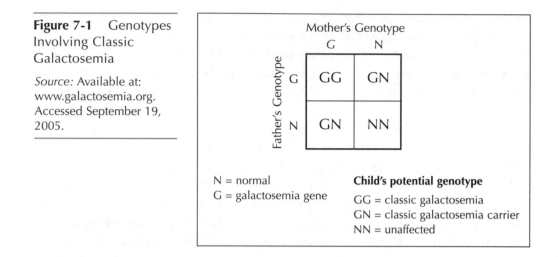

N = normal
G = galactosemia gene

Child's potential genotype

GG = classic galactosemia
GN = classic galactosemia carrier
NN = unaffected

forms the other half. When this metabolic process is interrupted, high levels of galactose-1-phosphate accumulate in the body, causing damage to the liver, kidney, brain, and eyes. Although there are more than 100 heritable mutations that can cause galactosemia, the three most common are

1. Galactose-1-phosphate uridyl transferase deficiency, the classic and most severe form, which causes the complete loss of the ability to process galactose

2. Galactokinase deficiency

3. Uridyl diphosphate galactose-4-empiridase deficiency

Diagnosis is usually made during the first week of life through blood analysis from a newborn screening test. Symptoms typically start about the third day of life and include jaundice, enlarged liver, vomiting, poor feeding, poor weight gain, lethargy, irritability, convulsions, and cataracts. When parents receive notice that the screening test indicates possible galactosemia, breastmilk feeding is stopped and replaced with a lactose-free formula. However, mothers should continue to pump and store their milk until a confirming test is done to determine if the infant has the classic form or a variant of galactosemia called Duarte galactosemia.

Duarte Galactosemia

Duarte galactosemia is a variant of the classic galactosemia, and infants with this form may have varying levels of enzyme activity depending on their genotype (Beutler et al., 1965). The child with Duarte galactosemia inherits a gene for classic galactosemia from one parent and a Duarte variant gene from the other parent. The possible variations include the following: a carrier of Duarte galactosemia may have approximately 75% enzyme activity, a homozygous carrier of Duarte would have about 50% enzyme activity, and a person with Duarte galactosemia may have about 25–50% enzyme activity. Depending on the levels of galactose-1-phosphate in the blood, some infants with the Duarte form of galactosemia may be able to partially or totally breastfeed. Mothers may be able to breastfeed every other feeding alternating with a lactose-free formula. Such enzyme levels should be confirmed before abandoning breastfeeding and ceasing breastmilk expression.

Congenital Heart Disease

Congenital heart disease (CHD) refers to any functional or structural defect in the heart or major blood vessels that is present at birth. Between 4.05 and 10.2 infants per 1,000 live births experience some form of CHD, with an overall incidence of about 1% (Botto, 2000; Hoffman, 1990). Women at high risk of having an infant with CHD include mothers with diabetes, a family history of CHD, exposure to certain medications such as indomethacin (Indocin), first-trimester exposure to rubella, and residing at high altitudes, which increases the incidence of patent ductus arteriosis (Allan, 1996; Mahoney, 1993). CHD is also part of many congenital birth defects and syndromes such as CHARGE, Down syndrome, fetal alcohol syndrome, Goldenhar syndrome, Turner syndrome, Rubinstein-Taybi syndrome, and velocardiofacial syndrome (Frommelt, 2004). Two classification systems describe CHD based on their cyanotic or acyanotic characteristics and based on their hemodynamic characteristics (Box 7-1).

Congestive heart failure is a syndrome associated with most CHD. Depending on the defect, the extent of involvement, and the existence of other problems, symptoms may manifest shortly after birth or weeks after discharge from the hospital. Symptoms may include eager sucking for only a few minutes followed by frequent pauses or rests, short sucking bursts, lethargy, fatigue, poor appetite, sweating while feeding, poor suck, uncoordinated suck-swallow-breathe patterns, weak suck, cyanosis, tachypnea (rapid breathing), heart murmur, and poor weight gain in older infants (Coffey, 1997). Although some infants may not become cyanotic, their coloring turns dusky. This is not to be confused with acrocyanosis, the normal bluish coloring of a newborn's hands and feet due to delayed capillary opening. Some infants may also demonstrate circumoral cyanosis (bluish coloring around the lips) when feeding.

BOX 7-1 Most Common Types of Congenital Heart Disease

ACYANOTIC

Increased Pulmonary Blood Flow

- Atrial septal defect—a hole in the wall between the atria (the two entry chambers of the heart)
- Ventricular septal defect—a hole in the wall between the ventricles (the pumping chambers of the heart); this is the most common CHD, accounting for 20–25% of CHD (Kenner et al., 1993)
- Patent ductus arteriosis—persistence of (failure to close) the connection between the pulmonary artery and the aorta after birth
- Atrioventricular canal—combination of atrial septal defect, ventricular septal defect, and common atrioventricular valve

Obstruction to Blood Flow From Ventricles

- Coarctation of the aorta—narrowing of the aorta
- Aortic stenosis—impairment of blood flow from left ventricle to the aorta due to aortic valve disease or obstruction
- Pulmonic stenosis—narrowing of the opening into the pulmonary artery from the right ventricle

CYANOTIC

Decreased Pulmonary Blood Flow

- Tetralogy of Fallot—a combination of four defects consisting of pulmonary stenosis, interventricular septal defect, dextraposed aorta that receives blood from both ventricles, and hypertrophy of the right ventricle
- Tricuspid atresia—narrowing of the opening to the tricuspid valve

Mixed Blood Flow

- Transposition of the great arteries—the aorta arises from the right ventricle and the pulmonary artery arises from the left ventricle (the exact opposite of where they should be located)
- Total anomalous pulmonary venous return
- Truncus arteriosis
- Hypoplastic left heart syndrome—underdevelopment of the left ventricle

Source: Adapted from: Coffey PM. Breastfeeding the Infant with Congenital Heart Disease. In: Dowling D, Danner SC, Coffey PM, Eds. *Breastfeeding the Infant with Special Needs.* March of Dimes Nursing Modules, March of Dimes Birth Defects Foundation; 1997. White Plains, NY.

Parents are sometimes discouraged from nursing their infant because of misconceptions regarding breastfeeding and human milk (Lambert & Watters, 1998). Some believe that breastfeeding is harder or more work for the infant than bottle-feeding. However, cardiorespiratory efforts during breastfeeding are less strenuous and more physiological than during bottle-feeding. Oxygen saturation levels during breastfeeding in infants with CHD are maintained at higher and less variable levels compared with feeding from a bottle (Marino et al., 1995). Data from oxygenation studies on preterm and full-term infants have shown that during bottle-feeding, transcutaneous oxygen pressure levels decrease and, for some infants, continue to drop for up to 10 minutes after feedings (Hammerman & Kaplan, 1995; Koenig et al., 1990; Meier, 1988). In infants with cyanotic lesions, it is extremely important to maintain their oxygen saturation as high as possible, and therefore it may be necessary to breastfeed to ensure this happens (Wheat, 2002).

Others believe that breastfeeding burns more calories, human milk has fewer calories, infants will have inadequate caloric intake, and infants will not be able to consume sufficient calories at the breast to meet increased metabolic and energy demands. Infants with CHD can suffer growth impairments due to anorexia, early satiety, mild gastrointestinal abnormalities, excess protein loss, fluid restriction, or frequent respiratory infections. After accounting for these and other effects on energy needs, infants with CHD may have only half as much energy available for growth as healthy infants (Weintraub & Menahem, 1993). However, it has been shown in a comparison between breastfed and formula-fed infants with CHD that breastfed infants gained weight more quickly and had shorter hospital stays than bottle-fed infants and that the severity of the cardiac defect was not predictive of the infant's ability to breastfeed or of breastfeeding duration (Combs & Marino, 1993). The higher concentrations of anti-infective factors in human milk are especially beneficial for infants with CHD, because these infants are more vulnerable to respiratory illness. These infants benefit from the incorporation into body tissues of components such as nucleotides that result in improved recovery after body injuries and surgery (Carver, 1999). Owens (2002) described an infant experiencing a heart transplant who successfully breastfed after transplantation, gained weight, showed no signs of organ rejection, and breastfed until 13 months of age.

CHD infants who require additional calories

- May receive higher caloric content feedings at breast when the mother uses alternate massage, when there are short intervals between feedings, and when the breasts have been well drained
- May receive expressed hindmilk through a supplementer device at the breast

- May have high-energy supplements added to breastmilk
- May be on fluid restrictions and benefit from fractionated human milk that delivers 28–30 calories per ounce
- May be gavage fed supplements (hindmilk or high-energy formula) after feedings at the breast
- May be breastfed during the day and placed on a continuous feeding pump at night

Mothers may experience a number of obstacles to breastfeeding an infant with CHD, including separations during procedures or surgeries, fasting protocols that interrupt breastfeeding, anxiety regarding feedings, difficulty establishing lactation, inconsistent or apathetic support from healthcare providers (Barbas & Kelleher, 2004), and lack of access to breast pumps and privacy for pumping (Lambert & Watters, 1998). Mothers also describe difficulty distinguishing the infant's satiation cues (when an infant stops breastfeeding because he or she is full) from fatigue (when an infant stops breastfeeding due to exhaustion) (Lobo, 1992).

Breastfeeding Management

Feeding plans must be individualized to the needs and conditions of both infant and mother. CHD does not preclude breastfeeding, and feedings at breast can begin at birth with modifications as needed.

Positioning

Positioning the infant at the breast may be more comfortable and efficient for the infant in an upright position because GERD is more common in infants with cardiac problems. Infants should be positioned such that the rib cage can fully expand and the head is just slightly extended to open the airway. Some infants feed better lying down in a side-lying position that avoids pressure on the abdomen.

Latch and Sucking

Many infants have a weak suck and fatigue easily at the breast. Alternate massage helps increase the caloric content of the feeding and assists the infant to sustain sucking. Some infants are capable of feeding on only one breast per feeding and others benefit from use of a nipple shield. Mothers may find that the dancer hand position helps support the infant and improve sucking.

Shorter and More Frequent Feedings

This pattern may meet the needs and limitations of many infants as well as increase the fat content of the milk. The feeding should be interrupted if the infant becomes tachypneic, short of breath, blue around the lips, pale, or fatigued. The infant may not wake spontaneously for feedings.

Mothers may need to pump their milk after feedings to provide milk that the infant is unable to extract as well as to maintain an abundant milk supply. The cream layer from this stored milk can be used as a high-calorie supplement. Mothers will also express milk during the times surrounding surgery.

Preoperative and Postoperative Fasting Times

These times vary considerably from one institution to another (American Society of Anesthesiologists, 1999), so please check with a mother's specific institution because fasting can cause significant disruption in breastfeeding and milk production.

During the perioperative period, mothers should be provided with

- A private, quiet place to pump milk
- A multiuser electric breast pump
- Sink, soap, and dishwashing liquid to wash hands and pump parts
- Refrigeration to store pumped milk (or she can use a cooler with blue ice brought from home)
- Nutritious food and water
- Unequivocal support for breastfeeding and pumping milk
- A place to rest and lie down; rooming-in accommodations

If other obligations preclude the mother from rooming-in or spending long periods of time with the infant, arrangements should be made for her pumped milk to be brought to the hospital and given to her infant.

Neurological Diseases, Deficits, Impairments, and Disorders

Neurological deficits, disorders, diseases, or impairments can affect breastfeeding to either a greater or a lesser extent. Some infants can feed well in spite of the problem or can learn over time, depending on the severity. Some neurological impairment occurs as a nervous system insult and may be temporary, such as with asphyxia, cranial bleeds, sepsis, birth trauma, or the effect of maternal medications or drugs.

The central nervous system could be abnormally developed or damaged during the prenatal or peripartum period, resulting in feeding difficulties either immediately after birth or gradually over a period of time. McBride and Danner (1987) divided sucking abnormalities related to neurological involvement into three categories:

1. Depressed sucking reflex (prematurity, Down syndrome [trisomy 21], trisomy 18, Prader-Willi syndrome, asphyxia, hypothyroidism)

2. Weak sucking reflex (Down syndrome, medullary lesions, congenital myasthenia gravis, muscle abnormalities)

3. Incoordinated sucking (cerebral bleeds, asphyxia, Arnold-Chiari malformation)

Other conditions such as neonatal/perinatal stroke, cerebral palsy, and neural tube defects can also contribute to ongoing feeding problems. Many of these conditions have common breastfeeding suggestions.

Down Syndrome

Down syndrome is a congenital condition caused by the duplication (a third copy) of chromosome 21. The chance of having an infant with Down syndrome is 1 in 1,000 births for mothers in their twenties, 1 in every 350 births for mothers over age 35, and 1 in 100 for women over 40 years of age. Many of these infants also have congenital heart defects, anomalies of the gastrointestinal tract, a large-appearing tongue with flaccid tone, and some degree of developmental delay. A number of characteristics present challenges to breastfeeding (Lewis & Kritzinger, 2004):

- Generalized hypotonia that impacts the amount of body and head support needed to position and stabilize the infant at the breast.

- Hypotonia of the perioral muscles, lips, and masseter muscle; milk may leak out the sides of the mouth because an adequate seal is not achieved.

- Passively or actively protruding tongue that may not form a central groove. A study on bottle-fed infants with Down syndrome showed that the tongue lacked the normal peristaltic movements and tended to fall to the back of the mouth, impairing the sucking motion (Mizuno & Ueda, 2001).

- Weak suck that may improve with time.

- The hard palate may be highly arched, narrow, and stair-like with acutely aligned palatine plates. The high palatal height is associated with a constricted palate that contributes to the commonly seen tongue projection and a smaller volume of the oral cavity (Bhagyalakshmi et al., 2007).

- Cardiac defects that, depending on the type and severity, contribute to excessive perspiring, fatigue during feeding, tachypnea, inadequate intake, long feeding sessions, and slow weight gain.
- Mid-face hypoplasia. The shape of the mid-face may narrow the nose passages, sinuses, middle and inner ear, and throat. Any congestion in the nasal passages makes breastfeeding more difficult as they are easily obstructed with mucus.

Breastfeeding Management

Pacifiers (and bottles if possible) should be avoided because pacifiers may mask hunger cues. Artificial nipples reinforce the narrowing of the palate, to which infants with Down syndrome are already prone. Some infants may not suck long enough or effectively enough to trigger the letdown reflex. Mothers may wish to cause the milk to let down before placing the infant at the breast.

Oral Stimulation

Oral stimulation before feedings may decrease dysfunctional sucking movements and patterns, ease mouth opening, and stimulate central grooving of the tongue (Genna, 2008).

Positioning

Positioning the infant should involve complete body support such that no part of the infant falls into extension, pulling down on the shoulder girdle and causing the infant to exert muscles in the neck or mouth to stay attached to the breast. Some of these infants do best when held in a nearly horizontal fashion with their hips almost at the same level as their head (Danner, 1992b). Flexing the infant's thighs and knees increases resting muscle tone throughout the body and reduces the tendency to hyperextension (Saenz, 2004).

Supporting the Jaw

Use of the dancer hand position provides jaw stability, decreases intraoral space, supports flaccid cheeks, and may assist the infant in generating and maintaining sufficient negative pressure to sustain milk transfer (Einarsson-Backes et al., 1994).

Latch and Sucking

Use of alternate massage, a supplementer device, and/or a nipple shield may improve milk transfer and overall intake at each feeding. Use of an asymmetrical latch while bringing the infant to the breast chin first may help achieve a deeper latch.

Tongue Protrusion

The infant's head should be brought into a neutral position to prevent neck extension from leading to an overly protruded tongue during latch attempts. Firm downward pressure, tapping with a finger to the midline of the tongue, and moving from tongue tip to tongue base may improve tone and central grooving (Wolf & Glass, 1992).

Referrals

Children with Down syndrome and any number of other conditions that significantly affect the capacity for oral feeding may need to be referred to specialists such as an occupational therapist, a physical therapist, or a speech-and-language pathologist for a more thorough evaluation of feeding impediments and an individualized therapeutic plan. Random orofacial exercises may not have the desired effects in solving breastfeeding problems unless tailored to the particular deficits and needs of the individual infant (Bovey et al., 1999).

Cerebral Palsy

Cerebral palsy describes a group of chronic conditions affecting motor control and postural abnormalities. It is caused by damage to differing areas of the brain often occurring during fetal development as well as during the perinatal or postnatal period. It is nonprogressive in nature, but clinical manifestations generally change over time. The estimated prevalence is 1.5 to 2.5 per 1,000 live births. Low-birth-weight infants comprise about 25% of all cases of cerebral palsy.

Spastic cerebral palsy, which is the most common type, is seen in 70–80% of affected individuals. It is characterized by stiff or permanently contracted muscles. A newborn with this type of cerebral palsy might have tremors or uncontrollable shaking that is limited to one side of the body. Athetoid (dyskinetic) cerebral palsy is seen in 10–20% of affected individuals. A newborn may drool or appear to be frowning, and there may be a slow, uncontrolled writhing of the arms, hands, feet, and legs. Symptoms tend to disappear when the infant is sleeping. Motor dysfunction becomes more evident as the infant matures. Weak sucking, difficulty swallowing, head lag, and hypotonia may be apparent at first with the infant displaying hypertonia 2–3 months later. Involvement ranges from mild to severe, but all children with cerebral palsy have a primary problem with the control of motor function (McMurray et al., 2002).

Cerebral palsy is often not diagnosed until after 1 year of age, but feeding difficulties have already manifested themselves and may vary over time. Poor sucking can impact weight gain and growth and may be an early sign of problems to come. Breastfeeding or the provision of breastmilk is important to this population of infants. Sacker et al. (2006) demonstrated that in a population of healthy term infants, those who were never breastfed had at least a 40% greater likelihood of fine motor delay than infants who were given breastmilk for a prolonged period. Any advantage that could improve motor activities of these infants is important to consider.

Breastfeeding Management

Many parents gradually become aware that there is something wrong with the infant. As developmental milestones fail to be achieved, difficulty with feeding may be one of a number of concerns that parents express. Positioning for breastfeeding is especially important to handle both hypotonia and hypertonia, which may both manifest at different ages in the same infant. Parents may wish to carry the infant in a sling between feedings to help reinforce a flexed position, especially if the infant tends to arch his or her back. Infants with tone abnormalities can take longer to establish a pattern of effective breastfeeding, with initiation and maintenance of maternal milk supply being a significant challenge. They may favor one side of their body, making positioning at breast a trial and error effort. Clinicians need to follow mothers closely to ensure that milk production is maintained under circumstances that include weak sucking, separation, and potential inadequate weight gain in the infant. Mothers may need to pump milk after or in between feedings to provide breastmilk supplements, preferably through a tube-feeding device at the breast. Feeding (and supplementing) at the breast provides opportunities for low-tone infants to stimulate their oral-facial muscles, helping with proper muscular development in preparation for handling solid foods and speech.

Rubinstein-Taybi Syndrome

Rubinstein-Taybi syndrome affects about 1 in 300,000 individuals and is similar to other syndromes and neurological disorders that have low muscle tone as a predominant characteristic. In addition to the distinctive hand and facial features, these infants also present with a small mouth, high arched palate, low muscle tone in the face and jaw, and GERD (Holland, 1996). Moe and coworkers (1998) surveyed the breastfeeding practices of mothers whose infants had Rubinstein-Taybi syndrome and reported that breastfeeding problems included poor sucking, inadequate weight gain, poor nipple grasp, failure to thrive, swallowing difficulties, infant fatigue, and GER—similar problems to those seen in many situations involving neurological conditions in infants. Most children experience poor weight gain in early life primarily due to feeding problems, including vomiting and swallowing difficulties. Frequent ear infections are seen in about half of children, with mild degrees of hearing loss being seen in 25% of infants. Recurrent upper respiratory infections are also common in infancy and childhood, making breastmilk an important contributor to reducing complications.

Breastfeeding Management

Small, frequent feedings may reduce vomiting and improve weight gain. Critical to maintaining lactation in situations where infants experience low tone is to ensure that mothers express their milk to stimulate their breasts in compensation for infants who cannot. Positioning infants with Rubinstein-Taybi syndrome is similar to that for infants with Down syndrome. Gartner (1996) recommended placing the infant on a near-level plane across the mother's lap or swaddled in a flexed position with the chin down and spine rounded. Weak sucking may also be compensated for by using alternate massage, supplementation of pumped milk with a tube-feeding device at the breast, use of a nipple shield, and use of the dancer hand position.

Neural Tube Defects

Neural tube defects are congenital deformities involving the coverings of the nervous system. They vary in severity and location; occur early in embryogenesis, usually by 23–28 days gestation; and may be caused by aberrant expression of a gene or family of genes, with the primary defect in all neural tube defects being the failure of the neural tube to close. Carbamazepine (Tegretol) and valproic acid (Depakote) are anticonvulsants that, when taken during pregnancy, have been definitively identified as acting as a teratogen for neural tube defects. A woman taking valproic acid has a 1–2% risk of having a child with a neural tube defect; therefore women taking antiepileptic medications during pregnancy often undergo prenatal screening tests such as alpha-fetoprotein. The mildest form is spina bifida aperta, and a very common form is spina bifida cystica or myelomeningocele. This defect involves a saclike casing filled with cerebrospinal fluid, spinal cord, and nerve roots that have herniated through a defect in the vertebral arches and dura. Certain neurological anomalies such as hydrocephalus and Chiari II malformation also accompany myelomeningoceles. Chiari II malformation is a herniation of the brainstem below the foramen magnum and can pose a life-threatening situation if it requires decompression. Symptomatic Chiari II is a neurosurgical emergency and may begin with signs such as stridor, poor suck, swallowing difficulties, central apnea, aspiration, and hypotonia. Spina bifida occulta involves the lesion being covered by skin without herniation through a bony defect. A skin lesion may be present such as a hairy patch, dermal sinus tract, dimple, hemangioma, or lipoma in the thoracic, lumbar, or sacral regions. If the brainstem is involved, feeding at the breast may not be possible.

There has been a dramatic reduction in the occurrence of neural tube defects due to the recommendation for women of childbearing age to consume 0.4 mg of folic acid per day. Surgical repair is sometimes accomplished in utero but usually within 24–72 hours after birth. Up to 50% of children with myelomeningocele may be latex sensitive, requiring clinicians to use latex-free products when working with these children. Infants benefit from breastfeeding with reduced overweight and obesity, improved pain management, reduced infection rates, decreased incidence of allergy, and improved cognitive development (Hurtekant & Spatz, 2007).

Breastfeeding Management

Most of these infants can be breastfed (unless the brainstem is significantly compromised), but mothers may encounter problems with reduced motor control and an infant who gags easily. Weakness may be present in the upper extremities. Most problems revolve around positioning the infant for feedings at the breast after surgery. Flexion of the spine may not be possible, and the infant is usually placed prone, flat on his or her back, or on his or her side for a number of days. The mother can lie on her side next to the infant to feed, slide the infant on pillows into the mother's lap, or, if the infant is supine (after a shunt placement for hydrocephalus), the mother can lean over the infant, bringing the breast to the infant rather than the infant to the breast (Merewood & Philipp, 2001). It is important that the clinician support the mother in her efforts to breastfeed her special infant because mothers have described hospital staff as another barrier to breastfeeding (Rivera et al., 2008).

Summary: The Design in Nature

A number of challenges are present when breastfeeding infants with major congenital malformations that include separation during the first week of life, surgeries, low birth weight, type of malformation (especially infants with digestive system malformations), suction and swallowing difficulties, inadequate weight gain, and real or perceived insufficient milk production (Rendon-Macias et al., 2002). All these issues should be addressed by clinicians working with affected families. Mothers are often in shock and emotionally upset or grieving when their infant is diagnosed with a congenital disorder of any kind. Establishing a nursing relationship may be fundamental to working through parenting the special child (Mojab, 2002).

References

Academy of Breastfeeding Medicine. Protocol Committee. Ballard, J., Chantry, C., & Howard, C. R. (2004). Clinical protocol number 11. Guidelines for the evaluation and management of neonatal ankyloglossia and its complications in the breastfeeding dyad. Retrieved September 18, 2005, from www.bfmed.org

Alaswad, B., Toubas, P. L., & Grunow, J. E. (1996). Environmental tobacco smoke exposure and gastroesophageal reflux in infants with apparent life-threatening events. *Journal of the Oklahoma State Medical Association, 89,* 233–237.

Alcantara, J., & Anderson, R. (2008). Chiropractic care of a pediatric patient with symptoms associated with gastroesophageal reflux disease, fuss-cry-irritability with sleep disorder syndrome and irritable infant syndrome of musculoskeletal origin. *Journal of the Canadian Chiropractic Association, 52,* 248–255.

Allan, L. D. (1996). Fetal cardiology. *Curr Opin Obstet Gynecol., 8,* 142–147.

American Academy of Pediatrics [AAP], Committee on Nutrition. (1998). Soy protein formulas: Recommendations for use in infant feeding. *Pediatrics, 101,* 148–153.

American Academy of Pediatrics [AAP], Newborn Screening Authoring Committee. (2008). Newborn screening expands: Recommendations for pediatricians and medical homes—implications for the system. *Pediatrics, 121,* 192–217.

American Academy of Pediatrics [AAP], Newborn Screening Task Force. (2000a). Newborn screening: A blueprint for the future—a call for a national agenda on state newborn screening programs. *Pediatrics, 106,* 389–422.

American Academy of Pediatrics [AAP] Task Force on Infant Positioning and SIDS. (2000b). Changing concepts of sudden infant death syndrome: Implications for infant sleeping environment and sleep position. *Pediatrics, 32,* 45–49.

American Academy of Pediatrics [AAP] Work Group on Breastfeeding. (1997). Breastfeeding and the use of human milk. *Pediatrics, 100,* 1035–1039.

American College of Medical Genetics. (2006). Newborn screening: Toward a uniform screening panel and system. *Genetics and Medicine, 8*(Suppl), 1S–252S.

American Society of Anesthesiologists. (1999). Practice guidelines for preoperative fasting and the use of pharmacologic agents to reduce the risk of pulmonary aspiration: Application to healthy patients undergoing elective procedures—a report by the American Society of Anesthesiologists task force on preoperative fasting. *Anesthesiology, 90,* 896–905.

American Society for Gastrointestinal Endoscopy. (1999). The role of endoscopy in the management of GERD: Guidelines for clinical application. *Gastrointest Endosc., 49,* 834–835.

Amir, L. H., James, J. P., & Donath, S. M. (2006). Reliability of the Hazelbaker assessment tool for lingual frenulum function. *Int Breastfeeding J., 1,* 3.

Aniansson, G., Svensson, H., Becker, M., & Ingvarsson, L. (2002). Otitis media and feeding with breast milk of children with cleft palate. *Scan J Plast Reconstr Surg Hand Surg., 36,* 9–15.

Anon. (1986). Milk fat, diarrhoea and the ileal brake. *Lancet, 1,* 658.

Anvenden-Hertzberg, L., Finkel, Y., Sandstedt, B., et al. (1996). Proctocolitis in exclusively breastfed infants. *Eur J Paediatr., 155,* 464–467.

Applegate, M. S., & Druschel, C. M. (1995). The epidemiology of infantile hypertrophic pyloric stenosis in New York State, 1983 to 1990. *Arch Pediatr Adolesc Med., 149,* 1123–1129.

Asnes, R. S., & Mones, R. L. (1982). Infantile colic: A review. *J Dev Behav Pediatr., 4,* 57–62.

Auer, C., & Gromada, K. K. (1998). A case report of breastfeeding quadruplets: Factors perceived as affecting breastfeeding. *J Hum Lact., 14,* 135–141.

Ault, D. L., & Schmidt, D. (1998). Diagnosis and management of gastroesophageal reflux in infants and children. *Nurs Pract., 23,* 78, 82, 88–89, 94, 99–100.

Axelsson, I., Jakobsson, I., Lindberg T., et al. (1986). Bovine beta-lactoglobulin in the human milk. A longitudinal study during the whole lactation period. *Acta Paediatr Scand., 75,* 702–707.

Bailey, D. J., et al. (1987). Lack of efficacy of thickened feeding as treatment for gastroesophageal reflux. *J Pediatr., 110,* 187–189.

Ballard, J. L., Auer, C. E., & Khoury, J. C. (2002). Ankyloglossia: Assessment, incidence, and effect of frenuloplasty on the breastfeeding dyad. *Pediatrics, 110,* e63.

Barbas, K. H., & Kelleher, D. K. (2004). Breastfeeding success among infants with congenital heart disease. *Pediatr Nurs., 30,* 285–289.

Barr, R. G. (1996). Colic. In W. A. Walker, P. Durie, J. Hamilton, et al. (Eds.), *Pediatric gastrointestinal disease: Pathophysiology, diagnosis, and management* (2nd ed.). St. Louis, MO: Mosby-Year Book.

Barr, R. G., & Rappaport, L. (1999). Infant colic and childhood recurrent abdominal pain syndromes: Is there a relationship? *J Dev Behav Pediatr., 20,* 315–317.

Belmont, J. R., & Grundfast, K. (1984). Congenital laryngeal stridor (laryngomalacia): Etiologic factors and associated disorders. *Ann Otol Rhinol Laryngol., 93,* 430–437.

Berg, K. L. (1990a). Two cases of tongue-tie and breastfeeding. *J Hum Lact., 6,* 124–126.

Berg, K. L. (1990b). Tongue-tie (ankyloglossia) and breastfeeding: A review. *J Hum Lact., 6,* 109–112.

Berkowitz, D., Naveh, Y., & Berant, M. (1997). "Infantile colic" as the sole manifestation of gastroesophageal reflux. *J Pediatr Gastroenterol Nutr., 24,* 231–233.

Berlin, C. M. Jr. (2007). "Exclusive" breastfeeding of quadruplets. *Breastfeeding Med., 2,* 125–126.

Bernard, H., Negroni, L., Chatel, J. M., et al. (2000). Molecular basis of IgE cross-reactivity between human beta-casein and bovine beta-casein, a major allergen of milk. *Mol Immunol., 37,* 161–167.

Beutler, E., Baluda, M. C., Sturgeon, P., & Day, R. (1965). A new genetic abnormality resulting in galactose-1-phosphate uridyltransferase (GALT) deficiency. *Lancet, 1,* 353–354.

Bhagyalakshmi, G., Renukarya, A. J., & Rajangam, S. (2007). Metric analysis of the hard palate in children with Down syndrome—A comparative study. *Down's Syndrome Research and Practice, 12,* 55–59.

Biancuzzo, M. (1994). Breastfeeding preterm twins: A case report. *Birth, 21,* 96–100.

Biancuzzo, M. (1998). Yes! Infants with clefts can breastfeed. *AWHONN Lifelines, 2,* 45–49.

Bibi, H., Khvolis, E., Shoseyov, D., et al. (2001). The prevalence of gastroesophageal reflux in children with tracheomalacia and laryngomalacia. *Chest, 119,* 409–413.

Botto, L. (2000). Occurrence of congenital heart defects in relation to maternal multivitamin use. *Am J Epidemiol., 151,* 878–884.

Bovey, A, Noble, R., & Noble, M. (1999). Orofacial exercises for babies with breastfeeding problems? *Breastfeeding Rev., 7,* 23–28.

Bowers, N. A., & Gromada, K. K. (2003). *Nursing management of multiple gestation: Preconception to postpartum* [nursing module]. White Plains, NY: March of Dimes.

Boyle, M., & Collopy, K. (2000). *Membership report 2000: An analysis of pregnancy, birth, and neonatal data from over 1000 higher order multiple pregnancies.* Brentwood, NY: Mothers of Supertwins.

Brown, J. E., & Carlson, M. (2000). Nutrition and multifetal pregnancy. *J Am Diet Assoc., 100,* 343–348.

Buckley, M. (2000). Some new and important clues to the causes of colic. *Br J Community Nurs., 5,* 462–465.

Businco, L., Bruno, G., & Giampietro, P. G. (1999). Prevention and management of food allergy. *Acta Paediatr Suppl., 88*(430), 104–109.

Byrnes, A. L., Berk, N. W., Cooper, M. E., & Marazita, M. L. (2003). Parental evaluation of informing interviews for cleft lip and/or palate. *Pediatrics, 112,* 308–313.

Campanozzi, A., Boccia, G., Pensabene, L., et al. (2009). Prevalence and natural history of gastroesophageal reflux: Pediatric prospective survey. *Pediatrics, 123,* 779–783.

Canani, R. B., Cirillo, P., Roggero, P., et al. (2006). Therapy with gastric acidity inhibitors increases the risk of acute gastroenteritis and community-acquired pneumonia in children. *Pediatrics, 117,* e817–e820.

Canifet, C., Jackobsson, I., & Hagander, B. (2002). Colicky infants according to maternal reports in telephone interviews and diaries: A large Scandinavian study. *J Dev Behav Pediatr., 23,* 1–8.

Canivet, C. A., Ostergren, P. O., Jakobsson, I. L., Dejin-Karlsson, E., & Hagander, B. M. (2008). Infantile colic, maternal smoking and infant feeding at 5 weeks of age. *Scan J Public Health, 36,* 284–291.

Cannella, P. C., Bowser, E. K., Guyer, L. K., et al. (1993). Feeding practices and nutrition recommendations for infants with cystic fibrosis. *J Am Diet Assoc., 93,* 297.

Cant, A., Marsden, R. A., & Kilshaw, P. J. (1985). Egg and cow's milk hypersensitivity in exclusively breastfed infants with eczema, and detection of egg protein in breast milk. *BMJ (Clinical Research Ed), 291,* 932–935.

Carpenter, R. O., Schaffer, R. L., Maeso, C. E., et al. (1999). Postoperative ad lib feeding for hypertrophic pyloric stenosis. *J Pediatr Surg., 34,* 959–961.

Carroll, A. E., Garrison, M. M., & Christakis, D. A. (2002). A systematic review of nonpharmacological and nonsurgical therapies for gastroesophageal reflux in infants. *Arch Pediatr Adolesc Med., 156,* 109–113.

Carver, J. (1999). Dietary nucleotides: Effects on the immune and gastrointestinal systems. *Acta Paediatr., 88*(Suppl), 83–88.

Chay, P., Genna, C. W., Gallagher, F., et al. (2007). *Breastfeeding multiples* (2nd ed.). East Islip, NY: Mothers of Supertwins.

Chen, D. C., Nommsen-Rivers, L., Dewey, K. G., & Lonnerdal, B. (1998). Stress during labor and delivery and early lactation performance. *Am J Clin Nutr., 68,* 335–344.

Chin, S. S., Brodsky, N. L., & Bhandari, V. (2003). Antenatal steroid use is associated with increased gastroesophageal reflux in neonates. *Am J Perinatol., 20,* 205–213.

Choi, B. H., Kleinheinz, J., Joos, U., & Komposch, G. (1991). Sucking efficiency of early orthopaedic plate and teats in infants with cleft lip and palate. *Int J Oral Maxillofac Surg., 20,* 167–169.

Choi, S. Y., Park, M. H., Choi, W. J., et al. (2005). Clinical features and the natural history of dietary protein induced proctocolitis: A study on the elimination of offending foods from the maternal diet. *Korean J Pediatr Gastroenterol Nutr., 8,* 21–30.

Clark, B. J. (1992). After a positive Guthrie—What next? Dietary management for the child with phenylketonuria. *Eur J Clin Nutr., 46*(Suppl I), S33.

Clark, D. (1999). Esophageal atresia and tracheoesophageal fistula. *Am Fam Physician, 59,* 910–916.

Clarren, S. K., Anderson, B., & Wolf, L. S. (1987). Feeding infants with cleft lip, cleft palate, or cleft lip and palate. *Cleft Palate Journal, 24,* 244–249.

Clifford, T. J., Campbell, M. K., Speechley, K. N., et al. (2002). Sequelae of infant colic: Evidence of transient infant distress and absence of lasting effects on maternal mental health. *Arch Pediatr Adolesc Med., 156,* 1183–1188.

Coffey, P. M. (1997). Breastfeeding the infant with congenital heart disease. In D. Dowling, S. C. Danner, & P. M. Coffey (Eds.), *Breastfeeding the infant with special need*s. March of Dimes Nursing Modules. White Plains, NY: March of Dimes Birth Defects Foundation.

Cohen, M., Marschall, M. A., & Schafer, M. E. (1992). Immediate unrestricted feeding of infants following cleft lip and palate repair. *J Craniofac Surg., 3*, 30–32.

Cohen, M. M., & Bankier, A. (1991). Syndrome delineation involving orofacial clefting. *Cleft Palate Craniofac J., 28*, 119–120.

Colombo, C., Costantini, D., Zazzeron, L., et al. (2007). Benefits of breastfeeding in cystic fibrosis: A single-centre follow-up survey. *Acta Paediatr., 96*, 1228–1232.

Combs, V. L., & Marino, B. L. (1993). A comparison of growth patterns in breast and bottle fed infants with congenital heart disease. *Pediatr Nurs., 19*, 175–179.

Cooper-Brown, L., Copeland, S., Dailey, S., et al. (2008). Feeding and swallowing dysfunction in genetic syndromes. *Dev Disabilities Res Rev., 14*, 147–157.

Corvaglia, L., Rotatori, R., Ferlini, M., Aceti, A., Ancora, G., & Faldella, G. (2007). The effect of body positioning on gastroesophageal reflux in premature infants: Evaluation by combined impedance and pH monitoring. *J Pediatr., 151*, 591–596.

Coryllos, E., Genna, C. W., & Salloum, A. C. (2004). Congenital tongue-tie and its impact on breastfeeding. American Academy of Pediatrics, Section on Breastfeeding. Breastfeeding: Best for baby and mother. Retrieved September 15, 2005, from www.aap.org/advocacy/bf/8–27newsletter.pdf

Coy, K., Speltz, M. L., & Jones, K. (2002). Facial appearance and attachment in infants with orofacial clefts: A replication. *Cleft Palate-Craniofac J., 39*, 66–71.

Crossman, K. (1998). Breastfeeding a baby with a cleft palate: A case report. *J Hum Lact., 14*, 47–50.

Curtin, G. (1990). The infant with cleft lip or palate: More than a surgical problem. *J Perinat Neonatal Nurs., 3*, 80–89.

Damato, E. G., Dowling, D. A., Madigan, E. A., & Thanattherakul, C. (2005). Duration of breastfeeding for mothers of twins. *JOGNN, 34*, 201–209.

Damato, E. G., Dowling, D. A., Standing, T. S., & Schuster, S. D. (2005). Explanation for cessation of breastfeeding in mothers of twins. *J Hum Lact., 21*, 296–304.

Danner, S. C. (1992a). Breastfeeding the infant with a cleft defect. *NAACOG's Clinical Issues in Perinatal and Women's Health Nursing: Breastfeeding, 3*, 634–639.

Danner, S. C. (1992b). Breastfeeding the neurologically impaired infant. *NAACOG's Clinical Issues in Perinatal and Women's Health Nursing: Breastfeeding, 3*, 640–646.

Danner, S. C. (1997). Breastfeeding infants with cleft defects. In D. Dowling, S. C. Danner, & P. M. Coffey (Eds.), *Breastfeeding the infant with special needs*. March of Dimes Nursing Modules. White Plains, NY: March of Dimes Birth Defects Foundation.

Darzi, M. A., Chowdri, N. A., & Bhat, A. N. (1996). Breastfeeding or spoon feeding after cleft lip repair: A prospective, randomised study. *Br J Surg., 49*, 24–26.

Dellert, S. F., Hyams, J. S., Treem, W. R., et al. (1993). Feeding resistance and gastroesophageal reflux in infancy. *J Pediatr Gastroenterol Nutr., 17*, 66–71.

Denk, M. J. (1998). Advances in neonatal surgery. *Pediatr Clin North Am., 45*, 1479–1506.

DeSantis, A., Coster, W, Bigsby, R., et al. (2004). Colic and fussing in infancy and sensory processing at 3–8 years of age. *Infant Mental Health Journal, 25*, 522–539.

Dewey, K. G. (2001). Maternal and fetal stress are associated with impaired lactogenesis in humans. *J Nutr., 131*, 3012S–3015S.

Dewey, K. G., Nommsen-Rivers, L., Heinig, M. J., & Cohen, R. J. (2003). Risk factors for suboptimal infant breastfeeding behavior, delayed onset of lactation, and excess neonatal weight loss. *Pediatrics, 112*, 607–619.

De Ybarrondo, L., & Mazur, L. J. (2000). Sandifer's syndrome in a child with asthma and cerebral palsy. *Southern Med J., 93,* 1019–1021.

Dobbelsteyn, C., Marche, D. M., Blake, K., & Rashid, M. (2005). Early oral sensory experiences and feeding development in children with CHARGE syndrome: A report of five cases. *Dysphagia, 20,* 89–100.

Dobbelsteyn, C., Peacocke, S. D., Blake, K., Crist, W., & Rashid, M. (2008). Feeding difficulties in children with CHARGE syndrome: Prevalence, risk factors, and prognosis. *Dysphagia, 23,* 127–135.

Dodge, J. A. (1975). Infantile hypertrophic pyloric stenosis in Belfast, 1957–1969. *Arch Dis Child., 50,* 171–178.

Dollberg, S., Botzer, E., Grunis, E., & Mimouni, F. B. (2006). Immediate nipple pain relief after frenotomy in breastfed infants with ankyloglossia: A randomized, prospective study. *J Pediatr Surg., 41,* 1598–1600.

Dombrowski, M., Anderson, G. C., Santori, C., et al. (2000). Kangaroo skin-to-skin care for premature twins and their adolescent parents. *MCN, 25,* 92–94.

Duncan, L. L., & Elder, S. B. (1997). Breastfeeding the infant with PKU. *J Hum Lact., 13,* 231–235.

Edmondson, R., & Reinhartsen, D. (1998). The young child with cleft lip and palate: Intervention needs in the first three years. *Infants and Young Children, 11,* 12–20.

Einarsson-Backes, L. M., Deitz, J., Price, R., et al. (1994). The effect of oral support on sucking efficiency in preterm infants. *Am J Occup Ther., 48,* 490–498.

El Amm, C. A., & Denny, A. (2008). Hyoid bone abnormalities in Pierre Robin patients. *J Craniofac Surg., 19,* 259–263.

Emmanouil-Nikoloussi, E. N., & Kerameos-Foroglou, C. (1992a). Developmental malformations of human tongue and associated syndromes [review]. *Bulletin du Groupement International Pour la Recherche Scientifique en Stomatologie & Odontologie, 35,* 5–12.

Emmanouil-Nikoloussi, E. N., & Kerameos-Foroglou, C. (1992b). Congenital syndromes connected with tongue malformations. *Bull Assoc Anat., 76,* 67–72.

Erkkila, A. T., Isotalo, E., Pulkkinen, J., & Haapanen, M. L. (2005). Association between school performance, breast milk intake and fatty acid profile of serum lipids in ten-year-old cleft children. *J Craniofacial Surg., 16,* 764–769.

Everett, K. V., Capon, F., Georgoula, C., et al. (2008). Linkage of monogenic infantile hypertrophic pyloric stenosis to chromosome 16q24. *Eur Jo of Hum Gene, 16,* 1151–1154.

Ewer, A. K., James, M. E., & Tobin, J. M. (1999). Prone and left lateral positioning reduce gastro-oesophageal reflux in preterm infants. *Arch Dis Child Fetal Neonatal Ed., 81,* F201–F205.

Feranchak, A. P., Orenstein, S. R., & Cohn, J. F. (1994). Behaviors associated with the onset of gastro-esophageal reflux episodes in infants: Prospective study using split screen video and pH probe. *Clin Pediatr., 33,* 654–662.

Ferguson, A., Bier, J. B., Cucca, J., et al. (1996). The quality of sucking in infants with colic. *Infant Mental Health, 17,* 161–169.

Fernando, C. (1998). *Tongue-tie: From confusion to clarity.* Sydney, Australia: Tandem Publications.

Finnegan, L. P. (1982). Substance abuse: Implication for the newborn. *Perinatol Neonatol., 6,* 17–24.

Fleiss, P. M., Burger, M., Ramkumar, H., et al. (1990). Ankyloglossia: A cause of breastfeeding problems? *J Hum Lact., 6,* 128–129.

Fletcher, S. G., & Meldrum, J. R. (1968). Lingual function and relative length of the lingual frenulum. *J Speech Lang Hear Res., 2,* 382–390.

Flidel-Rimon, O., & Shinwell, E. S. (2002). Breastfeeding multiples. *Sem Neonatol., 7,* 231–239.

Flidel-Romin, O., & Shinwell, E. S. (2006). Breastfeeding twins and high multiples. *Arch Dis Child Fetal Neonatal Ed., 91,* F377–F380.

Forrester, M. B., & Merz, D. (2004). Descriptive epidemiology of oral clefts in a multiethnic population, Hawaii, 1986–2000. *Cleft Palate Craniofac J., 41,* 622–628.

Freedman, S. B., Al-Harthy, N., & Thull-Freedman, J. (2009). The crying infant: Diagnostic testing and frequency of serious underlying disease. *Pediatrics, 123,* 841–848.

Friedman, S., Flidel-Rimon, O., Lavie, E., et al. (2004). The effect of prenatal consultation with a neonatologist on human milk feeding in preterm infants. *Acta Paediatr., 93,* 775–778.

Frommelt, M. A. (2004). Differential diagnosis and approach to a heart murmur in term infants. *Pediatr Clin North Am., 51,* 1023–1032.

Fuentes, A., & Goldkrand, J. W. (1987). Angiotensin-converting enzyme activity in hypertensive subjects after magnesium sulfate therapy. *Am J Obstet Gynecol., 156,* 1375–1379.

Fugimoto, T., Lane, G. J., Segawa, O., et al. (1999). Laparoscopic extramucosal pyloromyotomy versus open pyloromyotomy for infantile hypertrophic pyloric stenosis: Which is better? *J Pediatr Surg., 34,* 370–372.

Garcez, L. W., & Giugliani, E. R. (2005). Population-based study on the practice of breastfeeding in children born with cleft lip and palate. *Cleft Palate Craniofac J., 42,* 687–693.

Garrison, M., & Christakis, A. (2000). A systematic review of treatments for infantile colic. *Pediatrics, 106,* 184–190.

Gartner, S. L. (1996). Breastfeeding the infant with physical and developmental needs. *Nutrition Focus, 11,* 1–8.

Garza, J. J., Morash, D., Dzakovic, A., et al. (2002). Ad libitum feeding decreases hospital stay for neonates after pyloromyotomy. *J Pediatr Surg., 37,* 493–495.

Geddes, D. T., Langton, D. B., Gollow, I., Jacobs, L. A., Hartmann, P. E., & Simmer, K. (2008). Frenulotomy for breastfeeding infants with ankyloglossia: Effect on milk removal and sucking mechanism as imaged by ultrasound. *Pediatrics, 122,* e188–e194.

Genna, C. W. (2008). *Supporting sucking skills in breastfeeding infants.* Sudbury, MA: Jones and Bartlett.

Geraghty, S. R., Khoury, J. C., & Kalkwarf, H. J. (2004). Comparison of feeding among multiple birth infants. *Twin Research, 7,* 542–547.

Geraghty, S. R., Khoury, J. C., & Kalkwarf, H. J. (2005). Human milk pumping rates of mothers of singletons and mothers of multiples. *J Hum Lact., 21,* 413–420.

Geraghty, S. R., Pinney, S. M., Sethuraman, G., et al. (2004). Breast milk feeding rates of mothers of multiples compared to mothers of singletons. *Ambulatory Pediatrics, 4,* 226–231.

Ghaem, M., Armstrong, K. L., Trocki, O., et al. (1998). The sleep patterns of infants and young children with gastro-oesophageal reflux. *J Pediatr Child Health, 34,* 160–163.

Gibson, S. E. (2004). Laryngomalacia and its management: When to worry about the squeaky baby. *Medicine and Health, Rhode Island, 87,* 304–306.

Glass, R. P., & Wolf, L. S. (1994). Incoordination of sucking, swallowing, and breathing as an etiology for breastfeeding difficulty. *J Hum Lact., 10,* 185–189.

Glass, R. P., & Wolf, L. S. (1999). Feeding management of infants with cleft lip and palate and micrognathia. *Infant and Young Children, 12,* 70–81.

Gokcay, G., Baykal, T., Gokdemir, Y., & Demirkol, M. (2006). Breastfeeding in organic acidemias. *J Inherit Metab Dis., 29,* 304–310.

Gold, B. D. (2006). Is gastroesophageal reflux disease really a life-long disease: Do babies who regurgitate grow up to be adults with GERD complications? *Am J* Gastroenterol., *101,* 641–644.

Grady, E. (1977). Breastfeeding the baby with a cleft of the soft palate. *Clin Pediatr., 16,* 182–184.

Greve, L. C., Wheeler, M. D., Green-Burgeson, D. K., & Zorn, E. M. (1994). Breastfeeding in the management of the newborn with phenylketonuria: A practical approach to dietary therapy. *J Am Diet Assoc., 94,* 305–309.

Griffiths, D. M. (2004). Do tongue ties affect breastfeeding? *J Hum Lact., 20,* 409–414.

Gromada, K. (1981). Maternal-infant attachment: The first step toward individualizing twins. *Matern Child Nurs J., 6,* 129–134.

Gromada, K. K. (1992). Breastfeeding more than one: Multiples and tandem breastfeeding. *NAACOG's Clinical Issues in Perinatal and Women's Health Nursing: Breastfeeding, 3,* 656–666.

Gromada, K. K. (1999). *Mothering multiples: Breastfeeding and caring for twins or more!!* Schaumburg, IL: La Leche League International.

Gromada, K. K., & Spangler, A. K. (1998). Breastfeeding twins and higher-order multiples. *JOGNN, 27,* 441–449.

Guarino, N., Yoneda, A., Shima, H., & Puri, P. (2001). Selective neurotrophin deficiency in infantile hypertrophic pyloric stenosis. *J Pediatr Surg., 36,* 1280–1284.

Habbick, B. F., Khanna, C., & To, T. (1989). Infantile hypertrophic pyloric stenosis: A study of feeding practices and other possible causes. *CMAJ, 140,* 401–404.

Haberman, M. (1988). A mother of invention. *Nursing Times, 84,* 52–53.

Haldeman, W. (1993). Can magnesium sulfate therapy impact lactogenesis? *J Hum Lact., 9,* 249–252.

Hale, T. W. (2004). *Medications and mothers' milk.* Amarillo, TX: Pharmasoft.

Hale, T. W., & Ilett, K. F. (2002). *Drug therapy and breastfeeding: From theory to clinical practice.* New York: Parthenon.

Hammerman, C., & Kaplan, M. (1995). Oxygen saturation during and after feeding in healthy term infants. *Biology of the Neonate, 67,* 94–99.

Hattori, R., & Hattori, H. (199). Breastfeeding twins: Guidelines for success. *Birth, 26,* 37–42.

Hauben, M., & Amsden, G. W. (2002). The association of erythromycin and infantile hypertrophic pyloric stenosis: Causal or coincidental? *Drug Safety, 25,* 929–942.

Hazelbaker, A. K. (1993). The assessment tool for lingual frenulum function. Master's thesis. Pasadena, CA: Pacific Oaks College.

Heacock, H. J., Jeffery, H. E., Baker, J. L., & Page, M. (1992). Influence of breast versus formula milk on physiological gastroesophageal reflux in healthy, newborn infants. *J Pediatr Gastroenterol Nutr., 14,* 41–46.

Heine, R. G., Jordan, B., Lubitz, L., Meehan, M., & Catto-Smith, A. G. (2006). Clinical predictors of pathological gastroesophageal reflux in infants with persistent distress. *J Paediatr Child Health, 42,* 134–139.

Henly, S. J., Anderson, C. M., Avery, M. D., et al. (1995). Anemia and insufficient milk in first-time mothers. *Birth, 22,* 86–92.

Henry, S. M. (2004). Discerning differences: Gastroesophageal reflux and gastroesophageal reflux disease in infants. *Adv Neonatal Care, 4,* 235–247.

Hiimae, K. M., & Palmer, J. B. (2003). Tongue movements in feeding and speech. *Crit Rev Oral Biol Med., 14,* 413–429.

Hill, D. J., Hudson, I. L., Sheffield, L. J., et al. (1995). A low allergen diet is a significant intervention in infantile colic: Results of a community-based study. *J Allergy Clin Immunol., 96,* 886–892.

Hill, D. J., Roy, N., Heine, R. G., et al. (2005). Effect of a low-allergen maternal diet on colic among breastfed infants: A randomized, controlled trial. *Pediatrics, 116,* e709–e715.

Hill, P., Aldag, J., & Chatterton, R. (2001). Initiation and frequency of pumping and milk production in mothers of non-nursing preterm infants. *J Hum Lact., 17,* 9–13.

Hoffman, J. (1990). Congenital heart disease: Incidence and inheritance. *Pediatr Clin North Am., 37,* 25–43.

Hogan, M., Westcott, C., & Griffiths, M. (2005). Randomized, controlled trial of division of tongue-tie in infants with feeding problems. *J Paediatr Child Health, 41,* 246–250.

Holland, M. (1996). Rubenstein-Taybi syndrome. *Nutrition Focus, 11,* 1–4.

Holliday, K. E., et al. (1991). Growth of human milk-fed and formula-fed infants with cystic fibrosis. *J Pediatr., 118,* 77–79.

Howard, C. R., Lanphear, N., Lanphear, B. P., Eberly, S., & Lawrence, R. A. (2006). Parental responses to infant crying and colic: The effect on breastfeeding duration. *Breastfeeding Med., 1,* 146–155.

Huang, R.-C., Forbes, D. A., & Davies, M. W. (2003). *Feed thickener for newborn infants with gastroesophageal reflux* (Cochrane Review). Cochrane Library. Issue 2. Oxford: Update Software.

Huggins, K. (1990). Ankyloglossia—One lactation consultant's personal experience. *J Hum Lactation, 6,* 123–124.

Huhtala, V., Lehtonen, L., Uvnas-Moberg, K., & Korvenranta, H. (2003). Low plasma cholecystokinin levels in colicky infants. *J Pediatr Gastroenterol Nutr., 37,* 42–46.

Humenczuk, M. (1998). Feeding assistance for infants with cleft lip and palate. Presented at the annual meeting of the American Dietetic Association, October 10, Kansas City, Missouri.

Huner, G., Baykal, T., Demir, F., & Demirkol, M. (2005). Breastfeeding experience in inborn errors of metabolism other than phenylketonuria. *J Inherit Metab Dis., 28,* 457–465.

Hurtekant, K. M., & Spatz, D. L. (2007). Special considerations for breastfeeding the infant with spina bifida. *J Perinat Neonatal Nurs., 21,* 69–75.

Hwang, J.-B., Park, M. H., Kang, Y. N., Kim, S. P., Suh, S. I., & Kam, S. (2007). Advanced criteria for clinico-pathological diagnosis of food protein-induced proctocolitis. *J Korean Med Sci., 22,* 213–217.

Jadcherla, S. R. (2002). Gastroesophageal reflux in the neonate. *Recent Advances in Neonatal Gastro-enterology, 29,* 135–158.

Jain, E. (1995). Tongue-tie: Its impact on breastfeeding. *AARN News Letter, 51,* 18.

Jain, E. (1996). Tongue-tie: Impact on breastfeeding. Retrieved September 15, 2005, from www.drjain.com

Jakobsson, I., Borulf, S., Lindberg, T., et al. (1983). Partial hydrolysis of cow's milk proteins by human trypsins and elastases in vitro. *J Pediatr Gastroenterol Nutr., 2,* 613–616.

Jakobsson, I., & Lindberg, T. (1978). Cow's milk as a cause of infantile colic in breastfed infants. *Lancet, 2,* 437–439.

Jakobsson, I., & Lindberg, T. (1983). Cow's milk proteins cause infantile colic in breastfed infants: A double-blind crossover study. *Pediatrics, 71,* 268–271.

Jedd, M. B., Melton, L. J., Griffin, M. R., et al. (1986). Factors associated with infantile hypertrophic pyloric stenosis. *Am J Dis Child, 142,* 334–337.

Joanna Briggs Institute. (2008). The effectiveness of interventions for infant colic. *Best Practice: Evidence-Based Practice Information Sheets for Health Professionals, 12,* 1–4.

Jocelyn, L. J., Penko, M. A., & Rode, H. L. (1996). Cognition, communication, and hearing in young children with cleft lip and palate and in control children: A longitudinal study. *Pediatrics, 97,* 529–534.

Jones, E., Dimmock, P. W., & Spencer, S. A. (2001). A randomised controlled trial to compare methods of milk expression after preterm delivery. *Arch Dis Child Fetal Neonatal Ed., 85,* F91–F95.

Jung, A. D. (2001). Gastroesophageal reflux in infants and children. *Am Fam Physician, 64,* 1853–1860.

Kanufre, V., Starling, A. L. P., Leao, E., et al. (2007). Breastfeeding in the treatment of children with phenylketonuria. *J Pediatr., 83,* 447–452.

Karabulut, R., Sonmez, K., Turkyilmaz, Z., et al. (2008). Ankyloglossia and effects on breastfeeding, speech problems and mechanical/social issues in children. *B-ENT, 4,* 81–85.

Kenner, C., Brueggemeyer, A., & Porter-Gunderson, L. (1993). *Comprehensive neonatal nursing: A physiologic perspective.* Philadelphia: W.B. Saunders.

Kilshaw, P. .J, & Cant, A. J. (1984). The passage of maternal dietary proteins into human breast milk. *Int Arch Allergy Immunol., 75,* 8–15.

Koenig, J. S., Davies, A. M., & Thach, B. T. (1990). Coordination of breathing, sucking and swallowing during bottle feedings in human infants. *J Appl Physiol., 69*, 1623–1629.

Kogo, M., Okada, G., Ishii, S., et al. (1997). Breastfeeding for cleft lip and palate patients using the Hotz-type plate. *Cleft Palate Craniofac J., 34*, 351–353.

Koletzko, S., & Reinhardt, D. (2001). Nutritional challenges of infants with cystic fibrosis. *Early Human Development, 65*(Suppl), S53–S61.

Kotlow, L. A. (1999). Ankyloglossia (tongue-tie): A diagnostic quandary. *Quintessence International, 30*, 259–262.

Kramer, G. J. C., Hoeksma, J. B., & Prahl-Andersen, B. (1994). Palatal changes after lip surgery in different types of cleft lip and palate. *Cleft Palate Craniofac J., 31*, 376–384.

LaFleur, E., & Niesen, K. (1996). Breastfeeding conjoined twins. *JOGNN, 25*, 241–244.

Lake, A. M., Whitington, P. F., & Hamilton, S. R. (1982). Dietary protein-induced colitis in breastfed infants. *J Pediatr., 101*, 906–910.

Lalakea, M. L., & Messner, A. H. (2002). Frenotomy and frenuloplasty: If, when, and how. *Op Tech Otolaryngol., 13*, 96.

Lalakea, M. L., & Messner, A. H. (2003a). Ankyloglossia: Does it matter? *Pediatr Clin North Am., 50*, 381–397.

Lalakea, M. L., & Messner, A. H. (2003b). Ankyloglossia: The adolescent and adult perspective. *Otolaryngol Head Neck Surg., 128*, 746–752.

Lambert, J. M., & Watters, N. E. (1998). Breastfeeding the infant/child with a cardiac defect: An informal survey. *J Hum Lact., 14*, 151–155.

Lammer, E. J., & Edmonds, L. D. (1987). Trends in pyloric stenosis incidence, Atlanta, 1968 to 1982. *J Med Genet., 24*, 482–487.

Lawlor-Smith, C., & Lawlor-Smith, L. (1998). Lactose intolerance. *Breastfeeding Rev., 6*, 29–30.

Lawrence, R. A., & Lawrence, R. M. (2005). *Breastfeeding: A guide for the medical profession* (6th ed.). St. Louis, MO: Mosby.

Leonard, L. G. (1982). Twin pregnancy: Maternal-fetal nutrition. *J Obstet Gynecol Neonat Nurs., 11*, 139–145.

Leonard, L. G. (2000). Breastfeeding triplets: The at-home experience. *Public Health Nurs., 17*, 211–221.

Leonard, L. G. (2002). Breastfeeding higher order multiples: Enhancing support during the postpartum hospitalization period. *J Hum Lact., 18*, 386–392.

Leonard, L. G. (2003). Breastfeeding rights of multiple birth families and guidelines for health professionals. *Twin Research, 6*, 34–45.

Lewanda, A. F., & Jabs, E. W. (1994). Genetics of craniofacial disorders. *Curr Opin Pediatr., 6*, 690–697.

Lewis, E., & Kritzinger, A. (2004). Parental experiences of feeding problems in their infants with Down syndrome. *Down's Syndrome Research and Practice, 9*, 45–52.

Liang, R., Gunn, A. J., & Gunn, T. R. (1997). Can preterm twins breastfeed successfully? *New Zealand Medical Journal, 110*, 209–212.

Lobo, M. (1992). Parent-infant interaction during feeding when the infant has congenital heart disease. *J Pediatr Nurs., 7*, 97–105.

Loffredo, C. A., Wilson, P. D., & Ferencz, C. (2001). Maternal diabetes: An independent risk factor for major cardiovascular malformations with increased mortality of affected infants. *Teratology, 64*, 98–106.

Losee, J. E., Mason, A. C., Dudas, J., Hua, L. B., & Mooney, M. P. (2007). Nonsynostotic occipital plagiocephaly: Factors impacting onset, treatment, and outcomes. *Plast Reconstr Surg., 119*, 1866–1873.

Lothe, L., & Lindberg, T. (1989). Cow's milk whey protein elicits symptoms of infantile colic in colicky formula-fed infants: A double-blind crossover study. *Pediatrics, 83*, 262–266.

Lotle, L., Lindberg, T., & Jakobsson, I. (1982). Cow's milk formula as a cause of infantile colic: A double-blind study. *Pediatrics, 70,* 7–10.

Lucassen, P. L., Assendelft, W. J., van Eijk, J. T., et al. (2001). Systematic review of the occurrence of infantile colic in the community. *Arch Dis Child, 84,* 398–403.

Lucassen, P. L. B. J., Assendelft, W. J. J., Gubbels. J. W., et al. (1998). Effectiveness of treatments for infantile colic: Systematic review. *BMJ, 317,* 1563–1569.

Luder, E., Kattan, M., Tanzer-Torres, G., & Bonforte, R. J. (1990). Current recommendations for breast-feeding in cystic fibrosis centers. *Am J Dis Childhood, 144,* 1153–1156.

Luke, B., Hediger, M. L., Nugent, C., et al. (2003). Body mass index—Specific weight gains associated with optimal birth weights in twin pregnancies. *J Reprod Med., 48,* 217–224.

MacDonald, A., Depondt, E., Evans, S., et al. (2006). Breastfeeding in IMD. *J Inherit Metab Dis., 29,* 299–303.

Machida, H. M., Catto-Smith, A. G., Gall, D. G., et al. (1994). Allergic colitis in infancy: Clinical and pathological aspects. *J Pediatr Gastroenterol Nutr., 19,* 22–26.

Madlon-Kay, D. J., Ricke, L. A., Baker, N. J., & DeFor, T. A. (2008). Case series of 148 tongue-tied newborn babies evaluated with the assessment tool for lingual frenulum function. *Midwifery, 24,* 353–357.

Mahon, B. E., Rosenman, M. B., & Kleinman, M. B. (2001). Maternal and infant use of erythromycin and other macrolide antibiotics as risk factors for infantile hypertrophic pyloric stenosis. *J Pediatr., 139,* 380–384.

Mahoney, L. T. (1993). Acyanotic congenital heart disease. Atrial and ventricular septal defects, atrioventricular canal, patent ductus arteriosis, pulmonic stenosis. *Cardiol Clin., 11,* 603–616.

Mair, E. A., & Parsons, D. S. (1992). Pediatric tracheobronchomalacia and major airway collapse. *Ann Otol Rhinol Laryngol., 101,* 300–309.

Marcellus, L. (2001). The infant with Pierre Robin sequence: Review and implications for nursing practice. *J Pediatr Nurs., 15,* 23–33.

Marchini, G., Simoni, M. R., Bartolini, F., & Uvnas-Moberg, K. (1994). Plasma gastrin and somatostatin levels in newborn infants receiving supplementary formula feeding. *Acta Paediatr., 83,* 374–377.

Marino, B. L., O'Brien, P., & LoRe, H. (1995). Oxygen saturations during breast and bottle feedings in infants with congenital heart disease. *J Pediatr Nurs., 10,* 360–364.

Marmet, C., Shell, E., & Marmet, R. (1990). Neonatal frenotomy may be necessary to correct breast-feeding problems. *J Hum Lact., 6,* 117–121.

Marques, I. L., et al. (2001). Clinical experience with infants with Robin sequence: A prospective study. *Cleft Palate Craniofac J., 38,* 171–178.

Martin, J. A., Hamilton, B. E., Sutton, P. D., Ventura, S. J., et al. (2009). *Births: Final data for 2006.* National Vital Statistics Reports, vol. 57 no. 7. Hyattsville, MD: National Center for Health Statistics.

Masaitis, N. S., & Kaempf, J. W. (1996). Developing a frenotomy policy at one medical center: A case study approach. *J Hum Lact., 12,* 229–232.

Masarei, A. G., Sell, D., Habel, A., Mars, M., Sommerlad, B. C., & Wade, A. (2007). The nature of feeding in infants with unrepaired cleft lip and/or palate compared with healthy noncleft infants. *Cleft Palate Craniofac J., 44,* 321–328.

Mason, D. (2000). Gastroesophageal reflux in children: A guide for the advanced practice nurse. *Nurs Clin North Am., 35,* 15–36.

Masters, I. B., Chang, A. B., Patterson, L., et al. (2002). Series of laryngomalacia, tracheomalacia, and bronchomalacia disorders and their associations with other conditions in children. *Pediatr Pulmonol., 34,* 189–195.

Mathisen, B., et al. (1999). Feeding problems in infants with gastro-oesophageal reflux disease: A case controlled study. *J Paediatr Child Health, 35,* 163–169.

McBride, M. C., & Danner, S. C. (1987). Sucking disorders in neurologically impaired infants. *Clin Perinatol., 14,* 109–130.

McCabe, E., Leonard, C. O., Medici, F. N., et al. (1992). Issues in newborn screening. *Pediatrics, 89,* 345–349.

McCabe, L., Ernest, A. E., Neifert, M. R., et al. (1989). The management of breastfeeding among infants with phenylketonuria. *J Inherit Metab Dis., 12,* 467–474.

McMurray, J. L., Jones, M. W., & Khan, J. H. (2002). Cerebral palsy and the NICU graduate. *Neonatal Network, 21,* 53–57.

Mead, L. J., Chuffo, R., Lawlor-Klean, P., & Meier, P. P. (1992). Breastfeeding success with preterm quadruplets. *JOGNN, 21,* 221–227.

Medical Research Council Working Party on Phenylketonuria. (1993). Recommendations on the dietary management of phenylketonuria. *Arch Dis Child., 68,* 426–427.

Meier, P. (1988). Bottle and breastfeeding: Effect of transcutaneous oxygen pressure and temperature in premature infants. *Nurs Res., 37,* 36–41.

Mercado-Deane, M., Burton, E. M., Harlow, S. A., et al. (2001). Swallowing dysfunction in infants less than 1 year of age. *Pediatr Radiol., 31,* 423–428.

Merewood, A., & Philipp, B. L. (2001). *Breastfeeding: Conditions and diseases. A reference guide.* Amarillo, TX: Pharmasoft.

Merritt, L. (2005a). Part 1. Understanding the embryology and genetics of cleft lip and palate. *Adv Neonatal Care., 5,* 64–71.

Merritt, L. (2005b). Part 2. Physical assessment of the infant with cleft lip and/or palate. *Adv Neonatal Care., 5,* 125–134.

Messner, A. H., & Lalakea, M. L. (2000). Ankyloglossia: Controversies in management. *Int J Pediatr Otorhinolaryngol, 54,* 123–131.

Messner, A. H., & Lalakea, M. L. (2002). The effect of ankyloglossia on speech in children. *Otolaryngol Head Neck Surg., 127,* 539–545.

Messner, A. H., Lalakea, L., Aby, J., et al. (2000). Ankyloglossia: Incidence and associated feeding difficulties. *Arch Otolaryngol Head Neck Surg., 126,* 36–39.

Metcalf, T. J., Irons, T. G., Sher, L. D., & Young, P. C. (1994). Simethicone in the treatment of infant colic: A randomized, placebo-controlled, multicenter trial. *Pediatrics, 94,* 29–34.

Milczuk, H. A., & Johnson, S. M. (2000). Effect on families and caregivers of caring for a child with laryngomalacia. *Ann Otol Rhinol Laryngol., 109,* 348–354.

Miller, J. H. (1998). *The controversial issue of breastfeeding cleft-affected infants.* Innisfail, Alberta, Canada: InfoMed.

Miller-Loncar, C., Bigsby, R., High, P., et al. (2004). Infant colic and feeding difficulties. *Arch Dis Child., 89,* 908–912.

Mitchell, L. E., & Risch, N. (1991). The genetics of infantile hypertrophic pyloric stenosis: A reanalysis. *Am J Dis Child, 147,* 1203–1211.

Mizuno, K., & Ueda, A. (2001). Development of sucking behavior in infants with Down's syndrome. *Acta Paediatr., 90,* 1384–1388.

Moe, J. K., Holland, M. D., & Johnson, R. K. (1998). Breastfeeding practices of infants with Rubinstein-Taybi syndrome. *J Hum Lact., 14,* 311–315.

Mojab, C. G. (2002). *Congenital disorders in the nursling.* Unit 5/Lactation Consultant Series Two. Schaumburg, IL: La Leche League International.

Motzfeldt, K., Lilje, R., & Nylander, G. (1999). Breastfeeding in phenylketonuria. *Acta Paediatr Suppl., 88,* 25–27.

Moxley, S., & Haddon, L. (1999). Teaching breastfeeding to parents expecting multiple births. *Int J Childbirth Education, 14,* 22–27.

Mukai, S., Mukai, C., & Asaoka, K. (1991). Ankyloglossia with deviation of the epiglottis and larynx. *Ann Otol Rhinol Laryngol., 100,* 3–20.

Naimer, S. A., Biton, A., Vardy, D., & Zvulunov, A. (2003). Office treatment of congenital ankyloglossia. *Medical Science Monitor, 9,* CR432–CR435.

Nelson, S. P., Chen, E. H., Syniar, G. M., et al. (1997). Prevalence of symptoms of gastroesophageal reflux during infancy: A pediatric office based survey. *Arch Pediatr Adolesc Med., 151,* 569–572.

NIH Consensus Statement. (2000). *Phenylketonuria: Screening and management.* October 16–18, 17(3), 1–27. Washington, DC. Retrieved September 18, 2009, at http://consensus.nih.gov/2000/2000 Phenylketonuria113html.htm

Noble, R., & Bovey, A. (1997). Therapeutic teat use for babies who breastfeed poorly. *Breastfeeding Rev., 5,* 37–42.

Notestine, G. E. (1990). The importance of the identification of ankyloglossia (short lingual frenulum) as a cause of breastfeeding problems. *J Hum Lact., 6,* 113–115.

Nyqvist, K. H. (2002). Breastfeeding in preterm twins: Development of feeding behavior and milk intake during hospital stay and related caregiving practices. *J Pediatr Nurs., 17,* 246–256.

Nyqvist, K. H., & Lutes, L. M. (1998). Co-bedding twins: A developmentally supportive care strategy. *JOGNN, 27,* 450–456.

Odze, R. D., Bines, J., Leichtner, A. M., et al. (1993). Allergic proctocolitis in infants: A prospective clinico-pathologic biopsy study. *Hum Pathol., 24,* 668–674.

Ohshiro, K., & Puri, P. (1998). Pathogenesis of infantile hypertrophic pyloric stenosis: Recent progress. *Pediatr Surg Int., 13,* 243–252.

Oliver, R. G., & Jones, G. (1997). Neonatal feeding of infants born with cleft lip and/or palate: Parental perceptions of their experience in South Wales. *Cleft Palate Craniofac J., 34,* 526–532.

Omari, T. I., Barnett, C. P., Benninga, M. A., et al. (2002). Mechanisms of gastro-oesophageal reflux in preterm and term infants with reflux disease. *Gut, 51,* 475–479.

Orenstein, S. R. (1999). Gastroesophageal reflux. *Pediatr Rev., 20,* 24–28.

Orenstein, S. R., Shalaby, T. M., Kelsey, S. F., & Frankel, E. (2006). Natural history of infant reflux esophagitis: Symptoms and morphometric histology during one year without pharmacotherapy. *Am J Gastroenterol., 101,* 628–640.

Osuji, O. O. (1995). Preparation of feeding obturators for infants with cleft lip and palate. *J Clin Pediatr Dent., 19,* 211–214.

Owens, B. (2002). Breastfeeding an infant after heart transplant surgery. *J Hum Lact., 18,* 53–55.

Palmer, B. (2001). Frenum presentation. Retrieved December 14, 2004, from www.brianpalmerdds.com/frenum.htm

Palmer, B. (2003). Breastfeeding and frenulums. Retrieved December 14, 2004, from www.brianpalmerdds.com/bfeed_frenulums.htm

Paradise, J. L., Elster, B. A., & Tan, L. (1994). Evidence in infants with cleft palate that breast milk protects against otitis media. *Pediatrics, 94,* 853–860.

Parker, E. M., O'Sullivan, B. P., Shea, J. C., et al. (2004). Survey of breastfeeding practices and outcomes in the cystic fibrosis population. *Pediatr Pulmonol., 37,* 362–367.

Patenaude, Y., Bernard, C., Schreiber, R., & Sunsky, A. B. (2000). Cow's-milk-induced allergic colitis in an exclusively breastfed infant: Diagnosed with ultrasound. *Pediatr Radiol., 30,* 379–382.

Paulozzi, L. J. (2000). Is *Helicobacter pylori* a cause of infantile hypertrophic pyloric stenosis? *Medical Hypotheses, 55,* 119–125.

Perkins, J. A., Sie, K. C. Y., Milczuk, H., & Richardson, M. A. (1997). Airway management in children with craniofacial anomalies. *Cleft Palate Craniofac J., 34,* 135–140.

Persson, S., Ekborn, A., Granath, F., & Nordenskjold, A. (2001). Parallel incidences of sudden infant death syndrome and infantile hypertrophic pyloric stenosis: A common cause? *Pediatrics, 108*, 379–381.

Peter, C. S., Wiechers, C., Bohnhorst, B., et al. (2002). Influence of nasogastric tubes on gastroesophageal reflux in preterm infants: A multiple intraluminal impedance study. *J Pediatr., 141*, 277–279.

Pisacane, A., de Luca, U., Criscuolo, L., et al. (1996). Breastfeeding and hypertrophic pyloric stenosis: Population based case-control study. *BMJ, 312*, 745–746.

Practice Committee of the American Society for Reproductive Technology, the American Society for Reproductive Medicine. (2006). Guidelines on number of embryos transferred. *Fertility and Sterility, 86*(Suppl 5), S51–S52.

Prows, C. A., & Bender, P. L. (1999). Beyond Pierre Robin sequence. *Neonatal Network, 18*, 13–19.

Puapong, D., Kahng, D., Ko, A., & Applebaum, H. (2002). Ad libitum feeding: Safely improving the cost-effectiveness of pyloromyotomy. *J Pediatr Surg., 37*, 1667–1668.

Pumberger, W., Pomberger, G., & Geissler, W. (2001). Proctocolitis in breastfed infants: A contribution to differential diagnosis of haematochezia in early childhood. *Postgraduate Medical Journal, 77*, 252–254.

Purnell, H. (2001). Phenylketonuria and maternal phenylketonuria. *Breastfeeding Rev., 9*, 19–21.

Rawashdeh, M. A., & Jawdat Abu-Hawas, B. (2008). Congenital associated malformations in a sample of Jordanian patients with cleft lip and palate. *J Oral Maxillofac Surg., 66*, 2035–2041.

Redford-Badwal, D. A., Mabry, K., & Frassinelli, J. D. (2003). Impact of cleft lip and/or palate on nutritional health and oral-motor development. *Dent Clin North Am., 47*, 305–317.

Reid, J. (2004). A review of feeding interventions for infants with cleft palate. *Cleft Palate Craniofac J., 41*, 268–278.

Reid, J., Kilpatrick, N., & Reilly, S. (2006). A prospective, longitudinal study of feeding skills in a cohort of babies with cleft conditions. *Cleft Palate Craniofac J., 43*, 702–709.

Reid, J., Reilly, S., & Kilpatrick, N. (2007). Sucking performance of babies with cleft conditions. *Cleft Palate Craniofac J., 44*, 312–320.

Reijneveld, S. A., Brugman, E., & Hirasing, R. A. (2000). Infantile colic: Maternal smoking as potential risk factor. *Arch Dis Child., 83*, 302–303.

Reilly, S., Reid, J., Skeat, J., and the Academy of Breastfeeding Medicine Clinical Protocol Committee. (2007). ABM clinical protocol #17: Guidelines for breastfeeding infants with cleft lip, cleft palate, or cleft lip and palate *Breastfeeding Med., 2*, 243–248.

Reinthal, M., Andersson, S., Gustafsson, M., et al. (2008). Effects of minimal acupuncture in children with infantile colic—A prospective, quasi-randomised single blind controlled trial. *Acupuncture and Medicine, 26*, 171–182.

Rendon-Macias, M. E., Castaneda-Mucino, G., Cruz, J. J., et al. (2002). Breastfeeding among patients with congenital malformations. *Arch Med Res., 33*, 269–275.

Repucci, A. (1999). Resolution of stool blood in breastfed infants with maternal ingestion of pancreatic enzymes. *J Pediatr Gastroenterol Nutr., 29*, 500A.

Restani, P., Gaiaschi, A., Plebani, A., et al. (1999). Evaluation of the presence of bovine proteins in human milk as a possible cause of allergic symptoms in breastfed children. *Ann Allergy Asthma Immunol., 84*, 353–360.

Riaz, M., Porat, R., Brodsky, N. L., & Hurt, H. (1998). The effects of maternal magnesium sulfate treatment on newborns: A prospective controlled study. *J Perinatol., 18*, 449–454.

Richard, M. E. (1991). Feeding the newborn with cleft lip and/or palate: The enlargement, stimulate, swallow, rest (ESSR) method. *J Pediatr Nurs., 6*, 317–321.

Ricke, L. A., Baker, N. J., Madlon-Kay, D. J., & DeFor, T. A. (2005). Newborn tongue-tie: Prevalence and effect on breastfeeding. *J Am Board Fam Pract., 18*, 1–7.

Riva, E., Agostoni, C., Biasucci, G., et al. (1996). Early breastfeeding is linked to higher intelligence quotient scores in dietary treated phenylketonuric children. *Acta Paediatr., 85,* 56–58.

Rivera, A. F., Davilla Torres, R. R., Parilla Rodriguez, A. M., de Longo, I. M., & Gorrin Peralta, J. J. (2008). Exploratory study: Knowledge about the benefits of breastfeeding and barriers for initiation in mothers of children with spina bifida. *Maternal and Child Health Journal, 12,* 734–738.

Roem, K. (2003). Nutritional management of multiple pregnancies. *Twin Research, 6,* 514–519.

Rommel, N., De Meyer, A.-M., Feenstra, L., & Veereman-Wauters, G. (2003). The complexity of feeding problems in 700 infants and young children presenting to a tertiary care institution. *J Pediatr Gastroenterol Nutr., 37,* 75–84.

Rudolph, C. D., Mazur, L. J., Liptak, G. S., et al. (2001). Pediatric GE reflux clinical practice guidelines. *J Pediatr Gastroenterol Nutr., 32*(Suppl 2), S1–S31.

Ryckman, F. C., & Balistreri, W. F. (2002). Upper gastrointestinal disorders. In A. A. Fanaroff & R. J. Martin (Eds.), *Neonatal-perinatal medicine: Diseases of the fetus and infant* (7th ed.). St. Louis, MO: Mosby.

Sacker, A., Quigley, M. A., & Kelly, Y. J. (2006). Breastfeeding and developmental delay: Findings from the Millennium Cohort Study. *Pediatrics, 118,* e682–e689.

Saenz, R. B. (2004). *Helping a mother breastfeed her baby with Down syndrome.* Unit 9 Lactation Consultant Series Two. Schaumburg, IL: La Leche League International.

Saint, L., Maggiore, P., & Hartmann, P. E. (1986). Yield and nutrient content of milk in eight women breastfeeding twins and one woman breastfeeding triplets. *Br J Nutr., 56,* 49–58.

Salvatore, S., & Vandenplas, Y. (2002). Gastroesophageal reflux and cow milk allergy: Is there a link? *Pediatrics, 110,* 972–984.

Savino, F., Bailo, E., Oggero, R., et al. (2005a). Bacterial counts of intestinal *Lactobacillus* species in infants with colic. *Pediatr Allergy Immunol., 16,* 72–75.

Savino, F., Cresi, F., Castagno, E., Silvestro, L., & Oggero, R. (2005b). A randomized double-blind placebo-controlled trial of a standardized extract of *Matricariae recutita, Foeniculum vulgare* and *Melissa officinalis* (ColiMil) in the treatment of breastfed colicky infants. *Phytotherapy Research, 19,* 335–340.

Savino, F., Cresi, F., Pautasso, S., et al. (2004). Intestinal microflora in breastfed colicky and non-colicky infants. *Acta Paediatr., 93,* 825–829.

Savino, F., Pelle, E., Palumeri, E., Oggero, R., & Miniero, R. (2007). *Lactobacillus reuteri* (American Type Culture Strain 55730) versus simethicone in the treatment of infantile colic: A prospective randomized study. *Pediatrics, 119,* e124–e130.

Schach, B., & Haight, M. (2002). Colic and food allergy in the breastfed infant: Is it possible for an exclusively breastfed infant to suffer from food allergy? *J Hum Lact., 18,* 50–52.

Schwartz, K., d'Arcy, H., Gillespie, B., Bobo, J., Longeway, M., & Foxman, B. (2002). Factors associated with weaning in the first 3 months postpartum. *J Fam Pract., 51,* 439–444.

Segal, L. M., Stephenson, R., Dawes, M., & Feldman, P. (2007). Prevalence, diagnosis, and treatment of ankyloglossia. *Can Fam Physician, 53,* 1027–1033.

Shaw, G. M., Lammer, E. F., Wasserman, C. R., et al. (1995). Risks of orofacial clefts in children born to women using multivitamins containing folic acid periconceptually. *Lancet, 346,* 393–396.

Shaw, W. C., Bannister, R. P., & Roberts, C. T. (1999). Assisted feeding is more reliable for infants with clefts—A randomized trial. *Cleft Palate Craniofacial J., 36,* 262–268.

Sheffield, L. J., et al. (1987). A genetic follow-up study of 64 patients with the Pierre Robin complex. *Am J Med Genet., 28,* 25–36.

Shenassa, E. D., & Brown, M.-J. (2004). Maternal smoking and infantile gastrointestinal dysregulation: The case of colic. *Pediatrics, 114,* e497–e505.

Smedegaard, L., Marxen, D., Moes, J., Glassou, E. N., & Scientsan, C. (2008). Hospitalization, breastmilk feeding, and growth in infants with cleft palate and cleft lip born in Denmark. *Cleft Palate Craniofacial J., 45,* 628–632.

Smehilova, M., Vlkova, E., Nevoral, J., Flajsmanova, K., Killer, J., & Rada, V. (2008). Comparison of intestinal microflora in healthy infants and infants with allergic colitis. *Folia Microbiologica, 53,* 255–258.

Sollid, D. T., Evans, B. T., McClowry, S. G., & Garrett, A. (1989). Breastfeeding multiples. *J Perinat Neonatal Nurs., 3,* 46–65.

Solomons, N. B., & Prescot, C. A. J. (1987). Laryngomalacia: A review and the surgical management for severe cases. *Int J Pediatr Otorhinolaryngol., 13,* 31–39.

Sondergaard, C., et al. (2001). Smoking during pregnancy and infantile colic. *Pediatrics, 108,* 342–346.

Sorensen, H. T., Norgard, B., Pedersen, L., et al. (2002). Maternal smoking and risk of hypertrophic infantile pyloric stenosis: 10 year population based cohort study. *BMJ, 325,* 1011–1012.

Sorensen, H. T., Skriver, M. V., Pedersen, L., et al. (2003). Risk of hypertrophic pyloric stenosis after maternal postnatal use of macrolides. *Scand J Infect Dis., 35,* 104–106.

Spoon, J. M. (2003). VATER association. *Neonatal Network, 22,* 71–75.

Sprintzen, R. F., Siegel-Sadewitz, V. L., Amato, J., & Goldberg, R. B. (1985). Anomalies associated with cleft lip, cleft palate, or both. *Am J Med Genet., 20,* 585–595.

Srinivasan, A., Dobrich, C., Mitnick, H., & Feldman, P. (2006). Ankyloglossia in breastfeeding infants: The effect of frenotomy on maternal nipple pain and latch. *Breastfeeding and Medicine, 1,* 216–224.

Stang, H. (1986). Pyloric stenosis associated with erythromycin ingested through breastmilk. *Minnesota Medicine, 69,* 669–670, 682.

Stern, J. E., Cedars, M. I., Jail, T., Klein, N. A., et al. (2007). Assisted reproductive technology practice patterns and the impact of embryo transfer guidelines in the United States. *Fertility and Sterility, 88,* 27–82.

Stockdale, H. J. (2000). Long-term expressing of breastmilk. *Breastfeeding Review, 8,* 19–22.

Storr, G. (1989). Breastfeeding premature triplets: One woman's experience. *J Hum Lact., 5,* 74–77.

Stuart, C. A., Twiselton, R., Nicholas, M. K., et al. (1984). Passage of cow's milk protein in breast milk. *Clin Allergy, 14,* 533–535.

Styer, G. W., & Freeh, K. (1981). Feeding infants with cleft lip and/or palate. *JOGNN, 10,* 329–332.

Szucs, K. A., Axline, S. E., & Rosenman, M. B. (2009). Quintuplets and a mother's determination to provide human milk: It takes a village to raise a baby—how about five? *J Hum Lact., 25,* 79–84.

Tobin, J. M., McCloud, P., & Cameron, D. J. S. (1997). Posture and gastroesophageal reflux: A case for left lateral positioning. *Arch Dis Child., 7,* 254–258.

Tolarova, M., & Harris, J. (1995). Reduced recurrence of orofacial clefts after periconceptional supplementation with high-dose folic acid and multivitamins. *Teratology, 51,* 71–78.

Trenouth, M. J., & Campbell, A. N. (1996). Questionnaire evaluation of feeding methods for cleft lip and palate neonates. *Int J Paediatr Dent., 6,* 241–244.

Turner, L., Jacobsen, C., Humenczuk, M., et al. (2001). The effects of lactation education and a prosthetic obturator appliance on feeding efficiency in infants with cleft lip and palate. *Cleft Palate Craniofac J., 38,* 519–524.

Turner, L., & Moore, D. (1995). Use of feeding aids for cleft lip and palate infants. Presented at the International Lactation Consultant Association, Phoenix, Arizona.

Van Rijn, M., Bekhof, J., Dijkstra T., et al. (2003). A different approach to breastfeeding of the infant with phenylketonuria. *Eur J Paediatr., 162,* 323–326.

Vandenplas, Y., De Wolf, D., & Sacre, L. (1986). Influence of xanthines on gastroesophageal reflux in infants at risk for sudden infant death syndrome. *Pediatrics, 77,* 807–810.

Walker, M. (1989). Management of selected early breastfeeding problems seen in clinical practice. *Birth, 16,* 148–157.

Wang, J., Waller, D. K., Hwang, L. Y., Taylor, L. G., & Canfield, M. A. (2008). Prevalence of infantile hypertrophic pyloric stenosis in Texas, 1999–2002. *Birth Defects Res A Clin Mol Teratol., 82,* 763–767.

Ward, N. (1990). Ankyloglossia: A case study in which clipping was not necessary. *J Hum Lact., 6,* 126–127.

Weatherly-White, R. C. A., Kuehn, D. P., Mirrett, P., et al. (1987). Early repair and breastfeeding for infants with cleft lip. *Plast Reconstr Surg., 79,* 879–885.

Webb, A. R., Lari, J., & Dodge, J. A. (1983). Infantile hypertrophic pyloric stenosis in South Glamorgan 1970–9. *Arch Dis Child., 58,* 586–590.

Weintraub, R. G., & Menahem, G. (1993). Growth and congenital heart disease. *J Paediatr Child Health, 29,* 95–98.

Weissbluth, M. (1994). Melatonin increases cyclic guanosine monophosphate: Biochemical effects mediated by porphyrins, calcium and nitric oxide. Relationship to infant colic and the sudden infant death syndrome. *Medical Hypotheses, 42,* 390–392.

Wessel, M. A., Cogg, J. C., Jackson, E. B., et al. (1954). Paroxysmal fussing in infancy, sometimes called "colic." *Pediatrics, 14,* 421–434.

Wheat, J. C. (2002). Nutritional management of children with congenital heart disease. *Nutrition Bytes, 8*(2). Retrieved September 15, 2005, from http://repositories.cdlib.org/uclabiolchem/nutritionbytes/vol8/iss2/art5

White, B. P., Gunnar, M. R., Larson, M. C., et al. (2000). Behavioral and physiological responsivity, sleep, and patterns of daily cortisol production in infants with or without colic. *Child Development, 71,* 862–877.

White, D. R., Giambra, B. K., Hopkin, R. J., Daines, C. L., & Rutter, M. J. (2005). Aspiration in children with CHARGE syndrome. *Int J Pediatr Otorhinolaryngol., 69,* 1205–1209.

Willis, C. E., & Livingstone, V. (1995). Infant insufficient milk syndrome associated with maternal postpartum hemorrhage. *J Hum Lact., 11,* 123–126.

Wilson, A. C., Moore, D. J., Moore, M. H., et al. (2000). Late presentation of upper airway obstruction in Pierre Robin sequence. *Arch Dis Child., 83,* 435–438.

Wilton, J. M. (1990). Sore nipples and slow weight gain related to a short frenulum. *J Hum Lact., 6,* 122–123.

Wolf, L. S., & Glass, R. P. (1992). *Feeding and swallowing disorders in infancy.* Tucson, AZ: Therapy Skill Builders.

Wood, R. E. (1984). Spelunking in the pediatric airway: Exploration with the flexible fiberoptic bronchoscope. *Pediatr Clin North Am., 31,* 785–799.

Woolridge, M. W., & Fisher, C. (1988). Colic, "overfeeding," and symptoms of lactose malabsorption in the breastfed baby: A possible artifact of feed management. *Lancet, 2,* 382–384.

Wright, J. E. (1995). Tongue-tie. *J Paediatr Child Health, 31,* 276–278.

Yannicelli, S., Ernest, A., Heifert, M., & McCabe, E. (1988, October). Guide to breastfeeding the infant with PKU (2nd ed.). Department of Health and Human Services publication no. HRS-M-CH88-12. Washington, DC.

Young, J. L., O'Riordan, M., Goldstein, J. A., & Robin, N. H. (2001). What information do parents of newborns with cleft lip, palate, or both want to know? *Cleft Palate Craniofacial J., 38,* 55–58.

Zucchero, T. M., Cooper, M. E., Maher, B. S., et al. (2004). Interferon regulatory factor 6 (IRF6) gene variants and the risk of isolated cleft lip or palate. *N Eng J Med., 351,* 769–780.

Additional Reading/Resources

Twins and Higher-Order Multiples

National Organization of Mothers of Twins Clubs
www.nomotc.org

Mothers of Supertwins
www.mostonline.org

Triplet Connection
www.tripletconnection.org

The Center for Study of Multiple Birth
www.multiplebirth.com

Multiple Births Canada
www.multiplebirthscanada.org/english/booklets.php

Twins Magazine
www.twinsmagazine.com/twins-magazine

Chay P, Genna CW, Gallagher F, et al. *Breastfeeding Multiples.* 2nd ed. East Islip, NY: Mothers of Supertwins; 2007.

Ankyloglossia (Tongue-Tie)

Dr. Brian Palmer, DDS
www.brianpalmerdds.com/bfeed_frenulums.htm

Genna CW, Coryllos EV. Breastfeeding and tongue-tie. *J Hum Lact.* 2009;25:111–112.

ILCA's Inside Track patient handout

Academy of Breastfeeding Medicine. Protocol # 11: Guidelines for the evaluation and management of neonatal ankyloglossia and its complications in the breast-feeding dyad.
www.bfmed.org/Resources/Protocols.aspx

Frenotomy video
www.drjain.com/video.htm

Gastroesophageal Reflux Disease (GERD)

Gastroesophageal Reflux Disease and the Breastfeeding Baby
Susan Boekel, RD, CSP, LD, IBCLC

Independent Study Module
International Lactation Consultant Association
www.ilca.org

Breastfeeding Special Needs Infants

Breastfeeding the Infant with Special Needs. 2nd ed. March of Dimes, 2007.

Mojab CG. *Congenital Disorders in the Nursing.* Unit 5/Lactation Consultant Series Two. Schaumburg, IL: La Leche League International; 2002.

◖◗ PART III ◖◗

Maternal-Related Challenges to Breastfeeding

Chapter 8

Maternal Pathology:
Breast and Nipple Issues

Introduction

Breast and nipple problems are the bane of nursing mothers and have been reported in the medical literature since the 1500s (Fildes, 1986). Some of these problems may be related to underlying anatomical variations in a woman's breast, areola, and nipple. Problems may occur early or late in lactation, with some having a significant impact on the duration of exclusive breastfeeding and contributing to premature weaning. In this chapter we address maternal breastfeeding problems and issues related to the breast, areola, and nipple and inappropriate or ineffective breastfeeding guidelines.

Nipple Types

The following are common nipple descriptors:

- Inverted: This nipple type results from the failure of the mammary pit to elevate during embryonic development as a result of the lack of mesenchymal proliferation (Bland & Romnell, 1991). These are also referred to as tied, invaginated, or tethered.
- Retracted: These are described as occurring from adhesions at the base of the nipple.
- Nonprotractile: A type occurring from an anatomical fault that has been ascribed to short lactiferous ducts that tether the nipple and prevent it from projecting (McGeorge, 1994).

- Pseudoinverted: Also referred to as umbilicated (Terrill & Stapleton, 1991), these nipples appear inverted, but when the areola around them is compressed they evert. The connective tissue is thought to be deficient, but the length of the underlying ductwork is normal, and an adequately suckling infant will sufficiently elongate the nipple for proper latch.

Plastic surgeons have graded inverted nipples through evaluation and surgical confirmation relative to the degree of fibrosis (replacement of normal cells with connective tissue, similar to scar tissue) (Han & Hong, 1999):

> Grade I: The nipple is easily pulled out manually, maintains its protrusion or projection, and contains minimal fibrosis.

> Grade II: The nipple can be manually pulled out but does not maintain its protrusion, retreating back into the areola, and thought to have moderate fibrosis beneath the nipple.

> Grade III: The nipple can barely be manually pulled out, with severe fibrotic bands and less soft tissue underlying the nipple.

Inverted or nonprotractile nipples have been reported to occur in 7–10% of pregnant women who wish to breastfeed (Alexander, 1991; Hytten & Baird, 1958). Dewey, Nommsen-Rivers, Heinig, and Cohen (2003) reported a 9% incidence of flat or inverted nipples on the day the infant was born and a 7% incidence 7 days later. Although flat nipples are usually unable to be visually assessed, some inverted or dimpled nipples are easily seen during the prenatal period. A dimpled nipple folds back in on itself, with moist tissues adhering and setting the stage for skin breakdown after breastfeeding begins. The "pinch test" or compressing the areola can reveal flat or retracted nipples, because there is little protrusion and lack of definition between where the nipple ends and the areolar tissue begins. Nipples typically gain elasticity throughout the pregnancy, and the degree of inversion decreases with subsequent pregnancies.

Early data failed to find an association between an infant's ability to breastfeed successfully and the extent of maternal nipple protrusion (Inch, 1989). However, in a review of five infants admitted to the hospital with severe dehydration and hypernatremia, three of the mothers had inverted nipples and experienced problems with their infants attaining a proper latch (Cooper, Atherton, Kahana, & Kotagal, 1995). Dewey et al. (2003) showed that suboptimal infant breastfeeding behavior (defined as scoring less than or equal to 10 on the Infant Breastfeeding Assessment Tool) and delayed onset of lactation were significantly related to the presence of flat or inverted nipples on days 1, 3, and 7 postpartum. They specifically recommended that women with flat or inverted nipples be given special breastfeeding assistance until the infant is able to latch effectively.

Breastfeeding Recommendations Based on Nipple Type

Maternal nipples elongate two to three times their resting length when drawn into the infant's mouth (Smith, Erenberg, & Nowak, 1988) and present an expected and strong physical sucking signal to the infant when the teat reaches deep into the oral cavity. However, a nipple that retreats when stimulated may present a challenge for the infant who is unable to sufficiently elongate a nonprotractile nipple into a teat (composed of the nipple plus the underlying areola). Gunther (1955) described infants as becoming "apathetic" to the breast when flat or inverted nipples were present. She speculated that breastfeeding would be interrupted if the infant did not receive the proper physical signal (an elastic protrusive nipple–areola) to set an innate behavior in motion.

Antenatal Nipple Preparations

Three methods of antenatal nipple preparation were taught to women for decades in the belief that prenatal preparation would correct the defect and contribute to problem-free initiation of breastfeeding (Cadwell, 1981; Otte, 1975):

1. Nipple rolling involves pulling out the nipple to its outermost position and either holding it or rolling it, repeated 10 times twice a day to increase elasticity of the tissue (Applebaum, 1969).

2. In Hoffman's technique the thumbs are positioned to each side of the nipple and the areola is stretched sideways and then up and down (Hoffman, 1953).

3. Breast shells (also called Woolwich Shields, Netsy Cups, Hobbit Shells, Swedish Milk Cups) are a two-piece system consisting of a flat disk with a hole in the center through which the nipple protrudes. The disk is covered by a vented dome and placed under the bra to exert pressure on the base of the nipple "to gradually stretch and loosen its attachment to the deep structures of the breast" (Waller, 1946).

Two randomized trials comparing the use of Hoffman's exercises and breast shells showed little change in nipple anatomy from the use of either treatment and no increase in the duration of breastfeeding (Alexander, Grant, & Campbell,

1992; MAIN Trial Collaborative Group, 1994). The application of suction prenatally has been suggested as a nonsurgical method of everting nipples (Gangal & Gangal, 1978).

A device called the Niplette (Avent) uses the concept of tissue expansion through continuous long-term suction, derived from the disciplines of plastic and aesthetic surgery (McGeorge, 1994). This device consists of a transparent thimble-like nipple mold with a syringe port. The mold is placed over the flat nipple, air is evacuated from the mold by the connected syringe, and the nipple is slowly drawn out to the mother's comfort level and held in place while the device is worn. The device is worn 8 or more hours a day during the first 6 months of the pregnancy. Successful breastfeeding has been reported in a small number of mothers with the use of the device, but it has the potential for pain and nipple bleeding if too much suction is applied. It can be used briefly before each feeding in the first few days after birth, but the presence of milk in the mold impairs the device's suction.

After the infant is born, the flat or inverted nipple can be temporarily everted before each feeding such that enough nipple–areolar tissue is presented to the infant to enable latch. The application of a breast pump has been recommended and used for this purpose. However, a pump distributes vacuum over a relatively large area and has the potential to increase interstitial fluid pressure (Cotterman, 2004), causing nipple swelling (Wilson-Clay & Hoover, 2002): This creates another layer of fluid within the areola under the pump flange area that thickens the superficial areolar tissue and further impedes the infant's ability to latch (Cotterman, 2003). A simpler and less expensive tool can be fashioned from a 10-mL disposable plastic syringe. Kesaree, Banapurmath, Banapurmath, and Shamanur (1993) modified the syringe by removing the plunger, cutting off the end of the syringe 1/4-inch above where a needle would attach, and inserting the plunger through the end that was cut. The mother then places the smooth end of the syringe directly over her nipple and pulls back gently on the plunger to her comfort for 30 seconds to a minute before each feeding. This allows the nipple itself to be drawn out from the surrounding areola (Thorley, 1997). A commercial version of this device, called the Evert-It Nipple Enhancer, is also available.

Some nipples may appear flat but are actually enveloped by an edematous areola after labor and delivery. Large amount of intravenous fluids, use of Pitocin, or excessive water retention such as in preeclampsia (Cotterman, 2004; Miller & Riordan, 2004) may contribute to an areola that is so swollen it obliterates the nipple, erasing the definition or boundary between the nipple itself and the external areola.

This may remove the normally expected tactile stimulation that the infant's sensitive lips seek at latch-on, leading to a difficult or painful latching process.

Breastfeeding Management

A severely inverted or dimpled nipple may be obvious during pregnancy. A flat nipple may be apparent when the areola is gently squeezed (pinch test) and the nipple is seen flattening to the level of the areola. Nipple rolling, breast shells, and the Hoffman technique have not been shown to improve the elasticity or lengthen the nipple. The Niplette has been shown to evert nipples in a small number of women and can be worn during the first two trimesters of pregnancy. Many flat-appearing nipples may resolve by the end of the pregnancy and require no prenatal manipulation.

After the birth, to shape the nipple the mother can place a cold compress on the nipple, gently pull and roll it before feedings, or place her thumb and index finger above and below the nipple, pressing inward and together to help "pop" out the nipple. In addition, a modified syringe or the Evert-It Nipple Enhancer can be applied for 30 seconds to a minute before each feeding. Areolar compression can be done before latch attempts on an edematous areola (Miller & Riordan, 2004). The mother applies pressure with both thumbs and index fingers into the areola directly behind the nipple. Indentations are created as interstitial fluid is displaced and the fingers are then placed above and below the initial indentations, working their way up to the margins of the areola. The mother rotates her fingers to a new position behind the nipple and works her way to the outer margin of the areola again until the nipple becomes pliable and easily everted at which point the infant is brought to the breast.

Reverse pressure softening has a number of variations (Cotterman, 2004) using the mother's fingertips to create pits around the circumference of the nipple. The mother uses three or four fingertips of both hands encircling the base of the nipple and pushing inward for about 1–3 minutes firmly enough to form six to eight pits. This exposes the nipple and presents a better tactile stimulus for latching. A nipple shield can be applied either before or after areolar compression or reverse pressure softening if there appears no other way to effect a latch.

The "teacup" hold may be tried with a nonengorged breast and nonedematous areola. This involves shaping the nipple–areolar complex into a wedge whose long axis matches the long axis of the open mouth of the infant. The mother or clinician uses a thumb and index finger to grasp the areola directly above the nipple plus some of the breast tissue above it and form as much tissue as possible into a wedge, placing it as deep as possible into the infant's mouth. It is held in place until the infant is latched correctly and sucking well (Wilson-Clay & Hoover, 2002).

Caution should be exercised in placing a breast pump on swollen tissues. Hand expression may also aggravate an edematous areola.

Some mothers find that wearing breast shells under their bra between feedings everts flat nipples. This may result from the displacement of fluid from the continuous pressure exerted by the rim of the nipple opening. However, when the shells are worn for prolonged periods of time and there is significant areolar edema, potential for exacerbating edema and damaging underlying tissues exists from the strangulation of capillary circulation.

Both areolar compression and reverse pressure softening may have an added benefit, which is the stimulation of the milk ejection reflex. Compression directly on the center or core of the areola at the base of the nipple can have the effect of triggering milk letdown within a minute or 2, either from stimulation of the nerves converging in the center of the areola or as a reflex contraction of the myoepithelial cells caused by the pressure alone (Cotterman, 2004).

Sore Nipples

Because the concept of soreness or pain is subjective and studies on nipple pain vary in their methodology, reports in the literature of the incidence of sore nipples range from none at 6 days after delivery (Humenick & van Steenkiste, 1983) to 96% of breastfeeding mothers at some time during the first 6 weeks postpartum (Ziemer, Paone, Schupay, & Cole, 1990). Sore nipples are a frequent reason for early termination of breastfeeding (Neifert & Seacat, 1986; West, 1980; Yeung, Pennell, Leung, & Hall, 1981). Nipple pain (of any definition) has been reported to occur from the 2nd to the 15th postpartum day, continuing in some mothers through 90 days (Drewett, Kahn, Parkhurst, & Whiteley, 1987). It peaks in intensity from day 2 or 3 (Hewat & Ellis, 1987; Newton, 1952) to days 4 through 7 (Ziemer et al., 1990). There are also reported differences and many aspects of nipple pain, such as transient latch-on pain, sustained pain during a feeding, persistent nipple pain over a prolonged period of time, pain between feedings, burning pain, and degrees of pain, from mild sensitivity to excruciating.

In a study of the nipple pain experiences of 69 women, Heads and Higgins (1995) reported that about 75% of the mothers had pain at the outset of breastfeeding that declined sharply to 22% after letdown and the establishment of breastfeeding. Hill and Humenick (1993) described the daily occurrence of latch-on pain for the first 14 days in 155 first- and second-time breastfeeding mothers as well as the occurrence of pain severe enough to disrupt breastfeeding over the course of the first 6 weeks. Virtually all mothers experienced some level of discomfort when the infant first latched on (as also noted by L'Esperance, 1980). The maximum level of latch-on pain was reached by day 5 in 73.8% of mothers.

Latch-on pain and breast engorgement were positively correlated, showing that mothers experiencing more engorgement experienced more latch-on pain. The incidence of mothers experiencing nipple pain severe enough to interfere with breastfeeding ranged from 42.3% at week 1 to 12.4% at week 6. Mothers experiencing nipple pain severe enough to interfere with their desire to continue breastfeeding was significantly associated with latch-on pain at weeks 1 and 2. Up to one-third of mothers experiencing nipple pain and trauma may change to alternate feeding methods within the first 6 weeks postpartum (Briggs, 2003). Mothers who experience nipple pain also suffer from high levels of psychological distress (Amir et al., 1997), confirming that clinical support to improve nipple pain is important during the early days and weeks postpartum if breastfeeding is to continue. Pain or the anticipation of pain can delay or disrupt the milk ejection reflex, which can set in motion a cascade of undesirable side effects leading to ineffective milk transfer, residual milk build-up, and more or extended engorgement, coming full circle to more nipple pain (Newton & Newton, 1948).

Ziemer and Pigeon (1993) described nipple skin changes in 20 breastfeeding mothers during the first week of lactation. Changes and damage to the nipple skin was confined to the face or tip of the nipple, suggesting that normal changes and actual damage were due to suction. Ninety percent of the women experienced pain. Magnified photographs of the nipple tip in all women studied showed visible skin changes during the study period. The tip of the nipple before the start of breastfeeding was light pink and typically showed a papillar (small bumps) appearance with small lines and crevices uniquely distributed over the surface. Ten different changes were observed over time:

1. Erythema (reddening or inflamed areas): peaking on day 3

2. Edema (swelling) of the nipple and papillar bumps: occurred in all women and peaked on day 5

3. Fissures: for 65% of the mothers, some of the fissures widened and became raw, peaking on day 5

4. Blisters: 80% of the mothers had small blisters that could have been papillae that filled with fluid; occurred on day 3

5. Eschar (scabs)

6. White patches

7. Peeling

8. Dark patches

9. Pus

10. Ecchymosis (bruising or bleeding under the skin)

Positioning or proper nipple–areolar placement in the infant's mouth was not evaluated in this study; however, nipple skin changes were seen to occur right from the start of breastfeeding. These normal changes may be responsible for the common complaints of mothers describing some amount of nipple sensitivity or discomfort, whereas severe nipple pain may represent an exaggeration or extension of these changes.

Positioning: Proper Nipple–Areolar Placement

Gunther was one of the earliest authors to associate severe nipple pain and damage with the position of the infant at the breast. She described two common types of damage as erosive (petechial) and ulcerative (fissure) (Gunther, 1945). Woolridge (1986) described frictional trauma and suction lesions as the two main physical sources of nipple pain (as opposed to dermatological or infective causes). Frictional trauma is thought to be caused by inadequate amounts of breast tissue being drawn into the infant's mouth, resulting in poor milk transfer and distortion of the nipple. Rather than being compressed and extending to twice its resting length, the nipple–areolar complex is not formed into a teat, and the nipple skin can become abraded or actually pinched into a compression stripe. A nipple that is creased in a horizontal, vertical, or oblique manner has the potential for both significant pain and skin breakdown (contributed by both compression and suction concentrated on the distorted area).

Trauma from suction has been related to the application of continuous suction that is not relieved by periodic swallowing. Righard (1996) provided further insight into the effect of faulty sucking on nipple pain. Of the 52 mother–infant pairs referred for breastfeeding problems, 94% had a pattern of superficial nipple sucking where the infant sucked only on the nipple tip, failing to draw the nipple–areola complex deep into the mouth. Of the 94% of mother–infant pairs with the superficial sucking pattern, 33% of the mothers complained of sore nipples. An interesting finding in this study was that infants using pacifiers more often had a superficial sucking pattern at the breast than nonusers of pacifiers.

Nipple pain from faulty mechanics of infant sucking, either poor latch or failure to form a teat (Righard, 1998; Widstrom & Thingstrom-Paulsson, 1993) can occur quickly, with mothers experiencing nipple pain and damage before discharge from the hospital. Blair, Cadwell, Turner-Maffei, and Brimdyr (2003) studied 95 mothers reporting nipple pain within 10 days of giving birth. Their results showed that nipple pain was related to positioning and latching errors but that no single isolated part of the positioning and latch sequence was more related to pain than another. Clinicians therefore need to assess all elements of the positioning, latching, and sucking processes. Six specific types of nipple trauma were distributed among the mothers in this study: (1) 64.4% presented with fissures, (2) 53.3% with erythema, (3) 51.1% with crusting/scabs, (4) 32.2% with swelling, (5) 4.4% with blisters or blebs, and (6) 1.1% with exudate (oozing of fluid). It is interesting to note that Ziemer and Pigeon (1993) also reported a 65% rate of fissures in their description of causes of nipple pain. It could be speculated that faulty positioning, latching, and sucking mechanics could place enough stress on the normal anatomical features of the nipple (papillae and fissures on the face of the nipple) to cause erosion or a break in the skin integrity. The disruption of the skin surface by suction or friction, concomitant stretching or rupturing of the skin within the fissures, and destruction of the underlying skin layers may move the mother on a continuum from minor discomfort to macerated and bleeding nipple wounds if interventions do not rectify the problem.

After study infants painlessly drew the nipple–areola into their mouths, Jacobs, Dickinson, Hart, Doherty, and Faulkner (2007) measured by ultrasound the distance between the tip of the nipple and the junction of the hard and soft palates. Only 25% of correctly latched infants drew in the nipple as far as the hard–soft palate junction. The median distance between the tip of the nipple and this junction was 5 mm, and the nipple showed a range of movement during breastfeeding of 4.0 ± 1.3 mm. Nipple positioning and movements outside these ranges may be predictive of nipple pain.

Ankyloglossia (tongue-tie) can restrict the movement of the tongue, potentially inhibiting the nipple–areola from being drawn far enough into the mouth to prevent pain and promote optimal milk transfer. Geddes et al. (2008) reported that release of the frenulum altered tongue movement as imaged by ultrasound during breastfeeding. Infants with ankyloglossia showed two types of sucking dynamics. One type pinched the nipple tip, placing it a large distance from the junction of the hard and soft palates. The other type of sucking pinched the nipple at its base, placing the nipple tip in close proximity to the hard–soft palate junction. Frenotomy reduced the extent of nipple distortion and significantly relieved nipple pain experienced by mothers. This is in agreement with Dollberg, Botzer, Grunis, and Mimouni (2006) and Srinivasan, Dobrich, Mitnick, and Feldman (2006), who detailed the immediate relief from nipple pain after frenotomy.

Although most nipple pain may be relieved by correcting positioning and attachment at the breast, assessment and correction of technique may not always relieve all nipple pain (Cadwell, Turner-Maffei, Blair, Brimdyr, & McInerney, 2004; Henderson, Stamp, & Pincombe, 2001). McClellan et al. (2008) demonstrated that despite help with positioning and attachment, the infants of mothers with persistent nipple pain applied significantly stronger vacuums and transferred less milk than infants not causing pain. Their data revealed that infants causing pain exerted vacuums that were more than 50% stronger during active sucking and more than double during pausing when compared with infants not causing pain. Interventions to reduce these strong vacuums are unknown, but techniques of more frequent feeding to reduce strong sucking due to hunger or changes in positioning such as to ventral positioning could be tried.

When Extensive Interventions May Be Necessary

Bacterial Infection

Most early nipple discomfort and pain is due to physical forces on the nipple that can be remedied through correcting and optimizing the mechanics of breastfeeding (Renfrew, Woolridge, & McGill, 2000). However, if nipple pain persists or worsens and if a break in the skin surface occurs, other factors may become involved and more extensive interventions may be necessary. Once the integrity of the skin has been disrupted, there is a tendency for colonization by bacterial and fungal species.

Nipple wounds are frequently contaminated by *Staphylococcus aureus*, a common bacterial resident of the skin. Livingstone, Willis, and Berkowitz (1996) showed that mothers with infants younger than 1 month who presented with severe nipple pain and damage (cracks, fissures, ulcers, or exudates) had a 64% chance of having a positive bacterial skin culture and a 54% chance of having *S. aureus* impetigo vulgaris colonization. Impetigo vulgaris is a bacterial skin infection caused by staphylococci or streptococci with yellow to red weeping and crusted or pustular lesions, with the term "vulgaris" referring to the common form of this infection. Repetitive trauma to the nipple skin is thought to overcome the natural barriers to infection, and once bacterial contamination has occurred, a delay in wound healing may follow.

Livingstone and Stringer (1999) described a cascade of possible sequelae once a break in the integumentum occurs (Table 8-1). Eglash, Plane, and Mundt (2006) described a collection of physical and laboratory findings in a population of mothers with deep breast aching or pain, tender breasts upon palpation, and nipple lesions. Half of the mothers' nipples showed positive cultures for pathogenic bacteria. These symptoms may be suggestive of a bacterial lactiferous duct infection that responded to an average of 5 weeks of antibiotic treatment. Eglash and Proctor (2007) described a mother with a prolonged history of nipple cracks, dull throbbing of the breasts, sharp shooting pains, pain on palpation of the breasts, and redness and swelling of the left breast. Laboratory findings of the cultured milk showed viridans *Streptococcus* and coagulase-negative *Staphylococcus*. The authors postulated that the clinical and laboratory findings were descriptive of infections caused by small colony variants of *Staphylococci*. Small colony variants cause low-grade, persistent, antibiotic-resistant, chronic, and recurrent infections that take many weeks of antibiotics to clear. This type of infection may respond better to macrolides for 4–8 weeks.

Clinicians should be on the lookout for an ascending infection when a mother presents with severe nipple pain or a break of any sort in the nipple skin, because there is a significantly increased risk for mastitis in the presence of cracked nipples

---

TABLE 8-1 Cascade of Sequelae From *S. aureus* Colonization and Infection of the Nipple Skin

- A break in the skin facilitates a secondary infection due to bacterial or fungal contamination, delaying wound healing.
- Cracks, fissures, and ulcerations have a high risk of contamination.
- Strains of *S. aureus* can penetrate the superficial layers of the skin at the site of minor skin trauma.
- The toxins they produce can cause inflammation, skin separation, and the formation of blisters.
- The blisters break down, leaving erosions in the skin that become covered with a yellow crusted exudate.
- An ascending lactiferous duct infection can contribute to mastitis and abscess.

(Kinlay, O'Connell, & Kinlay, 2001). In a study of 28 mothers with nipple pain (Graves, Wright, Harman, & Bailey, 2003), 57% had nipple swabs positive for *S. aureus* and 48% had positive milk specimens, indicative of ascending infection of the lactiferous ducts. Mothers complaining of deep breast pain are frequently treated for fungal infections; however, Thomassen, Johansson, Wassberg, and Petrini (1998) found that bacteria were often found both on the nipple and in the milk of mothers who described deep breast pain during or after breastfeeding. Persistence or worsening of nipple pain requires careful history taking and direct observation to identify the etiology (Walker & Driscoll, 1989).

Eczema

Eczema can be present on the nipple itself or can extend onto and beyond the areola (Barankin & Gross, 2004). The clinical appearance can include erythema, papules, vesicles (fluid-filled blisters), oozing (Rago, 1988), crusts, lichenification (thickening and hardening of the skin), skin erosion, fissures, excoriations, and scaling (Ward & Burton, 1997). Burning and/or itching are typical symptoms of eczema (Bracket, 1988). Differentially, itching is not prominent in candidal infections.

Eczema is a general term for several types of dermatitis, including atopic, seborrheic, irritant contact, and allergic contact. These types usually respond to removing the irritant or allergen and/or the application of topical corticosteroids (Amir, 1993). In many instances atopic dermatitis is accompanied by high colony counts of *S. aureus*, necessitating treatment with a topical antibiotic also (Lever et al., 1988). Both nipples are commonly involved. When eczema appears on just one nipple, the clinician should consider referral to rule out the presence of Paget disease,[1] which has the appearance of a steadily progressing eczema.

Herpes Infection

Numerous discrete lesions at the junction of the nipple and areola and/or farther back on the areola can be a herpes simplex infection (Amir, 2004). The mother

---

[1] Paget disease of the nipple is a superficial manifestation of an underlying breast malignancy, thought to account for 1–3% of all breast cancers (Osther, Balslev, & Blichert-toft, 1990). The lesion appears as a well-demarcated, red, scaly plaque appearing on the nipple first and then spreading to the areola. Oozing, crusting, itching, burning, skin thickening, erythema, ulceration, and nipple retraction may be present superficially, with a 60% occurrence of an underlying breast mass. A small vesicular eruption on the nipple, persistent soreness, pain, or itching of the nipple–areolar complex in the absence of other clinical symptoms may be the early manifestations of this condition (Jamali, Ricci, & Deckers, 1996). A biopsy establishes the diagnosis.

usually has extreme pain, and cultures of the lesions generally show herpes simplex type 1. Herpes in the neonate can be serious or fatal and transmitted through direct contact with active lesions (Sullivan-Bolyai et al., 1983). The mother can continue to breastfeed on the nonaffected side, resuming on the infected side when the lesions have fully healed. Herpes can infect intact skin (Dekio, Kawasaki, & Jidoi, 1986) and originate in the infant's mouth from gingivostomatitis (Sealander & Kerr, 1989), a condition peaking in children between 6 months and 3 years of age. Older infants and toddlers with sores in the anterior portion of the mouth and refusal to eat should be checked for this condition. Mothers should take extra care in washing their hands.

Raynaud Phenomenon of the Nipple

Raynaud phenomenon was first described in 1862 as intermittent ischemia typically affecting the fingers and toes, but it can involve other parts of the body, including blood vessels supplying the heart, gastrointestinal system, genitourinary system, and placental vasculature. It is more common in women than men, affecting up to 20% of women aged 21–50 years (Olsen & Nielson, 1978). In a series of events in susceptible people, a precipitating event such as exposure to cold temperatures causes vasospasms of arterioles and intermittent ischemia to the affected body part. Clinically, this is seen as pallor or blanching, followed by a cyanotic coloring as oxygen is cut off from the venous blood, ending with erythema (redness) as reflex vasodilation occurs. These color changes may involve all three changes (triphasic) or just two changes (biphasic).

It is felt as a sensation of pain, burning, numbness, prickly, or stinging. Gunther (1970) described this type of vasospasm in the nipple but attributed it to psychosomatic causes. Coates (1992) described bilateral nipple vasospasms in a mother who complained of intense pain, biphasic color changes, and partial relief from heat applications to the nipples. Because heat provided some relief and the symptoms were bilateral, it was suggested that this particular set of conditions could be a variant of Raynaud phenomenon. Blanching of the nipples can occur not only during or just after a feeding but also between feedings, with or without a history of Raynaud phenomenon in other parts of the body and in conjunction with nipple trauma such as ulceration, cracking, or blistering (Lawlor-Smith & Lawlor-Smith, 1997). The pain associated with nipple vasospasm can be so throbbing and severe that some women may completely abandon breastfeeding. It can also occur with subsequent pregnancies.

Other causes of nipple blanching and pain arise from inappropriate positioning, faulty latching, and variations of infant sucking that cause mechanical trauma from biting the nipple. A diagnosis of Raynaud phenomenon requires that other factors be present, such as the biphasic or triphasic color changes and precipitation by a stimulus such as cold temperatures. Raynaud phenomenon has been misdiagnosed as it may mimic some of the symptoms of mastitis. Differentiation of Raynaud's from mastitis has been demonstrated by culturing milk samples, with milk from breasts with mastitis showing higher levels of bacteria (Delgado et al., 2009). Because of the nature of the pain, Raynaud phenomenon of the nipples may be misidentified as a *Candida albicans* infection and treated with medications that provide no relief from the symptoms (Morino & Winn, 2007).

Many of the options for treating this condition are extrapolated from interventions used for Raynaud phenomenon occurring in other parts of the body. The provision of warmth and the avoidance of cold stress are the first-line management options for Raynaud phenomenon of the nipples (Lawlor-Smith & Lawlor-Smith, 1996). Mothers may need to keep their entire body warm, use a heating pad over the breasts, wear warm clothing, wear warm coverings over the breasts, sleep under an electric blanket, or have warm packs available for application to the breast not being nursed on. If vasospasms occur between feedings, some mothers find relief by immersing the breasts in warm water. Mothers should avoid vasoconstricting drugs such as caffeine and nicotine. Mothers experiencing this acute pain during lactation require immediate relief if breastfeeding is to continue.

Nifedipine, a calcium channel blocker with vasodilating effects, has been used successfully to treat Raynaud phenomenon of the nipples (Anderson, Held, & Wright, 2004; Page & McKenna, 2006). Only small amounts are measurable in breastmilk (Ehrenkranz, Ackerman, & Hulse, 1989; Hale, 2008), and the American Academy of Pediatrics (2001) identified the drug as usually compatible with breastfeeding. Nifedipine can be prescribed for dosing of 5 mg three times per day or as 30–60 mg per day in slow-release formulations. Usually, one 2-week course eliminates the symptoms, but some mothers may require two or three courses of treatment for complete resolution.

Nipple Bleb

A nipple bleb typically represents a nipple pore that is blocked by milk seeping under the epidermis, causing a raised, opaque, shiny white bump on the tip of the nipple. The mother usually complains of extreme pinpoint pain when the infant feeds. The incidence is unknown, and speculation on its cause has mentioned a tendency in some people for epithelial overgrowth or the encouragement of epithelial growth by the epithelial growth factor in the mother's milk (Noble,

1991). If this tissue overgrowth obstructs milk flow from a nipple pore that drains a larger area of the breast, the possibility exists for milk stasis, a plugged duct farther back in the breast, or mastitis.

If the bleb does not open spontaneously, some mothers soften the skin with warm saline soaks and gently rub with a towel or scrape with sterilized tweezers. If these efforts are unsuccessful, the mother's healthcare provider can open it with a sterile needle and express out any material that has accumulated behind it. Some of this material may be thick and stringy, representing milk that has thickened as the water in it is reabsorbed by the body. Many mothers who experience continuous nipple blebs learn to open them at home. Whereas a nipple bleb presents on the face of the nipple, a sebaceous cyst has been reported on the shaft or side of the nipple, with relief obtained when the oily material was removed (Wilson-Clay & Hoover, 2002).

Glands of Montgomery

Because the glands of Montgomery have a secretory apparatus and capacity, they have the potential to become obstructed. The ductal system of the areola can also become infected (Al-Qattan & Robertson, 1990). A mother can experience a painful inflamed or infected Montgomery gland, appearing as a reddened raised bump or fluid-filled blister farther back on the areola. Although the condition is usually self-limiting, it can occasionally require interventions such as the application of warm compresses, the use of antibiotics (topical or systemic), and gentle squeezing to remove infected material. Mothers should be aware of equipment or irritants that could precipitate or aggravate Montgomery glands to the point of actual obstruction or damage. Use of pump flanges, breast shells, or nipple shields that could abrade these glands or the application of topical preparations that block the openings of the Montgomery glands should be investigated when mothers present with painful conditions on the areola rather than the nipple.

Nipple pain may originate from preparations applied to the nipples, misuse of breastfeeding equipment, allergies or sensitivity to chemicals or irritants, or other conditions such as psoriasis. Nipples may also swell during pumping. Clinicians should ask if the mother is pumping milk and make sure that she is correctly using a high-quality pump with the appropriate size flange.

Fungal Colonization

In addition to mechanical trauma of the nipple and bacterial infection, the fungal pathogen *Candida albicans* can contribute to nipple and breast pain in lactating women. Although the terms candidiasis, mammary candidosis, and thrush are used interchangeably, the old term monilia or moniliasis is not interchangeable because it refers to a different genus. *C. albicans* is an opportunistic, commensal, normally harmless organism residing on the skin and in the gastrointestinal and genitourinary tracts. Dry, healthy, intact skin and the presence of normal competing flora typically allow *C. albicans* to exist in harmony with its host. Stratified squamous epithelial cells lining the gastrointestinal and genitourinary tracts are easily colonized by *C. albicans*. Portions of the lining of the lactiferous ducts are also composed of layered squamous epithelial cells, posing the possibility that under the right circumstances these too could be vulnerable to fungal invasion (Heinig, Francis, & Pappagianis, 1999).

Laboratory evidence confirming the presence of *C. albicans* in the mammary ducts of humans is sparse (Amir, Garland, Dennerstein, & Farish, 1996; Thomassen et al., 1998), whereas ductal infections in dairy cattle and goats have been reported (Moretti et al., 1998; Singh et al., 1998). *C. albicans* has also been isolated from milk samples of dairy cows with mastitis and subclinical mastitis (dos Santos & Marin, 2005). This invites speculation that ductal colonization or infection in humans may be facilitated when the breast becomes susceptible through subclinical mastitis. Subclinical mastitis may render the ducts an easy target if they have become inflamed through a local adverse immune response to milk proteins that have remained in prolonged contact with them (Michie, Lockie, & Lynn, 2003). Opening of the tight junctions between luminal epithelial cells from milk stasis may increase the areas for colonization by pathogenic organisms.

Ultrasound imaging of the breasts has shown dilatation of the milk ducts by the milk ejection reflex, followed by a decrease in ductal diameter and a backflow of the milk that is not removed (Ramsay, Kent, Owens, & Hartmann, 2004). It could be speculated that the backward flow of milk away from the nipple and into the smaller collecting ducts and ductules could carry pathogens deeper into the breast. Hale, Bateman, Finkelman, and Berens (2009) evaluated the presence of *C. albicans* in the milk of breastfeeding women with and without breast pain suggestive of a clinical diagnosis of a fungal infection. An assay for beta-glucan, the presence of which is reflective of an active candidal infection, was performed on milk samples from mothers with and without symptoms. There was no significant difference in beta-glucan levels between the two groups, indicating that *Candida* was not present in the ductal system of the breasts.

C. albicans exists in at least three different morphologies (forms): yeast, pseudo-hyphae, and hyphae. By activating appropriate sets of genes, it can alter its form to adapt to its changing environment and increase its virulence, allowing it to colonize or infect virtually all body sites (Staib et al., 2000). *C. albicans* may appear as spherical yeast cells on the skin, and although they can change into filamentous forms that readily penetrate tissues, the organism has many other mechanisms to circumvent and take advantage of changing host conditions. The filamentous forms of hyphae and pseudohyphae adhere better to epithelial cells than spherical yeast cells. Their projections can follow surface discontinuities and penetrate through breaks in tissue, such as those occurring in nipple fissures (Odds, 1994). They can secrete enzymes that digest epidermal keratin, the tough top layer of skin, assisting hyphal filaments in their invasive process and inducing an inflammatory response.

A number of risk factors for mammary candidosis have been put forward:

- Between 22% (Cotch, Hillier, Gibbs, & Eschenbach, 1998) and 33% (Vidotto et al., 1992) of pregnant women test positive for vaginal candidosis by the end of their pregnancy, with the majority (95%) caused by *C. albicans* (Odds, 1994).

- Use of antibiotics during the peripartum period or while breastfeeding increases the risk factor (Amir et al., 1996; Chetwynd, Ives, Payne, & Edens-Bartholomew, 2002; Dinsmoor, Viloria, Lief, & Elder, 2005; Tanquay, McBean, & Jain, 1994).

- Sore or damaged nipples provide a route of entry for pathogens (Amir, 1991; Amir et al., 1996; Amir & Hoover, 2003; Livingstone et al., 1996; Tanquay et al., 1994).

- Colonization and development of oral thrush in infants occurs from the birth process (Remington & Klein, 1983) and other vectors, such as healthcare workers (Pfaller, 1994), as the infant gets older. Forty percent to 60% of infants carry the organism in their mouths, with 10–24% developing oral thrush within the first 18 months (Darwazeh & al-Bashir, 1995). Morrill, Heinig, Pappagianis, and Dewey (2005) reported oral colonization in 20% of infants studied, of whom 75% developed oral thrush by 9 weeks of age.

- Use of pacifiers in infants (Brook & Gober, 1997; Darwazeh & al-Bashir, 1995; Mattos-Graner, de Moraes, Rontani, & Birman, 2001) may facilitate oral colonization and contribute to persistence of candidal presence in the mouth (Manning, Coughlin, & Poskitt, 1985).

- The use of bottles has been demonstrated to be a key risk factor for *C. albicans* colonization in both mothers and infants. Morrill et al. (2005)

reported that of 52 mother–infant dyads that used bottles in the first 2 weeks postpartum, 44% of the mothers and 38% of the infants tested positive for *C. albicans*. They suggest that it may not be bottle use alone but the fluid contained in the bottle that provides the growth medium for facilitating *C. albicans* colonization. Infant formula contains large amounts of iron, with iron being known to increase growth of *C. albicans* in vitro (Andersson, Lindquist, Lagerqvust, & Hernell, 2000). Lactoferrin in human milk typically keeps *C. albicans* in check. However, the absence of lactoferrin in artificial infant milk plus its relatively heavy load of iron may combine to augment yeast proliferation in the infant's mouth. *C. albicans* adherence to epithelial surfaces can also be encouraged by the presence of sucrose or fructose (Pizzo, Giuliana, Milici, & Giangreco, 2000), such as seen in soy-based infant formulas. Some soy-based formulas can contain as much as 10% sucrose (table sugar).

The exact prevalence of *C. albicans* colonization in mothers in not known. Twenty-six percent of breastfeeding women referred to a clinic for nipple and breast pain fulfilled the clinical diagnosis for nipple candidosis (Tanquay et al., 1994). Thomassen et al. (1998) reported that 50% of women with superficial nipple pain and 20% of women with deep breast pain had positive cultures for *C. albicans*. Thus deep breast pain or shooting breast pain by itself may not be indicative of candidal infection within the breast (Carmichael & Dixon, 2002). In a healthy population of lactating women, Morrill et al. (2005) found 23% were colonized by *Candida* species on the nipple–areola or in their milk. The occurrence of mammary candidosis, defined as colonization plus symptoms, was 20% between 2 and 9 weeks postpartum. In the Morrill study, the rate of weaning by 9 weeks for this painful condition was 2.2 times higher in women who developed mammary candidosis. *C. albicans* was found more frequently in mothers who reported breastfeeding-associated pain (Andrews et al., 2007), possibly due to nipple alterations that predispose to candidal overgrowth.

Detecting *C. albicans* and diagnosing mammary candidosis can be difficult (Wiener, 2006). Accurate detection of candidal species in human milk is complicated by the action of lactoferrin. The lactoferrin in human milk inhibits yeast growth in vitro (Soukka, Tenovuo, & Lenander-Lumikari, 1992), often resulting in false-negative test results when the milk is cultured. Skin scrapings of the nipple–areola can be placed under a microscope in a 10% potassium hydroxide wet mount to identify the presence of yeast, yet few clinicians order any type of laboratory testing to identify and diagnose mammary candidosis (Brent, 2001).

A laboratory technique that uses the addition of iron to counteract the action of lactoferrin has been shown to reduce the likelihood of false-negative test results and provide a more accurate means of confirming the presence of *Candida* in human milk (Morrill et al., 2003). Accurate laboratory testing still takes about 3 days, leaving the mother in pain and validating the need for a more rapid means of determining when and how to treat the symptoms.

Mammary candidosis is most often diagnosed presumptively by signs and symptoms that are subjective, can be indicative of other problems, and are rarely confirmed by laboratory findings (Amir & Pakula, 1991; Johnstone & Marcinak, 1990). Signs include a nipple and/or areola that is red, shiny, or flaky, and symptoms include burning pain of the nipple–areola and deep, shooting, burning, or stabbing pain in the breast. In an effort to better delineate the signs and symptoms clinicians could use to determine treatment, Morrill, Heinig, Pappagianis, and Dewey (2004) used the measure of positive predictive value (PPV) for each sign and symptom. PPV was chosen as a measure because a PPV above 70% is considered to be of clinical value (Grimes & Schulz, 2002). The PPV was 50% or less for each of the signs and symptoms when they occurred individually. However, when certain combinations of signs and symptoms occurred, the PPV rose to over 70%, indicating that there was a high probability that the mother had *Candida*. These combinations of signs and symptoms are

- When the signs of shiny and flaky skin of the nipple–areola occurred together
- When either of the skin symptoms occurred together with nonstabbing or stabbing breast pain
- When combinations of three or more signs and symptoms occurred simultaneously, especially when the combination included either shiny or flaky skin of the nipple–areola

Treatment approaches should begin by assessing and correcting mechanical causes of nipple pain, including assessing for Raynaud phenomenon of the nipples (Amir, 2003), because sore nipples alone may not be indicative of *Candida*. If nipple pain persists after correction of breastfeeding techniques, bacterial infection may be present and can be treated with a topical antibiotic such as mupirocin (Bactroban). However, if the nipple pain worsens or is described as burning, a combined bacterial and fungal infection may be present to which a topical antifungal such as miconazole 2% can be added. Gentian violet, a strong purple dye that kills yeast on contact, can be painted on the nipples and areolae using a 0.5–1.0% strength aqueous solution for 4–7 days. At a higher concentration or used for a prolonged period of time, gentian violet has the potential for toxicity (Piatt & Bergeson, 1992). Therefore a dilution of 0.25–0.5% can be used in the infant's mouth once or twice daily for 3–7 days to avoid oral mucosal ulceration (Utter, 1990, 1992).

If signs and symptoms occur in any of the previous combinations or these treatments fail to address the problem, Newman's all-purpose nipple ointment (Newman, 2005) can be compounded in the following proportions:

Mupirocin 2% ointment (15 g)

Betamethasone 0.1% ointment (15 g)

Miconazole powder is added so that the final concentration is 2% miconazole

Newman's ointment should be applied sparingly after each feeding until the mother is pain free and then decreased over a week or 2 until the pain stops. If this topical treatment provides no pain relief in 3–4 days or is needed longer than 2–3 weeks to keep pain free, then the nipple–areolar skin and the milk should be tested.

Fluconazole (Diflucan) is a systemic agent that may be used when the previous treatments fail or when laboratory results confirm the presence of *Candida* in the milk. The loading dose is usually 400 mg followed by 100 mg twice daily for 2 weeks, until the mother is pain free for a week. It should be used in combination with Newman's topical nipple ointment, because fluconazole can take several days to start working. If there is no relief after 14–21 days of fluconazole treatment, the deep breast pain may have a different cause such as a bacterial infection. Some persistent or mismanaged cases of candidiasis may require a longer course of fluconazole, not only for the mother (Bodley & Powers, 1997) but also for the infant (Chetwynd et al., 2002). Both mother and infant should be treated simultaneously, even if thrush is not visible in the infant's mouth. There is a high correlation between oral and diaper candidosis among infants of mothers with nipple candidiasis (Tanguay et al., 1994). Mothers with deep breast pain may also benefit from anti-inflammatory pain medications such as ibuprofen.

Nystatin has long been used on both the nipples of the mother and the oral mucosa of the infant. However, its effective clinical cure rate for oral candidiasis has been reported to be only 54% in infants compared with a 99% cure rate when using miconazole (Hoppe & Hahn, 1996). Its effectiveness has been reduced over time, because almost 45% of *Candida* strains are resistant to nystatin (Hale & Berens, 2002). *C. albicans* persistently adheres to buccal mucosa and is less affected by nystatin than other *Candida* species (Ellepola, Panagoda, & Samaranayake, 1999). Nystatin is more fungistatic than fungicidal; thus it may reduce symptoms in some mothers and infants but can be ineffective in eradicating the infection.

Some mothers take acidophilus supplements (one tablet daily containing 40 million to 1 billion viable units) to help restore a balance of microorganisms in the body. Mothers may question if milk they expressed during a yeast infection can be given to the infant later. Under susceptible conditions, this milk may have the potential to infect or reinfect, because freezing does not kill yeast (Rosa et al., 1990), although lactoferrin may keep yeast levels low.

Panjaitan, Amir, Costs, Rudland, and Tabrizi (2008) demonstrated an association between *Candida* infection and nipple pain but identified other fungal species on sore nipples. This raised the possibility that nipple pain/thrush could be due to the presence of fungal organisms other than *C. albicans*.

Breastfeeding Management

Optimizing the mechanics of breastfeeding (positioning, latch, suck) continue to function as the first-line intervention for the prevention of both sore and damaged nipples (Morland-Schultz & Hill, 2005). Repetitive trauma from uncorrected faulty breastfeeding patterns may set the stage for breaks in skin integrity, which even when corrected may leave nipples in poor condition for healing.

Nipples that have been traumatized with breaks in skin integrity are easily colonized with bacterial and fungal species, are slow to heal, represent significant pain to the mother, and may lead to partial or total discontinuation of breastfeeding if therapeutic interventions do not provide quick relief. Topical antibiotics may be needed for rapid and effective resolution of pain and prevention of possible ascending infection into the breast itself. Because of the link between severe nipple soreness and colonization and infection of the nipple by *S. aureus* (Livingstone et al., 1996), careful washing of the nipple with soap and water and the application of mupirocin 2% ointment (Bactroban) may be effective in the early stages of the infection. Bacteria have the ability to grow in colonies and protect the colony with a coating called a biofilm. Biofilms may potentially be stimulated by saliva, such as when an infant feeds at the breast (Stewart & Costerton, 2001). To disrupt this protective biofilm, washing the nipple wound with soap and water once a day followed by a coating of mupirocin may penetrate the biofilm, promote wound healing, and prevent progression to an infection (Ryan, 2007). Because much nipple pain may stem from inflammation, topical application of low- to medium-strength steroids may provide welcome relief. No adverse effects have been reported when these types of preparations are used sparingly as thin coats to the nipples (Huggins & Billion, 1993). Systemic antibiotics may need to be added to the treatment regime if exudate is seen, erythema increases, or dry-scab formation is absent. Persistent sore nipples may be a combination of yeast and bacterial infection, causing difficulty in differentiating the offending organism. Some clinicians use miconazole 2% (Monistat) as the antifungal preparation in combination with the mupirocin and a topical steroid to ensure the best results (Porter & Schach, 2004). Tracing the source of infection when it persists or recurs may involve treating the infant with nasal mupirocin ointment if he or she is found to harbor the offending organism in the oropharynx (Livingstone & Stringer, 1999). Use of topical preparations on the nipple is consistent with the principles of moist wound healing.

Dry wound healing (air drying, sunlight, sun lamp, hair dryer, heat from a light bulb) has been advocated for many years. It was thought that continued tissue destruction and slower wound healing would occur if the nipples remained wet and that rapid drying would prevent this. However, close observation of damaged nipples usually reveals fissuring, which results from an insufficient amount of moisture in the stratum corneum (uppermost layer of the skin) and/or friction damage from the infant's sucking.

Treatment of nipple fissures is consistent with treating other types of skin fissures, which is to increase the moisture content of the skin and reduce further drying by applying an emollient to the damaged area (Sharp, 1992). An emollient is soothing and provides a moisture barrier that slows the evaporation of moisture naturally present in the skin, eliminating further drying and cracking. Scab formation does not occur when using moist wound healing. Rapid drying causes the stratum corneum to shrink in an irregular manner, placing tension on a layer of fragile tissue. The use of an emollient such as USP-modified anhydrous lanolin allows the contours of the stratum corneum to return to normal, enhancing the movement of cells across the wound as it heals. Sharp (1992) delineated a difference between surface skin moisture and internal moisture, stating that although a mother may pat the nipple area with a clean cloth to remove surface wetness, rapid drying can deplete the skin of internal moisture. He compared this with the act of licking dry chapped lips, which sets up a rapid wet-to-dry process that worsens the original condition. Some mothers or clinicians advocate the use of oils on the nipple skin (mineral, olive, other vegetable, vitamin E), which have not been shown to induce wound healing. Oils remain on the surface of the skin because they do not penetrate to deeper skin layers (dermis and subcutaneous) and are absorbed into the fabric of a nursing pad or bra. Fissured dry skin lacks moisture, not oil (Huml, 1994).

When observing treatment methods for wound healing on other parts of the body, occlusive or semiocclusive dressings are frequently used to cover the wound, maintain moisture, inhibit scab or crust formation, reduce pain, and enhance epithelial migration for wound repair (Ziemer, Cooper, & Pigeon, 1995). Ziemer et al. (1995) studied the prophylactic use of a polyethylene film dressing (BlisterFilm, Sherwood Medical) with an adhesive border on the occurrence of nipple skin damage during the first week of breastfeeding. Although significantly reducing pain, this dressing did not prevent skin changes and damage. A high dropout rate was seen due to skin pain and damage from the adhesive backing when the dressing was removed. No special breastfeeding instructions or corrections of feeding mechanics were provided for the mothers.

Building on the approach of using occlusive wound dressings for healing damaged nipples, Brent et al. (1998) randomized 42 mothers to receive a hydrogel wound dressing or a combination of breast shells and lanolin. The hydrogel dressing (Elasto-gel, Southwest Technologies, Inc.) was glycerine-based, highly absorbent, and nonadhesive with cooling properties. Breastfeeding technique was controlled for and help provided when needed. Mothers using the breast shells and lanolin experienced fewer breast infections and less pain than the group using the glycerin-based dressing. Cable, Stewart, and Davis (1997) used a water-based hydrogel dressing (ClearSite, New Dimensions in Medicine/ConMed) to avoid potential problems with breast infections associated with glycerin-based products. Mothers in their study experienced significant pain relief when the dressing was worn between feedings. The sheet was changed every 1–3 days until the nipple wound healed. Dodd and Chalmers (2003) compared the prophylactic use of lanolin with the water-based hydrogel dressing MaterniMates (Tyco Healthcare Group; currently marketed as Ameda ComfortGel, Ameda, Inc.). Mothers reported significantly lower pain scores when using the hydrogel dressing as a preventive measure, with no breast infections (vs. eight cases of mastitis in the lanolin group). Cadwell (2001) studied the use of a glycerin-based hydrogel dressing (Soothies, Puronyx, Inc.) compared with lanolin-application/breast-shell use in mothers presenting with established nipple pain and damage. Rates of healing between the two groups were similar, but the mothers using the hydrogel pads experienced markedly more relief from pain than the lanolin/shell group.

The moist wound healing options of lanolin and hydrogel dressings have been used both prophylactically to prevent nipple pain and damage and therapeutically as remedies. Lanolin may be a reasonable choice for sore or abraded nipples, whereas a hydrogel dressing may prove helpful for open sores or cracks with exudate. The dressing absorbs wound discharge and prevents the skin from adhering to the mother's bra. Lanolin use, however, has been associated with a longer healing time in mothers with sore nipples compared with the use of breastmilk (Mohammadzadeh, Farhat, & Esmaeily, 2005).

Prevention of sore, abraded, or cracked nipples is always preferable to treating the condition after the fact. Melli et al. (2007a) randomized 196 primiparous mothers to use either peppermint water or expressed breastmilk prophylactically on their nipples after feedings for the first 14 days after delivery. Nipple pain and damage were much less likely in the group of mothers using peppermint water compared with the group who used breastmilk, with peppermint water being three times more effective than expressed breastmilk. In a subsequent study, Melli et al. (2007b) randomized 163 primiparous mothers into three groups, one using purified lanolin, one using a peppermint gel, and one using a placebo gel after each feeding. The group using the peppermint gel had the lowest rates of nipple cracks; use of the peppermint gel was more effective than the use of peppermint water or any other of the interventions studied. Peppermint (*Mentha piperita*) has a calming and numbing effect and has been used to relieve skin irritations (Blumenthal, Goldberg, & Brinckmann, 2000). Peppermint also has antibacterial activity, increasing tissue flexibility and making tissue resistant to cracks (Schelz, Molnar, & Hohmann, 2006).

The best defense against *C. albicans* is healthy, intact skin and a robust immune system. Efforts should be made to ensure correct latch by the infant and assessment of any nipple pain reported by the mother. The longer incorrect sucking patterns persist, the greater the chance for both bacterial and fungal overgrowth of damaged nipple tissue. Pacifiers and bottles containing infant formulas should be avoided. Persistent nipple soreness, fissured nipples that are slow to heal, and nipples with obvious dermatological abnormalities must be addressed immediately. Clinicians may consider avoiding the use of nystatin, because it often prolongs the amount of time until the mother finds relief from the pain of a candidal infection. Unresolved nipple pain may cause untimely weaning (Schwartz et al., 2002). Both mother and infant should be treated if one or the other shows signs of candidiasis.

Engorgement[2]

Engorgement is a well-known but poorly researched aspect of lactation. Medical dictionaries define engorgement as congestion and/or distension with fluid. General lactation literature refers to engorgement as the physiological condition characterized by the painful swelling of the breasts associated with the sudden

---

[2]This section adapted with permission from Walker M. (2000). Breastfeeding and engorgement. *Breastfeeding Abstracts, 20*(2), 11–12.

increase in milk volume, lymphatic and vascular congestion, and interstitial edema during the first 2 weeks after birth. Engorgement is a normal physiological process with a progression of changes, not trauma or injury to tissues. When milk production increases rapidly, the volume of milk in the breast can exceed the capacity of the alveoli to store it. If the milk is not removed, overdistention of the alveoli can cause the milk-secreting cells to become flattened, drawn out, and even to rupture. The distention can partly or completely occlude the capillary blood circulation surrounding the alveolar cells, further decreasing cellular activity (Dawson, 1935). Congested blood vessels leak fluid into the surrounding tissue space, contributing to edema. Pressure and congestion obstruct lymphatic drainage of the breasts, stagnating the system that rids the breasts of toxins, bacteria, and cast-off cell parts, thereby predisposing the breast to mastitis (both inflammation and infection). In addition, a protein called the feedback inhibitor of lactation accumulates in the mammary gland during milk stasis, further reducing milk production (Prentice, Addey, & Wilde, 1989).

Accumulation of milk and the resulting engorgement are major triggers of apoptosis (programmed cell death) that causes involution of the milk-secreting gland, milk resorption, collapse of the alveolar structures, and the cessation of milk production (Marti, Feng, Altermatt, & Jaggi, 1997). A clinical sign of possible glandular involution may relate to descriptions of exceptionally thick or stringy milk being expressed from an engorged breast (Glover, 1998). This may represent milk inspissation (increased thickness or decreased fluidity) secondary to fluid resorption and an accumulation of fat cells in the gland (Weichert, 1980). Engorgement has also been classified as involving only the areola, only the body of the breast, or both. Areolar engorgement involves clinical observations of a swollen areola with tight, shiny skin, probably involving overfull lactiferous ducts. A puffy areola is thought to be tissue edema, possibly contributed by large amounts of intravenous fluids received by some mothers during labor.

Some degree of breast engorgement is normal. Minimal or no engorgement in the first week postpartum has been associated with insufficient milk (Neifert et al., 1990; Newton & Newton, 1951), early supplementation, and a higher percentage of breastfeeding decline in the early weeks (Humenick, Hill, & Anderson, 1994). Delayed onset of copious milk production, judged by mothers as breast fullness or engorgement, is of equal importance as the overfull breast. Excess infant weight loss was shown to be 7.1 times greater if the mother experienced delayed onset of lactation (Dewey et al., 2003). Rates of delayed engorgement (over 72 hours after birth) range between 22% (Dewey et al., 2003) and 31%

(Chapman & Perez-Escamilla, 1999) of breastfeeding mothers. Risk factors for this delay include primiparity (Chapman & Perez-Escamilla, 1999), cesarean section (Chapman & Perez-Escamilla, 1999; Vestermark et al., 1991), stress during labor and delivery (Chen, Nommsen-Rivers, Dewey, & Lonnerdal, 1998; Dewey, 2001), maternal diabetes (Hartmann & Cregan, 2001), and high maternal body mass index (Dewey et al., 2003; Rasmussen, Hilson, & Kjolhede, 2001). Presence of these risk factors should initiate intensive provision of lactation care and services to ensure adequate infant weight gain and the preservation of breastfeeding.

Also of concern are the moderate to severe degrees of engorgement, because painful breasts are concerns of new mothers (Hill, Humenick, & West, 1994). Objective methods to measure engorgement have appeared in the literature and include measurements of chest circumference changes (Newton & Newton, 1951), thermography (Menczer & Eskin, 1969), use of a pressure gauge to measure skin tension (Ferris, 1990, 1996; Geissler, 1967; Riedel, 1991), and mothers' self-ratings (Hill & Humenick, 1994; Moon & Humenick, 1989). Rates of engorgement between 20% and 85% have been reported in the literature, encompassing numerous definitions and usually limited to the first few days postpartum. Such reports described engorgement as peaking between days 3 and 6 and declining thereafter. However, data from two unpublished master's theses suggested that mothers actually experience more than one peak of engorgement (Csar, 1991) and that engorgement may continue for as long as 10 days or more (Riedel, 1991).

Four patterns of engorgement have been described: (1) firm, tender breasts followed by a resolution of symptoms; (2) multiple peaks of engorgement followed by resolution; (3) intense and painful engorgement lasting up to 14 days; and (4) minimal breast changes. These demonstrate that the experience of engorgement is not the same for all mothers (Humenick et al., 1994).

Predicting an individual mother's risk for and course of engorgement may not be possible, but some general principles may be of help in anticipating situations that predispose to a higher risk:

- A failure to prevent or resolve milk stasis resulting from infrequent or inadequate drainage of the breasts. The higher the cumulative number of minutes of sucking during the early days postpartum, the less pain from engorgement mothers describe (Evans, Evans, & Simmer, 1995; Moon & Humenick, 1989).

- Mothers with small breasts (other than hypoplastic and tubular). Although small breast size does not limit milk production, it can influence storage capacity and feeding patterns. Mothers with small breasts may need to engage in a greater number of breastfeedings over 24 hours than women with a larger milk storage capacity (Daly & Hartmann, 1995). Robson (1990) described a similar observation in engorged women who wore a significantly smaller bra cup size (34%) than women who did not become engorged (12.5%).

- Previous breastfeeding experience. Second-time breastfeeding mothers experience greater levels of engorgement sooner with faster resolution than do first-time breastfeeding mothers. Breast engorgement for multiparous mothers breastfeeding for the first time was similar to primiparous breastfeeding mothers (Hill & Humenick, 1994). Robson (1990) found that mothers in a nonengorged group were more likely to have never experienced engorgement after previous births than mothers in the engorged group. McLachlan, Milne, Lumley, and Walker (1993) found that 70% of multiparous mothers experiencing engorgement in a current lactation had also experienced engorgement with previous infants.

- Mothers with high rates of milk synthesis (hyperlactation) (Livingstone, 1996) or large amounts of milk. Mothers of multiples may see milk stasis magnified if infants consume less milk, if less milk is pumped, or whenever milk volume significantly exceeds milk removal.

- Limited mother–infant contact in the early days. Shiau (1997) demonstrated significantly less engorgement on day 3 in mothers who participated in skin-to-skin care of their full-term infants rather than standard nursery care.

Numerous strategies to reduce or prevent engorgement have been seen over the years. Mothers experience less-severe forms of engorgement with early frequent feedings (Newton & Newton, 1951), self-demand feedings (Illingworth & Stone, 1952), unlimited sucking times (Slaven & Harvey, 1981), thorough breast drainage (Evans et al., 1995), and with infants who demonstrate correct suckling techniques (Righard & Alade, 1992). Short, frequent feeds were shown to increase engorgement in one study (Moon & Humenick, 1989) probably because abbreviated feeds for as short as 2 minutes did not allow sufficient drainage of the breasts to prevent milk accumulation.

A more effective technique, called alternate breast massage, has been shown to significantly reduce the incidence and severity of engorgement while simultaneously increasing milk intake, increasing the fat content of the milk, and increasing infant weight gain (Bowles, Stutte, & Hensley, 1987; Iffrig, 1968; Stutte, Bowles, &

Morman, 1988). Alternate massage is a simple technique of massaging and compressing the breast during the infant's pause between sucking bursts. The technique alternates with the infant's sucking and is continued throughout the feeding on both breasts.

Treatment Modalities for Engorgement: Fact Versus Fiction

A plethora of treatment modalities for engorgement has been put forward, both anecdotally and in lactation literature. Some of the most commonly proposed treatments follow.

Heat Therapy

Heat application in the form of hot compresses, hot showers, or hot soaks is poorly researched and has usually been more of a comfort measure to activate the milk ejection reflex rather than a treatment for edema. Some mothers complain that heat exacerbates the engorgement and causes throbbing and an increased feeling of fullness (Robson, 1990).

Cold Therapy

Cold applications in the form of ice packs, gel packs, frozen bags of vegetables, frozen wet towels, and the like have been studied under various application conditions. Cold application triggers a cycle of vasoconstriction during the first 9–16 minutes in which blood flow is reduced, local edema decreases, and lymphatic drainage is enhanced (Hocutt, Jaffe, Rylander, & Beebe, 1982). This is followed by a deep-tissue vasodilation phase lasting 4–6 minutes that prevents thermal injury (Barnes, 1979). Robson (1990) discussed that the application of cold for 20 minutes would have a minimal vasoconstriction effect in the deeper breast tissue and that venous and lymphatic drainage would be enhanced in the deeper tissues due to the accelerated circulation to and from the superficial tissues. Sandberg (1998) reported on the application of cold packs for 20 minutes before each feeding on a small sample of women. Mothers reported increased comfort (compared with heat), decreased chest circumference, and no adverse effect on milk ejection or milk transfer.

Ultrasound

Thermal (continuous) ultrasound treatments of engorged breasts has not been shown to have objective beneficial effects on engorgement (McLachlan et al., 1993); however, mothers have found ultrasound to be comforting (Fetherston, 1997).

Lymphatic Breast Drainage Therapy

This is a gentle massage of the lymphatic drainage channels in the breast. Lymphatic drainage is thought to improve the movement of the stagnated fluid, to reduce edema, and to improve cellular function (Chikly, 1999; Upledger Institute, n.d.). Wilson-Clay and Hoover (2002) reported the relief of discomfort and better subsequent milk yields during pumping of three women with unrelieved severe engorgement after manual lymphatic drainage therapy. No data could be found regarding the remote possibility of moving cancer cells into lymphatic circulation by massaging the breast toward the axilla.

Chilled Cabbage Leaves

Rosier (1988) anecdotally described the use of chilled cabbage leaves applied to engorged breasts and changed every 2 hours in a small sample of women as having a rapid effect on reducing edema and increasing milk flow. Nikodem et al. (1993) showed a nonsignificant trend in reduced engorgement in mothers using cabbage leaves. Roberts (1995) compared chilled cabbage leaves and gel packs, showing similar significant reduction in pain with both methods, with two-thirds of the mothers preferring the cabbage due to a stronger, more immediate effect. Roberts, Reiter, and Schuster (1998) studied the use of cabbage extract cream applied to the breasts and found no more effect than the placebo cream.

Expressing Milk

Refraining from expressing milk because the mother will "just make more milk" cannot be justified. Hand expressing or pumping to comfort reduces the buildup of feedback inhibitor of lactation; decreases the mechanical stress on the alveoli, preventing the cell death process; prevents blood circulation changes; alleviates the impedance to lymph and fluid drainage; decreases the risk of mastitis and compromised milk production; and feels good to the mother. It is not known what degree of engorgement or duration of milk stasis poses an unrecoverable situation. The milk production in the alveoli not experiencing engorgement continues normally. The breast is capable of compensating to a point; future research will delineate this further.

Breastfeeding Management

Unrestricted, frequent, and effective breastfeedings contribute to the occurrence of lactogenesis II by 72 hours postpartum. Physiological engorgement is part of a continuum for abundant milk production. Efforts to relieve excessive congestion in the breast should not be delayed. Anti-inflammatory medication (the enzyme serrapeptase) has been shown to relieve some of the discomfort and symptoms of engorgement (Kee, Tan, & Salmon, 1989; Snowden, Renfrew, & Woolridge, 2001). An overfull breast with flattening of the areola may make latching difficult and painful. Mothers may need to hand express or pump milk before placing the infant at the breast. An edematous areola benefits from reverse pressure softening for easier latch. Most mothers find relief from the use of cold compresses, frequent milk removal, and anti-inflammatory medication for discomfort.

Plugged Ducts

Many breastfeeding women encounter tender small lumps in their breasts, usually related to the blockage of a milk duct. The lump may also have reddened skin over it and be warm to the touch. The exact cause is unknown. Clinicians have speculated that a large milk supply or pressure on the outside of the breasts, such as from purse straps, backpack straps, or an ill-fitting bra, could result in a physical obstruction of milk flow and a local collection of milk products that are too large to move down the small ductwork. Fetherston (1998) identified breastmilk that appeared thicker than normal as a predictor for blocked ducts in multiparous women. Eglash (1998) described a mother with repeated plugged ducts who routinely experienced a long delay in the milk ejection reflex at each feeding. Poor milk flow may subsequently ensue from the area of the breasts experiencing the blockage, contributing to milk stasis behind the plug. This focal area of engorgement used to be referred to as a caked breast.

Focal engorgement from a blocked duct may cause a segment of the breast to become swollen, firm, and tender. Milk secretions that remain blocked from exiting the breast may become inspissated (thickened by absorption of fluid). Milk expressed from the breast experiencing plugged ducts may contain the displaced material from the plug that is often of a fatty composition. Strings that resemble spaghetti or lengths of fatty-looking material have been described (Minchin, 1985). Ductal blockage from this material may account for the sometimes ropy texture of the breast upon palpation over the obstructed area. The observation of fatty material from the blockage has led clinicians to recommend the addition of lecithin to the maternal diet (Lawrence & Lawrence, 2005). Lecithin is a phospholipid and is used by the food industry as an emulsifier. An emulsifier keeps fat dispersed and suspended in water rather than aggregated in a fatty mass. One tablespoon per day of oral granular lecithin has been reported to relieve plugged ducts and to prevent their recurrence (Eglash, 1998; Lawrence & Lawrence, 2005).

Breastfeeding Management

Plugged ducts may also respond well to the use of a warm compress and direct massage over the lump while the infant is sucking. Ultrasound has been shown to be ineffective as a treatment for plugged ducts (Campbell & Smillie, 2003; Snowden et al., 2001). Massage over and/or behind the blockage has been a traditional recommendation to reduce and disperse the material obstructing the duct. A different approach has been recommended whereby the mother massages in front of the lump toward the nipple (Smillie, 2004). The mother begins the massage close to the nipple, repositions the massage farther back until she is massaging directly in front of the blockage (Campbell, 2006). This is thought to help clear the way through convoluted ductwork that may not be in straight alignment to the nipple. Plugged ducts require prompt attention, because they can start a cascade of events that leads to breast inflammation and breast infection (Kinlay, O'Connell, & Kinlay, 2001).

Mastitis

Mastitis is an inflammatory condition of the breast that may eventually or concurrently involve an infection (Walker, 2004). Confusion can arise in defining mastitis, because the words "mastitis" and "infection" are often used interchangeably. Mastitis the inflammation is often treated as if it were an infection. Thomsen, Espersen, and Maigaard (1984) microscopically examined milk to differentiate between milk stasis, inflammation, and infection. The diagnosis of an infection was made by observing and counting (not culturing) leukocytes and bacteria in milk samples to identify three clinical states, recommending antibiotics for the last classification only:

1. Milk stasis: $<10^6$ leukocytes and $<10^3$ bacteria/mL of milk
2. Noninfectious inflammation: $>10^6$ leukocytes and $<10^3$ bacteria/mL of milk
3. Infectious mastitis: $>10^6$ leukocytes and $>10^3$ bacteria/mL of milk

Most clinicians do not observe milk or use laboratory results but rely on a cluster of signs and symptoms to diagnose mastitis the infection (Freed, Landers, & Schanler, 1991; Lawrence & Lawrence, 2005; Niebyl, Spence, & Parmley, 1978):

- Fever of 101°F (38.4°C)
- Flu-like aching
- Nausea
- Chills
- Pain or swelling at the site
- Red, tender, hot area, often wedge shaped
- Red streaks extending toward the axilla (inflammation of the lymphatics may indicate a more generalized infection of the breast)
- Increased pulse rate
- Increased sodium levels in the milk; seen as the infant possibly rejecting the affected side due to the salty taste of the milk

Sometimes, signs and symptoms of breast complaints such as engorgement, plugged ducts, noninfectious mastitis, and infectious mastitis overlap, with each process having some element related to obstructed milk flow, making differential diagnosis difficult (Betzold, 2007). When drainage of breastmilk is blocked, paracellular pathways open, allowing for the leakage of cytokines that can induce fever chills, muscle aches, and general malaise. This state can provide the clinical impression of an infective process whether or not there is actual infection present.

The incidence of mastitis (of any definition) ranges between 1% and 33% (Inch, 1997), depending on the duration of the study. Studies that contained data up to 3 months postpartum showed the incidence of mastitis ranging from 2.9% to 24% (Evans & Heads, 1995; Hesseltine, Freundlich, & Hite, 1948; Jonsson & Pulkkinen, 1994; Kaufmann & Foxman, 1991; Nicholson & Yuen, 1995). Riordan and Nichols (1990) reported a 33% incidence of mastitis in a retrospective study that spanned the entire lactation period of the mothers, including durations exceeding 12 months.

Breast infections are the most common breast-related complaint seen by physicians during pregnancy and the postpartum period (Scott-Conner & Schorr, 1995). The highest occurrence of mastitis is generally at 2–3 weeks postpartum (Inch, 1997), with the bulk of cases developing within the first 12 weeks of breastfeeding (Riordan & Nichols, 1990). However, mastitis can occur at any time during the course of lactation, frequently occurring during the winter months (Evans & Heads, 1995). Bilateral mastitis occurs much less frequently than unilateral infection, ranging from 3% to 12% of cases (Evans & Heads, 1995; Inch & Fisher, 1995; Moon & Gilbert, 1935; Riordan, 1983; Riordan & Nichols, 1990). Although most cases of mastitis involve *S. aureus* as the causative organism (Osterman & Rahm, 2000), other organisms, such as beta-hemolytic streptococcus, may also be involved. Kenny (1977) described a case of recurrent group B beta-hemolytic streptococcal infection in an infant whose mother also presented with bilateral mastitis positive for group B beta-hemolytic streptococcal. Because bilateral mastitis is relatively rare, clinicians may wish to culture the milk from both breasts should this condition occur.

Human milk is not sterile (Carroll et al., 1979); the areolae, breast skin, and milk ducts are also not sterile. Bacterial counts of pathological and nonpathological bacteria have been noted to be indistinguishable between the mastitic and nonmastitic breast in women with unilateral mastitis (Matheson et al., 1988). The presence of bacteria does not necessarily indicate or precipitate a breast infection. Kvist, Larsson, Hall-Lord, Steen, and Schalen (2008) demonstrated that many healthy mothers have potentially pathogenic bacteria in their breastmilk and do not go on to develop mastitis. There generally needs to be some other condition or risk factor present for developing either a breast inflammation or infection. The following are some precipitating factors:

- Nipple damage/cracked nipple.
- Infant is a nasal carrier of *S. aureus* (Amir, Garland, & Lumley, 2006).
- Plugged milk ducts.
- Milk stasis.
- Blocked nipple pore.
- Hyperlactation or a high rate of milk synthesis.
- Insulin-dependent diabetes mellitus (IDDM): Neubauer, Ferris, and Hinckley (1990) studied milk from 67 breasts of mothers with IDDM and 114 breasts of non-IDDM lactating mothers. Mastitis was categorized according to leukocyte and bacteria counts according to the parameters established by Thomsen et al. (1984). Although the incidence of infectious mastitis was similar, significantly more mothers with IDDM (20.9% vs. 1.8%) tested positive for noninfectious inflammation. This may serve to remind the clinician that mothers with IDDM need to breastfeed frequently with no delays

in initiation of breastfeeding and usually require closer monitoring for correct breastfeeding management and techniques.

- Nipple piercing: In the months after this procedure, infection, mastitis, and abscess formation have been reported to be as high as 10–20%, with healing of the wound channel taking 6–12 months (Jacobs et al., 2003). Because some nipple piercings take up to 18 months to heal, the potential for scar tissue development could interfere with milk transfer, cause sore nipples, or contribute to plugged ducts and mastitis. Clinicians are reminded to check pierced nipples for numbness, discharge, hypersensitivity, healing, and scar tissue (Martin, 2004). Some mothers regret the piercing and seek to reverse it. A surgical procedure that excises the epithelial tunnel core can be performed with minimal damage to the surrounding tissue (Sadove & Clayman, 2008).

- Reduced concentration of secretory IgA: Secretory IgA is a defense component within the breast and has been shown to increase in concentration during mastitis (Fetherston, Lai, & Hartmann, 2006). Low levels of secretory IgA have been found in the milk of mothers with recurrent mastitis as well as in mothers with recurrent plugged ducts (Fetherston, 2001; Fetherston et al., 2006; Lawrence & Lawrence, 2005).

Other factors appear to be associated with mastitis rather than being causative, such as full-time employment (Kaufmann & Foxman, 1991), maternal stress or fatigue (Riordan & Nichols, 1990), poor nutrition, anemia (Dever, 1992), tight bra (Fetherston, 1998) or restrictive clothing, and use of nipple creams (Jonsson & Pulkkinen, 1994).

Subclinical Mastitis

Subclinical mastitis is usually described as an elevated milk sodium-to-potassium ratio that rises from 5–6 mmol/L of sodium in normal human milk to 12–20 mmol/L of sodium, often in association with the presence of inflammatory cytokines. Studies of subclinical mastitis in human mothers have shown that even though there may be no apparent clinical symptoms, biochemical changes occur in the milk. Increased sodium levels are also seen in colostrum, during weaning, in mastitis the infection, and in preterm mother's milk. Milk stasis may contribute to subclinical mastitis by promoting inflammation if there is a local adverse immune response to milk proteins left in contact with breast epithelium for prolonged periods of time (Michie et al., 2003). After that, changes might occur in the tight junctions between luminal epithelial cells, with a resultant leak of sodium, inflammatory cells, and other mediators into the milk.

The mammary gland has protective capabilities to modulate inflammation in the mammary alveoli (Semba et al., 1999c) and uses the natural defense mechanisms of nipple skin integrity and the flushing action of milk flow during the milk ejection reflex. However, bacteria may be able to resist or overcome these mechanisms by adhering to damaged epithelial cells lining the ducts and nipple pores, perhaps through trauma or the conditions presented by milk stasis (Fetherston, 2001). With ultrasound imaging of the lactating breast showing a reverse flow of breastmilk within the ducts after the end of a milk ejection reflex (Ramsay et al., 2004), backward milk flow (away from the nipple) into the smaller collecting ducts could possibly carry bacteria with it.

Subclinical mastitis has been associated with decreased milk production, slow infant weight gain (Filteau et al., 1999b; Morton, 1994), mixed feeding (breastmilk and formula) (Willumsen et al., 2000), and increased cell counts. In HIV-infected mothers, this increases the risk of elevated milk viral loads, a risk factor for vertical transmission of HIV (Semba et al., 1999a, 1999b; Willumsen et al., 2000). There appears to be a spectrum or continuum of pathology from mild changes initiated by milk stasis, which, if left unchecked or improperly treated, progresses through subclinical mastitis, clinically evident mastitis the inflammation, mastitis the infection, and, at its worst, abscess formation (Walker, 2004).

Interventions to prevent subclinical mastitis have been shown to significantly reduce the occurrence of elevated sodium-to-potassium ratios.

- Basic lactation counseling on exclusive breastfeeding for 4–6 months, correct position and latch, feeding on cue, and early breastfeeding after delivery resulted in a 14% decrease in sodium-to-potassium elevations in a group of 60 women counseled on simple lactation practices compared with a control group of 66 women who did not receive early breastfeeding counseling (Flores & Filteau, 2002).

- Because antioxidant micronutrient status in dairy cattle has been related to mastitis, studies have examined if supplementing human mothers with antioxidants might prevent subclinical mastitis. Supplementation with retinol and beta-carotene did not reduce inflammation (Filteau et al., 1999b), but supplementation with sunflower oil, a potent source of vitamin E, reduced the incidence of mastitis among women in a study from Tanzania (Filteau et al., 1999a).

- Although most attempts at vaccination against mastitis have met with little to no success, a vaccine based on newer technology has suggested some protection for those mothers at risk for recurrent mastitis (Shinefield et al., 2002).

- Antisecretory factor (AF) can be produced in the mammary gland and seems to have an anti-inflammatory effect by reducing fluid secretion (Hanson, 2004). AF has been found in samples of milk from mothers in developing countries, possibly because the mother herself was challenged with enterotoxin-producing bacteria (Hanson et al., 2000). A preliminary study showed a significant reduction in the prevalence of mastitis in Swedish women that resulted when AF was induced in their milk through the ingestion of a specially treated cereal (Svensson et al., 2004). Eventually, if AF can be shown to reliably prevent subclinical mastitis, it may be used to reduce the risk of transfer of HIV-1 from mother to infant via breastfeeding.

Recurrent Mastitis

Mastitis most frequently recurs when the bacteria are resistant or not sensitive to the prescribed antibiotic, when antibiotics are not continued long enough, when an incorrect antibiotic is prescribed, when the mother stopped nursing on the affected side, or when the initial cause of the mastitis was not addressed (such as milk stasis). *Staphylococcus epidermidis* is also a prevalent staphylococcal species isolated from breastmilk of women with mastitis, where it is present at a concentration notably higher than that present in milk of healthy women (Delgado et al., 2008). The percentage of strains showing biofilm production ability and resistance to mupirocin, erythromycin, clindamycin, and/or methicillin was significantly higher among those obtained from women with lactational mastitis than among those isolated from healthy women (Delgado et al., 2009). The resistance to many antibiotics and its propensity to form protective biofilms may help explain chronic or recurrent episodes of mastitis when this organism is present. Clinicians usually recommend that the mother continues to feed (or pump) on the affected side, that she rest, that she take a full 10- to 14-day course of antibiotics, and that the cause or precipitating factors be identified and remedied. If mastitis recurs, Lawrence and Lawrence (2005) recommended milk culture and sensitivity testing as well as cultures of the infant's nasopharynx and oropharynx to determine the offending organism and to what antibiotic it is sensitive. Milk cultures should be taken if the mastitis is unresponsive to antibiotics after 2 days (Spencer, 2008) because organisms can be resistant to multiple medications

(Betzold, 2005). Other family members may sometimes need to be cultured to determine the vector for transmission to keep it from reinfecting the mother. Infants who are nasal carriers of *S. aureus* should be identified and can be treated with mupirocin 2% (Bactroban nasal ointment) (Amir, 2002). If the infection seems to be chronic, low-dose antibiotics can be instituted for the duration of the lactation (erythromycin 500 mg/day) (Lawrence & Lawrence, 2005). If the locus of the infection occurs more than two or three times in the same location, a closer follow-up and evaluation must be done to rule out an underlying mass (Academy of Breastfeeding Medicine, 2004).

Identifying and treating the underlying cause of inflammatory signs and symptoms in the breast may halt the progression to an infection. If the mother has a low-grade fever, aching, red splotches, and a painful area in the breast, she may find relief from use of a nonsteroidal anti-inflammatory drug such as ibuprofen. Underlying causes should be explored and remedied (see Appendix 8-1). If there is no improvement within 8–24 hours, if the mother continues to run a fever, if the fever suddenly rises or spikes, if she develops flu-like symptoms, if she feels ill, or if she has obvious signs of a bacterial infection such as discharge of pus from the nipple, then she needs to call her care provider, who will usually prescribe a 10- to 14-day course of antibiotics.

Bacterial Pathogens

Because *S. aureus* is the most common organism associated with mastitis, penicillinase-resistant penicillins or cephalosporins are usually the initial drugs of choice. Antibiotic selection may include dicloxacillin (for non–methicillin-resistant *S. aureus*), clindamycin (for many community-acquired methicillin-resistant *S. aureus* [MRSA]), erythromycin and azithromycin for penicillin-allergic mothers, trimethoprim-sulfamethoxazole for some community-acquired MRSA, and cephalexin for methicillin-susceptible *S. aureus*. Mothers should take the antibiotic for the full course prescribed even if they start feeling better within 24 hours. Improvement in the mother's condition may be due to the antibiotics but not necessarily because they are eliminating an infection. Antibiotics are effective anti-inflammatory drugs (even though they are not used for that purpose). Mothers who are treated with antibiotics when they do not have a laboratory-confirmed infection experience improvement in their situation, but the underlying cause of the inflammatory process must be addressed because it will return if left unresolved. Repeated treatments with antibiotics of mastitis the inflammation can lead to bacterial resistance to antibiotics. Jimenez et al. (2008) treated mothers with mastitis with probiotics as an alternative.

More recently, community-acquired MRSA has emerged as an increasingly common pathogen in cases of mastitis and abscesses (Reddy, Qi, Zembower, Noskin, & Bolon, 2007; Saiman et al., 2003). Delayed nipple wound healing, stress, chronic engorgement, persistent breast pain, breast masses, with or without fever predispose mothers to mastitis and abscesses, making them easy prey to more virulent pathogens. Increased risk for hospital-acquired MRSA is seen in mothers with a cesarean delivery, administration of antibiotics in the peripartum period, mothers with multiple gestation, and mothers who have experienced in vitro fertilization (Behari, Englund, Alcasid, Garcia-Houchins, & Weber, 2004; Gastelum, Dassey, Mascola, & Yasuda, 2005; Morel et al., 2002). Delay in antibiotic therapy for mastitis, incorrect antibiotic choice, inadequate courses of antibiotics, and lack of culture and sensitivity testing of milk cultures and infant nasal swabs raise the risk of complications of mastitis such as abscesses (Wilson-Clay, 2008).

Milk production in the affected breast may decrease during the few days of florid symptoms (Wambach, 2003) and for a period of days beyond that time (Matheson et al., 1988). This may be due to the infant rejecting that breast or from a drop in lactose and problems with milk synthesis from alveolar tissue damage (Fetherston, 2001). Infants can consume milk from the mastitic breast because it contains the same anti-inflammatory components and characteristics found in normal milk. Elevations occur in certain factors that protect the infant from developing clinical illness due to consuming mastitic milk (Buescher & Hair, 2001).

Breasts that have undergone augmentation can also demonstrate signs of inflammatory or infective processes, such as swelling, tenderness, or induration around the prosthesis itself (Johnson & Hanson, 1996). *S. aureus* infections tend to be more localized and invasive. Streptococcus infections are often more diffuse with abscess formation in advanced stages (Sabate et al., 2007).

Breastfeeding Management

General breastfeeding guidelines during mastitis involve bed rest and increased fluids for the mother. Pain medication such as ibuprofen can be used because it also acts as an anti-inflammatory in conjunction with antibiotics. If antibiotics are prescribed, they should be taken for a full 10–14 days. Shorter courses or courses that are stopped by the mother because she feels better may lead to recurrence.

Some mothers find that hot compresses before feedings feel good and help elicit the milk ejection reflex. Mothers should continue breastfeeding on both sides, starting on the affected side and using alternate massage. If pain affects the let-down, the mother can start on the unaffected side to achieve milk ejection, then switch to and thoroughly drain the affected side. If the infant is unable or unwilling to feed from the affected side, then the infected breast should be pumped.

Complementary and alternative therapies have been recommended:

- Hot castor oil packs. Preheat a heating pad. A washcloth that has been dampened with hot water is placed on a sheet of plastic wrap. A table-spoonful of castor oil is poured on the cloth and spread around. This preparation is placed over the affected area of the breast with the heating pad over it while the mother lies down and rests for at least 20 minutes. The oil should be washed off of the nipple before the next feeding.

- Homeopathics. Phytolacca 30C every 3–4 hours; belladonna 30C every 3–4 hours; other homeopathic options include Hepar sulphuris and *Bellis perennis* (Barbosa-Cesnik, Schwartz, & Foxman, 2003).

- Acupuncture has been suggested as a potential remedy as has the use of oxytocin nasal spray to enhance the milk ejection reflex, which may be less effective due to distended milk ducts (Kvist, Hall-Lord, & Larsson, 2007).

Cracked nipples are frequently reported to accompany mastitis, either causative or co-existing (Amir, Forster, Lumley, & McLachlan, 2007; Kvist et al., 2007; Scott, Robertson, Fitzpatrick, Knight, & Mulholland, 2008), making it imperative that clinicians endeavor to provide guidance in their prevention or offer effective interventions for their timely resolution.

Breast Abscess

A breast abscess can be an infrequent complication of mastitis resulting from untreated, delayed, inadequate, or incorrect treatment of mastitis. An abscess is a walled-off localized collection of pus that lacks an outlet for the material from the affected area. Once encapsulated, it requires surgical drainage. Risk factors also include prior episodes of mastitis, avoiding breastfeeding on the affected side, or acute weaning. Estimates of the incidence of breast abscess among lactating women range from 0.04% (Waller, 1946) to 11% (Devereux, 1970). Calculation of the actual incidence is complicated by the varied definitions used for mastitis;

however, in laboratory-confirmed cases of mastitis the infection, 2.8% of mothers with mastitis went on to develop an abscess (Thomsen et al., 1984).

In an Australian study of women with mastitis, 3% of women were estimated to develop an abscess (Amir, Forster, McLachlan, & Lumley, 2004). Primiparous women appear to be at a greater risk for abscess as well as mothers over the age of 30 and those who give birth after term (Kvist & Rydhstroem, 2005). Benson and Goodman (1970) classified abscesses as subareolar 23% (superficial and near the nipple), intramammary unilocular 12% (a single area of pus deep in the breast and away from the nipple), and intramammary/multilocular 65% (having multiple sites of pus within the abscess). The most common offending organism is *S. aureus* (World Health Organization, 2000), although other organisms are occasionally cultured from an abscess, such as *Pseudomonas aeruginosa* (Bertrand & Rosenblood, 1991; Dixon, 1988; Karstrup et al., 1993).

Of abscesses containing *S. aureus*, over 50% can be MRSA, with trimethoprim-sulfamethoxazole (Proloprim) often being the antibiotic of choice (Moazzez et al., 2007). Lawrence and Lawrence (2005) reminded clinicians that any abscess drainage should be cultured and antibiotic sensitivities determined due to the increasing number of oxacillin-resistant *S. aureus* and MRSA infections occurring in hospitals. An infection with oxacillin-resistant *S. aureus* and MRSA may require the use of vancomycin, clindamycin, or rifampin therapy and may start as an inflammation of the lymphatics in the breast.

Delay in seeking treatment for a breast infection is consistently associated with poor lactation outcomes (Bertrand & Rosenblood, 1991; Devereux, 1970; Matheson et al., 1988; Thomsen et al., 1984; Walsh, 1949). However, antibiotic treatment of mastitis does not always prevent abscess formation (Rench & Baker, 1989). It is not always possible to confirm the existence of an abscess by clinical examination or mammography. Ultrasound is typically used to diagnose the presence of an abscess and to mark the site for either surgical drainage (Hayes, Michell, & Nunnerley, 1991) or needle or catheter aspiration and drainage. Surgical drainage of an abscess has been mostly replaced by needle drainage and appropriate antibiotics in abscesses less than 3 cm in diameter (Dener & Inan, 2003; Dixon, 1988; Hook & Ikeda, 1999; Karstrup et al., 1993; O'Hara, Dexter, & Fox, 1996) and catheter placement and drainage in abscesses 3 cm or larger (Ulitzsch, Nyman, & Carlson, 2004). Needle aspiration or catheter placement also has the advantage that mothers and infants are not separated because the condition is treated on an outpatient basis. Abscess treatment and resolution should be followed closely, because breast masses and inflammatory breast cancer can also masquerade as an abscess.

Breastfeeding Management

Breastfeeding can and should continue during and after the period of treatment (Cantile, 1988; Dixon, 1988; Karstrup et al., 1993) because it promotes drainage of the affected segment and helps resolve the infection. Weaning or inhibiting lactation may actually hinder the rapid resolution of the abscess by contributing to the production of increasingly viscid fluid that tends to promote rather than reduce breast engorgement (Benson, 1989). Breastfeeding should continue from the affected side unless the abscess is so close to the areola that the infant's mouth would cover it during feeding. If the infant will not feed from the affected side, the breast should be pumped. Changes in protein, carbohydrate, and electrolyte concentrations from an affected breast may decrease the level of lactose and cause a rise in sodium and chloride concentrations (Connor, 1979; Prosser & Hartmann, 1983), making the milk taste salty. The onset of mastitis can be rapid, with many negative emotions elicited surrounding the continuation of breastfeeding (Amir & Lumley, 2006). Mothers need close ongoing support for the resolution of mastitis and the prevention of its recurrence.

Additional Breast-Related Conditions

A number of other breast and nipple-related conditions may occur as a result of, or concurrently with, lactation.

Galactoceles and Other Breast Lumps

Galactoceles are localized collections of milk formed as a result of ductal obstruction (Stevens et al., 1997; Winkler, 1964). These tend to be smooth, mobile, tender masses that during and shortly after lactation are filled with milk. As time passes the water portion of the milk is reabsorbed by the body, leaving thickened, cheesy material that can be aspirated. Several aspirations may be required, because the cysts tend to refill with milk. The cysts form as a result of duct dilatation and may be surrounded by a fibrous capsule that can be associated with inflammation. Rare infections of the galactocele are possible. Surgical removal is seldom necessary.

Galactoceles can be painful but do not preclude breastfeeding. Bevin and Persok (1993) described a case study of a mother with a long-standing galactocele behind the left areola. This mother experienced multiple episodes of plugged ducts, mastitis, and ultimately an abscess, with antibiotics at one time causing temporary disappearance of the galactocele. Squeezing or compressing the galactocele can cause milk release from the nipple but does not completely evacuate the cyst. Clinicians need to be vigilant when a mother presents with breast lumps, ensuring they are benign in nature and helping the mother create a breastfeeding pattern that works for her.

A number of benign lesions in the breasts can occur during pregnancy and lactation. These include lipomas, lactating adenoma (a painless mass, usually in the upper outer quadrant composed of densely packed masses of acini or lobules), fibroadenoma or fibroid, and breast hamartoma (an overgrowth of many types of normal tissues). Differentiating one from another and benign from malignant can be challenging, with fine-needle aspiration used as a quick, safe, and simple method of diagnosis. Fibrocystic disease or fibrocystic changes involve proliferations of the alveolar system and may have a range of signs and symptoms from mild tenderness to pain, along with thickened areas of the breasts or nodules of various sizes. Depending on the size and location of the mass, milk flow may be obstructed due to compression of adjacent milk ducts and alveoli (Geddes, 2009). Women with type 1 diabetes are also prone to benign breast lumps, referred to as diabetic mastopathy or sclerosing lymphocytic lobulitis (Kudva, O'Brien, & Oberg, 2002). Although none are contraindications to breastfeeding, clinicians can help the mother remain observant that areas around, beneath, or behind these lesions are well drained of milk. Milk production within each breast is usually not affected.

The failure of one breast to produce abundant amounts of milk, along with the infant refusing to feed from that breast, and/or the presence of a mass indicates a need for further evaluation. Unilateral failure of lactation in a symptomatic breast may be associated with a malignancy (Makanjuola, 1998). Infant rejection of only one breast (as opposed to a nursing strike on both breasts or breast preference), either sudden or with no apparent reason, has been described as a possible indicator of breast carcinoma (Goldsmith, 1974; Makanjuola, 1998; Saber, 1996). Not all infants will reject the cancerous breast (Petok, 1995), but there are usually other signs and symptoms that would prompt an immediate referral to the mother's physician:

- A breast mass that shows no improvement within 72 hours of treatment
- Unilateral lactation failure combined with either infant rejection of the breast and/or a palpable mass
- Plugged duct or an area of milk stasis that repeatedly occurs in the same location
- Symptoms of mastitis unaccompanied by a fever that do not resolve after antibiotic treatment

The last of these indicators may serve as a cautionary flag for clinicians to further explore and to rule out inflammatory breast cancer that can mimic mastitis in its early stages. Inflammatory breast cancer may initially present with pain, tenderness, firmness, and an increase in breast size. This is followed in a few weeks by the skin becoming warm, pink or red in color, raised, heavy, hard, and edematous. The edema is sometimes described as a roughening or thickening of the skin with little pits (peau d'orange). The skin thickening is caused by direct tumor invasion along the subdermal lymphatics, resulting in a cutaneous lymphedema. The nipple may become flattened, red, and crusted over time. Mammography is generally supportive of a diagnosis, but fine-needle aspiration and cytology are needed to confirm the presence or absence of malignant cells (Dahlbeck, Donnelly, & Theriault, 1995).

Nipple Discharge

Both human milk and other types of nipple secretions and discharges are seen in a rainbow of colors. Colostrum may be light yellow to bright orange. Mother's milk may have a bluish tint when first expressed and when stored will have a thick white or yellow layer of cream on the top. Layered milk may take on colors from food that the mother consumes, such as a green layer of milk from the consumption of green vegetables. The most common cause of nipple discharge is a benign papilloma followed by duct ectasia (Hussain, Policarpio, & Vincent, 2006). Other common nipple discharges include the following:

- Green, yellow, brown, reddish brown, or gray discharges may be associated with manipulation of the nipple at the end of a pregnancy or in early lactation (O'Callaghan, 1981).

- Purulent (pus) discharge may be seen with mastitis or an abscess.

- Duct ectasia may produce a sticky discharge of various colors. Dilatation of the terminal ducts during pregnancy may start a process of the formation of an irritating lipid resulting in an inflammatory response and the resulting nipple discharge. Most often, the discharge is dark green or black, appearing to be blood but actually testing guaiac negative (Falkenberry, 2002). The discharge is more commonly multiductal, bilateral, and colored. Smoking may be associated with duct ectasia (Rahal, deFreitas-Junior, & Paulinelli, 2005). The nipple and areola may also be painful, burn, itch, and swell. Clinicians should be watchful for plugging of the nipple pores and the development of a mass in the breast.

- Approximately 15% of asymptomatic lactating mothers have blood in their early milk when cytologically tested (Lafreniere, 1990). Delicate capillary networks that are traumatized during the rapid cellular proliferation that takes place during pregnancy may result in early milk that is blood tinged (Kline & Lash, 1962).

- Intraductal papilloma is a common cause of blood in the milk. This is a tiny growth from the lining of the duct that protrudes into the lumen or duct channel and can bleed when disrupted by breastfeeding or breast pumping. Most women are not aware of these growths unless they see blood in their pumped milk or if their infant vomits blood-tinged milk. The bleeding usually stops spontaneously. If an infant vomits blood-tinged milk, clinicians need to determine the source of the blood. Testing for fetal or adult hemoglobin determines the origin of the blood. If the infant tolerates the milk, he or she can continue breastfeeding from the affected side. If the infant cannot tolerate the blood, because it acts as an emetic, the mother can pump her breast until the milk is clear of blood, usually from 3 to 7 days. Parents also need to know that they may see black flecks in the infant's stool, or the stool may at times be black or tarry as the blood passes through the infant's intestines. Bloody nipple discharge that persists must be evaluated by the mother's physician.

Additional Reasons for Breast Pain

Breast Pain (Mastalgia)

Breast discomfort or pain is one of the most common reasons that women seek urgent breast care (Givens & Luszczak, 2002). Clinicians may wish to explore these other sources of pain when breastfeeding mothers describe deep or shooting pains in their breasts.

- A source external to the breast such as costochondritis. This is an inflammation of the joints where the ribs attach to the sternum and is treated with a nonsteroidal anti-inflammatory agent.

- Breast discomfort may be felt with capsular contracture or if an implant ruptures. Along with pain, the clinician may observe breast deformity or skin changes (Brown, Todd, Cope, & Sachs, 2006).

- Postfeed breast pain or interfeeding deep breast pain has been reported and ascribed to pulling or tugging on the nipple by the infant (Ellis, 1993) and "internal injury" to the nipple during feeding (Hopkinson, 1992). Deep breast pain may relate to the relative diameter of the milk ducts. Peters, Diemer, Meeks, and Behnken (2003) described the positive relationship between breast pain and the width of milk ducts. The wider the milk ducts, the more severe the pain, with women correlating the site of the duct dilatation as seen on ultrasound with the site of the pain. Duct dilatation in these nonlactating women with noncyclical pain was similar to the duct dilatation seen in lactating women (Ramsay et al., 2004) following the milk ejection reflex. Extra wide ducts may provide a partial explanation of why some breastfeeding mothers describe such intense pain with milk letdown and increasing breast discomfort between feedings.

Summary: The Design in Nature

Nature provides an almost infinite variety of breasts and infants, each with their unique shape, size, and set of concerns and problems. Almost any breast and infant can be paired up to produce and receive human milk. However, it is the clinician's knowledge, skills, and empathy that facilitate optimal outcomes—whether the infant feeds directly from the breast or receives his or her mother's milk in another manner. Many breastfeeding problems can be chronic and discouraging to new mothers; clinicians should remember that the best therapeutic tool they can offer is themselves.

References

Academy of Breastfeeding Medicine. (2004). Clinical protocol number 4—mastitis. Retrieved September 15, 2005, from www.bfmed.org/protocol/.pdf

Al-Qattan, M. M., & Robertson, G. A. (1990). Bilateral chronic infection of the lactosebaceous glands of Montgomery. *Ann Plast Surg., 25,* 491–493.

Alexander, J. M. (1991). The prevalence and management of inverted and non-protractile nipples in antenatal women who intend to breastfeed. PhD dissertation. Southampton, UK: University of Southampton.

Alexander, J. M., Grant, A. M., & Campbell, M. J. (1992). Randomised controlled trial of breast shells and Hoffman's exercises for inverted and non-protractile nipples. *BMJ, 304,* 1030–1032.

American Academy of Pediatrics. (2001). The transfer of drugs and other chemicals into human milk. *Pediatrics, 108,* 776–789.

Amir, L. (1993). Eczema of the nipple and breast: A case report. *J Hum Lact., 9,* 173–175.

Amir, L. (2002). Breastfeeding and *Staphylococcus aureus*: Three case reports. *Breastfeeding Rev., 10,* 15–18.

Amir, L. (2004). Nipple pain in breastfeeding. *Aust Fam Physician, 33,* 44–45.

Amir, L., & Hoover, K. (2003). *Candidiasis and breastfeeding.* Lactation Consultant Series 2. Schaumburg, IL: La Leche League International.

Amir, L. H. (1991). Candida and the lactating breast: Predisposing factors. *J Hum Lact., 7,* 177–181.

Amir, L. H. (2003). Breast pain in lactating women: Mastitis or something else? *Aust Fam Physician, 32,* 392–397.

Amir, L. H., Dennerstein, L., Garland, S. M., et al. (1997). Psychological aspects of nipple pain in lactating women. *Breastfeeding Rev., 5,* 29–32.

Amir, L. H., Forster, D., McLachlan, H., & Lumley, J. (2004). Incidence of breast abscess in lactating women: Report from an Australian cohort. *BJOG, 111,* 1378–1381.

Amir, L. H., Forster, D. A., Lumley, J., & McLachlan, H. (2007). A descriptive study of mastitis in Australian breastfeeding women: Incidence and determinants. *BMC Public Health, 7,* 62.

Amir, L. H., Garland, S., Dennerstein, L., & Farish, S. (1996). *Candida albicans*: Is it associated with nipple pain in lactating women? *Gynecologic and Obstetric Investigation, 41,* 30–34.

Amir, L. H., Garland, S. M., & Lumley, J. (2006). A case-control study of mastitis: Nasal carriage of *Staphylococcus aureus. BMC Family Practice, 7,* 57.

Amir, L. H., & Lumley, J. (2006). Womens' experience of lactational mastitis. *Aust Fam Physician, 35,* 745–747.

Amir, L. H., & Pakula, S. (1991). Nipple pain, mastalgia and candidiasis in the lactating breast. *Aust N Z J Obstet Gynaecol., 31,* 378–380.

Anderson, J. E., Held, N., & Wright, K. (2004). Raynaud's phenomenon of the nipple: A treatable cause of painful breastfeeding. *Pediatrics, 113,* e360–e364. Retrieved September 15, 2005, from www.pediatrics. org/cgi/content/full/113/4/e360

Andersson, Y., Lindquist, S., Lagerqvust, C., & Hernell, O. (2000). Lactoferrin is responsible for fungistatic effect of human milk. *Early Hum Dev., 59,* 95–105.

Andrews, J. I., Fleener, D. K., Messer, S. A., Hansen, W. F., Pfaller, M. A., & Diekema, D. J. (2007). The yeast connection: Is *Candida* linked to breastfeeding associated pain? *Am J Obstet Gynecol., 197,* 424.e1–424.e4.

Applebaum, R. M. (1969). *Abreast of the times.* Miami: RM Applebaum.

Barankin, B., & Gross, M. S. (2004). Nipple and areolar eczema in the breastfeeding woman. *J Cutaneous Med Surg., 8,* 126–130.

Barbosa-Cesnik, C., Schwartz, K., & Foxman, B. (2003). Lactation mastitis. *JAMA, 289,* 1609–1612.

Barnes, L. (1979). Cryotherapy: Putting injury on ice. *Phys Sports Med., 7,* 130–136.

Behari, P., Englund, J., Alcasid, G., Garcia-Houchins, S., & Weber, S. (2004). Transmission of methicillin-resistant *Staphylococcus aureus* to preterm infants through breast milk. *Infect Control Hosp Epidemiol., 25,* 778–780.

Benson, E. A. (1989). Management of breast abscesses. *World J Surg., 13,* 753–756.

Benson, E. A., & Goodman, M. A. (1970). Incision with primary suture in the treatment of acute puerperal breast abscess. *Br J Surg., 57,* 55–58.

Bertrand, H., & Rosenblood, L. K. (1991). Stripping out pus in lactational mastitis: A means of preventing breast abscess. *CMAJ, 145,* 299–306.

Betzold, C. M. (2005). Infections of the mammary ducts in the breastfeeding mother. *J Nurs Pract., 1,* 15–21.

Betzold, C. M. (2007). An update on the recognition and management of lactational breast inflammation. *J Midwife Women Health, 52,* 595–605.

Bevin, T. H., & Persok, C. K. (1993). Breastfeeding difficulties and a breast abscess associated with a galactocele: A case report. *J Hum Lact., 9,* 177–178.

Blair, A., Cadwell, K., Turner-Maffei, C., & Brimdyr, K. (2003). The relationship between positioning, the breastfeeding dynamic, the latching process and pain in breastfeeding mothers with sore nipples. *Breastfeeding Rev., 11,* 5–10.

Bland, K. I., & Romnell, L. J. (1991). Congenital and acquired disturbances of breast development and growth. In K. I. Bland & E. M. Copeland III (Eds.), *The breast: Comprehensive management of benign and malignant diseases.* Philadelphia: Saunders.

Blumenthal, M., Goldberg, A., & Brinckmann, J. (2000). *Herbal medicine: Expanded Commission E monographs* (pp. 297–303). Newton, MA: Integrative Medicine Communications.

Bodley, V., & Powers, D. (1997). Long-term treatment of a breastfeeding mother with fluconazole-resolved nipple pain caused by yeast: A case study. *J Hum Lact., 13,* 307–311.

Bowles, B. C., Stutte, P. C., & Hensley, J. (1987). Alternate breast massage: New benefits from an old technique. *Genesis, 9,* 5–9.

Bracket, V. H. (1988). Eczema of the nipple/areola area. *J Hum Lact., 4,* 167–169.

Breier, B. H., Milsom, S. R., Blum, W. F., et al. (1993). Insulin-like growth factors and their binding proteins in plasma and milk after growth hormone-stimulated galactopoiesis in normally lactating women. *Acta Endocrinol., 129,* 427–435.

Brent, N., Rudy, S. J., Redd, B., et al. (1998). Sore nipples in breastfeeding women: A clinical trial of wound dressings vs conventional care. *Arch Pediatr Adolesc Med., 152,* 1077–1082.

Brent, N. B. (2001). Thrush in the breastfeeding dyad: Results of a survey on diagnosis and treatment. *Clin Pediatr., 40,* 503–506.

Briggs, J. (2003). The management of nipple pain and/or trauma associated with breastfeeding. *Best Practice, 7*(3), 1–6.

Brook, I., & Gober, A. E. (1997). Bacterial colonization of pacifiers of infants with acute otitis media. *J Laryngol Otol., 111,* 614–615.

Brown, S. L., Todd, J. F., Cope, J. U., & Sachs, H. C. (2006). Breast implant surveillance reports to the US Food and Drug Administration: Maternal-child health problems. *Journal of Long Term Effects of Medical Implants, 16,* 281–290.

Buescher, E. S., & Hair, P. S. (2001). Human milk anti-inflammatory components during acute mastitis. *Cell Immunol., 210,* 87–95.

Cable, B., Stewart, M., & Davis, J. (1997). Nipple wound care: A new approach to an old problem. *J Hum Lact., 13,* 313–318.

Cadwell, K. (1981, July–August). Improving nipple graspability for success at breastfeeding. *J Obstet Gynecol Neonat Nurs.,* 277–279.

Cadwell, K. (2001). Preliminary results: A comparison of treatment for sore nipples in nursing mothers: The use of Soothies glycerine gel therapy and the use of breast shells with Lansinoh lanolin cream. Retrieved September 15, 2005, from www.puronyx.com/html/soothies/latvia.html

Cadwell, K., Turner-Maffei, C., Blair, A., Brimdyr, K., & McInerney, Z. (2004). Pain reduction and treatment of sore nipples in nursing mothers. *J Perinat Med., 13,* 29–35.

Campbell, S. H. (2006). Recurrent plugged ducts. *J Hum Lact., 22,* 340–343.

Campbell, S. H., & Smillie, C. M. (2003, August). Recurrent plugged ducts: The effect of traditional therapy versus ultrasound therapy. *Proceedings of the Conference and Annual Meeting of the International Lactation Consultant Association,* Sydney, Australia.

Cantile, H. B. (1988). Treatment of acute puerperal mastitis and breast abscess. *Can Fam Physician, 34,* 2221–2227.

Carmichael, A. R., & Dixon, J. M. (2002). Is lactation mastitis and shooting breast pain experienced by women during lactation caused by *Candida albicans? Breast, 11,* 88–90.

Carroll, L., et al. (1979). Bacteriologic criteria for feeding raw breast milk to babies on neonatal units. *Lancet, 2*(8145), 732–733.

Chapman, D. J., & Perez-Escamilla, R. (1999). Identification of risk factors for delayed onset of lactation. *J Am Dietet Assn., 99*, 450–454.

Chen, D. C., Nommsen-Rivers, L., Dewey, K. G., & Lonnerdal, B. (1998). Stress during labor and delivery and early lactation performance. *Am J Clin Nutr., 68*, 335–344.

Chetwynd, E. M., Ives, T. J., Payne, P. M., & Edens-Bartholomew, N. (2002). Fluconazole for postpartum candidal mastitis and infant thrush. *J Hum Lact., 18*, 168–171.

Chikly, B. (1999). Lymph drainage therapy: Treatment for engorgement. Presented at International Lactation Consultant Association Conference, August 2, Scottsdale, Ariz. Audio tape.

Coates, M.-M. (1992). Nipple pain related to vasospasm in the nipple? *J Hum Lact., 8*, 153.

Connor, A. E. (1979). Elevated levels of sodium and chloride in milk from mastitic breasts. *Pediatrics, 63*, 910–911.

Cooper, W. O., Atherton, H. D., Kahana, M., & Kotagal, U. R. (1995). Increased incidence of severe breast-feeding malnutrition and hypernatremia in a metropolitan area. *Pediatrics, 96*, 957–960.

Cotch, M. F., Hillier, S. L., Gibbs, R. S., & Eschenbach, D. A. (1998). Epidemiology and outcomes associated with moderate to heavy *Candida* colonization during pregnancy. *Am J Obstet Gynecol., 178*, 374–380.

Cotterman, K. J. (2003, April/May). Too swollen to latch on? Try reverse pressure softening first. *Leaven*, 38–40.

Cotterman, K. J. (2004). Reverse pressure softening: A simple tool to prepare areola for easier latching during engorgement. *J Hum Lact., 20*, 227–237.

Csar, N. (1991). Breast engorgement: What is the incidence and pattern? Master's thesis. Chicago: University of Illinois.

Dahlbeck, S. W., Donnelly, J. F., & Theriault, R. L. (1995). Differentiating inflammatory breast cancer from acute mastitis. *Am Fam Physician, 52*, 929–934.

Daly, S. E. J., & Hartmann, P. E. (1995). Infant demand and milk supply. Part 2: The short-term control of milk synthesis in lactating women. *J Hum Lact., 11*, 27–37.

Darwazeh, A. M., & al-Bashir, A. (1995). Oral candidal flora in healthy infants. *J Oral Pathol Med., 24*, 361–364.

Dawson, E. K. (1935). Histological study of normal mamma in relation to tumour growth: Mature gland in lactation and pregnancy. *Edinburgh Medical Journal, 42*, 569.

Dekio, S., Kawasaki, Y., & Jidoi, J. (1986). Herpes simplex on nipples inoculated from herpes gingivo-stomatitis of a baby. *Clin Exp Dermatol., 11*, 664–666.

Delgado, S., Arroyo, R., Jimenez, E., et al. (2009). *Staphylococcus epidermidis* strains isolated from breast milk of women suffering infectious mastitis: Potential virulence traits and resistance to antibiotics. *BMC Microbiol., 9*, 82.

Delgado, S., Arroyo, R., Martin, R., Rodriguez, J. M. (2008). PCR-DGGE assessment of the bacterial diversity of breast milk in women with lactational infectious mastitis. *BMC Infect Dis., 8*, 51.

Dener, C., & Inan, A. (2003). Breast abscesses in lactating women. *World J Surg., 27*, 130–133.

Dever, J. (1992). Mastitis: Positive interventions. *Midwifery Today, 22*, 22–25.

Devereux, W. P. (1970). Acute puerperal mastitis: Evaluation of its management. *Am J Obstet Gynecol., 108*, 78–81.

Dewey, K. (2001). Maternal and fetal stress are associated with impaired lactogenesis in humans. *J Nutr., 131*, 3012S–3015S.

Dewey, K. G., Nommsen-Rivers, L. A., Heinig, M. J., & Cohen, R. J. (2003). Risk factors for suboptimal infant breastfeeding behavior, delayed onset of lactation, and excess neonatal weight loss. *Pediatrics, 112*, 607–619.

Dinsmoor, M. J., Viloria, R., Lief, L., & Elder, S. (2005). Use of intrapartum antibiotics and the incidence of postnatal maternal and neonatal yeast infections. *Obstet Gynecol., 106,* 19–22.

Dixon, J. M. (1988). Repeated aspiration of breast abscesses in lactating women. *BMJ, 297,* 1517–1518.

Dodd, V., & Chalmers, C. (2003). Comparing the use of hydrogel dressings to lanolin ointment with lactating mothers. *J Obstet Gynecol Neonat Nurs., 32,* 486–494.

Dollberg, S., Botzer, E., Grunis, E., & Mimouni, F. B. (2006). Immediate nipple pain relief after frenotomy in breastfed infants with ankyloglossia: A randomized, prospective study. *J Pediatr Surg., 41,* 1598–1600.

Dos Santos, R de C., & Marin, J. M. (2005). Isolation of *Candida* spp. from mastitic bovine milk in Brazil. *Mycopathologia, 159,* 251–253.

Drewett, R., Kahn, H., Parkhurst, S., & Whiteley, S. (1987). Pain during breastfeeding: The first three months. *J Repro Inf Psychol., 5,* 183–186.

Eglash, A. (1998). Delayed milk ejection reflex and plugged ducts: Lecithin therapy. *ABM News and Views, 4*(1), 4.

Eglash, A., Plane, M. B., & Mundt, M. (2006). History, physical and laboratory findings, and clinical outcomes of lactating women treated with antibiotics for chronic breast and/or nipple pain. *J Hum Lact., 22,* 429–433.

Eglash, A., & Proctor, R. (2007). A breastfeeding mother with chronic breast pain. *Breastfeeding Med., 2,* 99–103.

Ehrenkranz, R., Ackerman, B., & Hulse, J. (1989). Nifedipine transfer into human milk. *J Pediatr., 114,* 478–480.

Ellepola, A. N., Panagoda, G. J., & Samaranayake, L. P. (1999). Adhesion of oral *Candida* species to human buccal epithelial cells following brief exposure to nystatin. *Oral Microbiol Immunol., 14,* 358–363.

Ellis, D. (1993). Post-feed breast pain: A case report. *J Hum Lact., 9,* 182.

Evans, K., Evans, R., & Simmer, K. (1995). Effect of the method of breastfeeding on breast engorgement, mastitis, and infantile colic. *Acta Paediatr., 84,* 849–852.

Evans, M., & Heads, J. (1995). Mastitis: Incidence, prevalence and cost. *Breastfeeding Rev., 3,* 65–72.

Falkenberry, S. S. (2002). Nipple discharge. *Obstet Gynecol Clin N Am., 29,* 21–29.

Ferris, C. D. (1990). Instrumentation system for breast engorgement evaluation. *Biomed Instrum Technol., 90,* 227–229.

Ferris, C. D. (1996). Hand-held instrument for evaluation of breast engorgement. *Biomed Instrum Technol., 96,* 299–304.

Fetherston, C. (1997). Management of lactation mastitis in a Western Australian cohort. *Breastfeeding Rev., 5,* 13–19.

Fetherston, C. (1998). Risk factors for lactation mastitis. *J Hum Lact., 14,* 101–109.

Fetherston, C. (2001). Mastitis in lactating women: Physiology or pathology. *Breastfeeding Rev., 9,* 5–12.

Fetherston, C., Lai, C., & Hartmann, P. (2006). Relationships between symptoms and changes in breast physiology during lactation mastitis. *Breastfeeding Med., 1,* 136–145.

Fildes, V. (1986). *Breasts, bottles, and babies: A history of infant feeding.* Edinburgh: Edinburgh University Press.

Filteau, S. M., Liez, G., Mulokozi, G., et al. (1999a). Milk cytokines and subclinical breast inflammation in Tanzanian women: Effects of dietary red palm oil or sunflower oil supplementation. *Immunology, 97,* 595–600.

Filteau, S. M., Rice, A. L., Ball, J. J., et al. (1999b). Breast milk immune factors in Bangladeshi women supplemented postpartum with retinol or beta-carotene. *Am J Clin Nutr., 69,* 953–958.

Flores, M., & Filteau, S. (2002). Effect of lactation counseling on subclinical mastitis among Bangladeshi women. *Ann Trop Pediatr., 22,* 85–88.

Freed, G. L., Landers, S., & Schanler, R. J. (1991). A practical guide to successful breastfeeding management. *Am J Dis Child., 145,* 917–921.

Gangal, H. T., & Gangal, M. H. (1978). Suction method for correcting flat nipples or inverted nipples. *Plast Reconstr Surg., 61,* 294–296.

Gastelum, D. T., Dassey, D., Mascola, L., & Yasuda, L. M. (2005). Transmission of community-associated methicillin-resistant *Staphylococcus aureus* from breast milk in the neonatal intensive care unit. *Pediatr Infect Dis J., 24,* 1122–1124.

Geddes, D. T. (2009). Ultrasound imaging of the lactating breast: Methodology and application. *Int Breastfeeding J., 4,* 4.

Geddes, D. T., Langton, D. B., Gollow, I., Jacobs, L. A., Hartmann, P. E., & Simmer, K. (2008). Frenulotomy for breastfeeding infants with ankyloglossia: Effect on milk removal and sucking mechanism as imaged by ultrasound. *Pediatrics, 122,* e188–e194.

Geissler, N. (1967). An instrument used to measure breast engorgement. *Nurs Res., 16,* 130–136.

Givens, M. L., & Luszczak, M. (2002). Breast disorders: A review for emergency physicians. *J Emerg Med., 22,* 59–65.

Glover, R. (1998). The engorgement enigma. *Breastfeeding Rev., 6,* 31–34.

Goldsmith, H. S. (1974). Milk rejection sign of breast cancer. *Am J Surg., 1*(27), 280–281.

Graves, S., Wright, W., Harman, R., & Bailey, S. Painful nipples in nursing mothers: Fungal or staphylococcal? *Aust Fam Physician, 32,* 570–571.

Grimes, D. A., & Schulz, K. F. (2002). Uses and abuses of screening tests. *Lancet, 359,* 881–884.

Gunther, M. (1945). Sore nipples: Causes and prevention. *Lancet, 2,* 590–593.

Gunther, M. (1955). Instinct and the nursing couple. *Lancet, 1,* 575–578.

Gunther, M. (1970). *Infant feeding.* London: Metheun.

Hale, T. W. (2008). *Medications and mother's milk* (13th ed.). Amarillo, TX: Hale Publishing.

Hale, T. W., Bateman, T., Finkelman, M., & Berens, P. (2007). Detection of *Candida albicans* in control and symptomatic breastfeeding women using new technology [Abstract 26]. *Breastfeeding Med., 2,* 187–188.

Hale, T. W., Bateman, T. L., Finkelman, M. A., & Berens, P. D. (2009). The absence of *Candida albicans* in milk samples of women with clinical symptoms of ductal candidiasis. *Breastfeeding Med., 4,* 57–61.

Hale, T. W., & Berens, P. (2002). *Clinical therapy in breastfeeding patients* (2nd ed.). Amarillo, TX: Pharmasoft Publishing.

Han, S., & Hong, Y. G. (1999). The inverted nipple: Its grading and surgical correction. *Plast Reconstr Surg., 104,* 389–395.

Hanson, L. A. (2004). *Immunobiology of human milk: How breastfeeding protects babies.* Amarillo, TX: Pharmasoft Publishing.

Hanson, L. A., Lonnroth, I., Lange, S., et al. (2000). Nutrition resistance to viral propagation. *Nutr Rev., 58,* S31–S37.

Hartmann, P., & Cregan, M. (2001). Lactogenesis and the effects of insulin-dependent diabetes mellitus and prematurity. *J Nutr., 131,* 3016S–3020S.

Hayes, R., Michell, M., & Nunnerley, H. B. (1991). Acute inflammation of the breast—Role of breast ultrasound in diagnosis and management. *Clin Radiol., 44,* 253–256.

Heads, J., & Higgins, L. C. (1995). Perceptions and correlates of nipple pain. *Breastfeeding Rev., 3,* 59–64.

Heinig, M. J., Francis, J., & Pappagianis, D. (1999). Mammary candidosis in lactating women. *J Hum Lact., 15,* 281–288.

Henderson, A., Stamp, G., & Pincombe, J. (2001). Postpartum positioning and attachment education for increasing breastfeeding: A randomized trial. *Birth, 28,* 236–242.

Hesseltine, H. C., Freudlich, C. G., & Hite, K. E. (1948). Acute puerperal mastitis: Clinical and bacteriological studies in relation to penicillin therapy. *Am J Obstet Gynecol., 55,* 778–788.

Hewat, R., & Ellis, D. (1987). A comparison of the effectiveness of two methods of nipple care. *Birth, 14,* 41–45.

Hill, P. D., & Humenick, S. S. (1993). Nipple pain during breastfeeding: The first two weeks and beyond. *J Perinat Ed., 2,* 21–35.

Hill, P. D., & Humenick S. S. (1994). The occurrence of breast engorgement. *J Hum Lact., 10,* 79–86.

Hill, P. D., Humenick, S. S., & West, B. (1994). Concerns of breastfeeding mothers: The first six weeks postpartum. *J Perinat Ed., 3,* 47–58.

Hillervik-Lindquist, C. (1991). Studies on perceived breast milk insufficiency. *Acta Paediatr Scand., 80*(suppl 376), 6–27.

Hocutt, J. E., Jaffe, R., Rylander, C. R., & Beebe, J. K. (1982). Cryotherapy in ankle sprains. *Am J Sports Med., 10,* 317–319.

Hoffman, J. B. (1953). A suggested treatment for inverted nipples. *Am J Obstet Gynecol., 66,* 346.

Hook, G. W., & Ikeda, D. M. (1999). Treatment of breast abscesses with US-guided percutaneous needle drainage without indwelling catheter placement. *Radiology, 213,* 579–582.

Hopkinson, J. (1992). Interfeeding breast pain: A case report. *J Hum Lact., 8,* 149–151.

Hoppe, J. E., & Hahn, H. (1996). Randomized comparison of two nystatin oral gels with miconazole oral gel for treatment of oral thrush in infants. *Infection, 24,* 136–139.

Huggins, K. E., & Billion, S. F. (1993). Twenty cases of persistent sore nipples: Collaboration between lactation consultant and dermatologist. *J Hum Lact., 9,* 155–160.

Humenick, S., & van Steenkiste, S. (1983). Early indicators of breastfeeding progress. *Issues in Comprehensive Pediatric Nursing, 6,* 205–215.

Humenick, S. S., Hill, P. D., & Anderson, M. A. (1994). Breast engorgement: Patterns and selected outcomes. *J Hum Lact., 10,* 87–93.

Huml, S. C. (1994, January/February). Moist wound healing for cracked nipples in the breastfeeding mother. *Leaven,* 3–6.

Hussain, A. N., Policarpio, C., & Vincent, M. T. (2006). Evaluating nipple discharge. *Obstet Gynecol Survey, 61,* 278–283.

Hytten, F. E., & Baird, D. (1958). The development of the nipple in pregnancy. *Lancet, 1*(7032), 1201–1204.

Iffrig, M. C. (1968). Nursing care and success in breastfeeding. *Nurs Clin N Am., 3,* 345–354.

Illingworth, R., & Stone, D. (1952). Self-demand feeding in a maternity unit. *Lancet, 1,* 683–687.

Inch, S. (1989). Antenatal preparation for breastfeeding. In I. Chalmers, M. Enkin, & M. J. N. C. Keirse (Eds.), *Effective care in pregnancy and childbirth.* Oxford: Oxford University Press.

Inch, S. (1997). *Mastitis: A literature review.* Geneva: WHO, Division of Child Health & Development.

Inch, S., & Fisher, C. (1995). Mastitis: Infection or inflammation. *Practitioner, 239,* 472–476.

Jacobs, L. A., Dickinson, J. E., Hart, P. D., Doherty, D. A., & Faulkner, S. J. (2007). Normal nipple position in term infants measured on breastfeeding ultrasound. *J Hum Lact., 23,* 52–59.

Jacobs, V. R., Golombeck, K., Jonat, W., et al. (2003). Mastitis nonpuerperalis after nipple piercing: Time to act. *Int J Fertil Women Med., 48,* 226–231.

Jamali, F., Ricci, A., & Deckers, P. (1996). Paget's disease of the nipple-areola complex. *Surg Clin N Am., 76,* 365–381.

Jimenez, E., Fernandez, L., Maldonado, A., et al. (2008). Oral administration of *Lactobacillus* strains isolated from breast milk as an alternative for the treatment of infectious mastitis during lactation. *Applied and Environmental Microbiology, 74,* 4650–4655.

Johnson, P. E., & Hanson, K. D. (1996). Acute puerperal mastitis in the augmented breast. *Plast Reconst Surg., 98,* 723–725.

Johnstone, H. A., & Marcinak, J. F. (1990). Candidiasis in the breastfeeding mother and infant. *J Obstet Gynecol Neonat Nurs., 19,* 171–173.

Jonsson, S., & Pulkkinen, M. O. (1994). Mastitis today: Incidence, prevention and treatment. *Annales Chirurgiae et Gynaecologiae Supplementum, 208,* 84–87.

Karstrup, S., Khattar, S., et al. (1993). Acute puerperal breast abscess: US-guided drainage. *Radiology, 188,* 807–809.

Kaufmann, R., & Foxman, B. (1991). Mastitis among lactating women: Occurrence and risk factors. *Social Sci Med., 33,* 701–705.

Kee, W. H., Tan, S. L., & Salmon, Y. M. (1989). The treatment of breast engorgement with serrapeptase (Danzen): A double-blind controlled trial. *Singapore Med J., 30,* 48–54.

Kenny, J. F. (1977). Recurrent group B streptococcal disease in an infant associated with the ingestion of infected mother's milk. *J Pediatr., 91,* 158.

Kesaree, N., Banapurmath, C. R., Banapurmath, S., & Shamanur, K. (1993). Treatment of inverted nipples using a disposable syringe. *J Hum Lact., 9,* 27–29.

Kinlay, J. R., O'Connell, D. L., & Kinlay, S. (2001). Risk factors for mastitis in breastfeeding women: Results of a prospective cohort study. *Aust N Z J Public Health, 25,* 115–120.

Kline, T. S., & Lash, S. R. (1962). Nipple secretion in pregnancy: A cytologic and histologic study. *Am J Clin Pathol., 37,* 626.

Kudva, Y. C., O'Brien, T., & Oberg, A. L. (2002). "Diabetic mastopathy," or sclerosing lymphocytic lobulitis, is strongly associated with type 1 diabetes. *Diabetes Care, 25,* 121–126.

Kvist, L. J., Hall-Lord, M. L., & Larsson, B. W. (2007). A descriptive study of Swedish women with symptoms of breast inflammation during lactation and their perceptions of the quality of care given at a breastfeeding clinic. *Int. Breastfeeding J., 2,* 2.

Kvist, L. J., Larsson, B. W., Hall-Lord, M. L., Steen, A., & Schalen, C. (2008). The role of bacteria in lactational mastitis and some considerations of the use of antibiotic treatment. *Int Breastfeeding J., 3,* 6.

Kvist, L. J., & Rydhstroem, H. (2005). Factors related to breast abscess after delivery: A population-based study. *BJOG, 112,* 1070–1074.

Lafreniere, R. (1990). Bloody nipple discharge during pregnancy: A rationale for conservative treatment. *J Surg Oncol., 43,* 228.

Lawlor-Smith, L., & Lawlor-Smith, C. (1996). Nipple vasospasm in the breastfeeding woman. *Breastfeeding Rev., 4,* 37–39.

Lawlor-Smith, L., & Lawlor-Smith, C. (1997). Vasospasm of the nipple—A manifestation of Raynaud's phenomenon: Case reports. *BMJ 314,* 844–845.

Lawrence, R. A., & Lawrence, R. M. (2005). *Breastfeeding: A guide for the medical profession* (6th ed.). Philadelphia: Elsevier Mosby.

L'Esperance, C. (1980). Pain or pleasure: The dilemma of early breastfeeding. *Birth, 7,* 21–26.

Lever, R., Hadley, K., Downey, D., et al. (1988). Staphylococcal colonization in atopic dermatitis and the effect of topical mupirocin therapy. *Br J Dermatol., 119,* 189–198.

Livingstone, V. (1996). Too much of a good thing: Maternal and infant hyperlactation syndromes. *Can Fam Physician, 42,* 89–99.

Livingstone, V., & Stringer, L. J. (1999). The treatment of *Staphylococcus aureus* infected sore nipples: A randomized comparative study. *J Hum Lact., 15,* 241–246.

Livingstone, V. H., Willis, C. E., & Berkowitz, J. (1996). *Staphylococcus aureus* and sore nipples. *Can Fam Physician, 42,* 654–659.

MAIN Trial Collaborative Group. (1994). Preparing for breastfeeding: Treatment of inverted and non-protractile nipples in pregnancy. *Midwifery, 10,* 200–214.

Makanjuola, D. (1998). A clinico-radiological correlation of breast diseases during lactation and the significance of unilateral failure of lactation. *West African J Med., 17,* 217–223.

Manning, D. J., Coughlin, R. P., & Poskitt, E. M. E. (1985). Candida in mouth or on dummy? *Arch Dis Child., 60,* 381–382.

Marti, A., Feng, H. J., Altermatt, H. J., & Jaggi, R. (1997). Milk accumulation triggers apoptosis of mammary epithelial cells. *Eur J Cell Biol., 73,* 158–165.

Martin, J. (2004). Is nipple piercing compatible with breastfeeding? *J Hum Lact., 20,* 319–321.

Matheson, I., Aursnes, I., Horgen, M., et al. (1988). Bacteriological findings and clinical symptoms in relation to clinical outcome in puerperal mastitis. *Acta Obstetrica et Gynecologica Scandinavica, 67,* 23–726.

Mattos-Graner, R. O., de Moraes, A. B., Rontani, R. M., & Birman, E. G. (2001). Relation of oral yeast infection in Brazilian infants and the use of a pacifier. *ASDC Journal of Dentistry for Children, 68,* 33–36.

McClellan, H. L., Geddes, D. T., Kent, J. C., Garbin, C. P., Mitoulas, L. R., & Hartmann, P. E. (2008). Infants of mothers with persistent nipple pain exert strong sucking vacuums. *Acta Paediatr., 97,* 1205–1209.

McGeorge, D. D. (1994). The "niplette": An instrument for the non-surgical correction of inverted nipples. *Br J Plast Surg., 47,* 46–49.

McLachlan, Z., Milne, E. J., Lumley, J., & Walker, B. L. (1993, May). Ultrasound treatment for breast engorgement: A randomized double-blind trial. *Breastfeeding Rev.,* 316–321.

Melli, M. S., Rashidi, M. R., Delazar, A., et al. (2007a). Effect of peppermint water on prevention of nipple cracks in lactating primiparous women: A randomized controlled trial. *Int Breastfeeding J., 2,* 7.

Melli, M. S., Rashidi, M. R., Nokhoodchi, A., et al. (2007b). A randomized trial of peppermint gel, lanolin ointment, and placebo gel to prevent nipple crack in primiparous breastfeeding women. *Medicine and Science Monitor, 13,* CR406–CR411.

Menczer, J., & Eskin, B. (1969). Evaluation of postpartum breast engorgement by thermography. *Obstet Gynecol., 33,* 260–263.

Michie, C., Lockie, F., & Lynn, W. (2003). The challenge of mastitis. *Arch Dis Child., 88,* 818–821.

Miller, V., & Riordan, J. (2004). Treating postpartum breast edema with areolar compression. *J Hum Lact., 20,* 223–226.

Minchin, M. (1985). *Breastfeeding matters: What we need to know about infant feeding.* Victoria, Australia: Alma Publications and George Allen & Unwin Australia Pty Ltd.

Moazzez, A., Kelso, R. L., Towfigh, S., Sohn, H., Berne, T. V., & Mason, R. J. (2007). Breast abscess bacteriologic findings in the era of community-acquired methicillin-resistant *Staphylococcus aureus* epidemics. *Arch Surg., 142,* 881–884.

Mohammadzadeh, A., Farhat, A., & Esmaeily, H. (2005). The effect of breast milk and lanolin on sore nipples. *Saudi Med J., 26,* 1231–1234.

Moon, A. A., & Gilbert, B. (1935). A study of acute mastitis of the puerperim. *J Obstet Gynecol British Commonwealth, 42,* 268–282.

Moon, J. L., & Humenick, S. S. (1989). Breast engorgement: Contributing variables and variables amenable to nursing intervention. *J Obstet Gynecol Neonat Nurs., 18,* 309–315.

Morel, A., Wu, F., Dell-Latta, P., Cronquist, A., Rubenstein, D., & Saiman, L. (2002). Nosocomial transmission of methicillin-resistant *Staphylococcus aureus* from a mother to her preterm quadruplet infants. *Am J Infect Control, 30,* 170–173.

Moretti, A., Pasquali, P., Mencaroni, G., et al. (1998). Relationship between cell counts in bovine milk and the presence of mastitis pathogens (yeasts and bacteria). *Zentralblatt fur Veterinarmedizin, 45,* 129–132.

Morino, C., & Winn, S. M. (2007). Raynaud's phenomenon of the nipples: An elusive diagnosis. *J Hum Lact., 23,* 191–193.

Morland-Schultz, K., & Hill, P. D. (2005). Prevention of and therapies for nipple pain: A systematic review. *J Obstet Gynecol Neonat Nurs., 34,* 428–437.

Morrill, J. F., Heinig, M. J., Pappagianis, D., & Dewey, K. G. (2004). Diagnostic value of signs and symptoms of mammary candidosis among lactating women. *J Hum Lact., 20,* 288–295.

Morrill, J. F., Heinig, M. J., Pappagianis, D., & Dewey, K. G. (2005). Risk factors for mammary candidosis among lactating women. *J Obstet Gynecol Neonat Nurs., 34,* 37–45.

Morrill, J. M., Pappagianis, D., Heinig, M. J., et al. (2003). Detecting *Candida albicans* in human milk. *J Clin Microbiol., 41,* 475–478.

Morton, J. A. (1994). The clinical usefulness of breast milk sodium in the assessment of lactogenesis. *Pediatrics, 93,* 802–806.

Neifert, M., DeMarzo, S., Seacat, J., et al. (1990). The influence of breast surgery, breast appearance, and pregnancy-induced breast changes on lactation sufficiency as measured by infant weight gain. *Birth, 17,* 31–38.

Neifert, M., & Seacat, J. (1986). Medical management of successful breastfeeding. *Pediatr Clin N Am., 33,* 743–762.

Neubauer, S. H., Ferris, A. M., & Hinckley, L. (1990). The effect of mastitis on breast milk composition in insulin dependent diabetic and non-diabetic women. *FASEB Journal, 4,* A915.

Newman, J. (2005). *Candida* protocol. Retrieved September 15, 2005, from www.kellymom.com/newman/c-candida_protocol.html

Newton, N. (1952). Nipple pain and nipple damage. *J Pediatr., 41,* 411–423.

Newton, M., & Newton, N. R. (1948). The let-down reflex in human lactation. *J Pediatr., 33,* 698.

Newton, M., & Newton, N. (1951). Postpartum engorgement of the breast. *Am J Obstet Gynecol., 61,* 664–667.

Nicholson, W., & Yuen, H. P. (1995). A study of breastfeeding rates at a large Australian obstetric hospital. *Aust N Z J Obstet Gynaecol., 35,* 393–397.

Niebyl, J. R., Spence, M. R., & Parmley, T. H. (1978). Sporadic (non-epidemic) puerperal mastitis. *J Reprod Med., 20,* 97–100.

Nikodem, V. C., Danziger, D., Gebka, N., et al. (1993). Do cabbage leaves prevent breast engorgement? A randomized controlled study. *Birth, 20,* 61–64.

Noble, R. (1991). Milk under the skin (milk blister)—A simple problem causing other breast conditions. *Breastfeeding Rev., 2,* 118–119.

O'Callaghan, M. A. (1981). Atypical discharge from the breast during pregnancy and/or lactation. *Aust N Z J Obstet Gynaecol., 21,* 214–216.

O'Hara, R. J., Dexter, S. P., & Fox, J. N. (1996). Conservative management of infective mastitis and breast abscesses after ultrasonographic assessment. *Br J Surg., 83,* 1413–1414.

Odds, F. C. (1994). *Candida* species and virulence. *Am Soc Microbiol News, 60,* 313–318.

Olsen, N., & Nielson, S. L. (1978). Prevalence of primary Raynaud's phenomenon in young females. *Scand J Clin Lab Invest., 37,* 761–776.

Osterman, K. L., & Rahm, V. A. (2000). Lactation mastitis: Bacterial cultivation of breast milk, symptoms, treatment, and outcome. *J Hum Lact., 16,* 297–302.

Osther, P., Balslev, E., & Blichert-Toft, M. (1990). Paget's disease of the nipple: A continuing enigma. *Acta Chirurgiae Scandinavica, 156,* 343–352.

Otte, M, J. (1975). Correcting inverted nipples—An aid to breastfeeding. *MCN, 75,* 454–456.

Page, S. M., & McKenna, D. S. (2006). Vasospasm of the nipple presenting as painful lactation. *Obstet Gynecol., 108,* 806–808.

Panjaitan, M., Amir, L. H., Costs, A.-M., Rudland, E., & Tabrizi, S. (2008). Polymerase chain reaction in detection of *Candida albicans* for confirmation of clinical diagnosis of nipple thrush [letter]. *Breastfeeding Med., 3,* 185–187.

Peters, F., Diemer, P., Meeks, O., & Behnken, L. J. (2003). Severity of mastalgia in relation to milk duct dilatation. *Obstet Gynecol., 101,* 54–60.

Petok, E. S. (1995). Breast cancer and breastfeeding: Five cases. *J Hum Lact., 11,* 205–209.

Pfaller, M. A. (1994). Epidemiology and control of fungal infections. *Clin Infect Dis., 19*(suppl 1), S8–S13.

Piatt, J. P., & Bergeson, P. S. (1992). Gentian violet toxicity. *Clinical Pediatrics, 31,* 756–757.

Pizzo, G., Giuliana, G., Milici, M. E., & Giangreco, R. (2000). Effects of dietary carbohydrate on the in vitro epithelial adhesion of *Candida albicans, Candida tropicalis,* and *Candida krusei. New Microbiology, 23,* 63–71.

Porter, J., & Schach, B. (2004). Treating sore, possibly infected nipples. *J Hum Lact., 20,* 221–222.

Prentice, A., Addey, C. V. P., & Wilde, C. J. (1989). Evidence for local feedback control of human milk secretion. *Biochemical Society Transactions, 15,* 122.

Prosser, C. G., & Hartmann, P. E. (1983). Comparison of mammary gland function during the ovulatory menstrual cycle and acute breast inflammation in women. *Aust J Exp Biol Med Sci., 61,* 277–286.

Rago, J. L. (1988). Weeping areolar eczema. *J Hum Lact., 4,* 166–167.

Rahal, R. M., deFreitas-Junior, R., & Paulinelli, R. R. (2005). Risk factors for duct ectasia. *Breast Journal, 11,* 262–265.

Ramsay, D. T., Kent, J. C., Owens, R. A., & Hartmann, P. E. (2004). Ultrasound imaging of milk ejection in the breast of lactating women. *Pediatrics, 113,* 361–367.

Rasmussen, K. M., Hilson, J. A., & Kjolhede, C. L. (2001). Obesity may impair lactogenesis II. *J Nutr., 131,* 3009S–3011S.

Reddy, P., Qi, C., Zembower, T., Noskin, G. A., & Bolon, M. (2007). Postpartum mastitis and community-acquired methicillin-resistant *Staphylococcus aureus. Emerg Inf Dis., 13,* 298–301.

Remington, J. S., & Klein, J. O. (1983). *Infectious diseases of the fetus and newborn.* Philadelphia: WB Saunders.

Rench, M. A., & Baker, C. J. (1989). Group B streptococcal breast abscess in a mother and mastitis in her infant. *Obstet Gynecol., 73,* 875–877.

Renfrew, M. J., Woolridge, M. W., & McGill, H. R. (2000). *Enabling women to breastfeed: A review of practices which promote or inhibit breastfeeding—with evidence-based guidance for practice.* London: The Stationary Office.

Riedel, L. J. (1991). Breast engorgement: Subjective and objective measurements and patterns of occurrence in primiparous mothers. Master's thesis. Laramie, WY: Department of Nursing, University of Wyoming.

Righard, L. (1996). Early enhancement of successful breastfeeding. *World Health Forum, 17,* 92–97.

Righard, L. (1998). Are breastfeeding problems related to incorrect breastfeeding technique and the use of pacifiers and bottles? *Birth, 25,* 40–44.

Righard, L., & Alade, M. O. (1992). Sucking technique and its effect on success of breastfeeding. *Birth, 19,* 185–189.

Riordan, J. (1983). *A practical guide to breastfeeding.* St. Louis, MO: Mosby.

Riordan, J. M., & Nichols, F. H. (1990). A descriptive study of lactation mastitis in long-term breastfeeding women. *J Hum Lact., 6,* 53–58.

Roberts, K. L. (1995). A comparison of chilled cabbage leaves and chilled gelpaks in reducing breast engorgement. *J Hum Lact., 11,* 17–20.

Roberts, K. L., Reiter, M., & Schuster, D. (1998). Effects of cabbage leaf extract on breast engorgement. *J Hum Lact., 14,* 231–236.

Robinson, L. B. (2002). Olive oil: A natural treatment for sore nipples? *AWHONN Lifelines, 6,* 110–112.

Robson, B. A. (1990). Breast engorgement in breastfeeding women. PhD dissertation. Cleveland, OH: Case Western Reserve University.

Rosa, C., et al. (1990). Yeasts from human milk collected in Rio de Janeiro, Brazil. *Rev Microbiol., 21,* 361–363.

Rosier, W. (1988). Cool cabbage compresses. *Breastfeeding Rev., 12,* 28–31.

Ryan, T. J. (2007). Infection following soft tissue injury: Its role in wound healing. *Curr Op Infect Dis., 20,* 124–128.

Sabate, J. M., Clotet, M., Torrubia, S., et al. (2007). Radiologic evaluation of breast disorders related to pregnancy and lactation. *RadioGraphics, 27,* S101–S124.

Saber, A. (1996). The milk rejection sign: A natural tumor marker. *Am Surg., 62,* 998–999.

Sadove, R., & Clayman, M. A. (2008). Surgical procedure for reversal of nipple piercing. *Aesthetic Plastic Surgery, 32,* 563–565.

Saiman, L., O'Keefe, M., Graham, P., L., 3rd, et al. (2003). Hospital transmission of community-acquired methicillin-resistant *Staphylococcus aureus* among postpartum women. *Clin Infect Dis., 37,* 1313–1319.

Sandberg, C. A. (1998). Cold therapy for breast engorgement in new mothers who are breastfeeding. Master's thesis. St. Paul, MN: College of St. Catherine.

Schelz, Z., Molnar, J., & Hohmann, J. (2006). Antimicrobial and antiplasmid activities of essential oils. *Fitoterapia, 77,* 279–285.

Schwartz, K., D'Arcy, H. J., Gillespie, B., et al. (2002). Factors associated with weaning in the first 3 months postpartum. *J Fam Pract., 51,* 439–444.

Scott, J. A., Robertson, M., Fitzpatrick, J., Knight, C., & Mulholland, S. (2008). Occurrence of lactational mastitis and medical management: A prospective cohort study in Glasgow. *Int. Breastfeeding J., 3,* 21.

Scott-Conner, C. E., & Schorr, S. J. (1995). The diagnosis and management of breast problems during pregnancy and lactation. *Am J Surg., 170,* 401–405.

Sealander, J. Y., & Kerr, C. P. (1989). Herpes simplex of the nipple: Infant-to-mother transmission. *Am Fam Physician, 39,* 111–113.

Semba, R. D., Kumwenda, N., Hoover, D. R., et al. (1999a). Human immunodeficiency virus load in breast milk, mastitis, and mother-to-child transmission of human immunodeficiency virus type 1. *J Infect Dis., 180,* 93–98.

Semba, R. D., Kumwenda, N., Taha, T. E., et al. (1999b). Mastitis and immunological factors in breast milk of human immunodeficiency virus-infected women. *J Hum Lact., 15,* 301–306.

Semba, R. D., Kumwenda, N., Taha, T., et al. (1999c). Mastitis and immunological factors in breast milk of lactating women in Malawi. *Clinical and Diagnostic Laboratory Immunology, 6,* 671–674.

Sharp, D. A. (1992). Moist wound healing for sore or cracked nipples. *Breastfeeding Abstracts, 12*(2), 19.

Shiau, S.-H. H. (1997). Randomized controlled trial of kangaroo care with full term infants: Effects on maternal anxiety, breast milk maturation, breast engorgement, and breastfeeding status. PhD dissertation. Cleveland, OH: Case Western Reserve University.

Shinefield, H., Black, S., Fattom, A., et al. (2002). Use of a *Staphylococcus aureus* conjugate vaccine in patients receiving hemodialysis. *NEJM, 346,* 491–496.

Singh, P., Sood, P. P., Gupta, S. K., et al. (1998). Experimental candidal mastitis in goats: Clinical, haematological, biochemical and sequential pathological studies. *Mycopathologia, 140,* 89–97.

Slaven, S., & Harvey, D. (1981). Unlimited suckling time improves breastfeeding. *Lancet, 1,* 392–393.

Smillie, C. M. (2004). *The prevention and treatment of plugged ducts.* Clinical handout. Stratford, CT: Breastfeeding Resources.

Smith, W., Erenberg, A., & Nowak, A. (1988). Imaging evaluation of the human nipple during breast-feeding. *Am J Dis Child., 142,* 76–78.

Snowden, H. M., Renfrew, M. J., & Woolridge, M. W. (2001). Treatments for breast engorgement during lactation. *Cochrane Database of Systematic Reviews,* Issue 2.

Soukka, T., Tenovuo, J., & Lenander-Lumikari, M. (1992). Fungicidal effect of human lactoferrin against Candida albicans. *FEMS Microbiology Letters, 69,* 223–228.

Spencer, J. P. (2008). Management of mastitis in breastfeeding women. *Am Fam Physician, 78,* 727–731.

Srinivasan, A., Dobrich, C., Mitnick, H., & Feldman, P. (2006). Ankyloglossia in breastfeeding infants: The effect of frenotomy on maternal nipple pain and latch. *Breastfeeding Med., 1,* 216–224.

Staib, P., Kretschmar, M., Nichterlein, T., et al. (2000). Differential activation of a *Candida albicans* virulence gene family during infection. *Proceedings of the National Academy of Science USA, 97,* 6102–6107.

Stevens, K., et al. (1997). The ultrasound appearances of galactoceles. *Br J Radiol., 70,* 239–241.

Stewart, P. S., & Costerton, J. W. (2001). Antibiotic resistance of bacteria in biofilms. *Lancet, 358*(9276), 135–138.

Stutte, P. C., Bowles, B. C., & Morman, G. Y. (1988). The effects of breast massage on volume and fat content of human milk. *Genesis, 10,* 22–25.

Sullivan-Bolyai, J. Z., Fife, K. H., Jacobs, R. F., et al. (1983). Disseminated neonatal herpes simplex virus type 1 from a maternal breast lesion. *Pediatrics, 71,* 455–457.

Svensson, K., Lange, S., Lonnroth, I., et al. (2004). Induction of anti-secretory factor in human milk may prevent mastitis. *Acta Paediatr., 93,* 1228–1231.

Tanquay, K., McBean, M., & Jain, E. (1994). Nipple candidosis among breastfeeding mothers: A case control study of predisposing factors. *Can Fam Physician, 40,* 1407–1413.

Terrill, P. J., & Stapleton, M. J. (1991). The inverted nipple: To cut the ducts or not? *Br J Plast Surg., 44,* 372–377.

Thomassen, P., Johansson, V. A., Wassberg, C., & Petrini, B. (1998). Breastfeeding, pain and infection. *Gynecol Obstet Invest., 46,* 73–74.

Thomsen, A. C., Espersen, T., & Maigaard, S. (1984). Course and treatment of milk stasis, noninfectious inflammation of the breast, and infectious mastitis in nursing women. *Am J Obstet Gynecol., 149,* 492–495.

Thorley, V. (1997). Inverted nipple with fatty plaques on areola and nipple. *Breastfeeding Rev., 5,* 43–44.

Ulitzsch, D., Nyman, M. K., & Carlson, R. A. (2004). Breast abscess in lactating women: US-guided treatment. *Radiology, 232,* 904–909.

Upledger Institute, Inc. (n.d.). International Alliance of Healthcare Educators. Retrieved September 15, 2005, from http://upledger.com

Utter, A. R. (1990). Gentian violet treatment for thrush: Can its use cause breastfeeding problems [letter]? *J Hum Lact., 6,* 178–180.

Utter, A. R. (1992). Genital violet and thrush [letter]. *J Hum Lact., 8,* 6.

Verronen, P. (1982). Breastfeeding: Reasons for giving up and transient lactational crises. *Acta Paediatr Scand., 71,* 447–450.

Vestermark, V., Hogdall, C. K., Birch, M., et al. (1991). Influence of the mode of delivery on initiation of breastfeeding. *Eur J Obstet Gynecol Reprod Biol., 38,* 33–38.

Vidotto, B., Guevara-Ochoa, L., Ponce, L. M., et al. (1992). Vaginal yeast flora of pregnant women in the Cusco region of Peru. *Mycoses, 35,* 229–234.

Walker, M. (2004). *Mastitis in lactating women*. Unit 2/Lactation Consultant Series Two. Schaumburg, IL: La Leche League International.

Walker, M., & Driscoll, J. W. (1989). Sore nipples: The new mother's nemesis. *MCN, 14*, 260–265.

Waller, H. (1946). The early failure of breastfeeding—A clinical study of its causes and their prevention. *Arch Dis Child., 21*, 1–12.

Walsh, A. (1949). Acute mastitis. *Lancet, 2*, 635–639.

Wambach, K. A. (2003). Lactation mastitis: A descriptive study of the experience. *J Hum Lact., 19*, 24–34.

Ward, K. A., & Burton, J. L. (1997). Dermatologic diseases of the breast in young women. *Clin Dermatol., 15*, 45–52.

Weichert, C. E. (1980). Prolactin cycling and the management of breastfeeding failure. *Adv. Pediatr., 27*, 391–407.

West, C. (1980). Factors influencing the duration of breastfeeding. *J Biosoc Sci., 12*, 325–331.

Widstrom, A. M., & Thingstrom-Paulsson, J. (1993). The position of the tongue during rooting reflexes elicited in newborn infants before the first suckle. *Acta Paediatr Scand., 82*, 281–283.

Wiener, S. (2006). Diagnosis and management of *Candida* of the nipple and breast. *Journal of Midwifery and Women's Health, 51*, 125–128.

Willumsen, J. F., Filteau, S. M., Coutsoudis, A., et al. (200). Subclinical mastitis as a risk factor for mother-infant HIV transmission. *Adv Exp Med Biol., 478*, 211–223.

Wilson-Clay, B. (2008). Case report of methicillin-resistant *Staphylococcus aureus* (MRSA) mastitis with abscess formation in a breastfeeding woman. *J Hum Lact., 24*, 326–329.

Wilson-Clay, B., & Hoover, K. (2008). *The breastfeeding atlas* (4th ed.). Austin, TX: LactNews Press.

Wilson-Clay, B., & Hoover, K. (2002). *The breastfeeding atlas* (4th ed.). Austin, TX: LactNews Press.

Winkler, J. M. (1964). Galactocele of the breast. *Am J Surg., 108*, 357–360.

Woolridge, M. W. (1986). Aetiology of sore nipples. *Midwifery, 2*, 172–176.

World Health Organization. (2000). *Mastitis: Causes and management*. Geneva: World Health Organization.

Yeung, D., Pennell, M., Leung, M., & Hall, J. (1981). Breastfeeding: Prevalence and influencing factors. *Can J Public Health, 72*, 323–330.

Ziemer, M., Paone, J., Schupay, J., & Cole, E. (1990). Methods to prevent and manage nipple pain in breastfeeding women. *Western J Nurs Res., 12*, 732–744.

Ziemer, M. M., Cooper, D. M., & Pigeon, J. G. (1995). Evaluation of a dressing to reduce nipple pain and improve nipple skin condition in breastfeeding women. *Nurs Res., 44*, 347–351.

Ziemer, M. M., & Pigeon, J. G. (1993). Skin changes and pain in the nipple during the 1st week of lactation. *J Obstet Gynecol Neonat Nurs., 22*, 247–256.

Additional Reading/Resources

Academy of Breastfeeding Medicine
Protocol #4: Mastitis
Protocol #11: Neonatal ankyloglossia
Protocol #20: Engorgement
www.bfmed.org

Summary Questions for Breastfeeding Troubleshooting and Observation

Questions for Troubleshooting the Underlying Cause of Inflammatory or Infective Processes in the Breast

- Have there been skipped or hurried feedings that leave large amounts of residual milk in the breast?
- Is there a time limitation placed on the first breast so the infant will take the other side?
- Is an older infant sleeping longer at night?
- Are there restrictions on the number of times the infant is fed each 24 hours?
- Is the mother unable to express milk at her place of employment?
- Is there a plugged milk duct or blocked nipple pore?
- Are the nipples sore, cracked, or bleeding?
- Has the infant been given bottles or pacifiers?
- Has the infant started solid foods (either at the appropriate age of about 6 months or in a younger infant to urge him or her to sleep longer)?
- Does the mother use nipple shields?
- Is the infant an effective feeder and gaining weight appropriately?
- Has the mother been attending or hosting holiday or family functions?
- Has the mother been ill, stressed, or extremely fatigued?
- Does the mother have preexisting breast lesions such as fibroadenomas?
- Does the mother smoke?
- Has the mother previously had mastitis?

Checkpoints for Feeding Observation at the Breast

- Is the infant positioned and latched correctly?

- Is there milk transfer verified by audible swallowing or pre- and postfeed weight checks?

- Have all areas of the breast been drained after the feeding or can areas of stasis be felt upon palpation?

- Is there nipple pain during the feeding?

- Is the nipple creased, compressed, distorted, or in spasm when the infant comes off the breast?

- Does the infant suck in a weak or uncoordinated manner that leaves large milk residuals in the breast?

Chapter 9

Physical, Medical, Emotional, and Environmental Challenges to the Breastfeeding Mother

Introduction

A mother may encounter a variety of challenges to breastfeeding depending on her own health and the environment in which she lives. With support and good clinical management, most mothers are capable of breastfeeding in spite of these difficulties or conditions.

Physically Challenged Mothers

Physical challenges to mothers may include many types of impairments, including spinal cord injury, loss of limbs or loss of the use of limbs from accidents or disease, and visual or hearing impairments. Breastfeeding is usually possible and should be encouraged for both the empowerment of the mothers and the close mother–baby relationship it engenders. Breastfeeding is often more convenient, time-saving, economical, and safer than mixing bottles of formula, especially if a mother is visually impaired or has physical difficulty in mixing, measuring, and pouring. Holding a bottle for prolonged periods of time may be difficult with arm, wrist, or hand impairment or loss.

Spinal Cord Injury or Involvement

The course of lactation for mothers with spinal cord injury depends on the location and extent of the injury. The spinal column consists of 33 vertebrae: 7 cervical (neck), 12 thoracic (trunk), 5 lumbar (back), 5 sacral (lower back), and 4 coccygeal (tailbone). Thirty-one pairs of spinal nerves exit the spinal cord and surrounding vertebrae and innervate the trunk and limbs. Complete spinal cord injury means that there is loss of sensory and motor function at and below the level of injury, whereas an incomplete injury results in some sensory or motor function at and below the level of injury. Injury to cervical area (C1-3) results in the inability to breathe independently, whereas injury at C6-8 allows good upper extremity use; injury at T-1 results in paraplegia. For a breastfeeding woman, injury at the T-6 level and above may affect milk production because disruption occurs in the communication between the nipple, myoepithelial cells, and pituitary gland. A T-6 level injury or above may result in diminished milk production by 6 weeks postpartum due to disrupted sympathetic nervous system feedback (Craig, 1990) and cessation of lactation by 3 months or so from the concomitant lack of nipple stimulation (Sipski, 1991). Nipple stimulation is not effective in the feedback loop unless the injury is at or below the point of origin for the fourth, fifth, and sixth intercostal nerves (T-4–6) that innervate the breast and nipple (Cesario, 2002; Halbert, 1998). Sucking-induced afferent stimuli are absent in women with spinal cord injury above T-4 and reduced if the injury is between T-4 and T-6. A spinal cord injury at the T-6 level or higher places the mother at risk for autonomic dysreflexia, a condition caused by noxious stimuli below the level of injury that can result in headaches, severe high blood pressure, stroke, coma, or death. Mothers with a T-6 or higher injury usually receive an epidural during labor to avoid this. Although rare, breastfeeding has been reported as an unusual and unexpected cause of autonomic dysreflexia (Dakhil-Jerew, Brook, & Derry, 2008).

Breastfeeding Management

Positioning considerations depend on the level and extent of the injury. Nursing bras should be chosen with elastic or Velcro closures if the mother's arms are affected. Some mothers set up a "nursing nest" on the floor where feedings as well as diapering and other caretaking activities are done to avoid issues with lifting and transferring the infant. Breastfeeding guidelines should be directed toward maximizing milk production and even pumping and freezing surplus milk to extend the period of time for full breastmilk feeding. In a mother with lesions at T-6 or higher, every effort should be made to avoid sore, cracked, or damaged nipples because this can be a trigger for autonomic dysreflexia. Positioning, latch, and proper sucking are important right from the start and should be immediately corrected if causing sore nipples. If nipple pain becomes a significant problem at each feeding, the mother may need medications for autonomic dysreflexia or may need to pump or hand express breastmilk until the nipples are healed.

Weight gain should be watched closely in infants of mothers with spinal cord injury; occasionally, some mothers may not experience the milk ejection reflex when the infant is at the breast. Oxytocin nasal spray can be prescribed and obtained from a compounding pharmacy for use before each feeding. Some mothers find that mental imaging and relaxation techniques combined with oxytocin nasal spray help maintain long-term breastfeeding (Cowley, 2005).

Limb Deficiencies, Abnormalities, or Absence

Limb abnormalities may be congenital or occur as a result of disease or injury. Limited use of arms may also occur as a result of a cerebral vascular accident or stroke. A major problem for the breastfeeding mother with an above- or below-the-elbow limb absence is positioning the infant at the breast. Some mothers may use a prosthesis, whereas others may find it more difficult to position a wiggling infant and control the prosthesis simultaneously. The father of the infant and other helpers can be shown how to assist the infant to the breast. Mothers usually develop their own systems for positioning the infant at the breast. Although mothers are usually advised to bring the infant to the breast, a mother with a limb abnormality sometimes finds it more efficient to bring the breast to the infant. Thomson (1995) described a mother with the absence of her left forearm sitting upright, using a pillow on her lap, shaping the breast, and placing it in the infant's mouth by leaning forward. The infant can also be positioned straddled across the thigh. The infant could be seated and supported in an infant seat with the mother bringing each breast to the infant. Mothers with good leg flexibility can sit in bed, on the floor, or on a couch with their knees bent and the infant placed in their lap, facing the breasts. Some mothers find that a sling is easier for them to use for both feeding and transporting the infant. Breastfeeding for mothers with physical challenges provides a unique connection between the mother and infant. This helps avoid maternal–child distancing that could occur if someone else fed the infant by bottle (Dunne & Fuerst, 1995).

Limb function can also be disrupted by a cerebral vascular accident, either occurring before the birth of the infant or during the peripartum period. The occurrence of stroke has been estimated to be between 8.1 per 100,000 pregnancies (Kittner et al., 1996) and 26 per 100,000 deliveries (Jaigobin & Silver, 2000). The risk for stroke seems greatest during the postpartum period, possibly due to the large decrease in blood volume or rapid changes in hormonal status (Kittner et al., 1996). The presence of hypercoagulability, preeclampsia, eclampsia, cocaine use, HELLP syndrome (Kidner & Flanders-Stepans, 2004), and sickle cell disease (Kittner & Adams, 1996) adds to the risk.

Differing effects on sensory capacity and motor function may manifest themselves depending on the type of stroke and the location of the affected area within the brain. A stroke in the left hemisphere of the brain affects the right side of the body, with right-sided weakness or paralysis, right-sided visual problems, speech difficulty, emotional lability, possible attention difficulties, intellectual deficits, and poor judgment. A stroke on the right side of the brain can result in left-sided weakness or paralysis and left-sided visual deficits. Lactation itself should remain intact as long as the function of the hypothalamus and pituitary gland has not been compromised. Sensory interruption to either areola may remove the afferent arc necessary for the release of prolactin from areolar stimulation. However, because the nature of a stroke permits normal functioning on one side, complete function of one breast and its associated sensory pathways may remain intact (Halbert, 1998).

A number of medications, such as those used immediately during a stroke, antihypertensives, and anticoagulants, may remain compatible with breastfeeding. Early interventions may separate the mother and infant, necessitating the possibility of pumping milk when the mother is stabilized. Positioning for breastfeeding requires a creative look at what works best. Mothers may lie on the affected side while using the unaffected arm for support and positioning the infant. A nursing pillow, sling, or other supportive piece of equipment may be needed for the mother to safely hold the infant while breastfeeding. Oxytocin release may be beneficial to the mother with a stroke because it lowers blood pressure and exerts a calming effect. Close attention should also center on infant weight gain and adequacy of the milk supply if one breast does not produce an abundant amount of milk. Clinicians need to assess any deficits in the mother's field of vision because she may be unable to see the infant in certain nursing positions.

Epilepsy

Seizure disorders affect approximately 1.1 million women of reproductive age in the United States (Pschirrer, 2004), with about 20,000 of these women giving birth each year. Although most women with epilepsy can conceive and bear normal, healthy children, their pregnancies present a greater risk for complications. One-fourth to one-half of women with epilepsy may experience an exacerbation of their seizures during pregnancy, mostly toward the end of the pregnancy, but with about 31% experiencing this increase during their first trimester (Yerby, Kaplan, & Tran, 2004). This is frequently due to the decline in plasma concentrations of antiepileptic medications, even with correct or increasing doses. Maternal seizures increase the risk of injury, miscarriage, and of epilepsy and developmental delay in the children.

Many medications are used either singly or in combination to control the numerous types of seizures, with specific medications used for specific seizure types. First-generation antiepileptic drugs include carbamazepine (Tegretol), ethosuximide (Zarontin), phenobarbital (Liminal), phenytoin (Dilantin), primidone (Myidone), and valproic acid (Depakene, Depakote). Both seizure activity during pregnancy and some antiepileptic medications place infants at risk for a number of complications. Infants of mothers with epilepsy are at increased risk for congenital malformations (orofacial clefts and congenital heart disease) and anomalies (dysmorphic facial features), neural tube defects, neonatal hemorrhage, low birth weight, developmental delay, and childhood epilepsy. Several clinical syndromes have been described in infants of mothers with epilepsy, with learning and behavioral disturbances prominent aspects of these syndromes (Moore et al., 2000). The medication primidone (Myidone), especially when used in combination with other drugs, is associated with lower intelligence scores in school-aged children (Koch et al., 1999). Lower cognitive scores have also been seen in children whose mothers took valproate (Meador et al., 2009). This makes it extremely important that infants of mothers with epilepsy are breastfed or provided with as much mother's milk as possible. Meador (2008) demonstrated that children of mothers with epilepsy who had been breastfed had better cognitive scores than those who were bottle-fed.

There are no medical contraindications to breastfeeding when a mother has epilepsy (Crawford, 2009). A number of newer or second-generation antiepileptic drugs with limited data on their safety have been marketed in the United States since 1993, including gabapentin (Neurontin), felbamate (Felbatol), lamotrigine (Lamictal), levetiracetam (Keppra), oxcarbazepine (Trileptal), tiagabine (Gabitril), topiramate (Topamax), and zonisamide (Zonegran). Breastfeeding mothers taking phenobarbital or primidone may have infants who are sedated by the medications and should be monitored for adequate intake and weight gain. Taking antiepileptic medications is not considered a contraindication to breastfeeding (Delgado-Escueta & Janz, 1992), with infant reactions to maternal medications usually far outweighed by the benefits of breastfeeding and human milk (Ito, Moretti, Liau, & Koren, 1995).

Maternal Visual or Hearing Impairment

Visual or hearing impairment is not a contraindication to breastfeeding. Mothers with limited or no sight or with limited or no hearing use their intact senses to interact with their infant. The senses of touch, taste, and smell and intuitive sensitivity contribute to facilitate breastfeeding (Martin Cookson, 1992). Breastfeeding for visually impaired mothers avoids the problems of preparing and cleaning bottles of formula. Feeding cues are recognized easily when a mother carries her infant in a sling or front pack carrier. Breastfeeding consultation can be accomplished in sign language for hearing impaired mothers (Bowles, 1991), with materials written in Braille available from La Leche League International for mothers who have limited or no sight. Not all mothers with visual or hearing impairment are totally blind or totally deaf. If a mother appears to have trouble understanding what is being said to her, ask if she has a visual or hearing impairment. Some mothers are embarrassed or find it difficult to ask for help.

Insufficient Milk Supply

There are no specific diagnostic tests for lactation sufficiency. Insufficient milk supply, either real or perceived, remains the most frequent reason for the abandonment of breastfeeding (Ahluwalia, Morrow, & Hsia, 2005; Gatti, 2008; Li, Fein, Chen, & Grummer-Strawn, 2008; Segura-Millan, Dewey, & Perez-Escamilla, 1994; Verronen, 1982). Milk insufficiency has been classified by daily output and possible etiology (Box 9-1).

The perception of insufficient milk may begin within the first 48 hours after delivery when clinicians and mothers are unaware of the normal amounts of colostrum available to the infant as well as the infant's small stomach capacity. Attempts at pumping the breasts at this time often yield only drops of colostrum, further reinforcing the appearance of insufficient milk. Mothers' perceptions of insufficient milk commonly encompass the lack of fullness in the breasts, increased frequency of infant feeding, and an infant who continues to fuss after a feeding or does not settle between feeds. Measurement of infant intake and weight gain during the times of these perceptions (transient lactation crisis) revealed both parameters to be normal variations in infant appetite and behavior (Hillervik-Lindquist, 1991; Hillervik-Lindquist, Hofvander, & Sjolin, 1991). Mothers who describe insufficient milk supply most frequently do so because their infant was not satisfied after a feeding and, as a result, offer a bottle of formula as a complement after a breastfeeding (Hill & Aldag, 1991).

BOX 9-1 Classifications of Apparent Milk Insufficiency

Class I: Unsubstantiated Low Milk Supply

- Majority of insufficient milk supply cases.
- Typically controlled through routine breastfeeding management, i.e., positioning, latch, feed management (number of times, length of feed, etc.), and support and encouragement.

Class IIa: Physiological Low Milk Supply (output between 150 and 350 g/24 h)

- This class does not respond to normal routine advice and support.
- May require breastmilk removal via pump or hand expression to increase milk drainage from breast.

Class IIb: Iatrogenic Low Milk Supply (output < 450 g/24 h)

- May have had higher milk output prior, but output has decreased due to poor management, e.g., mother engorged and no one told her to pump, mother encouraged to allow infant to sleep through the night, mother was told to supplement unnecessarily, etc.

Class IIc: Behaviorally Induced Low Milk Supply (output < 450 g/24 h)

- Includes both mother's and infant's behaviors, e.g., infant being pushed on breast, sleepy infant, use of pacifiers, overactive letdown, etc.

Class III: Pathophysiological Lactation Failure (output < 150 g/24 h)

- Mammary hypoplasia—breasts do not undergo normal growth and development during pregnancy
- Asymmetric breasts, tubular shaped, lack sufficient glandular tissue
- Retained placental products (reversible)
- Necrosis of anterior pituitary due to hypotensive episode, postpartum hemorrhage (Sheehan syndrome)
- Endocrine deficiency—insufficient progesterone
- Low thyroid hormone
- Anemia
- History of chest tubes
- Breast surgery—including augmentation or reduction mammoplasty
- Polycystic ovary syndrome

Source: Woolridge MW. (1995). Breastfeeding: Physiology into practice. In D. P. Davies (Ed.), *Nutrition in child health. Proceedings of conference jointly organized by the Royal College of Physicians of London and the British Paediatric Association* (pp. 13–31). London, UK: RCPL Press.

Although mothers most commonly report infant crying as the cue used to determine insufficient milk (Huang et al., 2009), actual milk production is seldom assessed nor is the infant's efficiency at milk removal observed. Once crying is perceived as hunger, mothers and healthcare providers often turn to formula supplementation as a remedy to stop the crying and to fill up the infant (Sacco, Caulfield, Gittelsohn, & Martinez, 2006). Supplementing with bottles of formula has the potential to depress milk production and result in a real milk-supply problem. Maternal descriptions of insufficient milk are not only based on a perception of too little milk being produced for appropriate infant weight gain and infant dissatisfaction (Hill & Humenick, 1989) but also as doubts in maternal self-efficacy (McCarter-Spaulding & Kearney, 2001).

Overlapping etiologies exist for the development of real or perceived insufficient milk. The most common overarching contributors are mismanagement of breastfeeding (Powers, 1999) and lack of information (Hill, 1991):

- Breastfeeding mismanagement may include a limited number of feedings, short times at the breast, scheduled feedings that do not coincide with the infant's behavioral feeding readiness cues, poor latch, failure to assess for swallowing, inappropriate formula supplementation, unrelieved severe engorgement, use of artificial nipples, and pacifiers.

- Maternal conditions may include overweight/obesity and diabetes (Neubauer et al., 1993) that delay lactogenesis II, history of breast surgery or breast reduction (Hill, Wilhelm, Aldag, & Chatterton, 2004; Hughes & Owen, 1993), retained placental fragments, breast hypoplasia (Neifert et al., 1990; Neifert, Seacat, & Jobe, 1985), use of certain medications such as pseudoephedrine (Sudafed) (Aljazaf et al., 2003) or ergot alkaloids, maternal smoking (Hopkinson et al., 1992), oral contraceptives (Kennedy, Short, & Tully, 1997), inverted nipples, Sheehan syndrome (Sert, Tetiker, Kirim, & Kocak, 2003) or maternal postpartum hemorrhage (Willis & Livingstone, 1995), anemia (Henly et al., 1995), and endocrine problems such as hypothyroidism or polycystic ovary syndrome (Marasco, Marmet, & Shell, 2000).

- Situations where the mother must initiate lactation in the absence of the infant at the breast such as prematurity can place the mother at a 2.8 times increased risk for insufficient milk (Hill, Aldag, Chatterton, & Zinaman, 2005). Milk output during the first 6 weeks predicts feeding method at week 12 (Hill, Aldag, Zinaman, & Chatterton, 2007). Other contributors to insufficient milk production include infant conditions and diseases that preclude direct feeding from the breast or result in ineffective feedings, long-term pumping situations such as a hospitalized infant or a mother returning to employment, use of a poor breast pump or a poorly fitted flange on a breast pump, not enough pumping, exposure to acute or long-term stressors (Hill, Chatterton, & Aldag, 2003), and stressful labor and delivery (Chen, Nommsen-Rivers, Dewey, & Lonnerdal, 1998).

Indicators or signs and symptoms of insufficient milk may not be clearly evident. Assumptions of insufficient milk are often made if the infant loses more than 7% of birth weight and fails to regain birth weight by 2 weeks. However, this may also indicate an infant with poor breastfeeding skills who is unable to transfer milk even when there is an abundant supply. Weight gain of less than 5 oz per week, concentrated urine in the diapers, passing of dry hard stools, lethargy, and dry mucous membranes signal a potential problem with either milk transfer or milk supply and require assessment and intervention (Amir, 2006). Infants who sleep excessive amounts or who feed for longer than 45 minutes at a feed or appear to want to nurse continuously signal the need for a feeding observation. Mothers who have been pumping regularly and report a drop in the amount of milk pumped may be experiencing transient fluctuation in milk output, especially if their hospitalized infant's condition has deteriorated. This can happen early in lactation during the establishment of optimal milk production or later in lactation as a pump motor wears out.

Breastfeeding Management

Clinicians should first assess the infant during a breastfeeding to ascertain the status and amount of milk transfer. Pre- and postfeed weights can verify the amount of milk transfer. Faulty sucking skills, oral anomalies, and poor positioning may be recognized and remedied at this time.

Management options depend on the cause of the milk insufficiency. Clinicians could select options or combinations of options:

- Extra feedings (Decarvalho et al., 1983), extra pumpings, pumping after a feeding, improving infant positioning (Morton, 1992), and assisting milk transfer of the infant by using alternate massage (Lau & Hurst, 1999; Yokoyama et al., 1994) can be used.

- Mothers can use a tube-feeding device at the breast to deliver milk to the infant while the infant stimulates the breast.

- Mothers of preterm infants should be encouraged to engage in skin-to-skin care while their infant is hospitalized because this has been shown to improve milk output (Hurst et al., 1997). They can also pump next to their infant's bed while looking at or touching their infant.

- The increased use of an effective, electric, hospital-grade breast pump with double collection kit and properly fitted breast flange should be considered. Check the vacuum with a vacuum gauge to ensure the pump is operating efficiently.

- Consider the use of relaxation techniques such as listening to a guided imagery audio tape (Feher et al., 1989).

- Mothers who smoke should be encouraged to quit or reduce the number of cigarettes smoked per day. Smoking should not occur directly before a feeding as it may inhibit the letdown reflex.

- Medications have been used to improve milk production (Gabay, 2002); however, many studies on the use of metoclopramide and other medical galactagogues suffer from poor methodology and conflicting results, with some finding that pharmaceutical galactagogues made no difference in lactation success (Anderson & Valdes, 2007). Parity may also influence the effectiveness of these medications. Brown et al. (2000) administered single doses of two strengths of metoclopramide and a single dose of domperidone to nonpregnant women. Nulliparous women had the highest prolactin secretion with the 10-mg metoclopramide dose and multiparous women had prolactin secretion patterns that were equivalent between the medications. Medications can be selected for mothers who do not respond to other interventions:

  - Metoclopramide (Reglan), a dopamine antagonist, has been shown to stimulate basal prolactin levels, leading to increased milk production at doses of 30–45 mg/day (Budd et al., 1993; Ehrenkranz & Ackerman, 1986; Gupta & Gupta, 1985; Kauppila, Kivinen, & Ylikorkala, 1983). Metoclopramide is dose dependent, with some mothers not responding, especially if their prolactin levels are normal (Kauppila et al., 1983). Maternal side effects of metoclopramide include gastric cramping, diarrhea, and depression with longer term use (more than 4 weeks), but no untoward effects have been reported in infants (Hale, 2008). Abrupt discontinuation of the medication can result in a precipitous drop in milk production; tapering the dosage by decreasing it 10 mg/week is recommended.

  - Domperidone (Motilium) is a peripheral dopamine antagonist similar to metoclopramide. However, unlike metoclopramide it does not cross the blood–brain barrier. This feature reduces the likelihood of central nervous system side effects such as depression as seen in some mothers using metoclopramide. It produces significant increases in prolactin levels (Newman, 1998) and stimulates milk production at doses of 10–20 mg three to four times daily without maternal gastric side effects. Not all mothers respond to the use of domperidone, but for those who do there is somewhat of a dose-response relationship with higher doses resulting in more milk production (Wan et al., 2008). There have been no reported effects on the infant and it is considered a better choice as a galactagogue (Brouwers et al., 1980; Brown et al., 2000; da Silva, Knoppert, Angelini, & Forret, 2001; Hofmeyr & van Iddekinge, 1983; Hofmeyr, van Iddekinge, & Blott, 1985; Petraglia et al., 1985). Domperidone is contraindicated if the mother is taking other medications with anticholinergic properties because these may antagonize the effects on the gastrointestinal tract. The effects may not be seen for 3–4 days, with the maximum effect taking up to 2–3 weeks (Henderson, 2003a). Most mothers take the medication for 3–8 weeks. Although not widely available in the United States, compounding pharmacies can formulate domperidone with a physician's prescription.

- Human growth hormone has been used to successfully increase milk production in mothers of term and preterm infants, with (Gunn et al., 1996; Milsom, Rabone, Gunn, & Gluckman, 1998) and without (Breier et al., 1993; Milsom et al., 1992) lactation insufficiency. Results are dose dependent with no maternal or infant side effects reported over a 7-day study period.

- Oxytocin, although normally used to elicit the milk ejection reflex, has also been shown to improve milk production in older studies (Ruis et al., 1981). An appropriate dose of sublingual or buccal (not nasal) oxytocin may help improve milk output, especially in pump-dependent mothers, but should not replace proper breastfeeding and pumping guidelines (Renfrew, Lang, & Woolridge, 2000).

- Thyrotropin-releasing hormone has been minimally studied and shown to significantly improve milk production in mothers with lactation insufficiency with little effect on normally lactating mothers (Tyson, Perez, & Zanartu, 1976).

- Recombinant human prolactin was studied in non-postpartum women and showed expressible galactorrhea over a 7-day study period and may be a viable option for short-term lactation augmentation (Page-Wilson, Smith, & Welt, 2007).

- Acupuncture is an ancient and effective treatment used in China for insufficient milk (Zhao & Guo, 2006). Clavey (1996) discussed the procedure and reported over a 90% effectiveness rate when acupuncture is initiated within 20 days of birth but less than an 85% success rate after 20 days postpartum. The earlier postpartum the treatment is begun, the quicker the results and the more likely that milk production will significantly improve. Wei, Wang, Han, and Li (2008) described the very effective use of electroacupuncture at Shaoze (SI 1) in 46 mothers with insufficient milk.

- Herbal and botanical preparations have been used since antiquity to stimulate milk production. Although there is little science behind the use of most of these preparations or their effectiveness, many are widely recommended by clinicians for improving milk output. It is estimated that at least 15% of breastfeeding women use herbal galactagogues at some point (The National Children's Study, 2003). Some include fenugreek, milk thistle, raspberry leaf, and nettle; however, a number are unsafe for lactating women (Low Dog & Micozzi, 2005). Other herbal galactagogues frequently seen are goat's rue, fennel seed, chaste tree seed, fireweed, anise seed, blessed thistle, stinging nettle, and cotton root (Bingel & Farnsworth, 1994). Many of these herbs are combined in commercial galactagogue preparations such as Mother's Milk Blend Tea (chamomile, catnip, fennel, stinging nettle, and lavender), More Milk Plus (a tincture blend of fenugreek, blessed thistle, stinging nettle, and fennel), and Mother's Lactaflow (a tincture blend of fennel, blessed thistle, goat's rue, and fenugreek). Fenugreek (*Trigonella foenum-graecum*) is probably the most widely used herbal galactagogue. Fenugreek has been shown to have antianxiety effects, which may contribute to the herb's anecdotal effectiveness (Abascal & Yarnell, 2008). The dosage is usually a 1,200-mg capsule two to three times daily. Goat's rue (*Galega officinalis*) is a common galactagogue (Weiss, 2001) used historically for not only insufficient milk but also for symptoms of non–insulin-resistant diabetes. Several of the plant's constituents (guanidine and galegine) have been studied as antidiabetic agents, with metformin being a synthetic chemical based on galegine. Goat's rue is dosed as 1 teaspoon of dried herb steeped in 1 cup of water twice daily or 1–2 mL of tincture three times daily. Fennel seed (*Foeniculum vulgare*) is used to increase milk production at a dose of 5–7 g of seed per day as a tea. Chaste tree seed (*Vitex adnus-castus*) is used at a dosage of 1 teaspoon of the berries steeped in 1 cup of water three times daily or 2.5 mL of tincture three times daily. Milk thistle (*Silybum marianum*) was studied in a micronized 420-mg dose form in women with marginal milk production (Di Pierro, Callegari, Carotenuto, & Tapia, 2008). Fifty mothers (half in the experimental group and half in the placebo group) were treated for 63 days, with an increase of 85.94% of the daily milk production in the treatment group and a 32.09% increase in milk production in the placebo group. It is interesting to note that the herb was micronized before being administered, which improves its poor bioavailability.

Many authors disagree or provide completely contradictory information on the use of various preparations (Humphrey, 2003). Other "remedies" such as beer (hops) and brewer's yeast (vitamin B complex) are sometimes recommended rather than addressing the underlying cause of milk insufficiency. Although herbal and botanical preparations are commonly used, they require caution: Clinicians can refer to the German Commission E Monographs for safety profiles of botanicals (Blumenthal & Busse, 1998), to the American Herbal Products Association (www.ahpa.org) for information on manufacturing and labeling standards, and to the American Botanical Council (www.herbalgram.org) for information on the quality of herbal products.

Medications should not replace breastfeeding management guidelines tailored to each mother's situation. Any use of a galactagogue requires close follow-up by the clinician of both mother and infant (Academy of Breastfeeding Medicine, 2004).

Hyperlactation

Until the breasts calibrate the amount of milk to synthesize based on infant intake, it is possible for a mother to make amounts of milk far in excess of what the infant needs to consume. Milk production late in the first week of lactation ranges from 200 to 900 mL/day, with a milk synthesis rate of 11–58 mL/h. When mothers have a high rate of milk synthesis, 60 mL/h or more, a spectrum of breast and infant signs and symptoms may become apparent (Box 9-2) indicating hyperlactation and the need for clinical intervention (Livingstone, 1996).

This particular cluster of signs and symptoms in the infant, as listed in Box 9-2, may mimic lactose intolerance or an infant with uncoordinated sucking. Although lactose intolerance is unlikely, the high-volume, low-fat meals may experience a rapid transit through the gut, causing the green stools as mentioned in Box 9-2. Much of the gas may be the result of both fermentation of lactose and

---

BOX 9-2 Signs and Symptoms of Hyperlactation

Maternal Breast

- Breasts that never feel comfortable or drained and that refill very quickly
- Shooting pain deep in the breast
- Firm, lumpy, or tender areas
- Chronic plugged ducts or mastitis
- Intense pain with first milk ejection
- Forceful letdown
- Constant leaking between feedings
- Leaking milk prenatally

Infant

- Gulping, choking, or coughing while at the breast
- Milk leaking from the mouth
- Arching back off of the breast, thrashing, difficulty remaining latched to the breast
- Spitting up
- Excessive gas
- Green, frothy, explosive stools that may cause irritating diaper rash
- Poor weight gain or initial good weight gain with slow weight gain later

---

swallowed air from gulping during the fast flow of milk. Choking and sputtering at the breast are usually the result of an infant unable to swallow fast enough to accommodate a high flow of fluid into the throat. Mothers may describe the necessity of frequently burping the infant during each feeding as well as removing the infant from the breast several times during the feeding to allow the infant to breathe between periods of rapid milk flow. Oversupply can also mask real problems with sucking coordination, so clinicians should always look for improvement in the condition over time.

Galactorrhea can also have non-breastfeeding etiologies (Pena & Rosenfeld, 2001) that, although rare, should be considered:

- Neoplastic processes (prolactinoma)
- Hypothalamic-pituitary disorders

- Systemic diseases (hypothyroidism, Cushing disease)
- Medications (antidepressants, selective serotonin reuptake inhibitors [SSRIs], antihypertensives)
- Chest wall irritation (ill-fitting clothing or bra, herpes zoster, atopic dermatitis, esophageal reflux)

Breastfeeding Management

A number of options and combinations of interventions can be used to form individual feeding plans:

1. Reduce the rate of milk synthesis:
   - Offer one breast per feeding that the infant thoroughly drains (Smillie, Campbell, & Iwinski, 2005). If the infant wishes to return to the breast within an hour or so, the mother can use the same breast. Infants who are switched to the second breast before finishing the first may ingest a high volume of low-fat milk (Woolridge & Fischer, 1988).
   - If the other breast becomes uncomfortable, the mother should express just enough milk to soften the breast.
   - Decrease the frequency of feedings by allowing the infant to become satiated on the fat-rich milk available at the end of the feeding, which is assisted in its availability by the use of alternate massage.
   - Block feeding divides the day into equal time blocks starting with a 3-hour time block, where the same breast is offered for each feeding during the time block. At the start of the next time block, the other breast is offered for each feeding. Time blocks can be gradually lengthened if necessary if the condition does not improve after the first few time blocks. Van Veldhuizen-Staas (2007) recommended a protocol of full breast drainage and block feedings where the breasts are as fully drained as possible by pumping before the block feedings begin. They are fully drained/pumped again if they become overfull despite the block feedings.
   - Use of pseudoephedrine (Sudafed) (Aljazaf et al., 2003) can decrease but not eliminate milk production.
   - Herbal treatment includes the use of sage (Bisset, 1994).
   - Some mothers find that drinking peppermint tea lowers their milk output.
   - Cabbage leaves placed inside the bra for extended periods of time have been anecdotally reported to diminish milk production.

2. Management of feedings:
   - Have the mother place the infant in a semiprone position directly facing her breast with the mother leaning back or reclining.
   - The mother can express her milk until after the first milk ejection reflex, reducing the gush of milk and the forceful flow into the infant's mouth.
   - The mother may need to burp the infant frequently and pace the feeding by allowing the infant to rest between periods of strong milk flow.
   - The mother needs to make sure that any plugged milk ducts or areas of the breast that are not draining well are massaged during the feeding.

Induced Lactation and Relactation

Induced lactation is the initiation of milk production in a woman who has never been pregnant. Women who wish to induce lactation may be infertile, may be adopting an infant, or may be the intended mother of a surrogate pregnancy. Clinicians can help such mothers understand that they may be unable to produce all the milk necessary to meet the infant's needs without supplementation, but they will certainly meet the goal of a wonderful and unique nurturing experience (Wittig & Spatz, 2008). Numerous breast preparation techniques are used with varying amounts of milk being produced (L. Goldfarb & J. Newman, unpublished data, 2002; Newman & Pittman, 2000).

Adopting mothers typically start preparation several months ahead of the scheduled time for receiving the infant by using nipple stimulation (hand or breast pump) and a galactagogue such as metoclopramide (Cheales-Siebenaler, 1999). Oxytocin nasal spray is sometimes used before each pumping and breastfeeding session to enhance the milk ejection reflex and to stimulate milk flow. Protocols for induced lactation typically encourage nipple stimulation, estrogen and progesterone preparations to induce structural changes in the breast (as would happen during pregnancy), use of a dopamine antagonist to increase prolactin levels, and frequent breastfeeding when the infant is available (Bryant, 2006). If the mother is adopting an infant and has a long lead time or is the intended mother of a surrogate pregnancy, she may find the protocol in Box 9-3 helpful.

However, sometimes adopting mothers are given such short notice of the infant's arrival that neither partial nor full lactation is established and the process proceeds with the infant providing breast stimulation if he or she will latch. Often in this situation, mothers use a tube-feeding system to provide formula supplementation while the infant suckles at the breast. They may follow this with frequent breast pumping and/or the use of galactagogues. Mothers may find that

BOX 9-3 Selected Interventions From the Goldfarb and Newman Protocol for Inducing Lactation

Time frame	Intervention
6 mo before due date	Take one active birth control pill/day + 10 mg domperidone 4 times/day for 1 week. Increase dosage to 20 mg 4 times/day.
6 wk before due date	Stop the birth control pill and continue the domperidone and begin breast pumping ~8 times/day. Add Blessed Thistle herb (390 mg/capsule) and Fenugreek seed (610 mg/capsule). Take 3 capsules of each 3 times a day with meals.
After birth of infant	Breastfeed as often as possible, continue domperidone, maintain herbal intake and pumping after feedings.

Source: Complete protocols for inducing lactation with long and short lead times and for menopausal women can be found at http://asklenore.info/breastfeeding/induced_lactation/regular_protocol.html

power pumping helps increase milk production. Breastfeeding after a surrogate pregnancy allows a longer period of preparation time to induce lactation before the infant arrives (Biervliet et al., 2001). The composition of milk from an induced lactation is similar to and quite adequate for normal infant growth (Lawrence & Lawrence, 2005).

Relactation is a process of reestablishing lactation some time after it has ended. Mothers may choose to relactate if they change their mind about infant feeding, if they have an infant that cannot tolerate infant formula, if they have a preterm or ill infant and decide to breastfeed during the course of the infant's hospitalization (Thompson, 1996), or if they had experienced a life crisis that has been resolved. Infants in a relactation or induced lactation situation should be monitored closely for normal weight gain and their mothers closely supported and praised for their hard work and dedication to their infant's health and well-being (World Health Organization, 1998).

Overweight and Obese Mothers

The prevalence of obesity has continued to rise in women over 18 years of age, from 25.4% in 1994 to 33.4% in 2000 (Flegal, Carroll, Ogden, & Johnson, 2002) and up again to 52.2% in 2008 (Kaiser Family Foundation, 2008). Analysis of

2003–2004 NHANES (National Health and Nutrition Examination Survey) data showed 51.7% of nonpregnant women aged 20–39 years were overweight or obese (body mass index [BMI] $\geq$ 25 kg/m^2), 28.9% were obese (BMI $\geq$ 30 kg/m^2), and 8.0% were extremely obese (BMI $\geq$ 40 kg/m^2) (Ogden et al., 2006). Obesity can have numerous effects on health and reproduction, including an increased risk of diabetes mellitus, gestational diabetes, osteoarthritis, cardiovascular disease, miscarriage, hypertension in pregnancy, and cesarean delivery (Norman & Clark, 1998). Cesarean delivery risk is increased by 50% in overweight women and is more than double for obese women compared with women with a normal BMI (Poobalan, Aucott, Gurung, Smith, & Bhattacharya, 2009). Cesarean section increases the risk of delayed lactogenesis and low milk supply (Rowe-Murray & Fisher, 2002). Infants born to obese mothers have an increased risk of neural tube defects such as spina bifida, a higher rate of birth injuries, an increased incidence of low Apgar scores, and more admissions to neonatal intensive care units.

Excessive body weight and obesity can negatively influence the initiation and duration of breastfeeding (Donath & Amir, 2000; Li, Jewell, & Grummer-Strawn, 2003), with a higher BMI related to decreased initiation (Hilson, Rasmussen, & Kjolhede, 1997; Manios et al., 2009) and duration (Donath & Amir, 2008; Oddy, Landsborough, Kendall, Henderson, & Downie, 2006; Rutishauser & Carlin, 1992) of breastfeeding. The risk of early termination of any breastfeeding rises progressively with increasing BMI, with the greater the prepregnancy BMI, the earlier the termination of breastfeeding (Baker, Michaelsen, Sorensen, & Rasmussen, 2007). Perceived insufficient milk production, slow infant weight gain, and embarrassment to breastfeed in public have been reported to result in decreased exclusive breastfeeding rates in obese mothers (Mok et al., 2008).

Animal studies found that the timing of the onset of obesity affects lactation, with early-onset obesity (before menarche) resulting in lower milk production in Holstein heifers (Zanton & Heinrichs, 2005). Onset of obesity (before development of the breasts) has not been studied in humans relative to milk production effectiveness. Psychological, behavioral, and cultural influences also have a role in reduced lactation in overweight and obese women (Amir & Donath, 2007). Obese mothers may experience lower socioeconomic status (a group less likely to breastfeed), may be less likely to participate in preventive health behaviors, or may be embarrassed to breastfeed in public due to their discomfort with their body image.

Excessive body weight and obesity have been shown to be a risk factor for delayed lactogenesis II (Chapman & Perez-Escamilla, 1999a), with low milk transfer at 60 hours postpartum seen in obese women (Chapman & Perez-Escamilla, 2000). Part of this delay has been attributed to the tendency of overweight/obese mothers to have large areolas with flat nipples, contributing to a difficult latch, sore nipples, and resulting limited milk transfer.

For each 1-unit (1 kg/m^2) increase in prepregnant BMI, a 0.5-hour delay in onset of lactogenesis II has been calculated (Hilson, Rasmussen, & Kjolhede, 2004). Thus the difference in the onset of copious milk production can be up to 10 hours later in a mother with a BMI of 40 kg/m^2 compared with a mother with a BMI of 20 kg/m^2. This delay occurs at a time when the mother has been discharged from the hospital and is concerned about the delay in the onset of a copious milk supply. It is interesting to note that although increasing the frequency of breastfeeding in the early postpartum period is associated with an earlier onset of lactogenesis II in nonobese mothers, among obese women no benefit was seen from increasing breastfeeding frequency (Chapman & Perez-Escamilla, 1999b).

Animal models have also shown impaired lactogenesis in the presence of obesity. In the murine model, lipid accumulation in the secretory epithelial cells of obese mice was indicative of the absence of copious milk secretion, with the addition of marked abnormalities in the alveolar development of the mammary gland itself (Flint et al., 2005). Kamikawa et al. (2009) showed that obesity disrupts mammary ductal development in mice, with less dense distribution of ducts, reduced branching, and ducts that were incompletely lined with myoepithelium. It is not known if breast changes are associated with obesity in women.

The negative effect on breastfeeding of being overweight or obese is multifactorial, with hormonal alterations linked to lactation difficulties. Obesity may facilitate alterations in the hypothalamic-pituitary-gonadal axis and in fat metabolism that affects both milk production and composition (Bray, 1997; Rasmussen et al., 2001). Research has shown that overweight/obese women have a lower prolactin response to suckling during the early days when prolactin is more important to milk production than it is later in lactation (Hilson et al., 2004; Rasmussen & Kjolhede, 2004). At 48 hours postpartum, obese mothers compared with nonobese mothers showed a 45-ng/mL decrease in prolactin response to suckling that persisted over the first week. At 7 days postpartum excess body weight/obesity was associated with a reduction in the prolactin response to suckling of almost 100 ng/mL. The delay in lactogenesis II and the blunted prolactin response to suckling during the first 7 days may be contributors to the high proportion of obese mothers who abandon breastfeeding during this important period of time (Hilson et al., 1997).

With surgical management of obesity available for people with a BMI of 40 or more (or a BMI of 35–40 with other health problems), many women who were infertile as a result of extreme obesity become pregnant and deliver healthy infants. Breastfeeding is certainly recommended for overweight/obese mothers as well as mothers who have undergone gastric bypass or bariatric surgery. Breast-feeding may help with maternal weight control and may contribute to the prevention of overweight/obesity in their children. Breastfeeding has been shown to reduce postpartum weight retention in all but the heaviest of women (Baker et al., 2008). Mothers who have undergone bariatric surgery, however, should be closely followed postpartum. After gastric bypass surgery mothers may have difficulty absorbing vitamin B12 with consequently lower milk levels. B12 deficiencies in breastfeeding infants of mothers who have undergone bariatric surgery have been reported, manifesting as slow growth, developmental delays, apathy, hypotonia, hyperreflexive, and slow head growth (Granger & Finlay, 1994; Wardinsky et al., 1995). Mothers may be given monthly B12 injections and infants may be placed on supplemental vitamins to avoid adverse outcomes.

Breastfeeding Management

Although it has been shown that obese women are at an increased risk of delay in establishing lactation and for lactation failure, many clinicians do not manage obese mothers differently from normal weight women (Rasmussen, Lee, Ledkovsky, & Kjolhede, 2006). This could be a contributing factor to the less than optimal initiation and duration rates seen in obese mothers. If obese mothers experience a delay in lactogenesis, then the infant will be presented with a prolonged colostral phase during which time increased numbers of feedings are necessary to offset the low availability of a copious milk supply. Mothers should be encouraged to breastfeed about 10–12 times each day until lactogenesis II has been confirmed and the infant is gaining weight well. Increased numbers of feedings may not contribute to earlier lactogenesis II but will help keep the infant well hydrated, prevent weight loss, and avoid the need to supplement with infant formula. The infant should be monitored closely for sufficient weight gain.

Positioning for breastfeeding should include support for large breasts, such as a rolled-up towel or receiving blanket under the breast for support. If the infant is fed in a clutch or football position, care should be taken that the heavy breast does not rest on the infant's chest. If the nipples are flat, a modified syringe can be used to pull them out before each feeding. If a mother needs to use a breast pump, the clinician should make sure that the flange is properly fitted to the mother's breast and is not so small that the nipple strangulates in the flange's nipple tunnel. Both mother and infant may be supplemented with vitamin B12 if the mother has undergone gastric bypass surgery, especially if the mother's milk levels are very low. Intertrigo (inflammation of skinfolds due to skin-to-skin contact or friction from clothing) is commonly seen in obese breasts. Mothers should clean and dry breast skinfolds daily to prevent progression from the itching, burning, and pain to an infection (Jevitt, Hernandez, & Groer, 2007).

Peripartum Mood, Depressive, and Anxiety Disorders

Lifetime rates of depression in women range between 10% and 25% (Kessler et al., 1994), with the onset of depression peaking between the ages of 25 and 44, the prime childbearing years. Between 9% and 10% of pregnant women experience clinical depression (O'Hara, 1986). Overall postpartum depression (PPD) prevalence has been estimated to be 13% (one in eight women) (O'Hara & Swain, 1996). Many mood and anxiety disorders can occur before, during, or after a pregnancy, such as major depression, bipolar disorders, panic disorder, obsessive-compulsive disorder, general anxiety disorder, posttraumatic stress disorder, and PPD. Highly anxious mothers are less likely to exclusively breastfeed or breastfeed after delivery (Britton, 2007). Childbearing may coincide with the onset of a mood or anxiety disorder or the exacerbation of a preexisting one due to the synergistic effects of reproductive hormones, brain neurotransmitters, and stress (Driscoll, 2005). Sharma and Corpse (2008) described a case study of a mother who experienced three episodes of major depression, each of which closely followed the cessation of breastfeeding.

Holistic care for childbearing women with mood and anxiety disorders usually includes a number of modalities (psychotherapy, meditation, stress reduction, dietary interventions) constructed and based on the unique aspects of each woman's needs (Sichel & Driscoll, 1999). Breastfeeding can be very important in the realm of mood disorders. Breastfeeding women have lower depression, fatigue, anxiety and dysphoric moods, less perception of stress, and more positive life events than formula-feeding mothers (Groer, 2005). Breastfeeding mothers have an up-regulated inflammatory response system that helps protect them from infectious disease (Groer et al., 2005), a stressor that is certainly not welcome during the postpartum period. Formula-feeding mothers appear to have diminished cellular immunity when experiencing stress, placing them at higher risk for certain illnesses (Groer & Davis, 2006).

Postpartum Depression

PPD is the most common mood disorder after childbirth that emerges within several weeks of delivery. Rates of PPD can be as high as 26% among adolescent mothers (Troutman & Cutrona, 1990) and 38.2% among low-income first-time mothers (Hobfoll et al., 1995). PPD affects maternal–infant interactions, with descriptions that depressed mothers may be less affectionate and withdrawn or intrusive and hostile, and their infants may demonstrate behavior that is avoidant, discontent, and withdrawn (Horowitz & Goodman, 2005). PPD can affect the entire family, including exerting negative influences on fathers' mental health (Goodman, 2004a). Although PPD often remits within the first few months postpartum, depressive symptoms can continue for an extensive time beyond the postpartum period and well into the second year after childbirth (Goodman, 2004b).

Infant temperament has been linked to stable breastfeeding patterns in mothers with depressive symptoms; infants who demonstrate highly reactive temperaments generally had less-stable breastfeeding relationships (Jones, McFall, & Diego, 2004). Affective and physiological dysregulation in infants of depressed mothers may already be present when the clinician encounters such mother–infant pairs for breastfeeding interventions. Breastfeeding difficulties experienced by mothers with PPD have been described that include PPD's effects on mothers' high expectations for breastfeeding success, their difficulty in dealing with breastfeeding problems, problems with seeking professional lactation care and services, difficulties coping, and the feeling of guilt (Shakespeare, Blake, & Garcia, 2004). Although depression during pregnancy may not affect the initiation of breastfeeding, depressed breastfeeding mothers have a greater risk of early abandonment of breastfeeding before 4 weeks than do nondepressed new mothers (Akman et al., 2008; Henderson, 2003b; Pippins, Brawarsky, Jackson, Fuentes-Afflick, & Haas, 2006). Depressed mothers report more breastfeeding worries and difficulties, are more unsatisfied with their infant feeding method, and have decreased levels of breastfeeding confidence (Dennis & McQueen, 2007, 2009).

Exclusive breastfeeding is lower in depressed mothers than in nondepressed mothers (Hasselmann, Werneck, & Silva, 2008; McCarter-Spaulding & Horowitz, 2007). Some mothers with PPD (either the mild "infant blues" or those with more intense symptoms) may self-medicate with botanical preparations such as St. John's wort. With major depression, St. John's wort is no more effective in treating this condition than a placebo (Shelton et al., 2001) and should not be relied on if a mother is severely depressed or is suffering from postpartum psychosis. Studies on the efficacy of this herb for PPD are lacking, and there are no standardizations of the preparation. In a published case report of a mother taking 300 mg, three times a day, of a standardized extract of St. John's wort, low levels were detected in her milk and none in the infant's plasma (Klier et al., 2002).

Depressed mothers are in psychic pain, and they and their family require much support. Depressed mothers may feel lonely and isolated, may be unable to sleep or concentrate, may experience few positive emotions, may suffer from anxiety, and may describe experiencing an overwhelming loss of control (Beck, 1992, 1993). Many mothers with postpartum blues or mild PPD benefit from talking with a therapist and becoming involved in postpartum support groups. Mothers with severe PPD are generally medicated and engage in psychotherapeutic sessions with a psychiatrist, a psychologist, or an advanced practice clinical nurse specialist. Mothers who express irrational ideas, experience hallucinations, or threaten to harm themselves or the infant need immediate referral to a mental health specialist. If the mother is hospitalized, some psychiatric hospitals or psychiatric units within a hospital may also admit the infant but most will not.

Pharmacological Interventions

Pharmacological interventions are often used to normalize the brain chemistry based on the type of disorder present. Depressed breastfeeding mothers often have concerns about taking antidepressant medications due to concern about their effects on the infant. Breastfeeding mothers who take antidepressants often have more severe symptoms, greater functional impairment, and more extensive psychiatric histories (Battle et al., 2008). Depressive disorders are usually treated with SSRIs such as fluoxetine (Prozac), sertraline (Zoloft), and paroxetine (Paxil). Other antidepressants include bupropion (Wellbutrin), escitalopram (Lexapro, which can cause sleepiness in the infant), and venlafaxin (Effexor). Tricyclic antidepressants such as nortriptyline (Aventyl), amitriptyline (Elavil), and desipramine (Pertofrane) are older and still used but tend to have a greater number of side effects. Medications for mood swing disorders (bipolar) include mood stabilizers such as lithium (Lithobid), valproic acid (Depakene), divalproex, lamotrigine (Lamictal), and carbamazepine (Tegretol). Anxiety disorders are often treated with benzodiazepines such as lorazepam (Ativan), diazepam (Valium), and clonazepam (Klonopin). Although many, but not all, of these medications are safe for use during pregnancy and lactation, a number of possible side effects are relevant to breastfeeding of which the clinician should be aware.

Side Effects

Neonatal withdrawal syndrome may occur in some infants exposed to Paxil in utero, which includes jitteriness, vomiting, irritability, hypoglycemia, and necrotizing enterocolitis (Stiskal et al., 2001). Difficulty has been described in differentiating whether these symptoms are due to withdrawal or actual toxicity from the drug (Isbister et al., 2001). The extent of side effects in newborns from maternal use of a number of different SSRIs is linked to third trimester use of the medications. Fetal exposure to SSRIs during the third trimester has been reported to cause a number of symptoms in newborns such as irritability, constant crying, increased tone, shivering, feeding and sleeping difficulties, convulsions, and respiratory distress (Laine, Heikkinen, Ekblad, & Kero, 2003; Moses-Kolko et al., 2005; Nordeng, Lindemann, Perminov, & Reikvam, 2001; Oberlander et al., 2004). Although these symptoms may be transient and self-limiting, they pose a problem for early breastfeeding.

Lithium toxicity in a breastfed infant can cause floppiness and an infant who is unresponsive. Lithium use must be closely monitored, and often the medication is changed if possible to one less likely to cause side effects in the infant.

Clinicians should also be aware that benzodiazepine medications tend to have a long half-life and can be sedating in a breastfed infant if the mother is medicated over a long period of time. Shorter acting drugs from this family such as Ativan are sometimes substituted if their use is intermittent, short term, low dose, and after the first week of life (Maitra & Menkes, 1996).

Other reported side effects are as follows:

- Anecdotal reports of reduced milk supply in mothers taking Wellbutrin have been reported (Hale, 2004).

- Several side effects in infants of mothers receiving Prozac have been reported and include severe colic, fussiness, and crying (Lester et al., 1993), seizures (Brent & Wisner, 1998), and growth deficits (Chambers et al., 1999).

- Fluoxetine has been reported to induce a state of anesthesia in the vagina and nipples (Michael & Mayer, 2000). If this is so, anesthetized nipples may be unable to transmit signals for the milk ejection reflex, coming full circle to the reports of weight gain deficits in some infant as discussed.

Nonpharmacological Interventions

Research has found that inflammation plays a role in the etiology of depression (Kendall-Tackett, 2007). A function of cortisol is to keep inflammation in check, but depression down-regulates cortisol with abnormally low levels of cortisol seen in depressed women (Groer & Morgan, 2007). The immune system under psychological stress releases cytokines, but when levels are very high they increase the risk of depression (Maes, 2001). Many nonpharmacological interventions for depression are used for their anti-inflammatory properties, such as the fatty acids eicosapentaenoic acid and docosahexanoic acid, bright light therapy, exercise, social support, psychotherapy, and St. John's wort (which can interact with anti-depressants and should not be taken if the mother is also being treated with pre-scription antidepressants) (Kendall-Tackett, 2008). Vagal stimulation and massage therapy have been noted to reduce depression also (Field, 2008).

Breastfeeding Management

Early feeding problems, irritability, high tone (extensor reflexes are stronger than flexion), and the other side effects seen in some newborns of mothers who have taken prenatal SSRIs may mimic behaviors seen with other newborn conditions. The therapeutic intervention of skin-to-skin care may help the infant modulate and regain state control. Skin-to-skin care has also been reported to lessen post-partum blues in the mother by reengaging a blunted hypothalamic-pituitary-adrenal axis to its normal nonpregnant state (Dombrowski, Anderson, Santori, & Burkhammer, 2001). Every effort should be made to keep the mother and infant together to encourage a strong attachment between mother and child. Breastfeeding has been shown to be protective against maternal neglect with the odds for maternal maltreatment for non-breastfed children being 2.6 times higher than for children whose mothers breastfeed (Strathearn, Mamun, Najman, & O'Callaghan, 2009).

Infants of mothers taking psychotropic medications should be monitored closely for appropriate weight gain (Hendrick et al., 2003), sufficient nurturing, alterations in behavior or activity level, and achievement of developmental mile-stones (Burt et al., 2001). Infants who are irritable or not readily comforted can increase the stress in an already difficult situation. Restoring some control to the situation by suggesting the use of a sling, frequent suckling opportunities, and planned rest periods may reduce feelings of being overwhelmed. Mothers who are severely depressed and cannot handle placing the infant to the breast or fear they will harm the infant may be able to pump their milk and have it fed to the infant by the father or another caretaker. If a breastfeeding mother is hospitalized, she may or may not be able to pump her milk during the separation. Many mothers experience this depressed time as a period of just trying to survive. The preservation of milk production may be an accomplishment that the mother appreciates once she is feeling better, helping her to experience one less loss.

Endocrine, Metabolic, and Autoimmune Conditions

Diabetes

A number of forms of diabetes can occur in childbearing women:

- Insulin-dependent diabetes mellitus, or type 1 diabetes, is a polygenic autoimmune disorder resulting from destruction of the insulin-producing beta cells in the pancreas. It is thought to have a genetic component that is triggered by an environmental insult or event such as the early introduction of cow milk protein, viral infections, or exposure to toxins.

- Non–insulin-dependent diabetes mellitus, or type 2 diabetes, is typically associated with a metabolic syndrome that includes obesity and hypertension and is usually seen in adults (although with the rising rates of childhood overweight and obesity is now seen at an increased rate in children). Insulin is produced in the pancreas, but the cells' insulin receptors do not respond to it. Some mothers may be taking oral hypoglycemic agents such as glipizide (Glucotrol) or glyburide (Micronase) and should be encouraged to breastfeed because these medications are safe during lactation (Feig, Briggs, & Koren, 2007; Glatstein, Djokanovic, Garcia-Bournissen, Finkelstein, & Koren, 2009).

- Gestational diabetes mellitus (GDM) manifests itself as impaired glucose tolerance during pregnancy. The rates of GDM have risen from 1% to 2.5% in 1976 to 4% in 2000, with current rates of approximately 7% of all pregnancies being complicated by GDM (American Diabetes Association, 2004). This is primarily due to the increase in maternal overweight and obesity. Women with GDM are at increased risk for the development of diabetes, usually type 2, after pregnancy (Albareda et al., 2003; Schaefer-Graf, Buchanan, Xiang, Peters, & Kjos, 2002). Obesity enhances the risk of developing type 2 diabetes after GDM (American Diabetes Association, 2004). The recurrence rates for GDM in subsequent pregnancies range from 35% in predominantly white populations to greater than 50% in non-white populations (MacNeill et al., 2001). Women who experience GDM and do not breastfeed the infant from that pregnancy are twice as likely to develop type 2 diabetes (Kjos et al., 1993). Lifestyle modifications such as breastfeeding are an important intervention in efforts to prevent type 2 diabetes in women with a history of gestational diabetes (Bentley-Lewis, Levkoff, Stuebe, & Seely, 2008). Mothers whose weight is 190 lb or more at the start of the subsequent pregnancy are 70% more likely to have a recurrence of GDM, reinforcing the importance of breastfeeding as a potential contributor to reducing weight between pregnancies and helping lessen insulin resistance.

Breastfeeding has been reported to be less frequent and of a shorter duration in mothers with type 1 diabetes (Hummel et al., 2007). However, with optimal breastfeeding support, mothers with type 1 diabetes are quite capable of breast-feeding for prolonged periods of time, similar to mothers without diabetes (Schoen, Sichert-Hellert, Hummel, Ziegler, & Kersting, 2008). Breastfeeding can function as an important therapeutic intervention in the face of any type of diabetes (Taylor, Kacmar, Nothnagle, & Lawrence, 2005). Women with any type of diabetes should be actively encouraged to breastfeed (Gunderson, 2007; Metzger et al., 2007). Body fat accumulation after pregnancy is associated with alterations in insulin secretion; however, breastfeeding has a long-lasting protective effect on the insulin response (Diniz & da Costa, 2004).

Fasting blood glucose levels are significantly lower in type 1 diabetic mothers during the exclusively breastfeeding period compared with women with type 1 diabetes who stop breastfeeding or who have never breastfed (Ferris et al., 1988, 1993). Milk production could be limited in the presence of too much or too little insulin. Too much insulin causing hypoglycemia can potentially cause epinephrine to be released from the adrenal glands, inhibiting the release of milk (Asselin & Lawrence, 1987). After an initial episode of hypoglycemia after delivery, the ongoing metabolism of glucose into galactose and lactose during milk synthesis reduces the amount of insulin needed by a lactating mother. Mothers may find that insulin requirements are reduced between 27% (Davies et al., 1989) and 50% (Asselin & Lawrence, 1987). Insulin dosages will need to be adjusted during the early days of lactation. Riviello, Mello, and Jovanovic (2009) recommended that total daily basal insulin dosage for type 1 diabetic women who breastfeed be calculated as 0.21 units times the weight in kilograms per day. Once insulin dosage and diet are in balance, diabetic mothers are quite capable of synthesizing abundant amounts of milk and lactating successfully (Benz, 1992).

Women with type 1 diabetes have a 5–10% incidence of hyper- or hypothyroidism, with goiter and Hashimoto thyroiditis being common. Mothers with type 1 diabetes have three times the risk of developing postpartum thyroiditis

(Gallas et al., 2002). In women with type 2 diabetes where obesity is common, the clinician should be vigilant for the possibility of hypothyroidism (Jovanovic, 2000). This issue should be kept in mind if a diabetic mother reports problems with milk insufficiency.

Infants of diabetic mothers are at an increased risk for a number of conditions that can pose barriers to their breastfeeding such as prematurity, respiratory distress syndrome, congenital anomalies, hypoglycemia, large for gestation age (Cordero, Treuer, Landon, & Gabbe, 1998), hyperbilirubinemia (Sirota et al., 1992), hypocalcemia (Metcalfe & Baum, 1992), and being born by cesarean section. Many of these conditions result in separation of mother and infant during the important early time when breastfeeding is becoming established (Nigro et al., 1985). Delaying breastfeeding as the first feed reduces the chances of an infant being breastfed on discharge (Simmons, Conroy, & Thompson, 2005). Postponing the first feeding at the breast, lack of breast stimulation, and use of large amounts of formula contribute to cessation of breastfeeding by 7 days postpartum (Ferris et al., 1988). Further complicating the early days is a 15- to 28-hour delay in lactogenesis II typically accompanying maternal diabetes, which can result in low milk intake in the infant during the first few days of life (Arthur, Kent, & Hartmann, 1994; Bitman et al., 1989; Hartmann & Cregan, 2001; Miyake et al., 1989; Murtaugh, Ferris, Capacchione, & Reece, 1998; Ostrom & Ferris, 1993). Delayed lactogenesis seems more likely to occur in mothers with poor metabolic control (Neubauer et al., 1993), but good metabolic control (Whichelow & Doddridge, 1983) and intense breastfeeding support (Webster, Moore, & McMullan, 1995) work together to mitigate many potentially adverse effects on breastfeeding.

Because diabetic mothers can possibly have colostrum for 2–3 days longer than nondiabetic mothers, they may become discouraged if they feel unable to satisfy the hunger needs of their infants (Hutt, 1989). Clinicians may need to make extra efforts to ensure adequate infant intake in the early days and that optimal milk production takes place to avoid having the mother give her infant cow milk–based infant formula supplements or cereal to satisfy the infant's hunger. The relative risk of developing diabetes can be as much as 13 times higher when a genetically susceptible infant receives cow milk–based formula during the first 3–4 months of life (Perez-Bravo et al., 1996), putting cow milk–associated diabetes risk in the same range as the link between cigarette smoking and lung cancer, with a relative risk of approximately 10 (Hammond-McKibben & Dosch, 1997). Early introduction of cereal before 4 months of age also increases the infant's risk of developing type 1 diabetes (Norris et al., 2003; Ziegler et al., 2003).

Breastfeeding Management

Anticipating certain situations common to diabetic mothers and their infants in the immediate postpartum helps to avoid ongoing problems.

Infant Hypoglycemia

The incidence of hypoglycemia in the infant of a diabetic mother is 25–40% (Reece & Homko, 1994), usually occurring within 1–2 hours of birth. This is usually transient with spontaneous improvement. Persistent or recurrent hypoglycemia may require intravenous glucose infusions or pharmacological management. In asymptomatic infants who have blood glucose levels of 40 mg/dL or less, feeding practices should include the following (California Diabetes and Pregnancy Program, 2002):

- Breastfeed by 1 hour of age, hourly for three or four feedings until the blood glucose is stable, and then every 2–3 hours until 12 hours of age (stable is 40 mg/dL or more). Mothers may wish to use alternate breast massage to help transfer as much colostrum as possible when the infant is latched.

- Help from a lactation consultant may be necessary due to the infant's feeding difficulties, with supplementation to be considered if the infant is unable to feed directly at the breast.

- Glucose water should not be given due to its rapid absorption and resulting stimulation of insulin release.

Plans should be in place for how and what to feed an infant of a diabetic mother if he or she is placed in a special care nursery or is unable to transfer milk from the breast. Expressed colostrum should be the first choice. Mothers may express colostrum prenatally, freeze it, and bring it to the hospital for use if the infant is unable to breastfeed during the early hours. They can also hand express colostrum into a spoon and spoon-feed it to the infant if the infant is unable to feed directly from the breast. If the infant cannot tolerate oral feeds, the expressed colostrum can be refrigerated for use when the infant's condition has improved. Finally, banked human milk may be ordered before the birth by the infant's physician and kept frozen on the unit until needed.

Cow milk–based infant formula should be avoided because of its potential for sensitizing diabetes in a susceptible infant. If infant formula becomes temporarily necessary, a hydrolyzed formula can be used because it is less diabetogenic (Karges et al., 1997; Knip & Akerblom, 1998).

Mothers and infants should be kept in skin-to-skin contact as much as possible to keep the infant's blood sugar levels from dropping due to separation, thermal stress, or crying. This is especially important because it allows the mother to immediately respond to the infant's behavioral feeding cues, which can be difficult if an infant is near term with state-control difficulties.

Delayed Lactogenesis II

In anticipation of an extended colostral phase, infants of diabetic mothers should be breastfed 10–12 times each 24 hours. If the infant is unable to feed this frequently, mothers should pump their breasts. Milk production should be monitored during the first 2 weeks postpartum; diaper output in infants should be monitored as well for signs of jaundice and appropriate infant weight gain. If the infant was large at birth, positioning at the breast may need to be adapted to any birth injuries from shoulder dystocia such as a fractured clavicle, Erb's palsy, phrenic nerve palsy, temporomandibular joint misalignment, or latch problems from vacuum extraction.

Maternal Hypoglycemia

Mothers with type 1 diabetes may experience erratic blood glucose patterns. Hypoglycemia is most likely to occur within an hour after breastfeeding, making this an important time to measure blood glucose. Mothers should eat a snack containing carbohydrate and protein before or during nursing to avoid this problem rather than frequently changing insulin dosages. Nocturnal hypoglycemia is a common occurrence and can be avoided by addressing the nighttime insulin dose or eating a high-protein snack before sleep. Some mothers keep a nonperishable snack in locations where they breastfeed as well as glucose tablets or fast-acting sugars in case of a hypoglycemic emergency.

Mothers with type 2 diabetes who are unable to maintain normal glucose levels through exercise and diet may need to continue on insulin during the time they are lactating. Mothers with GDM may be transitioned from insulin over the first month of lactation to an oral hypoglycemic agent. Diabetic mothers should exercise caution in the use of herbal products because many have the potential to affect blood glucose levels.

Mastitis, Candidosis, Nipple Trauma

Every effort should be made to prevent or intervene promptly if a diabetic mother develops signs and symptoms of mastitis, candidosis, or nipple trauma that could lead to bacterial and yeast overgrowth of the damaged skin. Infections can raise blood glucose levels, and diabetic mothers are sometimes reported to be more susceptible to mastitis if blood sugars are not well controlled (Ferris et al., 1988; Gagne, Leff, & Jefferis, 1992).

Diabetic Mastopathy

This is a less common complication seen in premenopausal long-term type 1 or 2 diabetic women. The breast lesions consist of one or more hard lumps with irregular edges that are moveable and painless (Mak et al., 2003). It is a benign dense fibrous condition that can be easily confused with breast carcinoma. Surgical excision may be necessary to confirm the absence of malignancy (Boullu et al., 1998). Some long-standing diabetic mothers may have had biopsies or surgical incisions to remove small lumps. Any palpable lumps in the breasts of diabetic women should always be closely followed because the number and size of diabetic fibrous masses tend to increase with age.

Polycystic Ovary Syndrome

Insulin resistance and type 2 diabetes can be present in up to 12.6% of women with polycystic ovary syndrome (PCOS) (Talbott, Zborowski, & Boudreaux, 2004), with an even higher prevalence in obese women with PCOS. The prevalence of PCOS among women with type 2 diabetes is estimated to be from 21% (Conn, Jacobs, & Conway, 2000) to 26.7% (Peppard, Marfori, Iuorno, & Nestler, 2001). The clinician working with type 2 diabetic mothers should be aware that PCOS could affect approximately one-fourth of these women and may need to consider PCOS when diabetic mothers report perceived or real insufficient milk supplies or an infant with poor weight gain (Marasco et al., 2000).

Polycystic Ovary Syndrome

PCOS, formerly known as Stein-Leventhal syndrome, is a complex syndrome of ovarian, metabolic, and endocrine dysfunction of unknown cause. Its clinical manifestations usually include menstrual irregularities, signs of androgen excess (hirsutism), and obesity. Diagnostic criteria have recently been revised (Table 9-1), with no single diagnostic criterion being sufficient for a clinical diagnosis.

Women with PCOS may exhibit combinations of clinical and laboratory manifestations (Table 9-2) that may have started developing during adolescence. These women form the largest group of women at risk for the development of cardiovascular disease and diabetes (Polycystic Ovary Syndrome Writing Committee, 2005). PCOS occurs in 10% of reproductive-aged women, constituting the most common metabolic abnormality in young women (Azziz et al., 2004; Hart, Hickey, & Franks, 2004). Many women with PCOS experience quality-of-life issues that involve depression, anxiety, and low self-esteem, especially regarding their weight (McCook, Reame, & Thatcher, 2005). Galactorrhea with high serum prolactin levels has been reported in some women with PCOS (Isik et al., 1997), but it is insufficient milk supply that has brought PCOS to the attention of clinicians working with breastfeeding mothers. Hormonal aberrations are speculated to be associated with milk-supply problems (Table 9-3), but the exact mechanism is not known.

Although there is a typical set of clinical manifestation of PCOS (obesity, skin and hair alterations, and menstrual or infertility issues), not all women share all the many variations of the condition. Some mothers with less extensive hormonal alterations may produce abundant amounts of milk, whereas others may experience any number of symptoms (such as a combination of hypothyroidism, hypoplastic breasts, and insulin resistance) that collectively result in diminished milk production. Multiparous mothers may produce more milk under the same hormonal conditions due to an increase in prolactin receptors from the previous pregnancy (Zuppa et al., 1988). Hormonal medications that improve breast morphology such as progesterone therapy have been reported to improve lactation in infertile women (Bodley & Powers, 1999). Metformin (Glucophage) is a medication used to improve insulin sensitivity and reduce glucose levels in non–insulin-dependent diabetics while not altering glucose concentrations in healthy people. This property often

---

TABLE 9-1   Revised Diagnostic Criteria of PCOS

- Oligo- and/or anovulation
- Clinical and/or biochemical signs of hyperandrogenism
- Polycystic ovaries and the exclusion of other etiologies such as congenital adrenal hyperplasias, androgen-secreting tumors, or Cushing syndrome

Two of the three criteria need to be present for a diagnosis of PCOS.

Source: The Rotterdam ESHRE/ASRM-sponsored PCOS Consensus Workshop Group. (2004). Revised 2003 consensus on diagnostic criteria and long-term health risks related to polycystic ovary syndrome (PCOS). *Human Reproduction, 19,* 41–47.

TABLE 9-2   Clinical and Laboratory Manifestations of PCOS

- Excessive body hair growth, alopecia, balding
- Persistent acne, seborrhea, acanthosis nigricans (dark velvety plaques of thickened skin under the arms, in the groin, and at the nape of the neck usually associated with insulin excess)
- Obesity, elevated waist-to-hip ratio
- Reversed ratio of luteinizing hormone to follicle stimulating hormone
- Elevated free androgen index, elevated testosterone levels
- Elevated fasting insulin levels, insulin resistance
- Menstrual disturbances
    - Amenorrhea (lack of menstruation)
    - Oligomenorrhea (scanty or infrequent menstrual flow)
    - Anovulation (menstrual cycle in which ovulation is absent)
- Ovaries with increased cystic structures or increased ovarian volume
- History of infertility
- High triglycerides, low levels of high-density-lipoprotein cholesterol, increased blood pressure

TABLE 9-3   Hormonal Aberrations and Milk-Supply Problems

- High levels of androgens (testosterone and androstenedione) may down-regulate estrogen and prolactin receptors (Marasco et al., 2000).
- Elevated estrogen levels in obese women with PCOS postpartum may suppress prolactin.
- Insulin resistance may disrupt lactogenesis.
- Low progesterone levels may disrupt ductile and lobuloalveolar development in the breast, resulting in asymmetrical or hypoplastic breasts.
- Low estrogen levels or limited estrogen receptors may predispose to poor breast tissue development.
- Low prolactin or decreased prolactin receptors may interfere with breast growth during pregnancy and with lactogenesis after delivery.

influences it as a preferred choice for use in breastfeeding women (Hale et al., 2002). Metformin appears to have no adverse effects on the nursing infant (Glueck & Wang, 2007). Metformin has been used to increase milk production in mothers with insulin resistance (such as in PCOS) with mixed results (Gabbay & Kelly, 2003). Gabbay and Kelly described episodes of engorgement after dosage increases and a limited increase in milk output but speculated that starting the medication after lactation compromise has become apparent may be too late. However, even combinations of progesterone, metformin, domperidone (Motilium) or metoclopramide (Reglan) or additions of herbal galactagogues may be ineffective in increasing milk production with severe breast hypoplasia.

Breastfeeding Management

Mothers who present with a diagnosis of PCOS or delayed lactogenesis II and signs and symptoms associated with PCOS should be guided by the usual efforts to improve and increase milk production. Frequent feedings, use of alternate massage, additional milk expression, galactagogues, and whatever other medications her physician has placed her on for PCOS treatment may or may not result in adequate milk production. Infant weight must be monitored closely, and some mothers will need to supplement their infant with formula if they are unable to produce sufficient quantities of milk. Supplementation can be done at the breast with tube-feeding systems.

Mothers should be tested for hypothyroidism. Women need to be screened for depression before the use of metoclopramide, and herbal galactagogues that alter blood glucose levels should be used with caution in the presence of insulin resistance or diabetes. Mothers with PCOS should be encouraged to breastfeed, especially because this may help improve the chances for improved milk production with subsequent pregnancies. Many women with PCOS have difficulty conceiving or carrying a pregnancy to term and can be heavily invested in the health and care of the infant. Mothers should be helped to develop a feeding plan right from the start to maximize milk production. Clinicians should praise the mother for any amount of milk produced and help her understand that supplementation does not represent failure or inadequacy on her part.

Hyperreactio Luteinalis

Although more common in pregnancies complicated by hydatidiform mole, fetal hydrops, and multiple pregnancies (Bakri, Bakhashwain, & Hugosson, 1994), hyperreactio luteinalis (theca lutein cysts) can occasionally occur in normal pregnancies. These types of cysts result in ovaries that are enlarged by multiple cysts, producing high levels of testosterone. Mothers may notice hirsutism and limited breast growth during pregnancy. As with PCOS, this hormonal alteration has the potential to disrupt lactogenesis II and delay the establishment of a full milk supply. As the cysts resolve postpartum and the testosterone levels drop, milk production usually increases, leading to full lactation in most situations, but this can take up to a month to happen (Betzold, Hoover, & Snyder, 2004). The normal female adult value of testosterone is 62 ng/dL or less. Case reports in the literature have reported values up to 711 ng/dL, with mothers describing their milk coming in when levels fell to approximately 300 ng/dL (Hoover, Barbalinardo, & Platia, 2002).

Breastfeeding Management

If the presence of theca lutein cysts has been confirmed prenatally, breastfeeding mothers should be encouraged to breastfeed their infant often and monitor the infant's weight closely until the infant is gaining adequately and consistently. Clinicians should schedule frequent weight checks and may need to recommend supplementation with either pumped breastmilk or infant formula until testosterone levels fall and the mother's milk production rebounds. Any needed supplementation should be done at the breast. If undiagnosed in the prenatal period, theca lutein cysts may present postpartum as delayed lactogenesis II, limited milk production, infant weight-gain problems, and lack of breast changes in the prenatal period. In the presence of these conditions, the clinician might wish to ask the mother if she has experienced excess body hair growth or other signs of virilization during her pregnancy. If so, the clinician may wish to have testosterone levels measured and pelvic ultrasound to confirm the presence of theca lutein cysts.

Thyroid Disorders

The thyroid gland is a butterfly-shaped endocrine gland located in the lower front of the neck whose hormones are actively involved in controlling metabolic functions, energy use, heat generation, and the activity of the brain, heart, muscles, and other organs. The thyroid gland produces the hormones thyroxine (T_4), triiodothyronine (T_3), and calcitonin.

Thyroid disease is more common in women than in men, with about 2–3% of Americans having pronounced hypothyroidism and about 10–15% having subclinical or mild hypothyroidism. A breastfeeding mother can present with one of several types of thyroid diseases: hypothyroidism, hyperthyroidism, or postpartum thyroiditis.

Hypothyroidism

Hypothyroidism is an underactive thyroid gland resulting from a number of causes, including Hashimoto disease or Hashimoto thyroiditis. This is an auto-immune thyroiditis in which the immune system's attack on the thyroid causes a goiter (swelling) and a possible resulting hypothyroidism. Disruptions in communication with the pituitary gland, which directs the thyroid in how much hormone to produce, could lead to low thyroid levels with a resulting diminished milk supply. In the dairy cow, low thyroid levels have been associated with low fat content of the milk, low prolactin levels, and decreased milk production and poor weight gain in the calves (Thrift et al., 1999), further implicating a thyroid-pituitary axis involvement. Because the thyroid is responsible for cellular activity, diminished milk production could also result from a slow down in milk-secreting cell activity.

Undiagnosed and/or untreated hypothyroidism during the first trimester of pregnancy places the fetus at increased risk for intellectual impairment, abnormal neuropsychological development, and impaired psychomotor functioning (Berbel et al., 2009; Morreale, Obregon, & Escobar, 2000; Pop et al., 1999), and as much as a 10-point lower IQ in the presence of autoimmune thyroiditis (Muller, Drexhage, & Berghout, 2001). Many common symptoms of hypothyroidism mimic those of the normal postpartum period, such as fatigue, sleepiness, decreased energy, hair loss, poor concentration, weight gain, carpal tunnel syndrome, muscle aches, constipation, and dry skin. If low milk production is also present, the clinician may wish to have the mother's thyroid function tested (Shames & Youngkin, 2002). Many people with low thyroid levels also complain of being cold and demonstrate periorbital edema and hoarseness. Hypothyroidism is generally treated with synthetic thyroxine or levothyroxine (Synthroid, Levothyroid, Thyroid, Unithyroid, Levoxyl), including during pregnancy and lactation. Oral levothyroxine transfer into milk is extremely low (Hale, 2004).

Hyperthyroidism

Hyperthyroidism, commonly called Graves disease, is the production of excess thyroid hormone. It is characterized by weight loss despite increased appetite, nervousness, sweating, heat intolerance, heart palpitations, and possibly bulging eyes and goiter. The main concern during lactation is the safety of the medications used to treat the mother. Medications may be used to treat both the symptoms of the disease and the high thyroid levels. Propranolol (Inderal) is a beta-blocker and may be used to treat hypertension and cardiac arrhythmias. Propylthiouracil is usually the drug of choice in breastfeeding mothers to suppress maternal thyroid function (Hale & Berens, 2002). Many endocrinologists still do not recommend breastfeeding during propylthiouracil therapy (Lee et al., 2000), even though the American Academy of Pediatrics (2001) has classified this drug as usually compatible with breastfeeding and has done so for many years. Methimazole (Tapazole) has also been shown safe to use during lactation with no adverse outcomes reported in infants, including changes in thyroid function or physical or intellectual development (Azizi, Khoshniat, Bahrainian, & Hedayati, 2000).

Mothers should be aware that their infant's thyroid may be monitored periodically to ensure adequate functioning. The use of radioactive diagnostic material such as technetium-99m pertechnetate is compatible with breastfeeding with a 12- to 24-hour interruption of nursing until the material is cleared, but radioactive ablation of the thyroid gland with iodine-131 requires cessation of breastfeeding (Nuclear Regulatory Commission, 1996). The breast tissue itself acts as a repository for almost 40% of the iodine-131 dose, which may increase the risk of breast cancer. For maximal protection of the mother, Hale and Berens (2002) recommended that the mother cease breastfeeding several weeks before the ablation procedure to reduce deposition of iodine-131 material into the breast tissue.

Postpartum Thyroiditis

Postpartum thyroiditis occurs in approximately 5–10% of women. Inflammation of the thyroid gland is not uncommon in the postpartum woman. The risk is greater in women with autoimmune disorders, positive antithyroid antibodies, or a history of previous thyroid dysfunction, with 20% of women having a recurrence of thyroiditis with subsequent pregnancies. Thyroiditis includes two phases: initial thyrotoxicosis (high thyroid hormone levels), occurring 1–3 months after delivery, followed by a hypothyroid phase, occurring 4–8 months after delivery and lasting up to 1 year. Not all women experience both phases. Treatment of the thyrotoxicosis phase is usually with beta-blockers to reduce the palpitations, tremors, and shakes, not antithyroid medication, because this phase is transient. The hypothyroid phase is treated with thyroid hormone replacement and gradually tapered off, because 80% of mothers regain normal thyroid function.

Although primary thyroid dysfunction is associated with mood disorders (Harris, 1999), PPD has been shown to be associated with positive thyroid antibody status and an increase in depressive symptoms in antibody-positive mothers (Harris et al., 1992). Clinicians may wish to ask mothers with thyroid dysfunction or mothers encountering lactation problems thought to occur in association with thyroid problems if they are experiencing "infant blues" or new-onset depression. Symptoms of thyroid dysfunction can mimic normal postpartum adjustment and fatigue and should be distinguished from these so that treatment may commence (Pereira & Brown, 2008). Lawrence and Lawrence (2005) recommended screening for thyroid disease before prescribing antidepressants. In addition, mothers should be asked if they are self-medicating with herbal products, such as St. John's wort, which could mask the thyroid disease.

Breastfeeding Management

Good initial breastfeeding guidelines are always important. Mothers with milk production problems, infants who experience weight-gain difficulties, and mothers with a predisposing history for thyroid problems should be followed closely. Hypothyroid mothers have been shown to produce significantly less milk during the first 6 days postpartum (Miyake et al., 1989). Lactation deficiency has been reported in association with infant weight gain problems due to reduced milk production (Buckshee et al., 1992; Stein, 2002). Animal studies in rats revealed a reduction in circulating oxytocin in hypothyroid mothers resulting in less milk release, poor milk transfer, and reduced litter growth (Hapon et al., 2003). Similar problems have been reported in both animal and human mothers who are hyperthyroid.

When lactogenesis has occurred yet there seems to be little milk transfer and other explanations have been ruled out, hyperthyroid should be considered as a possibility (Marasco, 2006). Insufficient milk supplies that do not improve by standard corrective measures should alert the clinician to a possible endocrine problem and recommend diagnostic testing. Diminished milk output between 4 and 8 months postpartum, although certainly related to other issues, may also have an endocrine origin, with the clinician wishing to possibly check thyroid hormone levels at this time. Breastfeeding should not be interrupted unless radioactive diagnostic procedures are needed nor abandoned unless ablation of the thyroid gland is indicated. It is especially important for mothers with a history of thyroid problems to continue breastfeeding because lack of breastfeeding has been associated with an increased risk for thyroid cancer (Mack et al., 1999).

Both hypothyroidism and hyperthyroidism seem to impair milk release, not milk synthesis. Without adequate milk removal, milk production decreases, placing the infant at a higher risk for insufficient weight gain. Efforts to improve milk release include the use of oxytocin nasal spray to induce milk ejection, use of alternate massage/breast compressions, and stimulation of the nipple–areola complex.

Fibromyalgia

Fibromyalgia affects as many as 8 million people in the United States, occurring mainly in women of childbearing age. Symptoms usually arise between the ages of 20 and 55 years, but the condition also may be diagnosed in childhood. Symptoms of fibromyalgia typically include

- Feeling of pain, burning, aching, and soreness in the body
- Headaches, tenderness of the scalp, pain in the back of the skull
- Pain in the neck, shoulder, shoulder blades, and elbows
- Pain in hips, top of buttocks, outside the lower hip, below buttocks, and the pelvis
- Pain in the knees and kneecap area
- Fatigue, unrefreshing sleep, waking up tired, morning stiffness
- Insomnia, frequent waking, difficulty falling asleep, or falling asleep immediately
- Raynaud phenomenon
- Irritable bowel syndrome, diarrhea and constipation, bloating, cramping
- Balance problems
- Neurally mediated hypotension; balance problems
- Restless leg syndrome
- Sense of tissues feeling swollen
- Numbness, tingling, and feeling of cold in the hands and feet
- Chest pain, palpitations
- Shortness of breath
- Anxiety, depression, and "fibrofog"—term used to describe the confusion and forgetfulness, inability to concentrate and difficulty recalling simple words and numbers, and transposing words and numbers

Fibromyalgia can negatively affect breastfeeding by making it very difficult to stay in one position for very long during breastfeeding sessions. Mothers may experience extreme pain or stiffness when holding their infant for extended periods of time in the same position. Breastfeeding mothers with fibromyalgia may experience sore nipples, insufficient milk supply, and depression (Schaefer, 2004).

Breastfeeding Management

Mothers need help in finding comfortable nursing positions and may need to switch positions several times during each breastfeeding session. Lying down while breastfeeding and semireclining with ventral positioning of the infant are relaxing positions. Mothers may find that the use of a sling or breastfeeding pillow reduces strain on muscles. Adaptive infant care equipment may be needed in severe situations (see Physically Challenged Mothers, above). Clinicians need to remain vigilant regarding sore nipples, Raynaud phenomenon of the nipples, and milk production. Warm compresses or heating pads may be helpful for sore neck and back muscles.

Cystic Fibrosis

Cystic fibrosis (CF) is an autosomal recessive disease involving multiple body organs and systems including the lungs, pancreas, urogenital system, skeleton, and skin. CF is the most common genetic disease among whites. It affects about 30,000 children and adults in the United States and about 70,000 people worldwide. Although CF is more commonly found in the white population, the disease affects all racial groups. CF occurs in about 1 in every 3,500 white births, 1 in every 17,000 black births, and 1 in every 90,000 Asian births. About 12 million people (about 1 in 30 people) in the United States carry one CF gene mutation. Dysfunction in exocrine glands and chronic lung problems are typical manifestations of the condition. With improved diagnostic and therapeutic interventions, many young women with CF bear children and breastfeed, whereas in the past, few people with CF lived to adulthood. The median age of survival is 35 years (Cystic Fibrosis Foundation, n.d.).

Some mothers with CF choose or are advised not to breastfeed due to real or perceived concerns for maternal health or fear of potential harm to the infant from maternal medications. Breastfeeding decisions should be based on the overall health and wishes of the mother (Edenborough et al., 2008). Possible side effects of medications are a common reason in women's decisions not to breastfeed (Gilljam et al., 2000), but most medications needed for the treatment of CF are safe to take while breastfeeding. Festini et al. (2006) reported a mother who underwent intravenous tobramycin (Tobrex) therapy while breastfeeding with no detectable medication found in her milk. An increasing number of women with CF choose to breastfeed (Luder et al., 1990), with breastmilk composition quite capable of adequately nourishing their infants (Michel & Mueller, 1994), even if the fat content is slightly lower than normal (Bitman et al., 1987). Shiffman et al. (1989) reported that concentrations of milk macronutrients were decreased during exacerbations of the pulmonary aspect of CF and that mothers and infants should be monitored more closely during these times.

As long as the mother remains healthy, maintaining her weight and respiratory status, breastfeeding benefits both her and her infant. Breastfeeding increases maternal nutritional requirements for energy, calcium, and many other vitamins and minerals. Mothers with CF may or may not be able to sustain exclusive breastfeeding for the recommended period of time but should be encouraged to continue for as long as possible (Odegaard et al., 2002). Breastfeeding after transplantation is possible with needed medications reviewed by the CF and transplant teams. Infants of breastfeeding mothers with CF are protected against many of the pathogens that the mother chronically carries, reducing the incidence and severity of illness in the infant (Parker et al., 2004).

Breastfeeding Management

Clinicians should monitor the caloric requirements of both the mother and infant, ensuring that each partner maintains adequate weight under conditions of increased need. Mothers with mild CF usually do quite well with breastfeeding but should receive close support during the establishment of lactation. Maternal diabetes and gestational diabetes are common in women with CF during pregnancy, so close monitoring for infant hypoglycemia and hyperglycemia is important. Infants may need to be weighed more frequently, especially during times of maternal disease exacerbations. The most common complication for the infant born to a mother with CF is prematurity, with about 25% of these infants born preterm. Some clinicians occasionally monitor the mother's milk for sodium, chloride, and total fat and routinely do so when the mother experiences pulmonary infections or disease flare-ups.

Phenylketonuria

Phenylketonuria (PKU) is an autosomal recessive inherited metabolic disorder arising from a defect in the enzyme phenylalanine hydroxylase that converts phenylalanine (PHE) to tyrosine. Women with PKU can breastfeed quite successfully, produce milk with normal levels of components, and should maintain their special PKU diet throughout their lifetime (Matalon, Michals, & Gleason, 1986). It is vital that nonpregnant women and mothers with PKU be on their special diet before conception and throughout the entire pregnancy (Lee, Ridout, Walter, & Cockburn, 2005; Maillot, Lilburn, Baudin, Morley, & Lee, 2008). High levels of PHE can be present in the fetus from very early in the pregnancy (Purnell, 2001). High PHE levels during pregnancy can result in maternal PKU effects on the developing fetus that include facial dysmorphism, microcephaly, intrauterine growth retardation, developmental delays, and congenital heart disease. The longer it takes to achieve metabolic control during pregnancy the lower developmental scores are in the infant (Waisbren et al., 2000). High serum and milk levels of PHE in mothers with PKU do not result in abnormal PHE levels in their non-PKU breastfeeding infants (Fox-Bacon et al., 1997). Breastfeeding mothers with PKU usually remain on a modified diet during breastfeeding, avoiding aspartame, an artificial sweetener made from PHE. A neurological assessment of the infant is usually done at 4 and 8 weeks and an echocardiogram for infants conceived off diet (Maillot, Cook, Lilburn, & Lee, 2007).

Breastfeeding Management

Good breastfeeding management practices are important as usual. After the infant is born, he or she is no longer at risk for side effects from high maternal PHE levels. Infants of mothers with PKU should be breastfed and should be tested for PKU during their routine newborn screening. It is important to breastfeed right from the start, because even if this infant eventually tests positive for PKU, breastfeeding during the early days until dietary intervention begins has been linked to higher intelligence quotient scores in dietary-treated phenylketonuric children (Riva et al., 1996).

Multiple Sclerosis

Multiple sclerosis (MS) is a progressive autoimmune demyelinating disease of the central nervous system. It is one of the most common causes of neurological disability in young adults, affecting females two to three times more frequently than males, with onset between the ages of 20 and 40 years. Approximately 70% of those with MS are women. The prevalence of MS has been reported as 46 per 100,000 in the United States and 90 per 100,000 in Canada (Pugliatti, Sotgiu, & Rosati, 2002). The condition is unpredictable, has periods of exacerbations and remissions, has no cure, and has an unknown cause. Symptoms may be erratic and progressive and include numbness and tingling, urinary tract problems, difficulty walking, visual disturbances, weakness, profound fatigue, vertigo, loss of balance, incoordination, speech difficulties, and paralysis. Women may experience relief from relapses of the condition during pregnancy followed by an increased relapse rate after delivery (Lorenzi & Ford, 2002), especially during the first 3 months postpartum (Worthington et al., 1994).

Breastfeeding does not adversely affect the health of mothers with MS (Birk & Rudick, 1986), does not cause an increase in relapse rate postpartum (Nelson, Franklin, & Jones, 1988), and has been shown to promote their health by decreasing MS relapse rates by between 10% and 50% during the first 6 months postpartum (Confavreux et al., 1998; Gulick & Halper, 2002). Exclusive breastfeeding is extremely important, because women with MS who breastfeed exclusively during the first 2 months are approximately five times less likely to relapse in the first year postpartum than women who did not breastfeed or began supplemental formula feedings during that time (Langer-Gould et al., 2009). Breastfeeding the infant of a mother with MS is very important because human-milk feeding appears to decrease the risk of developing MS (Pisacane et al., 1994). Breastfed infants of mothers with MS experience reduced rates of otitis media, lower respiratory illness, constipation, milk intolerance, and allergy during the first year of life (Gulick & Johnson, 2004), sparing a fatigued mother the further burden of caring for a sick infant.

Women with MS have numerous concerns regarding their own health as well as that of the fetus and newborn. These include the fear of transmitting MS to their infant, relapses in the postpartum period and how to handle an infant during those times, effects of medications on the infant while breastfeeding, effects of profound fatigue on child care and lactation (Eggum, 2001; Halbert, 1998), and concern that breastfeeding would be more exhausting than preparing bottles of formula. Many mothers receive conflicting advice from healthcare providers regarding breastfeeding in the presence of MS and become confused by differing opinions of the specialists caring for them (Coyle et al., 2004; Smeltzer, 1994). MS is not transmitted through breastmilk but may have a familial tendency. The lifetime risk of MS developing in a child whose mother has MS is 0.5–3%, compared with the general population risk of 0.1%. The nature of the condition creates uncertainty regarding if and when relapses will occur and if the symptoms will abate without treatment. This results in a high level of emotional distress (Kroencke & Denney, 1999). Mothers are particularly distressed by fatigue, limb weakness, balance problems, vision disturbances, tingling and numbness, and urinary incontinence (Gulick & Kim, 2004), which without appropriate interventions could lead to depression (Harrison & Stuifbergen, 2002).

Numerous medications may be prescribed for the mother, such as glatiramer (Copaxone), a mixture of polymers of four amino acids that is similar to myelin basic protein; adrenocorticotropic hormone; and interferon beta-1A (Avonex) and interferon beta-1B (Betaseron), which are immunomodulators and appear to be moderately safe, with transport into human milk being limited (Hale, 2004). Methylprednisolone (Solu-Medrol, Medrol) or other corticosteroids are used to treat a number of MS symptoms but can be prescribed in high-dose courses either intravenously or orally over a period of up to 2 weeks. High doses and prolonged administration of these types of medications could affect an infant when exposed through breastmilk. Hale (2004) recommended a brief period of pumping and discarding milk (8–24 hours) after intravenous administration of methylprednisolone at doses up to 1 g.

Breastfeeding Management

It is most helpful for the clinician to meet with the mother before the birth of her infant to determine the extent of the MS progression and begin preparations for social and lactation support postpartum. Prenatal preparations can include the following:

- A plan should be developed for household help and help with the care of the infant and other children.

- Family and friends who provide care and support should be educated about why breastfeeding is important to both the mother and infant. Caregivers should understand that breastfeeding does not exacerbate the disease. They should not take over complete care of the infant, especially the feeding of the infant, so that the mother can rest (Siebenaler, 2002). Helpers can bring the infant to the mother and help her assume a comfortable supported position for breastfeeding.

- Mothers should purchase or rent a high-grade electric breast pump with a double collection kit (Jacobson, 1998). Mothers use the pump to express milk during disease remission periods and store it for use if necessary during times when exacerbations occur and/or breastfeeding must be interrupted for drug therapy. Mothers also may need to pump during interruptions in breastfeeding to ensure an abundant milk supply once the infant is back on the breast.

- Mothers may desire a special nursing pillow, a sling, and a small footstool. These can be used if needed for help with positioning.

- If the mother is in a wheelchair, the home should be arranged for unobstructed access to the infant and an area set up where the mother can comfortably nurse the infant.

- Resting and sleeping arrangements can be prepared before delivery. Mothers may find it easier to breastfeed if the infant is kept within arm's reach next to the bed in a small crib designed to attach to the adult bed.

- Arrangements should be made for community support services as well as lactation support for the postpartum period.

In-hospital support during the initial stay after birth should center on the creation of an individualized breastfeeding plan for both the time spent in the hospital and for feedings after discharge. Many suggestions are designed to minimize the fatigue associated with MS. For instance, positioning for breastfeeding may need to be modified depending on the extent of the MS progression. Before hospital discharge mothers should be documented as being able to position their infant for breastfeeding or a helper should be documented as capable to assist for proper positioning. Mothers breastfeeding in the sitting position may benefit from strategically placed pillows or the use of a pillow designed for breastfeeding to provide support for both the infant and the mother's arms (Figure 9-1).

Some mothers find that use of a sling helps stabilize and support the weight of the infant if the mother's arms have muscular weakness, lack coordination, or are painful (Figure 9-2). In addition, a wheelchair-bound mother will need to use pillows or a tray across her lap (Figure 9-3).

Mothers should be taught how to breastfeed while lying down. Mothers who nurse in the reclining position have reported fewer fatigue-related symptoms after nursing in the side-lying position as opposed to the sitting position (Milligan, Flenniken, & Pugh, 1996). An alternative position might be reclining the mother to a 30-degree angle with the infant placed in a ventral or biological nurturing position that avoids strain from gravity when seated upright.

Systemic Lupus Erythematosus

Systemic lupus erythematosus (SLE) is a chronic autoimmune inflammatory disease distinguished by the presence of non–organ-specific autoantibodies. SLE can affect almost any part of the body, including the joints, kidneys, skin, heart, lungs, brain, and blood vessels. It most often affects young adults under 40 years of age and has a three times higher incidence in African Americans and African Caribbeans.

Figure 9-1   Multiple Pillows Supportive positioning for mothers with MS.

Figure 9-2   A Baby Sling Support Suggestions for mothers with muscular weakness.

Figure 9-3   Pillows and Tray Support Suggestions for wheelchair-bound mothers.

Source: Figures this page, reprinted with permission from Walker, *Core Curriculum for Lactation Consultant Practice.* Sudbury, MA: Jones and Bartlett; 2005.

Approximately 85% of people with SLE are women, and SLE may be familial (see www.lupus.org). This makes it especially important that all women, and especially if there is a family history of SLE, are encouraged and assisted with breastfeeding because breastfeeding is associated with a decreased risk of developing SLE (Cooper et al., 2002). There are little data regarding disease flares during lactation. One case study (Mok, Wong, & Lau, 1998) reported a disease flare with hyper-prolactinemia during breastfeeding, but because other hormones were not assayed, it remains important for mothers to understand that breastfeeding will not exacerbate their disease.

Of the different types of lupus SLE is the most common, with varying signs and symptoms that alternate between remissions and flares. More frequently seen symptoms include a butterfly-like rash across the nose and cheeks, skin rashes on body parts exposed to the sun, sores in the mouth or nose, painful or swollen joints, fatigue, chest pain during deep breathing, Raynaud phenomenon, kidney inflammations, depression, headaches, memory and thinking problems, strokes, and blood clots.

Preeclampsia, prematurity, and intrauterine growth retardation are more common in mothers with SLE. A number of medications are used to treat SLE depending on the extent of organ involvement and frequency and types of disease flares. Aspirin, subcutaneous heparin, nonsteroidal anti-inflammatory drugs (NSAIDs), and corticosteroids may be used during the pregnancy to improve the chances of carrying the infant to term and for reducing joint and muscle pain and inflammation. Antimalarial medications such as hydroxy-chloroquine (Plaquenil) and chloroquine (Aralen) are sometimes used to treat joint pain, skin rashes, and ulcers.

High doses of aspirin and NSAIDs are generally avoided in the last weeks of pregnancy to avoid any unwanted effects on uterine contraction, platelet function, or closure of the ductus arteriosis. Medication use during lactation can involve the use of aspirin but not in large doses. Most but not all NSAIDs are compatible with breastfeeding; however, NSAIDs can displace bilirubin and are contraindicated in jaundiced infants. Small amounts of corticosteroids can be found in breastmilk. When the dose exceeds 20 mg/day, some clinicians recommend that mothers wait at least 4 hours before nursing to reduce infant exposure (Ost et al., 1985).

Immunosuppressive agents/chemotherapy medications are used in serious cases of SLE when major organs are losing their ability to function (Mok & Wong, 2001). Azathioprine (Imuran) and cyclosporin A are not teratogenic and may be considered in situations of severe lupus, whereas cyclophosphamide (Cytoxan) is a teratogen in humans and is not used during pregnancy.

About 3% of infants born to mothers with lupus have neonatal lupus. This lupus consists of a temporary rash and abnormal blood counts. Neonatal lupus usually disappears by the time the infant is 3–6 months old and does not recur. About one-half of infants with neonatal lupus are born with a heart condition. This condition is permanent but can be treated with a pacemaker.

Breastfeeding Management

Mothers with SLE may also experience chronic fatigue syndrome and fibro-myalgia, compounding the major problem of fatigue. Because most mothers with SLE are taking some type of medication or multiple medications, the clinician should be aware of and ensure the safety of all drugs taken during lactation. Anecdotal reports of insufficient milk supply in breastfeeding mothers with SLE may alert the clinician to ensuring a good start to breastfeeding with steps taken to maximize milk production. It is not known whether the SLE itself, high blood pressure/preeclampsia, or some combination of medications inhibits sufficient milk production. The infant should be closely monitored for normal weight gain and any possible side effects from maternal medications. Planned rest periods and breastfeeding in the side-lying or ventral position may help with SLE-related fatigue. Because people with SLE may experience Raynaud phenomenon, breast-feeding mothers and their healthcare providers should be vigilant for this condi-tion in the nipple. Some infants of mothers with SLE are preterm, intrauterine growth retarded, or separated from their mother during the early days of life. If the infant is not available to be put directly to the breast, mothers need to begin pumping as soon as possible after delivery. Breastfeeding management guidelines should be incorporated into an individualized feeding plan for this mother.

Rheumatoid Arthritis

Rheumatoid arthritis (RA) is a chronic inflammatory condition with autoimmune, genetic predisposition and familial clustering properties. Some researchers are uncertain if RA is just one disease or several different diseases with common fea-tures. Prevalence estimates range from 0.3% to 1.5% in North America (Silman & Pearson, 2002), with prevalence increasing with age and 2.5 times higher in women than in men. Researchers believe that female reproductive hormones may have an influence on the greater incidence of RA seen in women. Evidence regarding reproductive hormones, pregnancy, and breastfeeding as risk factors for RA is conflicting. Because RA has both genetic and familial clustering trends, mothers who have a family history of RA should be encouraged and supported to breastfeed. Karlson, Mandl, Hankinson, and Grodstein (2004) showed that women who breastfed for 13–23 months had a 20% reduction in risk for development of RA, whereas those breastfeeding for at least 24 months during their childbearing years increased their risk reduction to 50%.

Many women with RA enjoy a remission in their condition during pregnancy, when levels of the proinflammatory hormone prolactin are reduced, but experience flares postpartum, especially in the presence of breastfeeding (Barrett, Brennan, Fiddler, & Silman, 2000). However, the onset of RA and flares of the condition postpartum in susceptible mothers (Hampl & Papa, 2001) may also be related to limited durations of breastfeeding as well as the cumulative effects of the number of total months spent breastfeeding. Brennan and Silman (1994) looked at 187 women who had developed RA within 12 months of a pregnancy. Eighty-eight women (47%) with RA developed it after their first pregnancy, and 71 of these 88 mothers had breastfed. However, breastfeeding by the third pregnancy posed no increased risk of developing RA.

The duration of breastfeeding has been shown to be inversely related to the risk of RA, with the protective effect of longer breastfeeding remaining significant even after adjustment for other environmental influences (Liao, Alfredsson, & Karlson, 2009; Pikwer et al., 2009). Cortisol levels are increased during lactation, with a long-term association seen between the cumulative duration of breastfeeding and elevated cortisol playing protective roles in the acquisition of certain autoimmune diseases such as RA long after the childbearing years (Lankarani-Fard, Kritz-Silverterin, Barrett-Connor, & Goodman-Gruen, 2001). Other confounding factors could also place first-time mothers at an increased risk for development of RA including irregular menstrual cycles (Karlson et al., 2004). Such subfertility may be a marker for women at increased risk for development of RA, as could states of hyperprolactinemia or abnormal responses to prolactin. It is known that pregnant women with SLE have significantly elevated prolactin levels (Jara, Lavelle, & Espinoza, 1992), as do patients with RA, osteoarthritis, and fibromyalgia. Problems with the pituitary regulation of prolactin may contribute to RA in susceptible populations, whereas a high cumulative duration or "dose" of breastfeeding is related to a decreased risk of RA, perhaps because lactation provides a regulatory mechanism.

Drug therapy usually involves a combination of medications depending on the extent of the disease, exacerbations, and tolerance. Some drugs are safe for use during lactation, some are not, and some have effects that are simply unknown. The main categories of drugs used to treat RA are as follows:

- NSAIDs are used to reduce inflammation and relieve pain. These may include aspirin, ibuprofen (Advil, Motrin), acetaminophen (Tylenol, Paracetamol), flurbiprofen (Ansaid, Froben), diclofenac (Cataflam, Voltaren), indomethacin (Indocin), and piroxicam (Feldene). NSAIDs have many gastrointestinal side effects and should not be used in the presence of a jaundiced infant. Their use requires closer monitoring of the infant for potential side effects.

- Analgesic drugs used to relieve pain but not inflammation include acetaminophen, propoxyphene (Darvocet N, Darvon), and ketorolac (Toradol).

- Glucocorticoids or prednisone are used in low doses to prevent joint damage.

- Disease-modifying antirheumatic drugs, used along with NSAIDs and/or prednisone, slow joint destruction over time. Examples include methotrexate (Folex, Rheumatrex), injectable gold (Myochrysine, Solganal), penicillamine (Cuprimine, Depen), azathioprine (Imuran), chloroquine (Aralen, Novochloroquine), hydroxychloroquine (Plaquenil), sulfasalazine (Azulfidine), and oral gold (Ridura). Hydroxychloroquine has been safely used, but methotrexate can be stored in the mucosal cells of the gastrointestinal tract in infants and could be problematic. Gold has a very long half-life and would expose an infant for long periods of time to a very toxic product. These drugs can suppress the immune system, so it is important to practice good breastfeeding management to prevent infections such as mastitis.

- Biological-response modifiers directly modify the immune system by inhibiting cytokines that contribute to inflammation. These include etanercept (Enbrel), infliximab (Remicade), adalimumab (Humira), anakinra (Kineret), abatacept (Orencia), and rituximab (Rituxan).

- Protein-A immunoadsorption therapy is a process that filters the blood to remove antibodies and immune complexes that promote inflammation.

- Steroids such as triamcinolone (Aristocort) can be directly injected into affected joints.

Breastfeeding Management

Prenatal preparation for breastfeeding should include the promotion of breastfeeding for women with RA and plans for handling any relapse or flares after delivery. Medications are often given in combination and should be chosen based on their safety profile and urgency of need. Along with good breastfeeding management guidelines, special attention may need to be directed to help the mother with RA assume a comfortable position for breastfeeding depending on which joints are affected. Any adaptive equipment or special household arrangements should be made at this time. Mothers should ensure that any forms of anemia are corrected and that they will follow good nutritional guidelines to prevent anemia from interfering with the establishment and maintenance of an abundant milk supply.

Cervical Spine

A mother with pain, stiffness, or a limited range of motion in the neck may be unable to look down for any length of time while placing her infant to the breast or while using a breast pump. A heating pad or application of warm compresses to the neck before breastfeeding or pumping may be soothing. The mother may find that breastfeeding in front of a mirror (Drazin, 1995) provides a mechanism to visualize positioning, latch, suck, and swallowing of the infant and allows the proper placement and use of a breast pump. Some mothers may find the side-lying position or ventral positioning of the infant to be effective and comfortable.

Spinal Column

Mothers with back pain usually need to experiment with positions and supporting pillows to see what feels best for them. Some mothers find that placing their feet on a small footstool when in a seated position removes strain from the lower back and tips the infant slightly toward the mother's body. With the infant tipped toward the mother, she will not need to provide as much support with her arm, lessening the strain on the shoulder girdle and upper back. Reclining at a 30-degree angle with ventral positioning of the infant may ease back strain.

Wrist, Hand, and Fingers

Some mothers with RA find a nursing pillow that allows the infant to maintain a position that does not require extended use of the wrist can be helpful. The side-lying positioning eases strain on the wrist and hands and can reduce the need to reposition the infant if the mother shifts her position to present the upper breast to the infant while still lying on her side. A small rolled towel can be placed under the breast if a large breast requires support throughout the feeding.

If a mother requires the use of a breast pump, the clinician should consider the use of an electric pump with a double collection kit. Use of a cylinder pump, especially with the wrist pronated, can provoke or exacerbate lateral epicondylitis (tennis elbow) and strain on the wrist (Williams, Auerbach, & Jacobi, 1989). Use of a manual pump with a squeeze handle places considerable stress on the wrist, as will any pump that requires repetitive hand motion. Even holding the collection kits of an electric pump in place may place a strain on painful joints. Mothers can consider the use of a nursing bra with special openings constructed to hold pump flanges in place for hands-free pumping. She may also consider using a hands-free pump that fits under each bra cup.

Fatigue remains a primary problem for women with RA or any chronic pain and can be quite overwhelming to a mother (Carty, Connie, & Wood-Johnson, 1986). Planned rest periods along with braces or splints may help reduce fatigue and improve joint mobility (Carty, Connie, & Hall, 1990).

Maternal Employment

In 2008 the labor force participation rate of mothers with children under 6 years old was 64.0%. The participation rate of mothers with infants under a year old was 56.4% (U.S. Bureau of Labor Statistics, 2009). Employment outside the home is associated with a shorter duration of breastfeeding, with intention to work full time significantly related to lower rates of breastfeeding initiation and shorter duration (Fein & Roe, 1998). Low-income women are more likely to return to work earlier than higher income earners and are more likely to be employed in jobs that present numerous challenges to the continuation of breastfeeding (Lindberg, 1996). Mothers who believe that breastfeeding while employed cannot be done without a considerable amount of additional work and stress may not even consider breast-feeding (Stewart-Glenn , 2008). Mothers with professional jobs are similar to stay-at-home mothers in terms of breastfeeding duration (Kimbro, 2006). Changes in federal welfare policy that require work by women with young infants has contributed significantly to lower national breastfeeding rates. Women on WIC (the Special Supplemental Nutrition Program for Women, Infants, and Children) living in states with the most stringent work laws showed a reduced breastfeeding rate of 22% relative to imposing no work requirements on new mothers. Estimates for all mothers (not just WIC participants) imply that if welfare reform had not been enacted, national breastfeeding rates 6 months after birth would have been 5.5% higher than they were in 2000 (Haider, Jacknowitz, & Schoeni, 2003).

The duration of work leave contributes significantly to the duration of breast-feeding, with each week of work leave increasing breastfeeding duration by approximately half a week (Roe, Kritz-Silverterin, Barrett-Connor, & Goodman-Gruen, 1999). Returning to work within the first 12 weeks after birth is related to the greatest decrease in breastfeeding duration. Guendelman et al. (2009) found that a maternity leave of less than or equal to 6 weeks or from 6 to 12 weeks after delivery was associated, respectively, with fourfold and twofold higher odds of failure to establish breastfeeding and an increased probability of cessation after successful establishment, relative to women not returning to work, after adjusting for covariates. The impact of short postpartum leave on breastfeeding cessation was stronger among nonmanagers, women with inflexible jobs, and with high psychosocial distress. However, for low-income women a long maternity leave is usually not an option, especially if welfare benefits are tied to work requirements. The greater the number of hours worked each day, the fewer breastmilk feedings an infant receives, placing infants whose mothers return to work within 4–6 weeks of birth at high risk of partial or no breastmilk intake. Employment is significantly associated with breastfeeding cessation as early as 2–3 months postpartum, with working no more than 20 hours per week protective for continued breastfeeding (Gielen et al., 1991).

Many mothers continue to experience childbirth-related symptoms at 5 weeks postpartum, such as fatigue, low hemoglobin levels, pain, breast symptoms in lactating mothers, role limitations, and incomplete recovery, especially mothers who delivered by cesarean section (McGovern et al., 2006). Mothers may wish to use intermittent rather than straight-time leave under the Family and Medical Leave Act, which allows a gradual, part-time return to work over a longer period of time. Physicians must certify mothers for intermittent leave under Family and Medical Leave Act regulations (McGovern et al., 2006). Many mothers cannot afford to take uncompensated maternity leave or may have a short-term disability policy that provides a partial salary for 4 to 6 weeks.

In addition to work-leave issues, employed breastfeeding mothers face a number of conflicts (Cardenas & Major, 2005) and challenges from the worksite itself, including lack of flexibility in work schedules or alternative work options, difficulty arranging breaks for pumping, breaks that are too short or lactation rooms that are located too far from the mother's area of work, inappropriate or no locations for pumping, and lack of support from coworkers and supervisors (Bar-Yam, 1998; Johnston & Esposito, 2007; Rojjanasrirat, 2004). Employers may believe that breastfeeding is a personal choice and not a matter of employer responsibility (Dunn et al., 2004) with little understanding how the health benefits of breastfeeding (Bridges, Frank, & Curtin, 1997) translate into employer cost savings

(Cohen & Mrtek, 1994; Cohen, Mrtek, & Mrtek, 1995). Coworkers may believe that breastfeeding accommodation is unfair (Seijts, 2004) even though monetary costs for the employer to put in place such accommodations tend to be minimal (Prince, 2002). Working mothers who do not breastfeed have higher absentee rates and health costs than those who do. Employers may be unaware that lactation support can be a relatively inexpensive boost to the company's bottom line (Tyler, 1999), especially since a $15-per-hour employee who is absent for just 1 day costs a company $160 (Faught, 1994). Employee retention is less costly than hiring new employees and a supportive work environment strengthens employee commitment to the company (Bond, Galinsky, & Swanberg, 1998).

A major reason companies with lactation support programs continue to offer such accommodation is that mothers remain with the company, even through two or more births (Ortiz, Galinsky, & Swanberg, 2004). Lactation accommodation by an employer can have a positive effect on the employee recruitment process, with potential employees being more likely to submit a resume and accept a job offer (Seijts, 2002). Mothers can express their milk two to three times per day, spending less than an hour total, often coinciding with their already allotted break time (Slusser et al., 2004). Lack of time to pump milk and the resulting diminishing milk supply are common causes of premature weaning (Arthur, Saenz, & Replogle, 2003). A hostile work environment that forces mothers to secretly breastfeed or to experience negative feedback from coworkers and management may result in untimely weaning (Gatrell, 2007). Poor or expensive child care options reduce breastfeeding success. Some child care providers sabotage breastfeeding by feeding formula when mothers are away at work or are uneasy handling breastmilk. When child care is onsite or nearby, working mothers report increased breastfeeding success (Thompson & Bell, 1997).

Breastfeeding Management

Preparation in advance is most important to the continuation of breastfeeding after the return to work (Meek, 2001). Unanticipated fatigue, anxiety, role conflict/overload, competing demands, household chores, and child care issues challenge the new mother and should be addressed before a mother returns to work (Nichols & Roux, 2004). Clinicians should help mothers address the following issues:

- Length of maternity leave, options for full-time work, flex time, use of earned time, job sharing, phased-back work schedule, part-time work, compressed work week, telecommuting, and onsite or near-site child care

(Bar-Yam, 1998). Use of these options may allow the mother to spend more time with her infant, increasing the amount of breastfeeding and breast-milk feedings per day. Fein, Mandal, and Roe (2008) found that feeding the infant from the breast during the workday is the most effective strategy for combining breastfeeding and work. Ways to enable direct feeding include onsite child care, telecommuting, keeping the infant at work, allowing the mother to leave work to go to the infant, and having the infant brought to the worksite.

- What options exist for expressing milk at the workplace. Discuss with the employer the use of break times, a location for pumping, coworker and supervisor support, and how pumped milk will be stored.

Based on the age of the infant when the mother returns to work, the clinician and mother can create a breastfeeding plan for the times before and after resumption of employment (Biagioli, 2003). For instance, mothers returning to work at 6 months postpartum may find that expressing milk twice each workday is suffi-cient to keep up with the infant's needs because the infant is likely to start solid foods around this age. Mothers with a 3-month maternity leave should plan to have breastfeeding well established, address any early breastfeeding problems, have an infant gaining weight adequately, and consider pumping milk several times per week to have a supply in the freezer for times of fluctuating milk supply. Mothers should secure a high-quality personal-use electric pump with a double collection kit, a small cooler or insulated bag, "blue ice" to keep the milk cool during storage and transport, and bottles or bags in which to store the milk. Expressed milk is safe and stable when stored for 24 hours in a little cooler case at 59°F (15°C) (Hamosh et al., 1996).

Mothers generally need to pump two to three times each day depending on the length of their workday. Mothers can plan how the infant will be fed in their absence. Infants at this age can be given a bottle; however, some breastfed infants may refuse a bottle. Starting infants on a bottle in the early days does not guar-antee that an infant will take one at 3 months and can interfere with breastfeeding and milk production. An infant can be started on a bottle about 7–10 days before the return to work at the times when the mother is usually gone. Many mothers begin a gradual introduction of the infant to the bottle and child care environ-ment at this time such that a bottle is given by someone other than the mother in the location where such feedings will take place. Infants who refuse a bottle can be fed with a small cup or a child's sippy cup with a spout. Some mothers in this situation use a reverse-cycle feeding technique whereby the infant's sleep patterns are encouraged to change to longer sleep periods during the time the mother is at work, minimizing milk intake, and then remaining awake for longer periods in the evening for clustered feeds at the breast.

Mothers with a 4- to 6-week maternity leave can experience a more difficult course, especially if any early breastfeeding problems continue unresolved. Faltering milk production is often the most pressing problem once a mother starts back to work at this early time. Using the model of initiating and maintaining abundant milk production in the preterm mother, mothers returning to work this early can follow a plan to maximize milk output by the 6-week mark through 10–12 feedings each 24 hours for the first 14 days. After this time (or during the first 2 weeks if the mother has a large supply or if the infant is not effectively stimulating the supply), mothers can pump milk after each feeding such that the breasts calibrate to a 50% oversupply of milk to be stored in the freezer. This oversupply compensates for the natural falloff in milk production when a mother returns to work and ensures that breastmilk is available for growth spurts, supply fluctuations, missed pumping sessions, or other unforeseen circumstances.

Mothers should be encouraged to breastfeed right before dropping off the infant at child care or just before leaving for work and then breastfeed again at the child care setting or immediately upon arrival at home, frequently during the evening, and frequently on her days off.

To avoid faltering milk production, it is not only important to calibrate the breasts to an initial very-high milk volume but also to express milk on a thorough and regular basis with a high-quality personal use or multiuser quality breast pump with a double collection kit. Mothers prefer high-quality electric pumps over nonelectrical pumps that take longer to express milk and use up short pumping times (Stevens & Janke, 2003). Some employers provide a multiuser pump that is shared among the breastfeeding employees who each use their own collection kit. Some employers give their breastfeeding employees a personal collection kit as an employee benefit. Some mothers have jobs that leave little to no time for pumping and find that other types of pumps might work better in their situation. This might include pumps that are battery operated, worn under the bra, and leave the hands free for work activities.

Some mothers find it difficult to pump under time constraints and may experience a delayed letdown reflex or minimal volumes of milk per pumping session. Mothers can be encouraged to elicit the milk ejection reflex first, before applying the pump, by looking at a picture of the infant or by massaging and hand expressing until milk spurts or sprays. If this is ineffective, oxytocin nasal spray can be used to hasten the letdown reflex. The pump flanges should then be put in place and the mother can continue to massage and compress each breast while pumping to maximize output, minimize pumping time, and avoid leaving milk residuals that can contribute to diminished milk production, focal engorgement, and mastitis. Mothers can hold the flanges in place with one arm placed across the collection kits or use a bra that is specially made with openings to secure the flanges in place for hands-free pumping.

Clinicians may wish to help employed mothers by writing a letter to the employer detailing the importance of accommodations in the workplace (Angeletti, 2009) or may wish to work with employers to create an onsite lactation program (Click, 2006). Physicians and advanced practice nurses may write a prescription for breastmilk that mothers can show to employers. Many states have legislation regarding workplace accommodation for breastfeeding mothers with which clinicians should be familiar. Mothers should be encouraged to ask for breastfeeding accommodation, because one reason for the lack of such employer support is the absence of employee demand. Clinicians should be vocal proponents of paid maternity leave (Calnen, 2007).

Summary: The Design in Nature

Except under the most extraordinary circumstances, mothers should be encouraged and supported to breastfeed or provide expressed milk for their infants.

References

Abascal, K., & Yarnell, E. (2008). Botanical galactagogues. *Altern Complement Ther., 14,* 288–294.

Academy of Breastfeeding Medicine. (2004). Clinical protocol number 9—Use of galactagogues in initiating or augmenting maternal milk supply. Retrieved September 15, 2005, from www.bfmed.org/protocol/galactogogues.pdf

Ahluwalia, I. B., Morrow, B., & Hsia, J. (2005). Why do women stop breastfeeding? Findings from the Pregnancy Risk Assessment and Monitoring System. *Pediatrics, 116,* 1408–1412.

Akman, I., Kuscu, M. K., Yurdakul, Z., et al. (2008). Breastfeeding duration and postpartum psychological adjustment: Role of maternal attachment styles. *J Pediatr Child Health, 44,* 369–373.

Albareda, M., Caballero, A., Badell, G., et al. (2003). Diabetes and abnormal glucose tolerance in women with previous gestational diabetes. *Diabetes Care, 26,* 1199–1205.

Aljazaf, K., Hale, T. W., Ilett, K. F., et al. (2003). Pseudoephedrine: Effects on milk production in women and estimation of infant exposure via breastmilk. *Br J Clin Pharmacol., 56,* 18–24.

American Academy of Pediatrics, Committee on Drugs. (2001). The transfer of drugs and other chemicals into human milk. *Pediatrics, 108,* 776–788.

American Diabetes Association. (2004). Gestational diabetes mellitus. Position statement. *Diabetes Care,* *27*(Suppl 1), S88–S90.

Amir, L. H. (2006). Breastfeeding: Managing supply difficulties. *Aust Fam Physician, 35,* 686–689.

Amir, L. H., & Donath, S. (2007). A systematic review of maternal obesity and breastfeeding intention, initiation, and duration. *BMC Pregnancy and Childbirth, 7,* 9.

Anderson, P. O., & Valdes, V. (2007). A critical review of pharmaceutical galactagogues. *Breastfeeding Med., 2,* 229–242.

Angeletti, M. A. (2009). Breastfeeding mothers returning to work: Possibilities for information, anticipatory guidance and support from US health care professionals. *J Hum Lact., 25,* 226–232.

Arthur, C., Saenz, R. B., & Replogle, W. H. (2003). The employment-related breastfeeding decisions of physician mothers. *Journal of the Mississippi State Medical Association, 44,* 383–387.

Arthur, P. G., Kent, J. C., & Hartmann, P. E. (1994). Metabolites of lactose synthesis in milk from diabetic and nondiabetic women during lactogenesis II. *J Pediatr Gastroenter Nutr., 19,* 100–108.

Asselin, B. L., & Lawrence, R. A. (1987). Maternal disease as a consideration in lactation management. *Clin Perinatol., 14,* 71–87.

Azizi, F., Khoshniat, M., Bahrainian, M., & Hedayati, M. (2000). Thyroid function and intellectual development of infants nursed by mothers taking methimazole. *J Clin Endocrinol Metabol., 85,* 3233–3238.

Azziz, R., Woods, K. S., Reyna, R., et al. (2004). The prevalence and features of the polycystic ovary syndrome in an unselected population. *J Clin Endocrinol Metabol., 89,* 2745–2749.

Baker, J. L., Gamborg, M., Heitmann, B. L., Lissner, L., Sorenses, T. I., & Rasmussen, K. M. (2008). Breastfeeding reduces postpartum weight retention. *Am J Clin Nutr., 88,* 1543–1551.

Baker, J. L., Michaelsen, K. F., Sorensen, T. I., & Rasmussen, K. M. (2007). High prepregnant body mass index is associated with early termination of full and any breastfeeding in Danish women. *Am J Clin Nutr., 86,* 404–411.

Bakri, Y. N., Bakhashwain, M., & Hugosson, C. (1994). Massive theca-lutein cysts, virilization, and hypothyroidism associated with normal pregnancy. *Acta Obstetricia et Gynecologica Scandinavica, 73,* 153–155.

Bar-Yam, N. B. (1998). Workplace lactation support, part 1: A return-to-work breastfeeding assessment tool. *J Hum Lact., 14,* 249–254.

Barrett, J. H., Brennan, P., Fiddler, M., & Silman, A. (2000). Breastfeeding and postpartum relapse in women with rheumatoid arthritis. *Arthritis and Rheumatism, 43,* 1010–1015.

Battle, C. L., Ziotnick, C., Pearlstein, T., et al. (2008). Depression and breastfeeding: Which postpartum patients take antidepressant medications? *Depression and Anxiety, 25,* 888–891.

Beck, C. T. (1992). The lived experience of postpartum depression: A phenomenological study. *Nurs Res., 41,* 166–170.

Beck, C. T. (1993). Teetering on the edge: A substantive theory of postpartum depression. *Nurs Res., 42,* 42–48.

Bentley-Lewis, R., Levkoff, S., Stuebe, A., & Seely, E. W. (2008). Gestational diabetes mellitus: Postpartum opportunities for the diagnosis and prevention of type 2 diabetes mellitus. *Nat Clin Pract Endocrinol Metabol., 4,* 552–558.

Berbel, P., Mestre, J. L., Santamaria A., et al. (2009). Delayed neurobehavioral development in children born to pregnant women with milk hypothyroxinemia during the first month of gestation: The importance of early iodine supplementation. *Thyroid, 19,* 511–519.

Betzold, C. M., Hoover, K. L., & Snyder, C. L. (2004). Delayed lactogenesis II: A comparison of four cases. *Journal of Midwifery and Womens Health, 49,* 132–137.

Benz, J. (1992). Antidiabetic agents and lactation. *J Hum Lact., 8,* 27–28.

Biagioli, F. (2003). Returning to work while breastfeeding. *Am Fam Physician, 68,* 2201–2208, 2215–2217.

Biervliet, F. P., Maguiness, S. D., Hay, D. M., et al. (2001). Induction of lactation in the intended mother of a surrogate pregnancy. *Hum Reprod., 16,* 581–583.

Bingel, A. S., & Farnsworth, N. R. (1994). Higher plants as potential sources of galactagogues. *Econ Med Plant Res., 6,* 1–54.

Birk, K., & Rudick, R. (1986). Pregnancy and multiple sclerosis. *Arch Neurol., 43,* 719–726.

Bisset, N. G. (1994). *Herbal drugs and phytopharmaceuticals.* London: CRC Press.

Bitman, J., Hamosh, M., Hamosh, P., et al. (1989). Milk composition and volume during the onset of lactation in a diabetic mother. *Am J Clin Nutr., 50,* 1364–1369.

Bitman, J., Hamosh, M., Wood, D. L., et al. (1987). Lipid composition of milk from mothers with cystic fibrosis. *Pediatrics, 80,* 927–932.

Blumenthal, M., & Busse, W. R. (Eds.). (1998). *The complete German Commission E monographs: Therapeutic guide to herbal medicine* (trans. S. Klein & R. S. Rister). Austin, TX: American Botanical Council.

Bodley, V., & Powers, D. (1999). Patient with insufficient glandular tissue experiences milk supply increase attributed to progesterone treatment for luteal phase defect. *J Hum Lact., 15,* 339–343.

Bond, J., Galinsky, E., & Swanberg, J. (1998). *The 1997 national study of the changing workforce.* New York: Families and Work Institute.

Boullu, S., Andrac, L., Piana, L., et al. (1998). Diabetic mastopathy, complication of type 1 diabetes mellitus: Report of two cases and a review of the literature. *Diabetes and Metabolism, 24,* 448–454.

Bowles, B. C. (1991). Breastfeeding consultation in sign language. *J Hum Lact., 7,* 21.

Bray, G. A. (1997). Obesity and reproduction. *Hum Reprod., 12* (Suppl 1), 26–32.

Breier, B. H., Milsom, S. R., Blum, W. F., et al. (1993). Insulin-like growth factors and their binding proteins in plasma and milk after growth hormone-stimulated galactopoiesis in normally lactating women. *Acta Endocrinologica, 129,* 427–435.

Brennan, P., & Silman, A. (1994). Breastfeeding and the onset of rheumatoid arthritis. *Arthritis and Rheumatism, 37,* 808–813.

Brent, N. B., & Wisner, K. L. (1998). Fluoxetine and carbamazepine concentrations in a nursing mother/infant pair. *Clin Pediatr., 37,* 41–44.

Bridges, C. B., Frank, D. I., & Curtin, J. (1997). Employer attitudes toward breastfeeding in the workplace. *J Hum Lact., 13,* 215–219.

Britton, J. R. (2007). Postpartum anxiety and breastfeeding. *J Reprod Med., 52,* 689–695.

Brouwers, J. R., Assies, J., Wiersinga, W. M., et al. (1980). Plasma prolactin levels after acute and subchronic oral administration of domperidone and of metoclopramide: A cross-over study in healthy volunteers. *Clin Endocrinol., 12,* 435–440.

Brown, T. E., Fernandes, P. A., Grant, L. J., et al. (2000). Effect of parity on pituitary prolactin response to metoclopramide and domperidone: Implications for the enhancement of lactation. *J Soc Gynecol Investig., 7,* 65–69.

Bryant, C. A. (2006). Nursing the adopted infant. *J Am Board Fam Med., 19,* 374–379.

Buckshee, K., Kriplani, A., Kapil, A., et al. (1992). Hypothyroidism complicating pregnancy. *Aust N Z J Obstet Gynaecol., 32,* 240–242.

Budd, S. C., Erdman, S. H., Long, D. M., et al. (1993). Improved lactation with metoclopramide: A case report. *Clin Pediatr., 32,* 53–57.

Burt, V. K., Suri, R., Altshuler, L., et al. (2001). The use of psychotropic medications during breastfeeding. *Am J Psychiatr., 158,* 1001–1009.

California Diabetes and Pregnancy Program. (2002). *Guidelines for care: Sweet success express.* Sacramento, CA: Maternal and Child Health Branch, Department of Health Services.

Calnen, G. (2007). Paid maternity leave and its impact on breastfeeding in the United States: An historic, economic, political, and social perspective. *Breastfeeding Med., 2,* 34–44.

Cardenas, R. A., & Major, D. A. (2005). Combining employment and breastfeeding: Utilizing a work-family conflict framework to understand obstacles and solutions. *Journal of Business Psychology, 20,* 31–51.

Carty, E., Connie, T. A., & Hall, L. (1990). Comprehensive health promotion for the pregnant woman who is disabled. *J Nurse Midwifery, 35,* 133–142.

Carty, E., Connie, T. A., & Wood-Johnson, F. (1986). Rheumatoid arthritis and pregnancy: Helping women to meet their needs. *Midwives Chronicles, 99,* 254–257.

Cesario, S. K. (2002). Spinal cord injuries. *AWHONN Lifelines, 6,* 225–232.

Chambers, C. D., Anderson, P. O., Thomas, R. G., et al. (1999). Weight gain in infants breastfed by mothers who take fluoxetine. *Pediatrics, 104*(5), e61.

Chapman, D. J., & Perez-Escamilla, R. (1999a). Identification of risk factors for delayed onset of lactation. *J Am Dietet Assn., 99,* 450–454.

Chapman, D., & Perez-Escamilla, R. (1999b). Maternal perception of delayed onset of lactogenesis (OL): A useful marker of delayed onset of lactogenesis stage II (OLII). Presented at the 9th International Conference of the International Society of Research in Human Milk and Lactation, October, Irsee, Germany.

Chapman, D. J., & Perez-Escamilla, R. (2000). Maternal perception of the onset of lactation is a valid, public health indicator of lactogenesis stage II. *J Nutr., 130,* 2972–2980.

Cheales-Siebenaler, N. J. (1999). Induced lactation in an adoptive mother. *J Hum Lact., 15,* 421–423.

Chen, D. C., Nommsen-Rivers, L., Dewey, K. G., & Lonnerdal, B. (1998). Stress during labor and delivery and early lactation performance. *Am J Clin Nutr., 68,* 335–344.

Clavey, S. (1996). The use of acupuncture for the treatment of insufficient lactation (Que Ru). *American Journal of Acupuncture, 24,* 35–46.

Click, E. R. (2006). Developing a worksite lactation program. *MCN, 31,* 313–317.

Cohen, R., & Mrtek, M. B. (1994). The impact of two corporate lactation programs on the incidence and duration of breastfeeding by employed mothers. *Am J Health Promotion, 8,* 436–441.

Cohen, R., Mrtek, M. B., & Mrtek, R. G. (1995). Comparison of maternal absenteeism and infant illness rates among breastfeeding and formula-feeding women in two corporations. *Am J Health Promotion, 10,* 148–153.

Confavreux, C., Hutchinson, M., Hours, M. M., et al. (1998). Rate of pregnancy-related relapse in multiple sclerosis. *N Eng J Med., 339,* 285–291.

Conn, J. J., Jacobs, H. S., & Conway, G. S. (2000). The prevalence of polycystic ovaries in women with type 2 diabetes mellitus. *Clin Endocrinol., 52,* 81–86.

Cooper, G. S., Dooley, M. A., Treadwell, E. L., et al. (2002). Hormonal and reproductive risk factors for development of systemic lupus erythematosus. *Arthritis and Rheumatism, 46,* 1830–1839.

Cordero, L., Treuer, S. H., Landon, M. B., & Gabbe, S. G. (1998). Management of infants of diabetic mothers. *Arch Adolesc Med., 152,* 249–254.

Cowley, K. C. (2005). Psychogenic and pharmacologic induction of the let-down reflex can facilitate breastfeeding by tetraplegic women: A report of 3 cases. *Arch Phys Med Rehabil., 86,* 1261–1264.

Coyle, P. K., Christie, S., Fodor, P., et al. (2004). Multiple sclerosis gender issues: Clinical practices of women neurologists. *Multiple Sclerosis, 10,* 582–588.

Craig, D. (1990). The adaptation to pregnancy of spinal cord injured women. *Rehabil Nurs., 15,* 6–9.

Crawford, P. M. (2009). Managing epilepsy in women of childbearing age. *Drug Safety, 32,* 293–307.

Cystic Fibrosis Foundation. (n.d.). Retrieved September 15, 2005, from www.cff.org

Dakhil-Jerew, F., Brook, S., & Derry, F. (2008). Autonomic dysreflexia triggered by breastfeeding in a tetraplegic mother. *J Rehabil Med., 40,* 780–782.

da Silva, O. P., Knoppert, D. C., Angelini, M. M., & Forret, P. A. (2001). Effect of domperidone on milk production in mothers of premature newborns: A randomized, double-blind, placebo-controlled trial. *CMAJ, 164,* 17–21.

Davies, H. A., Clark, J. D. A., Dalton, K. J., et al. (1989). Insulin requirements of diabetic women who breastfeed. *BMJ, 298,* 1357–1358.

DeCarvalho, M., Robertson, S., Friedman, A., et al. (1983). Effect of frequent breastfeeding on early milk production and infant weight gain. *Pediatrics, 72,* 307.

Delgado-Escueta, A. V., & Janz, D. (1992). Consensus guidelines: Preconception counseling, management, and care of the pregnant women with epilepsy. *Neurology, 42*(Suppl 5), 149–160.

Dennis, C. L., & McQueen, K. (2007). Does maternal postpartum depressive symptomatology influence infant feeding outcomes? *Acta Paediatr., 96,* 590–594.

Dennis, C. L., & McQueen, K. (2009). The relationship between infant-feeding outcomes and postpartum depression: A qualitative systematic review. *Pediatrics, 123,* e736–e751.

Diniz, J. M., & da Costa, T. H. (2004). Independent of body adiposity, breastfeeding has a protective effect on glucose metabolism in young adult women. *Br J Nutr., 92,* 905–912.

Di Pierro, F., Callegari, A., Carotenuto, D., & Tapia, M. M. (2008). Clinical efficacy, safety and tolerability of BIO-C (micronized Silymarin) as a galactagogue. *Acta Biomedica, 79,* 205–210.

Dombrowski, M. A., Anderson, G. C., Santori, C., & Burkhammer, M. (2001). Kangaroo (skin-to-skin) care with a postpartum woman who felt depressed. *Am J Matern Child Nurs., 26,* 214–216.

Donath, S., & Amir, L. (2000). Does maternal obesity adversely affect breastfeeding initiation and duration? *J Paediatr Child Health, 36,* 482–486.

Donath, S. M., & Amir, L. H. (2008). Maternal obesity and initiation and duration of breastfeeding: Data from the longitudinal study of Australian children. *Matern Child Nutr., 4,* 163–170.

Drazin, P. (1995). Use of a mirror to assist breast pumping. *J Hum Lact., 11,* 219.

Driscoll, J. W. (2005). Recognizing women's common mental health problems: The earthquake assessment model. *J Obstet Gynecol Neonat Nurs., 34,* 246–254.

Dunn, B. F., Zavela, K. J., Cline, A. D., & Cost, P. A. (2004). Breastfeeding practices in Colorado businesses. *J Hum Lact., 20,* 170–177.

Dunne, G., & Fuerst, K. (1995). Breastfeeding by a mother who is a triple amputee: A case report. *J Hum Lact., 11,* 217–218.

Edenborough, F. P., Borgo, G., Knoop, C., et al. (2008). Guidelines for the management of pregnancy in women with cystic fibrosis. *Journal of Cystic Fibrosis, 7,* S2–S32.

Eggum, M. (2001). Breastfeeding with multiple sclerosis: Helping women confront their fears. *AWHONN Lifelines, 5,* 36–40.

Ehrenkranz, R. A., & Ackerman, B. A. (1986). Metoclopramide effect on faltering milk production by mothers of premature infants. *Pediatrics, 78,* 614–620.

Faught, L. (1994, September/October). Lactation programs benefit the family and the corporation. *Journal of Compensation Benefits,* 44–47.

Feher, D. K., Berger, L. R., Johnson, D., et al. (1989). Increasing breast milk production for preterm infants with a relaxation/imagery audiotape. *Pediatrics, 83,* 57.

Feig, D. S., Briggs, G. G., & Koren, G. (2007). Oral antidiabetic agents in pregnancy and lactation: A paradigm shift? *Ann Pharmacother., 41,* 1174–1180.

Fein, S. B., Mandal, B., & Roe, B. E. (2008). Success of strategies for combining employment and breastfeeding. *Pediatrics, 122*(Suppl 2), S56–S62.

Fein, S. B., & Roe, B. (1998). The effect of work status on initiation and duration of breastfeeding. *Am J Public Health, 88*, 1042–1046.

Ferris, A. M., Dalidowitz, C. K., Ingardia, C. M., et al. (1988). Lactation outcome in insulin-dependent diabetic women. *J Am Dietet Assn., 88*, 317–322.

Ferris, A. M., Neubauer, S. H., Bendel, R. R., et al. (1993). Perinatal lactation protocol and outcome in mothers with and without insulin-dependent diabetes mellitus. *Am J Clin Nutr., 58*, 43–48.

Festini, F., Ciuti, R., Taccetti, G., Repetto, T., Campana, S., & De Martino, M. (2006). Breastfeeding in a woman with cystic fibrosis undergoing antibiotic intravenous treatment. *J Matern Fetal Neonat Med., 19*, 375–376.

Field, T. (2008). Breastfeeding and antidepressants. *Infant Behavior and Development, 31*, 481-487.

Flegal, K. M., Carroll, M. D., Ogden, C. L., & Johnson, C. L. (2002). Prevalence and trends in obesity among U.S. adults, 1999–2000. *JAMA, 288*, 1723–1727.

Flint, D. J., Travers, M. T., Barber, M. C., et al. (2005). Diet-induced obesity impairs mammary development and lactogenesis in murine mammary gland. *Am J Physiol Endocrinol Metabol., 288*(6), E1179–E1187.

Fox-Bacon, C., et al. (1997). Maternal PKU and breastfeeding: Case report of identical twin mothers. *Clin Pediatr., 36*, 539–542.

Gabay, M. P. (2002). Galactagogues: Medications that induce lactation. *J Hum Lact., 18*, 274–279.

Gabbay, M., & Kelly, H. (2003). Use of metformin to increase breastmilk production in women with insulin resistance: A case series. *ABM News and Views, 9*, 20–21.

Gagne, M. G., Leff, E. W., & Jefferis, S. C. (1992). The breastfeeding experience of women with type 1 diabetes. *Health Care Wom Int., 13*, 249–260.

Gallas, P. R., Stolk, R. P, Bakker, K., Endert, E., & Wiersinga, W. M. (2002). Thyroid dysfunction during pregnancy and in the first postpartum year in women with diabetes mellitus type 1. *Eur J Endocrinol., 147*, 443–451.

Gatrell, C. J. (2007). Secrets and lies: Breastfeeding and professional paid work. *Soc Sci Med., 65*, 393–404.

Gatti, L. (2008). Maternal perceptions of insufficient milk supply in breastfeeding. *J Nurs Scholarship, 40*, 355–363.

Gielen, A. C., Faden, R. R., O'Campo, P., et al. (1991). Maternal employment during the early postpartum period: Effects on initiation and continuation of breastfeeding. *Pediatrics, 87*, 298–305.

Gilljam, M., Antoniou, M., Shin J., et al. (2000). Pregnancy in cystic fibrosis: Fetal and maternal outcome. *Chest, 118*, 85–91.

Glatstein, M. M., Djokanovic, N., Garcia-Bournissen, F., Finkelstein, Y., & Koren, G. (2009). Use of hypoglycemic drugs during lactation. *Can Fam Physician, 55*, 371–373.

Glueck, C. J., & Wang, P. (2007). Metformin before and during pregnancy and lactation in polycystic ovary syndrome. *Exp Op Drug Safety, 6*, 191–198.

Goodman, J. H. (2004a). Paternal postpartum depression, its relationship to maternal depression, and implications for family health. *J Adv Nurs., 45*, 26–35.

Goodman, J. H. (2004b). Postpartum depression beyond the early postpartum period. *J Obstet Gynecol Neonat Nurs., 33*, 410–420.

Granger, D. K., & Finlay, J. L. (1994). Nutritional vitamin B_{12} deficiency in a breastfed infant following maternal gastric bypass. *Pediatr Hematol Oncol., 11*, 311–318.

Groer, M. (2005). Relationships among naturalistic stress, mood, lactational status, and endocrine variables. *Biol Res Nurs., 7*, 106–117.

Groer, M. W., & Davis, M. W. (2006). Cytokines, infections, stress, and dysphoric moods in breastfeeders and formula feeders. *J Obstet Gynecol Neonat Nurs., 35*, 599–607.

Groer, M. W., Davis, M., Casey, K., Smith, K., Kramer, V., & Bukovsky, E. (2005). Immunity and infection: Differences between breastfeeders, formula feeders and controls. *Am J Reprod Immunol., 54,* 222–231.

Groer, M. W., & Morgan, K. (2007). Immune, health and endocrine characteristics of depressed postpartum mothers. *Psychoneuroendocrinology, 32,* 133–139.

Guendelman, S., Kosa, J. L., Pearl, M., Graham, S., Goodman, J., & Kharrazi, M. (2009). Juggling work and breastfeeding: Effects of maternity leave and occupational characteristics. *Pediatrics, 123,* e38–e46.

Gulick, E. E., & Halper, J. (2002). Influence of infant feeding method on postpartum relapse of mothers with multiple sclerosis. *International Journal of Multiple Sclerosis Care, 4,* 183–191.

Gulick, E. E., & Johnson, S. (2004). Infant health of mothers with multiple sclerosis. *West J Nurs Res., 26,* 632–649.

Gulick, E. E., & Kim, S. (2004). Postpartum emotional distress in mothers with multiple sclerosis. *J Obstet Gynecol Neonat Nurs., 33,* 729–738.

Gunderson, E. P. (2007). Breastfeeding after gestational diabetes pregnancy: Subsequent obesity and type 2 diabetes in women and their offspring. *Diabetes Care, 30*(Suppl 2), S161–S168.

Gunn, A. J., Gunn, T. R., Rabone, D. L., et al. (1996). Growth hormone increases breast milk volumes in mothers of preterm infants. *Pediatrics, 98,* 279–282.

Gupta, A. P., & Gupta, P. K. (1985). Metoclopramide as a lactogogue. *Clin Pediatr., 24,* 269–272.

Haider, S. J., Jacknowitz, A., & Schoeni,.R. F. (2003). Welfare work requirements and child well-being: Evidence from the effects on breastfeeding. *Demography, 40,* 479–497.

Halbert, L.-A. (1998). Breastfeeding in the woman with a compromised nervous system. *J Hum Lact., 14,* 327–331.

Hale, T. W. (2008). *Medications and mothers' milk.* Amarillo, TX: Pharmasoft Publishing.

Hale, T. W., & Berens, P. (2002). *Clinical therapy in breastfeeding patients.* Amarillo, TX: Pharmasoft Publishing.

Hale, T. W., Kristensen, J. H., Hackett, L. P., et al. (2002). Transfer of metformin into human milk. *Diabetologia, 45,* 1509–1514.

Hammond-McKibben, D., & Dosch, H.-M. (1997). Cow milk, BSA and IDDM: Can we settle the controversies? *Diabetes Care, 20,* 897–901.

Hampl, J. S., & Papa, D. J. (2001). Breastfeeding-related onset, flare, and relapse of rheumatoid arthritis. *Nutrition Reviews, 59,* 264–268.

Hamosh, M., Ellis, L. A., Pollock, D. R., Henderson, T. R., & Hamosh, P. (1996). Breastfeeding and the working mother: Effect of time and temperature of short-term storage on proteolysis, lipolysis, and bacterial growth in milk. *Pediatrics, 97,* 492–498.

Hapon, M., Simoncini, M., Via, G., et al. (2003). Effect of hypothyroidism on hormone profiles in virgin, pregnant and lactating rats, and on lactation. *Reproduction, 126,* 371–382.

Harris, B. (1999). Postpartum depression and thyroid antibody status. *Thyroid, 9,* 699–703.

Harris, B., Othman, S., Davies, J. A., et al. (1992). Association between postpartum thyroid dysfunction and thyroid antibodies and depression. *BMJ, 305,* 152–156.

Harrison, T., & Stuifbergen, A. (2002). Disability, social support, and concern for children: Depression in mothers with multiple sclerosis. *J Obstet Gynecol Neonat Nurs., 31,* 444–453.

Hart, R., Hickey, M., & Franks, S. (2004). Definitions, prevalence and symptoms of polycystic ovaries and polycystic ovary syndrome. *Best Pract Res Clin Obstet Gynaecol., 18,* 671–683.

Hartmann, P., & Cregan, M. (2001). Lactogenesis and the effects of insulin-dependent diabetes mellitus and prematurity. *J Nutr., 131,* 3016S–3020S.

Hasselmann, M. H., Werneck, G. L., & Silva, C. V. (2008). Symptoms of postpartum depression and early interruption of exclusive breastfeeding in the first two months of life. *Cad Saude Publica*, 24(Suppl 2), S341–S352.

Henderson, A. (2003a). Domperidone: Discovering new choices for lactating mothers. *AWHONN Lifelines, 7*, 55–60.

Henderson, J. (2003b). Impact of postnatal depression on breastfeeding duration. *Birth, 30*, 175–180.

Hendrick, V., Smith, L. M., Hwang, S., et al. (2003). Weight gain in breastfed infants of mothers taking antidepressant medications. *J Clin Psychiat., 64*, 401–412.

Henly, S., Anderson, C., Avery, M., et al. (1995). Anemia and insufficient milk in first-time mothers. *Birth, 22*, 87–92.

Hill, P. D. (1991). The enigma of insufficient milk supply. *MCN, 16*, 31–316.

Hill, P. D., & Aldag, J. (1991). Potential indicators of insufficient milk supply syndrome. *Res Nurs Health, 14*, 11–19.

Hill, P. D., Aldag, J. C., Chatterton, R. T., & Zinaman, M. (2005). Comparison of milk output between mothers of preterm and term infants: The first 6 weeks after birth. *J Hum Lact., 21*, 22–30.

Hill, P. D., Aldag, J. C., Zinaman, M., & Chatterton, R. T. (2007). Predictors of preterm infant feeding methods and perceived insufficient milk supply at week 12 postpartum. *J Hum Lact., 23*, 32–38.

Hill, P. D., Chatterton, R. T. Jr., & Aldag, J. C. (2003). Neuroendocrine responses to stressors in lactating and nonlactating mammals: A literature review. *Biol Res Nurs., 5*, 79–86.

Hill, P. D., & Humenick, S. S. (1989). Insufficient milk supply. *Journal of Nursing Scholarship, 21*, 145–148.

Hill, P. D., Wilhelm, P. A., Aldag, J. C., & Chatterton, R. T. Jr. (2004). Breast augmentation and lactation outcome: A case report. *MCN, 29*, 238–242.

Hillervik-Lindquist, C. (1991). Studies on perceived breast milk insufficiency. *Acta Paediatrica Scandinavica, 80*(Suppl 376), 6–27.

Hillervik-Lindquist, C., Hofvander, Y., & Sjolin, S. (1991). Studies on perceived breast milk insufficiency. *Acta Paediatrica Scandinavica, 80*, 297–303.

Hilson, J. A., Rasmussen, K. M., & Kjolhede, C. L. (1997). Maternal obesity and breastfeeding success in a local population of Caucasian women. *Am J Clin Nutr., 66*, 1371–1378.

Hilson, J. A., Rasmussen, K. M., & Kjolhede, C. L. (2004). High prepregnant body mass index is associated with poor lactation outcomes among white, rural women independent of psychosocial and demographic correlates. *J Hum Lact., 20*, 18–29.

Hobfoll, S. E., Ritter, C., Lavin, J., et al. (1995). Depression prevalence and incidence among inner-city pregnant and postpartum women. *Journal of Consulting and Clinical Psychology, 63*, 445–453.

Hofmeyr, G. J., & van Iddekinge, B. (1983). Domperidone and lactation. *Lancet, 1*(8325), 647.

Hofmeyr, G. J., van Iddekinge, B., & Blott, J. A. (1985). Domperidone: Secretion in breast milk and effect on puerperal prolactin levels. *Br J Obstet Gynaecol., 92*, 141–144.

Hoover, K. L., Barbalinardo, L. H., & Platia, M. P. (2002). Delayed lactogenesis II secondary to gestational ovarian theca lutein cysts in two normal singleton pregnancies. *J Hum Lact., 18*, 264–268.

Hopkinson, J., Schanler, R., Fraley, J., et al. (1992). Milk production by mothers of premature infants: Influence of cigarette smoking. *Pediatrics, 90*, 934–938.

Horowitz, J. A., & Goodman, J. H. (2005). Identifying and treating postpartum depression. *J Obstet Gynecol Neonat Nurs., 34*, 264–273.

Huang, Y. Y., Lee, J. T., Huang, C. M., Gau, M. L. (2009). Factors related to maternal perception of milk supply while in the hospital. *J Nurs Res., 17*, 179–188.

Hughes, V., & Owen, J. (1993). Is breastfeeding possible after breast surgery? *MCN, 18*, 213–217.

Hummel, S., Winkler, C., Schoen, S., et al. (2007). Breastfeeding habits in families with type 1 diabetes. *Diabetes and Medicine, 24*, 671–676.

Humphrey, S. (2003). *The nursing mother's herbal*. Minneapolis, MN: Fairview Press.

Hurst, N. M., Valentine, C. J., Renfro, L., et al. (1997). Skin-to-skin holding in the neonatal intensive care unit influences maternal milk volume. *J Perinatol., 17*, 213.

Hutt, P. (1989). The effect of diabetes on lactation. *Breastfeeding Review, 14*, 21–25.

Isbister, G. K., Dawson, A., Whyte, I. M., et al. (2001). Neonatal paroxetine withdrawal syndrome or actually serotonin syndrome? *Arch Dis Child. Fetal and Neonatal Edition, 85*, F147–F148.

Isik, A. Z., Gulekli, B., Zorlu, C. G., et al. (1997). Endocrinological and clinical analysis of hyperprolactinemic patients with and without ultrasonically diagnosed polycystic ovary syndrome. *Gynecol Obstet Invest., 43*, 183–185.

Ito, S., Moretti, M., Liau, M., & Koren, G. (1995). Initiation and duration of breastfeeding in women receiving antiepileptics. *Am J Obstet Gynecol., 173*, 881–886.

Jacobson, P. M. (1998). Multiple sclerosis: A supportive approach for breastfeeding. *Mother and Baby Journal, 3*, 13–17.

Jaigobin, C., & Silver, F. L. (2000). Stroke and pregnancy. *Stroke, 31*, 2948–2951.

Jara, L. J., Lavelle, C., & Espinoza, L. R. (1992). Does prolactin have a role in the pathogenesis of systemic lupus erythematosus? *J Rheumatol., 19*, 1333.

Jevitt, C., Hernandez, I., & Groer, M. (2007). Lactation complicated by overweight and obesity: Supporting the mother and newborn. *Journal of Midwifery and Womens Health, 52*, 606–613.

Johnston, M. L., & Esposito, N. (2007). Barriers and facilitators for breastfeeding among working women in the United States. *J Obstet Gynecol Neonat Nurs., 36*, 9–20.

Jones, N. A., McFall, B. A., & Diego, M. A. (2004). Patterns of brain electrical activity in infants of depressed mothers who breastfeed and bottle feed: The mediating role of infant temperament. *Biological Psychology, 67*, 103–124.

Jovanovic, L. (Ed.). (2000). *Medical management of pregnancy complicated by diabetes* (3rd ed.). Alexandria, VA: American Diabetes Association.

Kaiser Family Foundation. Overweight and Obesity Rates for Adults by Sex (2008). Retrieved September 26, 2009, from www.statehealthfacts.kff.org/comparebar.jsp?ind=90&cat=2

Kamikawa, A., Ichii, O., Yamaji, D., et al. (2009). Diet-induced obesity disrupts ductal development in the mammary glands of nonpregnant mice. *Developmental Dynamics, 238*, 1092–1099.

Karges, W., Hammond-McKibben, D., Cheung, R. K., et al. (1997). Immunological aspects of nutritional diabetes prevention in NOD mice: A pilot study for the cow's milk based IDDM prevention trial. *Diabetes, 46*, 557–564.

Karlson, E. W., Mandl, L. A., Hankinson, S. E., & Grodstein, F. (2004). Do breastfeeding and other reproductive factors influence future risk of rheumatoid arthritis? Results from the Nurses' Health Study. *Arthritis and Rheumatism, 50*, 3458–3467.

Kauppila, A., Arvela, P., Koivisto, M., et al. (1983). Metoclopramide and breastfeeding: Transfer into milk and the newborn. *Eur J Clin Pharmacol., 25*, 819–823.

Kendal-Tackett, K. (2008). *Non-pharmacologic treatments for depression in new mothers*. Amarillo, TX: Hale Publishing.

Kennedy, K. I., Short, R. V., & Tully, M. R. (1997). Premature introduction of progestin-only contraceptive methods during lactation. *Contraception, 55*, 347–350.

Kessler, R. C., McGonagle, K. A., Zhao, S., et al. (1994). Lifetime and 12 month prevalence of DSM-IVR psychiatric disorders in the United States: Results from the National Comorbidity Survey. *Archives of General Psychiatry, 51*, 8–19.

Kidner, M. C., & Flanders-Stepans, M. B. (2004). A model for the HELLP syndrome: The maternal experience. *J Obstet Gynecol Neonat Nurs., 33*, 44–53.

Kimbro, R. T. (2006). On-the-job moms: Work and breastfeeding initiation and duration for a sample of low-income women. *Matern Child Health J., 10,* 19–26.

Kittner, S., & Adams, R. (1996). Stroke in children and young adults. *Curr Op Neurol., 9,* 53–56.

Kittner, S. J., Stern, B. J., Feeser, B. R., et al. (1996). Pregnancy and the risk of stroke. *N Eng J Med., 335,* 768–774.

Kjos, S. L., Henry, O., Lee, R. M., et al. (1993). The effect of lactation on glucose and lipid metabolism in women with recent gestational diabetes. *Obstet Gynecol., 82,* 451–455.

Klier, C. M., Schaefer, M. R., Schmid-Siegel, B., et al. (2002). St. John's wort (*Hypericum perforatum*): Is it safe during breastfeeding? *Pharmacopsychiatry, 35,* 29–30.

Knip, M., & Akerblom, H. K. (1998). IDDM prevention trials in progress: A critical assessment. *J Pediat Endocrinol Metabol., 11,* 371.

Koch, S., Titze, K., Zimmermann, R. B., et al. (1999). Long-term neuropsychological consequences of maternal epilepsy and anticonvulsant treatment during pregnancy for school age children and adolescents. *Epilepsia, 40,* 1237–1243.

Kroencke, D. C., & Denney, D. R. (1999). Stress and coping in multiple sclerosis: Exacerbation, remission and chronic subgroups. *Multiple Sclerosis, 5,* 89–93.

Laine, K., Heikkinen, T., Ekblad, U., & Kero, P. (2003). Effects of exposure to selective serotonin reuptake inhibitors during pregnancy on serotonergic symptoms in newborns and cord blood monoamine and prolactin concentrations. *Arch Gen Psychiatr., 60,* 720–726.

Langer-Gould, A., Huang, S. M, Gupta, R., et al. (2009). Exclusive breastfeeding and the risk of postpartum relapses in women with multiple sclerosis. *Arch Neurol., 66*(8), 958–963.

Lankarani-Fard, A., Kritz-Silverterin, D., Barrett-Connor, E., & Goodman-Gruen, D. (2001). Cumulative duration of breastfeeding influences cortisol levels in postmenopausal women. *Journal of Womens Health and Gender-Based Medicine, 10,* 681–687.

Lau, C., & Hurst, N. (1999). Oral feeding in infants. *Curr Probl Pediatr., 29,* 101.

Lawrence, R. A., & Lawrence, R. M. (2005). *Breastfeeding: A guide for the medical profession* (6th ed.). Philadelphia: Elsevier Mosby.

Lee, A., Moretti, M. E., Collantes, A., et al. (2000). Choice of breastfeeding and physicians' advice: A cohort study of women receiving propylthiouracil. *Pediatrics, 106,* 27–30.

Lee, P. J., Ridout, D., Walter, J. H., & Cockburn, F. (2005). Maternal phenylketonuria: Report from the United Kingdom Registry 1978–97. *Arch Dis Child., 90,* 143–146.

Lester, B. M., Cucca, J., Andreozzi, L., et al. (1993). Possible association between fluoxetine hydrochloride and colic in an infant. *J Am Acad Child Adolesc Psychiatr., 32,* 1253–1255.

Li, R., Fein, S. B., Chen, J., & Grummer-Strawn, L. M. (2008). Why mothers stop breastfeeding: Mothers' self-reported reasons for stopping during the first year. *Pediatrics, 122*(Suppl 2), S69–S76.

Li, R., Jewell, S., & Grummer-Strawn, L. (2003). Maternal obesity and breastfeeding practices. *Am J Clin Nutr., 77,* 931–936.

Liao, K. P., Alfredsson, L., & Karlson, E. W. (2009). Environmental influences on risk for rheumatoid arthritis. *Curr Op Rheumatol., 21,* 279–283.

Lindberg, L. D. (1996). Trends in the relationship between breastfeeding and postpartum employment in the United States. *Social Biology, 43,* 191–202.

Livingstone, V. (1996). Too much of a good thing: Maternal and infant hyperlactation syndromes. *Can Fam Physician, 42,* 89–99.

Lorenzi, A. R., & Ford, H. L. (2002). Multiple sclerosis and pregnancy. *Postgraduate Medical Journal, 78,* 460–464.

Low Dog, T., & Micozzi, M. S. (2005). *Women's health in complementary and integrative medicine: A clinical guide.* St. Louis, MO: Elsevier.

Luder, E., Kaltan, M., Tanzer-Torres, G., et al. (1990). Current recommendations for breastfeeding in cystic fibrosis centers. *Am J Dis Child.*, *144*, 1153.

Mack, W. J., Preston-Martin, S., Bernstein, L., et al. (1999). Reproductive and hormonal risk factors for thyroid cancer in Los Angeles County females. *Cancer Epidemiology, Biomarkers and Prevention, 8*, 991–997.

MacNeill, S., Dodds, L., Hamilton, D. C., et al. (2001). Rates and risk factors for recurrence of gestational diabetes. *Diabetes Care, 24*, 659–662.

Maes, M., Editorial Board. (2001). Psychological stress and the inflammatory response system. *Clin Sci (Lond). 101*, 193–194

Maillot, F., Cook, P., Lilburn, M., & Lee, P. J. (2007). A practical approach to maternal phenylketonuria management. *Journal of Inherited Metabolic Disease, 30*, 198–201.

Maillot, F., Lilburn, M., Baudin, J., Morley, D. W., & Lee, P. J. (2008). Factors influencing outcomes in the offspring of mothers with phenylketonuria during pregnancy: The importance of variation in maternal blood phenylalanine. *Am J Clin Nutr., 88*, 700–705.

Maitra, R., & Menkes, D. B. (1996). Psychotropic drugs and lactation. *N Z Med J., 109*, 217–218.

Mak, C. W., Chou, C. K., Chen, S. Y., et al. (2003). Diabetic mastopathy. *Br J Radiol., 76*, 192–194.

Manios, Y., Grammatikaki, E., Kondaki, K., Ioannou, E., Anastasiadou, A., & Birbilis, M. (2009). The effect of maternal obesity on initiation and duration of breastfeeding in Greece: The GENESIS study. *Public Health and Nutrition, 12*, 517–524.

Marasco, L. (2006). The impact of thyroid dysfunction on lactation. *Breastfeeding Abstracts, 25*, 9–12.

Marasco, L., Marmet, C., & Shell, E. (2000). Polycystic ovary syndrome: A connection to insufficient milk supply? *J Hum Lact., 16*, 143–148.

Martin Cookson, D. (1992). La Leche League and the mother who is blind. *Leaven, 5*, 67–68.

Matalon, R., Michals, K., & Gleason, L. (1986). PKU: Strategies for dietary treatment and monitoring compliance. *Ann N Y Acad Sci., 477*, 223.

McCarter-Spaulding, D. E., & Kearney, M. H. (2001). Parenting self-efficacy and perception of insufficient breast milk. *J Obstet Gynecol Neonat Nurs., 30*, 515–522.

McCook, J. G., Reame, N. E., & Thatcher, S. S. (2005). Health-related quality of life issues in women with polycystic ovary syndrome. *J Obstet Gynecol Neonat Nurs., 34*, 12–20.

McGovern, P., Dowd, B., Gjerdingen, D., et al. (2006). Postpartum health of employed mothers 5 weeks after childbirth. *Ann Fam Med., 4*, 159–167.

Meador, K. J., Baker, G. A., Browning, N., Clayton-Smith, J., Combs-Cantrell, D. T., Cohen, M., et al. (2009). Cognitive function at 3 years of age after fetal exposure to antiepileptic drugs. *N Engl J Med., 360*, 1597–1605.

Meador K., et al. (2008). Effects of breastfeeding in women taking antiepileptic drugs on their children's cognitive outcomes. AAN meeting 2008; Abstract S45.001. Retrieved September 26, 2009, from www.medpagetoday.com/MeetingCoverage/AAN/9183

Meek, J. Y. (2001). Breastfeeding in the workplace. *Pediatr Clin N Am., 48*, 461–474.

Metcalfe, M. A., & Baum, J. D. (1992). Family characteristics and insulin dependent diabetes. *Arch Dis Child., 67*, 731.

Metzger, B. E., Buchanan, T. A., Coustan, D. R., et al. (2007). Summary and recommendations of the Fifth International Workshop-Conference on Gestational Diabetes Mellitus. *Diabetes Care, 30*(Suppl 2), S251–S260.

Michael, A., & Mayer, C. (2000). Fluoxetine-induced anesthesia of vagina and nipples. *Br J Pschiatr., 176*, 299.

Michel, S. H., & Mueller, D. H. (1994). Impact of lactation on women with cystic fibrosis and their infants: A review of five cases. *J Am Dietet Assn., 94*, 159–165.

Milligan, R. A., Flenniken, P. M., & Pugh, L. C. (1996). Positioning intervention to minimize fatigue in breastfeeding women. *Appl Nurs Res., 9*, 67–70.

Milsom, S. R., Breier, B. H., Gallaher, B. W., et al. (1992). Growth hormone stimulates galactopoiesis in healthy lactating women. *Acta Endocrinologica, 127,* 337–343.

Milsom, S. R., Rabone, D. L., Gunn, A. J., & Gluckman, P. D. (1998). Potential role for growth hormone in human lactation insufficiency. *Hormone Research, 50,* 147–150.

Miyake, A., Tahara, M., Koike, K., Tanizawa O., et al. (1989). Decrease in neonatal suckled milk volume in diabetic women. *Eur J Gynecol Reprod Biol., 33,* 49–53.

Mok, C. C., & Wong, R. W. S. (2001). Pregnancy in systemic lupus erythematosus. *Postgraduate Medical Journal, 77,* 157–165.

Mok, C. C., Wong, R. W. S., & Lau, C. S. (1998). Systemic lupus erythematosus exacerbated by breast-feeding. *Lupus, 7,* 569–570.

Mok, E., Multon, C., Piguel, L., et al. (2008). Decreased full breastfeeding, altered practices, perceptions, and infant weight change of prepregnant obese women: A need for extra support. *Pediatrics, 121,* e1319–e1324.

Moore, S. J., Turnpenny, P., Quinn, A., et al. (2000). A clinical study of 57 children with fetal anticonvulsant syndromes. *Journal of Medical Genetics, 37,* 489–497.

Morreale, D. E., Obregon, M. J., & Escobar, D. R. (2000). Is neuropsychological development related to maternal hypothyroidism or to maternal hypothroxinemia? *J Clin Endocrinol Metabol, 85,* 3975–3987.

Morton, J. A. (1992). Ineffective suckling: A possible consequence of obstructive positioning. *J Hum Lact., 8,* 83–85.

Moses-Kolko, E. L., Bogen, D., Perel, J., et al. (2005). Neonatal signs after late in utero exposure to serotonin reuptake inhibitors: Literature review and implications for clinical applications. *JAMA, 293,* 2372–2383.

Muller, A. F., Drexhage, H. A., & Berghout, A. (2001). Postpartum thyroiditis and autoimmune thyroiditis in women of childbearing age: Recent insights and consequences for antenatal and postnatal care. *Endocrine Reviews, 22,* 605–630.

Murtaugh, M. A., Ferris, A. M., Capacchione, C. M., & Reece, E. A. (1998). Energy intake and glycemia in lactating women with type 1 diabetes. *J Am Dietet Assn., 98,* 642–648.

National Children's Study. (2003, December 16). Use of herbal products in pregnancy, breastfeeding, and childhood workshop. Retrieved June 1, 2009, from www.nationalchildrensstudy.gov/research/workshops/Pages/herbal_122003.aspx

Neifert, M., DeMarzo, S., Seacat J., et al. (1990). The influence of breast surgery, breast appearance, and pregnancy-induced breast changes on lactation sufficiency as measured by infant weight gain. *Birth, 17,* 31–38.

Neifert, M. R., Seacat, J. M., & Jobe, W. E. (1985). Lactation failure due to insufficient glandular development of the breast. *Pediatrics, 76,* 823–828.

Nelson, L. M., Franklin, G. M., & Jones, M. C. (1988). Risk of multiple sclerosis exacerbation during pregnancy and breastfeeding. *JAMA, 259,* 3441–3443.

Neubauer, S. H., Ferris, A. M., Chase, C. G., et al. (1993). Delayed lactogenesis in women with and without insulin-dependent diabetes mellitus. *Am J Clin Nutr., 58,* 54–60.

Newman, J. (1998, January). Domperidone. Retrieved September 26, 2009, from http://bflrc.com/newman/lbreastfeeding/domperid.htm

Newman, J., & Pittman, T. (2000). *The ultimate breastfeeding book of answers.* Roseville, CA: Prima Publishing.

Nichols, M. R., & Roux, G. M. (2004). Maternal perspectives on postpartum return to the workplace. *J Obstet Gynecol Neonat Nurs., 33,* 463–471.

Nigro, G., Campea, L., DeNovellis, A., et al. (1985). Breastfeeding and insulin-dependent diabetes mellitus. *Lancet, 1,* 467.

Nordeng, H., Lindemann, R., Perminov, K. V., & Reikvam, A. (2001). Neonatal withdrawal syndrome after in utero exposure to selective serotonin reuptake inhibitors. *Acta Paediatrica, 90,* 288–291.

Norman, R., & Clark, A. (1998). Obesity and reproductive disorders: A review. *Reproduction, Fertility, and Development, 10,* 55–63.

Norris, J. M., Barriga, K., Klingensmith, G., et al. (2003). Timing of initial cereal exposure in infancy and risk of islet autoimmunity. *JAMA, 290,* 1713–1720.

Nuclear Regulatory Commission. (1996). Activities of radiopharmaceuticals that require instructions and records when administered to patients who are breastfeeding an infant or child. NRC Regulatory Guide 8.39, 1996. Retrieved September 15, 2005, from www.nrc.gov/NRC/RG/08/08-039.htm and from http://neonatal.ama.ttuhsc.edu/lact/radioactive.html

Oberlander, T. F., Misri, S., Fitzgerald, C. E., et al. (2004). Pharmacologic factors associated with transient neonatal symptoms following prenatal psychotropic medication exposure. *J Clin Psychiatr., 65,* 230–237.

Oddy, W. H., Landsborough, L., Kendall, G. E., Henderson, S., & Downie, J. (2006). The association of maternal overweight and obesity with breastfeeding duration. *J Pediatr., 149,* 185–191.

Ogden, C. L., Carroll, M. D., Curtin, L. R., McDowell, M. A., Tabak, C. J., & Flegal, K. M. (2006). Prevalence of overweight and obesity in the United States, 1999–2004. *JAMA, 295,* 1549–1555.

O'Hara, M. W. (1986). Social support, life events, and depression during pregnancy and the puerperium. *Arch Gen Psychiatr., 43,* 569–573.

O'Hara, M. W., & Swain, A. M. (1996). Rates and risk of postpartum depression: A meta-analysis. *Int Rev Psychiatr., 8,* 37–54.

Ortiz, J., McGilligan, K., & Kelly, P. (2004). Duration of breast milk expression among working mothers enrolled in an employer-sponsored lactation program. *Pediatr Nurs., 30,* 111–119.

Ost, L., Wettrell, G., Bjorkhem, I., et al. (1985). Prednisone excretion in human milk. *J Pediatr., 106,* 1008–1011.

Ostrom, K. M., & Ferris, A. M. (1993). Prolactin concentrations in serum and milk of mothers with and without insulin-dependent diabetes mellitus. *Am J Clin Nutr., 58,* 49–53.

Page-Wilson, G., Smith, P. C., & Welt, C. K. (2007). Short-term prolactin administration causes express-ible galactorrhea but does not affect bone turnover: Pilot data for a new lactation agent. *International Breastfeeding Journal, 2,* 10.

Parker, E. M., O'Sullivan, B. P., Shea, J. C., et al. (2004). Survey of breastfeeding practices and outcomes in the cystic fibrosis population. *Pediatr Pulmonol., 37,* 362–367.

Pena, K. S., & Rosenfeld, J. A. (2001). Evaluation and treatment of galactorrhea. *Am Fam Physician, 63,* 1763–1770,1775.

Peppard, H. R., Marfori, J., Iuorno, M. J., & Nestler, J. E. (2001). Prevalence of polycystic ovary syndrome among premenopausal women with type 2 diabetes. *Diabetes Care, 24,* 1050–1052.

Pereira, K., & Brown, A. (2008). Postpartum thyroiditis: Not just a worn out mom. *Journal of Nurse Practitioner, 4,* 175–182.

Perez-Bravo, F., Carrasco, E., Gutierrez-Lopez, M. D., et al. (1996). Genetic predisposition and environ-mental factors leading to the development of insulin-dependent diabetes mellitus in Chilean chil-dren. *Journal of Molecular Medicine, 74,* 105–109.

Petraglia, F., De Leo, V., Sardelli, S., et al. (1985). Domperidone in defective and insufficient lactation. *Eur J Obstet Gynecol Reprod Biol., 19,* 281–287.

Pikwer, M., Bergstrom, U., Nilsson, J. A., Jacobsson, L., Berglund, G., & Turesson, C. (2009). Breastfeeding, but not use of oral contraceptives, is associated with a reduced risk of rheumatoid arthritis. *Ann Rheumat Dis., 68,* 526–530.

Pippins, J. R., Brawarsky, P., Jackson, R. A., Fuentes-Afflick, E., & Haas, J. S. (2006). Association of breast-feeding with maternal depressive symptoms. *J Womens Health, 15*(6), 754–762.

Pisacane, A., Impagliazzo, N, Russon, M., et al. (1994). Breastfeeding and multiple sclerosis. *BMJ, 308,* 1411–1412.

Polycystic Ovary Syndrome Writing Committee. (2005). American Association of Clinical Endocrinologists position statement on metabolic and cardiovascular consequences of polycystic ovary syndrome. *Endocrine Practice, 11,* 126–134.

Poobalan, A. S., Aucott, L. S., Gurung, T., Smith, W. C., & Bhattacharya, S. (2009). Obesity as an independent risk factor for elective and emergency cesarean delivery in nulliparous women—Systematic review and meta-analysis of cohort studies. *Obesity Reviews, 10,* 28–35.

Pop, V. J., Kuijpens, J. L., van Barr, A., et al. (1999). Low maternal free thyroxine concentrations during early pregnancy are associated with impaired psychomotor development in infancy. *Clin Endocrinol., 50,* 149–155.

Powers, N. G. (1999). Slow weight gain and low milk supply in the breastfeeding dyad. *Clin Perinatol., 26,* 399–430.

Prince, M. (2002, April 22). More employers are offering lactation rooms for new moms. *Business Insurance,* 6.

Pschirrer, E. R. (2004). Seizure disorders in pregnancy. *Obstet Gynecol Clin N Am., 31,* 373–384.

Pugliatti, M., Sotgiu, S., & Rosati, G. (2002). The worldwide prevalence of multiple sclerosis. *Clin Neurol Neurosurg., 104,* 182–191.

Purnell, H. (2001). Phenylketonuria and maternal phenylketonuria. *Breastfeeding Rev., 9,* 19–21.

Rasmussen, K. M., Hilson, J. A., & Kjolhede, C. L. (2001). Obesity may impair lactogenesis II. *J Nutr., 131,* 3009S–3011S.

Rasmussen, K. M., & Kjolhede, C. L. (2004). Prepregnant overweight and obesity diminish the prolactin response to suckling in the first week postpartum. *Pediatrics, 113,* e465–e471.

Rasmussen, K. M., Lee, V. E., Ledkovsky, T. B., & Kjolhede, C. L. (2006). A description of lactation counseling practices that are used with obese mothers. *J Hum Lact., 22,* 322–327.

Reece, E. A., & Homko, C. J. (1994). Infant of the diabetic mother. *Sem Perinatol., 18,* 459–469.

Renfrew, M. F., Lang, S., & Woolridge, M. (2000). Oxytocin for promoting successful lactation (Cochrane Review). In *The Cochrane Library* (Issue 3). Oxford, UK: Update Software.

Riva, E., Agostini, C., Biasucci, G., et al. (1996). Early breastfeeding is linked to higher intelligence quotient scores in dietary treated phenylketonuric children. *Acta Paediatrica, 85,* 56–58.

Riviello, C., Mello, G., & Jovanovic, L. G. (2009). Breastfeeding and the basal insulin requirement in type 1 diabetic women. *Endocr Pract., 15,* 187–193.

Roe, B., Whittington, L. A., Fein, S. B., & Teisl, M. F. (1999). Is there competition between breastfeeding and maternal employment? *Demography, 36,* 157–171.

Rojjanasrirat, W. (2004). Working women's breastfeeding experiences. *MCN Am J Matern Child Nurs., 29,* 222–227.

Rowe-Murray, H. J., & Fisher, J. R. (2002). Baby friendly hospital practices: Cesarean section is a persistent barrier to early initiation of breastfeeding. *Birth, 29,* 124–131.

Ruis, H., Rolland, R., Doesburg, W., et al. (1981). Oxytocin enhances onset of lactation among mothers delivering prematurely. *BMJ, 283,* 340–342.

Rutishauser, I. H. E., & Carlin, J. B. (1992). Body mass index and duration of breastfeeding: A survival analysis during the first six months of life. *J Epidemiol Community Health, 46,* 559–565.

Sacco, L. M., Caulfield, L. E., Gittelsohn, J., & Martinez, H. (2006). The conceptualization of perceived insufficient milk among Mexican mothers. *J Hum Lact., 22,* 277–286.

Schaefer, K. M. (2004). Breastfeeding in chronic illness: The voices of women with fibromyalgia. *MCN, 29,* 248–253.

Schaefer-Graf, U. M., Buchanan, T. A., Xiang, A. H., Peters, R. K., & Kjos, S. L. (2002). Clinical predictors for a high risk for the development of diabetes mellitus in the early puerperium in women with recent gestational diabetes mellitus. *Am J Obstet Gynecol., 186,* 751–756.

Schoen, S., Sichert-Hellert, W., Hummel, S., Ziegler, A. G., & Kersting, M. (2008). Breastfeeding duration in families with type 1 diabetes compared to non-affected families: Results from BABYDIAB and DONALD studies in Germany. *Breast Medicine, 3,* 171–165.

Segura-Millan, S., Dewey, K. G., & Perez-Escamilla, R. (1994). Factors associated with perceived insufficient milk in a low-income urban population in Mexico. *J Nutr., 124,* 202–212.

Seijts, G. H. (2002). Milking the organization? The effect of breastfeeding accommodation on perceived fairness and organizational attractiveness. *Journal of Business Ethics, 40,* 1–13.

Seijts, G. H. (2004). Coworker perceptions of outcome fairness of breastfeeding accommodation in the workplace. *Employee Responsibility and Rights Journal, 16,* 149–166.

Sert, M., Tetiker, T., Kirim, S., & Kocak, M. (2003). Clinical report of 28 patients with Sheehan's syndrome. *Endocrine Journal, 50,* 297–301.

Shakespeare, J., Blake, F., & Garcia, J. (2004). Breastfeeding difficulties experienced by women taking part in a qualitative interview study of postnatal depression. *Midwifery, 20,* 251–260.

Shames, K. H., & Youngkin, E. Q. (2002). The thyroid dance . . . nursing approaches to autoimmune low thyroid. *AWHONN Lifelines, 6,* 53–59.

Sharma, V., & Corpse, C. S. (2008). Case study revisiting the association between breastfeeding and postpartum depression. *J Hum Lact., 24,* 77–79.

Shelton, R. C., et al. (2001). Effectiveness of St. John's wort in major depression: A randomized controlled trial. *JAMA, 285,* 1978–1986.

Shiffman, M. L., Seale, T. W., Flux, M., et al. (1989). Breast milk composition in women with cystic fibrosis: Report of two cases and a review of the literature. *Am J Clin Nutr., 49,* 612–617.

Sichel, D. A., & Driscoll, J. W. (1999). *Women's moods: What every woman must know about the hormones, the brain, and emotional health.* New York: William Morrow.

Siebenaler, N. (2002). Maternal physical impairments. In M. Walker (Ed.), *Core curriculum for lactation consultant practice.* Sudbury, MA: Jones and Bartlett.

Silman, A. J., & Pearson, J. E. (2002). Epidemiology and genetics of rheumatoid arthritis. *Arthritis Research, 9*(Suppl 3), S265–S272.

Simmons, D., Conroy, C., & Thompson, C. F. (2005). In-hospital breastfeeding rates among women with gestational diabetes and pregestational type 2 diabetes in South Auckland. *Diabetes Medicine, 22,* 177–181.

Sipski, M. L. (1991). The impact of spinal cord injury on female sexuality, menstruation, and pregnancy: A review of the literature. *Journal of American Paraplegia Society, 14,* 122–126.

Sirota, L., Ferrera, M., Lerer, N., et al. (1992). Beta glucuronidase and hyperbilirubinemia in breastfed infants of diabetic mothers. *Arch Dis Child., 67,* 120.

Slusser, W. M., Lange, L., Dickson, V., et al. (2004). Breast milk expression in the workplace: A look at frequency and time. *J Hum Lact., 20,* 164–169.

Smeltzer, S. (1994). The concerns of pregnant women with multiple sclerosis. *Quality of Health Research, 4,* 480–502.

Smillie, C. M., Campbell, S. H., & Iwinski, S. (2005). Hyperlactation: How left-brained "rules" for breastfeeding can wreak havoc with a natural process. *Newborn Infant Nurs Rev., 5,* 49–58.

Stein, M. (2002). Failure to thrive in a four-month-old nursing infant. *Dev Behav Pediatrics, 23,* S69–S73.

Stevens, K. V., & Janke, J. (2003). Breastfeeding experiences of active duty military women. *Military Medicine, 168,* 380–384.

Stewart-Glenn, J. (2008). Knowledge, perceptions, and attitudes of managers, coworkers, and employed breastfeeding mothers. *AAOHN Journal, 56,* 423-429.

Stiskal, J. A., Kulin, N., Koren, G., et al. (2001). Neonatal paroxetine withdrawal syndrome. *Arch Dis Child. Fetal and Neonatal Edition, 84,* F134–F135.

Strathearn, L., Mamun, A. A., Najman, J. M., & O'Callaghan, M. J. (2009). Does breastfeeding protect against substantiated child abuse and neglect? A 15-year cohort study. *Pediatrics, 123,* 483–493.

Talbott, E. O., Zborowski, J. V., & Boudreaux, M. Y. (2004). Do women with polycystic ovary syndrome have an increased risk of cardiovascular disease? Review of the evidence. *Minerva Ginecologica, 56,* 27–39.

Taylor, J. S., Kacmar, J. E., Nothnagle, M., & Lawrence, R. A. (2005). A systematic review of the literature associating breastfeeding with type 2 diabetes and gestational diabetes. *J Am Coll Nutr., 24,* 320–326.

Thompson, N. M. (1996). Relactation in a newborn intensive care setting. *J Hum Lact., 12,* 233–235.

Thompson, P., & Bell, P. (1997). Breastfeeding in the workplace: How to succeed. *Issues in Comprehensive Pediatric Nursing, 20,* 1–9.

Thomson, V. M. (1995). Breastfeeding and mothering one-handed. *J Hum Lact.,* 1995 *11,* 211–215.

Thrift, T. A., Bernal, A., Lewis, A. L., et al. (1999). Effects of induced hypothyroidism on weight gains, lactation and reproductive performance of primiparous Brahman cows. *Journal of Animal Science, 77,* 1844–1850.

Troutman, B., & Cutrona, C. (1990). Nonpsychotic postpartum depression among adolescent mothers. *J Ab Psychol., 99,* 69–78.

Tyler, K. (1999). Got milk? *HR Magazine, 44*(3), 68–73.

Tyson, J. E., Perez, A., & Zanartu, J. (1976). Human lactational response to oral thyrotropin releasing hormone. *J Clin Endocrinol Metab., 43,* 760–768.

U.S. Bureau of Labor Statistics. (2009, May). Employment characteristics of families in 2008. News release USDL 09-0568. Retrieved September 26, 2009, from www.bls.gov/news.release/pdf/famee.pdf

van Veldhuizen-Staas, C. G. A. (2007). Overabundant milk supply: An alternative way to intervene by full drainage and block feeding. *Int Breastfeeding J., 2,* 11.

Verronen, P. (1982). Breastfeeding: Reasons for giving up and transient lactational crises. *Acta Paediatrica Scandinavica, 71,* 447–450.

Waisbren, S. E., Hanley, W., Levy, H. L., et al. (2000). Outcome at age 4 years in offspring of women with maternal phenylketonuria: The Maternal PKU Collaborative Study. *JAMA, 283,* 756–762.

Wan, E. W., Davey, K., Page-Sharp, M., Hartmann, P. E., Simmer, K., & Ilett, K. F. (2008). Dose-effect study of domperidone as a galactagogue in preterm mothers with insufficient milk supply, and its transfer into milk. *Br J Clin Pharmacol., 66,* 283–289.

Wardinsky, T. D., Montes, R. G., Friederich, R. L., et al. (1995). Vitamin B_{12} deficiency associated with low breast milk vitamin B_{12} concentration in an infant following maternal gastric bypass surgery. *Arch Pediatr Adolesc Med., 149,* 1281–1284.

Webster, J., Moore, K., & McMullan, A. (1995). Breastfeeding outcomes for women with insulin dependent diabetes. *J Hum Lact., 11,* 195–200.

Wei, L., Wang, H., Han, Y., & Li, C. (2008). Clinical observation on the effects of electroacupuncture at Shaoze (SI 1) in 46 cases of postpartum insufficient lactation. *Journal of Traditional Chinese Medicine, 28,* 168–172.

Weiss, R. F. (2001). *Weiss's herbal medicine* (classic ed.). New York: Thieme.

Whichelow, M. J.,& Doddridge, M. C. (1983). Lactation in diabetic mothers. *BMJ, 287,* 649–650.

Williams, J., Auerbach, K., & Jacobi, A. (1989). Lateral epicondylitis (tennis elbow) in breastfeeding mothers. *Clin Pediatr., 28,* 42–43.

Willis, C., & Livingstone, V. (1995). Infant insufficient milk syndrome associated with maternal post-partum hemorrhage. *J Hum Lact., 11,* 123–126.

Wittig, S. L., & Spatz, D. L. (2008). Induced lactation: Gaining a better understanding. *MCN, 33,* 76–81.

Woolridge, M. W., & Fischer, C. (1988). Overfeeding and symptoms of lactose malabsorption in the breastfed baby: A possible artifact of feeding management? *Lancet, 2,* 382–384.

World Health Organization. (1998). Relactation: Review of experience and recommendations for practice. Geneva. Retrieved June 3, 2009, from http://whqlibdoc.who.int/hq/1998/WHO_CHS_CAH_98.14.pdf

Worthington, J., Jones, R., Crawford, M., et al. (1994). Pregnancy and multiple sclerosis—A three year prospective study. *J Neurol., 241,* 228–233.

Yerby, M. S., Kaplan, P., & Tran, T. (2004). Risks and management of pregnancy in women with epilepsy. *Cleveland Clinic Journal of Medicine, 71*(Suppl 2), S25–S37.

Yokoyama, Y., Ueda, T., Irahara, M., et al. (1994). Releases of oxytocin and prolactin during breast massage and suckling in puerperal women. *Eur J Obstet Gynecol Reprod Biol., 53,* 17.

Zanton, G. I., & Heinrichs, A. J. (2005). Meta-analysis to assess effect of prepubertal average daily gain of Holstein heifers on first-lactation production. *J Dairy Sci., 88,* 3860–3867.

Zhao, Y., & Guo, H. (2006). The therapeutic effects of acupuncture in 30 cases of postpartum hypogalactia. *Journal of Traditional Chinese Medicine, 26,* 29–30.

Ziegler, A. G., Schmid, S., Huber, D., et al. (2003). Early infant feeding and risk of developing type 1 associated antibodies. *JAMA, 290,* 1721–1728.

Zuppa, A. A., Tornesello, A., Papacci, P., et al. (1988). Relationship between maternal parity, basal prolactin levels and neonatal breast milk intake. *Biology of the Neonate, 53,* 144–147.

Additional Reading/Resources

Resources for Physically Challenged Mothers

Disabled Woman's Guide to Pregnancy and Birth
Judi Rogers, OTR/L
Demos Press, 2005

Insufficient Milk

Mothers Overcoming Breastfeeding Issues (MOBI Motherhood)
www.mobimotherhood.org/

Low Milk Supply

www.lowmilksupply.org/

West, D., & Hirsch, E. M. (2008). *Breastfeeding after breast and nipple procedures: A guide for healthcare professionals.* Amarillo, TX: Hale Publishing.

West, D., & Marasco, L. The breastfeeding mothers guide to making more milk. Retrieved September 26, 2009, from www.makingmoremilk.com

Mood Disorders

Depression after Delivery, Inc., is an online resource for parents and professionals dealing with antepartum and postpartum mood disorders. www.depressionafterdelivery.com

Beck, C. T., & Driscoll, J. W. (2005). *Postpartum mood and anxiety disorders: A clinician's guide.* Sudbury, MA: Jones and Bartlett.

Kendall-Tackett, K. (2008). *Non-pharmacologic treatments for depression in new mothers.* Amarillo, TX: Hale Publishing.

Sichel, D., & Driscoll, J. W. (1999). *Women's moods: What every woman should know about hormones, the brain, and emotional health.* New York: William Morrow.

Medications and Breastfeeding

Journals

Akus, M., & Bartick, M. (2007). Lactation safety recommendations and reliability compared in 10 medication resources. *Annals of Pharmacotherapy, 41,* 1352–1360.

American Academy of Pediatrics, Committee on Drugs. (2001). The transfer of drugs and other chemicals into human milk. *Pediatrics, 108,* 776–789.

Books

Briggs, G. R., Freeman, R. K., & Yaffe, S. J. (2005). *Drugs in pregnancy and lactation: A reference guide to fetal and neonatal risk* (7th ed.). Baltimore: Lippincott, Williams & Wilkins.

Hale, T. W. (2002). *Clinical therapy in breastfeeding patients* (2nd ed.). Amarillo, TX: Pharmasoft.

Hale, T. W. (2008). *Medications and mothers' milk* (13th ed.). Amarillo, TX: Hale Publishing.

Hale, T. W., & Ilett, K. F. (2002). *Drug therapy and breastfeeding: From theory to clinical practice.* New York: Parthenon.

Lawrence, R. A., & Lawrence, R. W. (2005). *Breastfeeding: A guide for the medical profession* (6th ed.). St. Louis, MO: Mosby.

Telephone Resources

Breastfeeding and Human Lactation Study Center
University of Rochester School of Medicine and Dentistry
Box 777, Rochester, NY 14642
(585) 275-0088 8 am to 5 pm EST M–F

Health ONE Lactation Program
4500 East 9th Ave, Suite 320 South, Denver, CO 80220
(303) 320-7081 8:30 am–12:00 and 1:00 pm–5:00 pm MT M–F

La Leche League International Center for Breastfeeding Information
1400 North Meachum Rd, Schaumburg, IL 60173-4826
(847) 519-7730
www.lalecheleague.org

Philip Anderson, PharmD, UCSD Breastfeeding and Drugs Information
UCSD 1-619-543-6971

Rocky Mountain Poison and Drug Center
(303) 739-1100
Subscriber service only

Yale-New Haven Hospital Lactation Center
(716) 275-0088 9 am to 5 pm EST weekdays

Internet Resources

Case Western Reserve University
www.breastfeedingbasics.org

Dr. Hale's Breastfeeding Pharmacology Page
http://neonatal.ttuhsc.edu/lact

Maternal Employment

Breastfeeding and working
www.workandpump.com

Healthy Mothers, Healthy Babies, USA
The Workplace Models of Excellence series
Single copies of each publication are free.
www.hmhb.org/pub_breast.html

Parenting in the Workplace Institute
www.parentingatwork.org

U.S. Breastfeeding Committee
www.usbreastfeeding.org

Department of Health, Oregon
www.ohd.hr.state.or.us/bf/working.cfm

Vermont
http://healthvermont.gov/family/breastfeed/employer_project.aspx

Wisconsin
http://dhs.wisconsin.gov/health/Nutrition/Breastfeeding/bffriendlycomm.htm

Texas
www.dshs.state.tx.us/wichd/lactate/mother.shtm

Washington
www.breastfeedingwa.org/working_packet

New Hampshire
www.dhhs.state.nh.us/NR/rdonlyres/euomaqezvninsn55ulepvt56vsweof
qvkovhcybyokhof3ydxtyqbmwos2tjtcsq6g2gesyhig2ahtgvnucrt7n7u2c/worksite
breastfeeding.pdf

Massachusetts Breastfeeding Coalition
http://massbfc.org/workplace/

Healthy Mothers, Healthy Babies Coalition of Washington State
www.hmhbwa.org/forprof/materials/BCW_packet.htm

The Business Case for Breastfeeding
Health Resources and Services Administration
www.4woman.gov/breastfeeding/programs/business-case/

Working without Weaning
Kirsten Berggren
Hale Press, 2006
www.ibreastfeeding.com

Child Care

"Breastfed Babies Welcome Here": This informational packet by the USDA promotes breastfeeding in child care settings. It offers advice on feeding the breastfed infant; preparing for child care; and collecting, storing, and handling breastmilk.

Supplemental Food Programs
Food and Nutrition Service—USDA
3101 Park Center Drive
Alexandria, VA 22302
Telephone: (703) 305-2746
www.wicworks.ca.gov/breastfeeding/EmployeeResources/ReadyforChildcare.html

Massachusetts Department of Public Health
www.eec.state.ma.us/docs/TABreastFeedingDayCareBrochure.pdf

Vermont Department of Health
http://healthvermont.gov/family/breastfeed/childcare.aspx

U.S. Department of Agriculture
http://healthymeals.nal.usda.gov/nal_display/index.php?info_center=14&tax_level=4&tax_subject=264&topic_id=1364&level3_id=5168&level4_id=10015

New York State Department of Health
www.health.state.ny.us/prevention/nutrition/cacfp/breastfeedingspon.htm

Sample childcare center breastfeeding policy
http://dhs.wisconsin.gov/health/Nutrition/Breastfeeding/BF_FriendlyComm/SampleChildcareCenterBFPolicy.pdf

Relactation/Induced Lactation/Adoptive Breastfeeding

The Protocols for Induced Lactation
Lenore Goldfarb and Jack Newman
www.asklenore.info/breastfeeding/induced_lactation/gn_protocols.html

Polycystic Ovary Syndrome

Glueck, C. J., Salehi, M., Aregawi, D., Sieve, L., & Wang, P. (2008). *Polycystic ovary syndrome: Pathophysiology, endocrinopathy, treatment, and lactation.* Independent Study Module, Hale Publishing. Retrieved from www.ibreastfeeding.com/catalog/product_info.php?cPath=15&products_id=173

Diabetes

Guidelines for managing diabetes with a section on breastfeeding
http://sweetsuccessexpress.com/guidelines.htm

Slide presentation on diabetes and breastfeeding
http://lomalindahealth.org/medical-center/our-services/diabetes-treatment-center/
resources/sweet-success/slides/growth-spurts/index.html

❧ Index ❧

Italicized page locators indicate a photo/figure; tables are noted with a *t*.

C

M

Upright positioning, isolated cleft of bony palate and, 462
Urea, in human milk, 28
Uric acid, in human milk, 28
Uric acid crystals in diaper
    dehydration and, 222*t*
    weight loss monitoring and, 220
Uridine diphosphoglucuronosyl transferase, 348
Uridyl diphosphate galactose-4-empiridase deficiency, 488
Urinary tract infections, excessive crying and, 475
Urine output, dehydration issues and, 221, 221*t*
Urobilinogen, 349
U.S. Breastfeeding Committee, 656
U.S. Department of Agriculture, Food and Nutrition Service, 657
U.S. Food and Drug Administration, 20, 24, 89, 198, 199
    vacuum extraction warning and, 207–208
U-shaped cleft palate, 155
Uvula, 136
    cleft of, 165

V

Vaccine responses, enhanced, breastfeeding and, 27
Vaccines, recurrent mastitis and, 556
Vacuum, milk ejection reflex and, 148, 151
Vacuum extraction
    epidural use and, 206
    hyperbilirubinemia and, 355
    infant and maternal injuries related to, 206–207
    latch and, 285
    life-threatening complications related to, 207–208
Vagal tone imbalance, in colicky infants, 475
Vaginal candidosis, 537
Vaginal delivery, oxytocin pulses and, 100
Vaginally born infants
    gastrointestinal tract of, 6
    sleep patterns of, 298
Vagus nerve (cranial nerve X), 141*t*
    jugular foramina and, 286
Valium, 603
Vallone, S., 286
Valproic acid, 498, 585, 603
Vancomycin, breast abscesses and, 560
van Veldhuizen-Staas, C. G. A., 595
Vasoactive intestinal peptide, pyloric stenosis and, 482
Vasopressin, 15, 101
    increased production of, fluid retention and, 205
    prolactin secretion and, 99

Vasospasm, nipple, 93, 533, 534
VATER (or VACTERL) association, 470, 471
Vegan diet, maternal, vitamin B12 concerns and, 32
Velocardiofacial syndrome, congenital heart disease and, 489
Velum (soft palate), 138–139
Venlafaxin, 603
Ventral positioning, 274
    for late preterm infants, 404
Ventricular septal defect, congenital heart disease and, 490 (box 7–1)
Vermont, maternal employment website in, 656
Vermont Department of Health, 657
V-hold, 266–267
Via Christi Breastfeeding Assessment Tool, 174–175, 174*t*
Video conferencing capabilities, multiple births and use of, 439
Video resources, for mothers of multiples, 435
Vieth, R., 36
Vio, F., 25
Visual acuity, delayed, formula feeding and, 24
Visual impairment, maternal, 586
Vitamin A, in colostrum, 5, 33
Vitamin B1 (thiamin), in human milk, 32
Vitamin B2 (riboflavin), in human milk, 32
Vitamin B6 (pyridoxine)
    growth faltering and deficiency of, 373
    in human milk, 32
Vitamin B12, in human milk, 32
Vitamin B12 deficiencies, in breastfeeding infants of mothers who underwent bariatric surgery, 600, 601
Vitamin C (ascorbic acid), in human milk, 32
Vitamin D
    deficiency of, health consequences related to, 33–34
    in human milk, 33–37
        details on, 34 (box 1–1)
        status of, in infants, 35–36
    maternal maintenance of, 71
Vitamin D2 (ergocalciferol), 33
Vitamin D3 (cholecalciferol), 33
Vitamin E (alpha-tocopherol)
    in colostrum, 5
    in human milk, 37
Vitamin K, in human milk, 33, 37
Vitamins
    in human milk, 32–37
        anti-inflammatory components, 44t
Vocal cord anomalies or paralysis, 165